Mechanisms of Carcinogenesis

Contributions of Molecular Epidemiology

Edited by Patricia Buffler, Jerry Rice, Robert Baan,
Michael Bird and Paolo Boffetta

IARC Scientific Publications No. 157

International Agency for Research on Cancer, Lyon

2004

Published by the International Agency for Research on Cancer,
150 cours Albert Thomas, 69372 Lyon Cedex 08, France

©**International Agency for Research on Cancer**, 2004

Distributed by

IARC*Press*
Worldwide except US and Canada: Fax: +33 472 738 302; E-mail: press@iarc.fr;
For the US and Canada: Fax: +1 (202) 223 1782; E-mail: iarcpress@who.int

The World Health Organization, Marketing and Dissemination,
CH-1211 Geneva 27: Fax: +41 227 914 857; E-mail: bookorders@who.int and

Oxford University Press, Walton Street,
Oxford OX2 6DP, UK: Fax: +44 1 536 454 518; E-mail: bookorders.uk@oup.com.

IARC Library Cataloguing in Publication Data

Mechanisms of Carcinogenesis: Contributions of Molecular Epidemiology / editors,
    Patricia Buffler, Jerry Rice, Robert Baan, Michael Bird and Paolo Boffetta

    (IARC scientific publications ; 157)

    1. Carcinogenicity 2. Molecular epidemiology I. Buffler, Patricia A. II. Rice, Jerry M.
    III. Baan, Robert IV. Bird, Michael G. V. Boffetta, Paolo VI. Series

    ISBN 92 832 2157 5   (NLM Classification: W1)

Printed in France

Preface

During the last two decades, molecular epidemiology has become an important discipline in cancer research. The early contributions came from the application of markers of exposure, such as measurements of adducts in blood and urine, in population-based studies. The investigation of aflatoxin exposure markers in cohorts at high risk for liver cancer remains a paradigm of the potential of these new approaches. Over the years, molecular cancer epidemiology has evolved towards the development, validation and application of markers of susceptibility and, more recently, markers of mechanisms of cancer development.

The International Agency for Research on Cancer (IARC) has a long tradition of collaboration between epidemiological and laboratory research, and has been an important leader in the growth of molecular cancer epidemiology. Previous IARC Scientific Publications have addressed specific aspects of molecular epidemiology such as the development and application of biomarkers to cancer epidemiology (Toniolo P. *et al.*, eds, IARC Sci. Publ. No. 142, Lyon, IARC, 1997) and the use of genetic polymorphisms as markers of cancer susceptibility (Vineis P. *et al.*, eds, IARC Sci. Publ. No. 148, Lyon, IARC, 1999).

This volume, which originates from a workshop jointly organized by IARC and the University of Vermont and held in Lyon during 14–17 November 2001 covers, from an interdisciplinary perspective, the contribution of molecular epidemiology to the understanding of mechanisms of carcinogenesis, and represents a further contribution to the development of molecular epidemiology as a major cancer research domain.

Paul Kleihues
Director, IARC
Lyon, December 2003

Acknowledgement

This Scientific Publication contains manuscripts submitted by participants in the Workshop on Mechanisms of Carcinogenesis: Contributions of Molecular Epidemiology, which was held 14–17 November 2001 in Lyon, France.

The International Agency for Research on Cancer is grateful for financial support of this meeting by the US National Institute of Environmental Health Sciences, the University of California at Berkeley (USA), the University of Vermont Center of Molecular Epidemiology (USA) and the European Chemical Industry Council (CEFIC).

Workshop on Mechanisms of Carcinogenesis:
Contributions of Molecular Epidemiology
Lyon, 14–17 November 2001

List of Participants

John F. Acquavella
Epidemiology, Monsanto
Company/A2NE, 800 North
Lindbergh Boulevard,
St Louis, MO 63167, USA

Richard Albertini
Genetic Toxicology Labora-
tory, University of Vermont,
32 North Prospect Street,
Burlington,
VT 05401, USA

Hermann M. Bolt
Institute for Occupational
Physiology, University of
Dortmund, Ardeystrasse 67,
Dortmand 44139, Germany

James Bond
Chemico-Biological Inter-
actions, 5505 Frenchman's
Creek, Durham, NC 27713,
USA

Paul Brennan
Unit of Environmental
Cancer Epidemiology,
International Agency for
Research on Cancer,
150 cours Albert Thomas,
69372 Lyon Cedex 08,
France

Pelayo Correa
Department of Pathology,
Louisiana State University
Medical Center, 1901
Perdido Street, New Orleans,
LA 70012, USA

David M. De Marini
Environmental Carcino-
genesis Division (MD-68),
US Environmental Protection
Agency, 86 Alexander Drive,
Research Triangle Park, NC
27711, USA

Peter B. Farmer
MRC Toxicology Unit,
Hodgkin Building, Univer-
sity of Leicester, Lancaster
Road, PO Box 138, Leicester
LE1 9HN, UK

John E. French
Transgenic Carcinogenesis,
Laboratory of Molecular
Toxicology, DIR, National
Institute of Environmental
Health Sciences, PO Box
12233, MD F1-05, Research
Triangle Park, NC 27709,
USA

Seymour Garte
Genetics Research Institute,
Strada della Carità 10,
20135 Milan, Italy

Mel F. Greaves
Leukaemia Research Fund
Centre, Institute of Cancer
Research, Chester Beatty
Laboratories, 237 Fulham
Road, London SW3 6JB, UK

Lars Hagmar
Department of Occupational
and Environmental Medi-
cine, University Hospital,
221 85 Lund, Sweden

Pierre Hainaut
Molecular Carcinogenesis
Group, International Agency
for Research on Cancer, 150
cours Albert Thomas, 69372
Lyon Cedex 08, France

Kari Hemminki
Department of Biosciences at
Novum, Karolinska Institute,
Hälsovagen 7, 141 57
Huddinge, Sweden

Rogene Henderson
Lovelace Respiratory
Research Institute, 2425
Ridgecrest Drive SE,
Albuquerque, NM 87108,
USA

Jun-Yan Hong
School of Public Health and
EOHSI, University of Medi-
cine & Dentistry of New
Jersey, Room 340, EOHSI
Building, 170 Frelinghuysen
Road, Piscataway, NJ 08854,
USA

S. Perwez Hussain*
Laboratory of Human
Carcinogenesis, Division of
Cancer Etiology, National
Cancer Institute, NIH,
Building 37, Room 2C04,
37 Convent Drive, Bethesda,
MD 20892, USA

Karl T. Kelsey
Department of Cancer Cell
Biology, Harvard School of
Public Health, 665 Hun-
tington Avenue, Boston, MA
02115-6021, USA

R. Jeffrey Lewis
ExxonMobil Biomedical
Sciences, Inc., Occupational
Health and Epidemiology,
1545 Route 22 East, PO Box
971, Room LF 264,
Annandale, NJ 08801-0971,
USA

Julian Little
Epidemiology Group,
Department of Medicine and
Therapeutics, University of
Aberdeen, Foresterhill House
Annex, Foresterhill,
Aberdeen AB25 2ZD, UK

Stephanie J. London
NIEHS, PO Box 12333,
Mail Drop A3-05, Research
Triangle Park, NC 27709,
USA

Ruggero Montesano
(Emeritus Scientist),
International Agency for
Research on Cancer,
150 cours Albert Thomas,
69372 Lyon Cedex 08,
France

Robert Newton
Imperial Cancer Research
Fund, Cancer Epidemiology
Unit, Gibson Building,
Radcliffe Infirmary, Oxford
OX2 6HE, UK

Hannu Norppa
Department of Industrial
Hygiene and Toxicology,
Finnish Institute of
Occupational Health,
Topeliuksenkatu 41 aA,
00250 Helsinki, Finland

Julian Peto
Section of Epidemiology,
Institute of Cancer
Research, Block D,
15 Cotswold Road,
Belmont, Sutton, Surrey
SM2 5NG, UK

Martyn Plummer
Unit of Field and Interven-
tion Studies, International
Agency for Research on
Cancer, 150 cours Albert
Thomas, 69372 Lyon
Cedex 08, France

* Unable to attend

Charles Poole
Department of Epidemiology
(CB 7435), University of
North Carolina, School of
Public Health, Chapel Hill,
NC 27599-7435, USA

Timothy R. Rebbeck
University of Pennsylvania,
School of Medicine, 904
Blockley Hall, 423 Guardian
Drive, Philadelphia,
PA 19104-6021, USA

Kyndaron Reinier
Division of Epidemiology,
University of California, 220
East Avenue, Burlington,
VT 05401, USA

Nathaniel Rothman*
Occupational Epidemiology
Branch, National Cancer
Institute, NIH/NCI/EPS
8116, Bethesda, MD 20892,
USA

Regina M. Santella
Mailman School of Public
Health, Columbia University,
701 West 168th Street
(Room 505), New York,
NY 10032, USA

Christine F. Skibola
Division of Environmental
Health Sciences, School of
Public Health, 217 Earl
Warren Hall, University of
California, Berkeley,
CA 94720-7360, USA

Martyn T. Smith
Division of Environmental
Health Sciences, School of
Public Health, 216 Earl
Warren Hall, University of
California, Berkeley,
CA 94720-7360, USA

Robert Snyder
Environmental Occupational
Health Sciences Institute,
Rutgers University, 170
Frelinghuysen Road,
Piscataway, NJ 08854, USA

Margaret R. Spitz
Department of Epidemio-
logy, UT MD Anderson
Cancer Center, Box 189,
1515 Holcombe Boulevard
Houston, TX 77030, USA

Radim J. Šrám
Laboratory of Genetic Eco-
toxicology, Institute of
Experimental Medicine,
Academy of Sciences of the
Czech Republic, Videnska
1083, 142 20 Prague 4,
Czech Republic

Jim A. Swenberg*
School of Medicine
CB 7400, University of
North Carolina, Rosenau
Hall, Room 357, Chapel Hill,
NC 27599-7525, USA

Eiichi Tahara*
Radiation Effects Research
Foundation Hiroshima-
Nagasaki, 5-2 Hijiyama
Park, Minami-ku, Hiroshima
732-0815, Japan

M. Jane Teta
Exponent Health Group,
234 Old Woodbury Road,
Southbury, CT 06488, USA

Duncan C. Thomas
Biostatistics Division, Verner
Richter Chair in Cancer
Research, Department of
Preventive Medicine,
University of Southern
California, 1540 Alcazar
Street, CHP-220,
Los Angeles, CA 90089-
9011, USA

Pamela M. Vacek
Medical Biostatistics,
University of Vermont, 25D
Hills Building, Burlington,
VT 05405, USA

Paolo Vineis
Unit of Cancer Epidemio-
logy, Department of Bio-
medical Science and Human
Oncology, University of
Turin, Via Santena 7, 10126
Torino, Italy

Joseph Wiemels
Laboratory for Molecular
Epidemiology, Department
of Epidemiology & Bio-
statistics, University of
California, 500 Parnassus
Avenue MU-W 420, San
Francisco, CA 94143-0560,
USA

John K. Wiencke
Department of Epidemiology
& Biostatistics, University of
California, MU-420 West,
San Francisco, CA 94143-
0560, USA

IARC Secretariat
Robert Baan
Alain Barbin
Franca Bianchini
Michael Bird[1]
Paolo Boffetta[2]
Patricia Buffler[3]
David Evered
Silvia Franceschi
Yann Grosse
Hiroshi Ohshima
Christiane Partensky
Jerry Rice[4]
Annie Sasco
Leslie Stayner[5]
Kurt Straif
Eero Suonio
Harri Vainio[6]

Technical Editor
Kathleen Lyle, 43 Brighton
Terrace Road, Sheffield S10
1NT, UK

* Unable to attend
[1] Present address: ExxonMobil Biomedical Sciences, Inc., 1545 Route 22 East, Annandale, NJ 08801-0971, USA
[2] Present address: Division of Clinical Epidemiology, German Cancer Research Centre (DKFZ), Im Neuenheimer Feld 280, 69120 Heidelberg, Germany
[3] Present address: School of Public Health, University of California, Berkeley, CA 94720, USA
[4] Present address: Department of Oncology, Lombardi Cancer Center, Georgetown University School of Medicine, 3970 Reservoir Road NW, Washington, DC 20057, USA
[5] Present address: Division of Epidemiology and Biostatistics (MD 923), School of Public Health, 1603 West Taylor Street, Room 971, Chicago, IL 60612, USA
[6] Present address: Finnish Institute of Occupational Health, Topeliuksenkatu 41 aA, 00250 Helsinki, Finland

Contents

Mechanisms of Carcinogenesis: Contributions of Molecular Epidemiology
Patricia Buffler, Jerry Rice, Robert Baan, Michael Bird and Paolo Boffetta, eds
IARC Scientific Publications No. 157
International Agency for Research on Cancer, Lyon, 2004

Workshop Report

1 Molecular epidemiology
1.1 Definition

Molecular epidemiology is the study of the distribution and determinants of disease in human populations using techniques of molecular biology and epidemiology.

Molecular epidemiology has found many domains of application, in particular in cancer epidemiology, environmental epidemiology and the epidemiology of infectious disease. This Workshop was devoted to providing guidelines for the use of molecular techniques in cancer epidemiology, in particular with respect to the study of the mechanisms of cancer. Molecular cancer epidemiology is often defined in terms of biomarkers, which are found internally within biological systems as indicators of exposure, effects or susceptibility to disease. However, the traditional distinction between biomarkers of exposure, effect and susceptibility is no longer necessary. For example, DNA adducts are markers that integrate exposure, effect and susceptibility.

1.2 Historical developments

Since the beginning of its development some 20 years ago (Perera & Weinstein, 1982), molecular epidemiology has benefited from the technical developments in its related or contributing disciplines: molecular biology, molecular genetics and molecular pathology. The nature and complexity of the techniques applied has depended on the availability of suitable markers. Early studies were based primarily on markers of carcinogenic exposure such as DNA and protein adducts, and the analysis of acquired genetic alterations in neoplastic and preneoplastic tissue samples represented an area of important development in the late 1980s. During the 1990s, large-scale analyses of somatic mutations and polymorphisms were developed, as well as a wide range of phenotypic assays, to assess important aspects of carcinogenesis such as DNA repair, gene expression and genomic instability. Early molecular epidemiological studies of cancer were based on the distinction between markers of 'exposure', markers of 'effect' and markers of 'susceptibility'. With increasing knowledge of the mechanisms of carcinogenesis, the distinction between the first two groups of markers has become blurred, and the results of current molecular epidemiological studies are more and more often interpreted in terms of elucidation of mechanisms of carcinogenesis. A key contribution to this change in paradigm has been made by studies that integrated different types of biomarkers such as adducts in target or surrogate tissues, acquired alterations and single nucleotide polymorphisms (SNPs). For example, in a study of lung cancer among women, an interaction was detected between the level of tobacco-related polycyclic aromatic hydrocarbon (PAH)–DNA adducts and glutathione S-transferase M1 null genotype, but not between either biomarker and the presence of sister chromatid exchanges in leukocytes (Tang et al., 1998). In this situation, an elevated PAH–DNA adduct level is no longer considered only to reflect the biologically effective dose of a carcinogen, but rather to contribute to the identification of sensitive subpopulations.

1.3 Examples of the application of biomarkers to cancer epidemiology

In many cases, the application of a molecular or even a general biologically-based approach has represented an important component of causal evidence in addition to that obtained from traditional epidemiological methods (Table 1). Assessment of exposure to aflatoxins, enhanced sensitivity and specificity of assessment of past viral infection and detection of protein and DNA adducts in workers exposed to reactive chemicals, such as ethylene oxide, are among the examples in which molecular epidemiology has greatly contributed to the understanding of human cancer. In many other cases, however, promising initial results have not been confirmed by subsequent,

Table 1. Examples of important contributions of molecular epidemiology to cancer research

Class of biomarkers	Agent, exposure	Reference
Dose marker	Aflatoxin	IARC (1993)
Viral infection	HPV	IARC (1995)
Adducts	Ethylene oxide	IARC (1994)
Acquired *TP53* mutations	Tobacco	Hernandez & Hainaut (1999)
Chromosomal aberrations	Individual susceptibility	Bonassi *et al.* (2000)
Metabolic polymorphisms	NAT2	Vineis *et al.* (1999)

usually methodologically sounder, investigations. For example, in the search for susceptibility to environmental carcinogens by looking at polymorphisms for a number of metabolic enzymes, early studies of genetic polymorphisms were not replicated (Vineis *et al.*, 1999; Lohmueller *et al.*, 2003).

If biomarkers offer new opportunities to overcome some of the limitations of epidemiology, their added value over traditional approaches should be assessed systematically. Biomarkers should be validated; consideration of sources of bias and confounding in molecular epidemiology studies should be as stringent as in other types of epidemiological studies. Similarly, other aspects of the study (e.g. determination of required sample size, statistical analysis, reporting and interpretation of results) should be approached with the same rigour as that used in epidemiology in general. Molecular epidemiology will have reached its maturity when studies are conducted according to state-of-the-art methods for design, analysis and interpretation.

2   Scope and aims of the Workshop

The goals of the Workshop were to provide useful guidelines for investigators on the design and interpretation of future epidemiological studies of cancer which employ molecular techniques, and to provide guidance to the *IARC Monographs* Programme on the use of molecular data from epidemiological studies in the identification and evaluation of carcinogenic hazards.

An understanding of the underlying biological mechanisms that are associated with certain biological responses (biomarkers) is essential in the design and interpretation of epidemiological studies that incorporate molecular approaches. For example, selection of a particular biomarker requires knowledge of the expression time of the relevant genetic marker or knowledge of the functional isozymes (which may be polymorphic) in the metabolism of the xenobiotic agent. The validation necessary for a biomarker will depend on its specificity in the cancer process. Furthermore, circumstances of exposure such as timing, duration and intensity may affect the metabolic pathways that induce molecular changes.

To achieve these goals, the two major objectives of the Workshop were to examine critically the impact of mechanistic and toxicological knowledge on the major categories of biomarker currently used in epidemiological studies of cancer and to identify mechanistic and toxicological principles related to the use of biomarkers of exposure, effect, repair and susceptibility that could provide guidance in the design and interpretation of epidemiological studies of cancer that employ molecular approaches. Genetic variations in the metabolism of xenobiotic agents and differences in mechanistic responses may alter markedly the response of an individual to these exposures.

This Workshop was intended to expand the earlier work of IARC in examining the application of molecular techniques in cancer epidemiology and the study of mechanisms of carcinogenesis (Vainio *et al.*, 1992; Toniolo *et al.*, 1997; Miller *et al.*, 2001).

Three groups of neoplasm were selected as models for discussion at the Workshop, on the basis of current knowledge of their sequence of identified pathological and genetic events and the relevance of biomarkers or molecular data to the study of their epidemiology. These were head and neck cancers, gastric cancer and haematopoietic malignancies, which represent three groups for which different markers have been developed and applied in recent years. Their discussion (Newton *et al.*, Little *et al.*, Spitz *et al.*, this volume) therefore offers an overview of the spectrum of markers currently available.

3 Relevance of biomarkers to the study of mechanisms and the evaluation of carcinogenesis

The remarkable advances in cellular and molecular biology over the past two decades have transformed the scope and methods of cancer epidemiology. In fact, modern epidemiological studies often depend on genetic, biochemical and viral assays that were not available 20 years ago (Peto, 2001).

It is widely agreed that the predominant forces of carcinogenesis are mutation, clonal expansion and selection. These concepts have been incorporated into a wide range of theories of carcinogenic processes, both qualitative and quantitative. Recent research has revealed the extraordinary degree of complexity in terms of the cancer process (Cortessis & Thomas, this volume). For decades, the Armitage–Doll model has served as the dominant mathematical paradigm for epithelial tumours. Here, cancer is modelled as the result of the single cell undergoing a series of discrete, heritable events in a particular sequence (Peto, 2001). However, this model is less successful in describing the epidemiological features of the haematopoietic neoplasms.

Moolgavkar and Knudson (1981) proposed a two-event clonal-expansion model, in part to account for such features as the distinctive age distribution of leukaemias, initiation–promotion and the genetics of cancer: in this model, cancer arises from a single cell undergoing two rate-limiting events (mutations), with the intermediate cells (those which have undergone the first mutation) being subject to a stochastic birth-and-death process that can lead to clonal expansion.

However, as in the Armitage–Doll model, the pools of normal, intermediate and fully malignant cells are treated as if they were homogeneous. The genetic diversity of many cancers suggests the need for a new concept, in which there might be many different paths to cancer, involving an accumulation of a wide variety of possible genetic changes, each affecting the dynamics of the resulting clone (e.g. birth, death and mutation rates) in a random fashion. This will lead to a proliferation of clones with differing characteristics, many dying out rapidly and a few expanding until they encounter some bottleneck, leading to a selection that favours clones with a proliferative advantage. Ultimately, the first of these clones to attain the molecular characteristics that confer uncontrolled proliferation will lead to the appearance of a frank malignancy. The greater the genomic instability is early in the process, the more branching may be involved.

Although not yet developed formally, the stochastic theory of branching processes may be helpful in describing this phenomenon (Tsao *et al.*, 2000). Even without a well-developed mathematical theory, the basic concept may be useful as an organizing principle for the discussion to follow about mechanisms of carcinogenesis and the ways in which biomarkers can be used to understand the process and to study etiology.

3.1 Biomarkers of internal dose

The measurement of biomarkers of internal dose is a method of assessing exposures to carcinogens and other toxicants that accounts for inter-individual variations in uptake, metabolism, bioaccumulation or excretion of the compound. Such a method provides an estimate of the actual levels of the compound within the body, compared with an imprecise or potentially inaccurate estimate provided by questionnaire data or external monitoring devices. Two strategies for the use of biomarkers to determine prior exposures are described below.

Physiologically based toxicokinetic modelling is one strategy for linking biomarkers of exposure with prior exposures (Cortessis & Thomas, this volume). To develop such models, information must be obtained on the rate of formation or change of a biomarker following exposure to a toxic agent or its active metabolites and the rate of removal of the marker from the body, as well as the factors (age, sex, species, repeated versus single exposures) that influence these rates. In addition, physiological parameters must be known, such as the breathing rate, blood flow, cardiac output and other parameters depending on the target organ of interest. The physicochemical characteristics of the chemical and its metabolites must also be known, to determine the partition coefficients between air and blood and between blood and tissues. Such detailed metabolic and toxicokinetic information must normally be obtained in animal studies. A mathematical model based on animal studies can then be modified to take into account human differences in physiological parameters and in metabolism of the compound. The modified model can be used to predict the concentration of various markers following various exposure regimens. An example of successful use of this strategy is the physiologically based toxicokinetic model for styrene developed by Ramsey and Andersen (1984).

A second, simpler strategy is the use of single or a battery of biological markers of different half-lives to obtain information on prior exposures (Henderson, 1995; Ward & Henderson, 1996). The relative amounts of biomarkers having a short half-life compared with markers with longer half-lives can be used to determine whether the prior exposure was a brief, high-level exposure or a low-level, continuous exposure occurring over an extended period of time. Animal studies can be used to determine the relative half-lives of bio-markers. For example, when an organic vapour such as benzene or 1,3-butadiene is inhaled, most of the internal dose will be excreted in some form in the urine (Bond et al., 1986; Sabourin et al., 1987). The half-life of the urinary metabolites may be only a few hours. Some of the parent compound will be exhaled unchanged in the breath, and this biomarker of exposure will also last only a few hours. Markers with a longer half-life can be detected as adducts to the blood proteins with half-lives of weeks or months depending on the protein (albumin or haemoglobin). Finally, a small amount of the inhaled compound will form DNA adducts

with widely varying half-lives, depending on the degree of DNA repair and cell turnover. It should be noted, however, that most of the successful examples of exposure biomarkers concern specific chemicals in fairly simple exposure circumstances, typically in the occupational setting.

Although the use of biomarkers of internal dose plays a vital role in the accurate assessment of exposures in individuals, they do not provide information on the extent to which the agent has affected the target tissues or cells. The measurement of protein or DNA adducts as biomarkers of biologically effective dose can provide further insight into the mechanistic properties of the carcinogenic effects of certain exposures.

3.2 Biomarkers of biologically effective dose

An important question to be addressed for individuals who have a biomarker of exposure to a chemical is whether the amount of the marker indicates that any adverse health effect related to cancer will develop from the exposure. Unfortunately, very little information is usually available to answer such a question. However, techniques have been developed that allow the measurement of the 'biologically effective dose' of a compound. The detection of specific protein or DNA adducts as biomarkers is an indication that a compound has reacted with critical cellular targets. Strategies must be developed to extend our knowledge, beyond noting the existence of a biomarker of a chemical exposure, to determining the significance of the markers. The first question that must be considered is which markers are associated with the disease process of interest. Biomarker studies of vinyl chloride (VC) offer a good example of the types of study that are helpful in linking biomarkers in the form of DNA adducts with the disease of interest, liver cancer.

VC is a known human and animal liver carcinogen (Swenberg et al., 1990); preweaning rats are more susceptible than adults to VC-induced liver cancer (Fedtke et al., 1990). Four DNA adducts have been identified from the livers of rats exposed to VC (Ciroussel et al., 1990). Of these, by far the largest amount formed is the oxyethyldeoxyguanosine adduct, but it also has the shortest half-life of all the adducts identified. In addition, this adduct has no activity in DNA fidelity replication assays (Hall *et al.*, 1981; Barbin *et al.*, 1985). Thus, the adduct formed to the greatest extent does not appear to be indicative of risk for disease.

The three other adducts, which are all etheno adducts formed on different deoxynucleotides, have longer half-lives in the body and are active in inducing mutations in DNA fidelity replication assays (Singer *et al.*, 1987). A study of adducts in VC-exposed newborn versus adult rats indicates that the ethenodeoxyguanosine adduct is more prevalent in young rats, suggesting that it is the marker that would be more predictive of risk than the others (Fedtke *et al.*, 1990). In this strategy, animal studies were used to identify the DNA adducts that are formed by exposure to a chemical and to determine their half-lives. In-vitro studies were used to determine their mutagenic potential. Comparison of levels of adducts in animals known to be at greater risk for liver cancer with those in less sensitive animals was used to select the adduct that is most predictive of risk. A similar strategy could be used with other chemicals to select DNA adducts that represent markers of risk for disease.

In the strategy described above, additional steps are required to determine whether the marker of risk in rats is also a marker of risk in humans. It is also obvious that, from a practical point of view, adducts in the liver are not acceptable biological markers for screening humans for potential health effects, and that adducts in circulating white blood cells would be more appropriate. In such a case, the quantitative relationship between adducts in blood cells and those in the relevant target organ should be determined in order to validate the usefulness of the former in assessing the risk for health effects. An excellent example of such an approach is found in the work on biological markers of exposure to aflatoxin as reviewed by Groopman *et al.* (1996).

Epidemiological studies have shown a strong association between the ingestion of aflatoxins (AFBs) from moulds growing on a poorly preserved food supply and the development of liver cancer, a disease of high incidence in some regions

of Africa and Asia (Groopman *et al.*, 1996). Quantitative relationships between selected biomarkers of exposure to AFB and the induction of cancer were first determined in animal studies. The quantitative relationship between exposure to AFB, biomarkers of internal dose (urinary metabolites) and the biologically effective dose (AFB–liver DNA adducts) was studied. It was found that one biomarker (AFB–N7-guanine) in 24-h urine samples reflects dietary intake of AFB, and the urinary concentration of AFB–N7-guanine is correlated with the concentration of the AFB–liver DNA adducts. Subsequently, it was found that levels of serum albumin adducts, a biomarker with a longer half-life than the urinary adducts, correspond well with both dietary intake and levels of liver DNA adducts. When the studies were extended to exposed human populations in Africa and China, it was found that, as in animals, urinary AFB–N7-guanine reflected the dietary intake of AFB. In several prospective studies, increased levels or the presence of such biomarkers of AFB intake were strongly associated with risk for liver cancer (Ross *et al.*, 1992; Chen *et al.*, 1996).

A number of reports have been published on the detection of DNA adducts in human tissues using different methods such as ELISA, ^{32}P-post-labelling and mass spectrometry (Swenberg, this volume). These studies measured adducts arising from exogenous chemical exposures, as well as DNA adducts that arise endogenously. The exogenous chemicals include such groups as PAHs, aromatic amines, heterocyclic amines, industrial chemicals and drugs. Both endogenous processes and redox cycling of chemicals have been shown to result in oxidative DNA damage. In addition, several exocyclic DNA adducts arising from products of lipid peroxidation represent secondary forms of DNA damage that result from oxidative stress. Studies on endogenous forms of DNA damage arising from lipid peroxidation, such as malondialdehyde and etheno adducts, are just beginning and may provide additional insights into the influence of diet and lifestyle factors, as well as interactions between the known risk factors.

Most studies of DNA adduct in humans have used blood as a surrogate for the target tissue, with little information on correlations between the two. Experimental studies in animals may help establish these relationships. Care needs to be taken in the selection of white blood cells as a source of DNA, since lymphocytes have a much longer lifespan than neutrophils and are preferable for such studies. Some studies have been carried out on easily available epithelial tissues such as skin and genital or oral mucosa. For neoplasms arising in these organs, studies can be performed correlating target to non-target tissue. In conclusion, chemical-specific DNA adducts provide evidence of exposure; however, it is more difficult to establish causal relationships between these adducts and cancer.

3.3 Biomarkers of preclinical biological effects in surrogate and target tissues

Biomarkers of preclinical biological effects provide valuable information regarding genotoxic events that are thought to be critical in the multistep sequence of carcinogenesis, and are important in helping to elucidate mechanisms of carcinogenesis. In addition, these biomarkers may serve as surrogate end-points to cancer in epidemiological studies.

3.3.1 Cytogenetic biomarkers

Chromosomal aneuploidy was identified early as a distinct feature of the 'cancer phenotype' (Boveri, 1914). As chromosome staining techniques improved, scientists recognized that aberrations were not random but selective for certain cancer types, and were present in every type of cancer, representing a key event in carcinogenesis (Rowley, 2001). The recognition that specific genes were the targets of certain types of alterations, such as translocation, deletion and amplification, has led to specific diagnostic tools as well as molecular markers that are used in epidemiological studies. Cytogenetic biomarkers can be used as markers of susceptibility, markers of early effect and markers of disease.

In prospective studies, an association was observed between the levels of chromosomal aberration in cultured peripheral lymphocytes and increased overall risk for cancer. This association was observed in smokers and nonsmokers and in

individuals with occupational exposure or with no apparent occupational exposure to carcinogens (Hagmar et al., this volume). The reasons for these findings are at present unclear, but they probably reflect individual susceptibility to genotoxic carcinogens in the common environment or diet. Such susceptibility factors may include genetic polymorphisms affecting carcinogen metabolism, cellular response to genotoxic damage (DNA repair) and genomic integrity (Norppa, this volume).

Aberrations induced by mutagens in culture have also been shown to correlate with cancer risk in case–control studies (Bondy et al., 2001; Xiong et al., 2001). Again, such alterations are markers of susceptibility that could indicate defects in, for example, DNA repair and carcinogen metabolism, but lack specific mechanistic information. Other assays have been developed, such as the sister chromatid exchange and micronucleus assays, which are used as biomarkers of exposure or early effect (Waters et al., 1999). An association could not be established between cancer risk and the frequency of sister chromatid exchange or micronuclei in peripheral lymphocytes (Hagmar et al., Norppa, this volume). As the genetic basis of variable response in cytogenetic biomarkers is revealed, these assays may be replaced or supplemented in the future by the use of panels of genetic susceptibility markers that will not be subject to the vagaries of sample collection, processing, storage and cell culture conditions that may affect cytogenetic markers.

The past decade has seen significant advances in the specificity and throughput of cytogenetic assays that assess structural biomarkers of effect and disease. Visual assays have been enhanced by fluorescence in-situ hybridization (FISH) to include entire chromosomes (e.g. centromeric probes, chromosome painting, SKY cytogenetics). In addition, when specific fusion genes are involved, molecular assays can replace visual ones (Greaves, Gunn & Smith, this volume). These assays assess the presence of fusion gene products of translocations, and may be used as markers in the classification of tumours or early biological effects (Smith et al., 1998; Wiemels et al., 2001). Chromosome translocations that initiate childhood leukaemia occur (and produce clonally expanded populations) at a frequency that is 100-fold that of the disease itself (Mori *et al.*, 2002). It is likely that similar biomarkers will become available for most paediatric and adult cancers. The implications of biomarker studies are considerable. In addition, newer methods, including arrays, that allow the scanning of the entire genome (Snijders *et al.*, 2001) have just begun to impact on cancer epidemiology studies. Many studies, however, now include the collection of specimens from study subjects, which allows wholesale use of such assays.

3.3.2 *Alterations in reporter genes*
Another potentially useful biomarker that can serve as a pre-disease mechanistic probe is somatic mutation in specific reporter genes. Although these mutations do not play a direct role in the disease process, they may serve as an accurate method of quantifying and characterizing mutational events *in vivo*. Individuals exposed to carcinogens are expected to show higher frequencies of somatic mutations than non-exposed individuals (Albertini, this volume). Currently, somatic mutations are measured in four gene systems, including the glycophorin-A (*GPA*) gene, the hypoxanthine-guanine phosphoribo-syltransferase (*HPRT*) gene, the human leukocyte antigen (*HLA*) genes and the T-cell receptor (*TCR*) genes. Of the four genes described for human monitoring, only *GPA* and *HPRT* have been used to any extent.

3.3.3 *Alterations in cancer-related genes*
The activation of proto-oncogenes and inactivation of tumour-suppressor genes, often by mutations in the somatic cells from which tumours arise, are considered to be core events that provide selective growth advantage to the affected cells. Mutations in the *TP53* tumour-suppressor gene occur, with loss of function, in about half of all human cancers. The frequency of *TP53* mutations, the specific sites within the *TP53* DNA sequence at which mutations occur and the kinds of mutations seen vary from cancer to cancer. Patterns of mutation in cancers of a given organ site and pathological type contribute to the generation of hypotheses about the etiology and pathogenesis of

these neoplasms. Sometimes, *TP53* mutations are sufficiently characteristic to identify the environmental carcinogen associated with a specific tumour, notably aflatoxins with hepatocellular carcinoma and solar/ultraviolet radiation with non-melanoma skin cancer (Olivier *et al.*, this volume). In most cases, *TP53* mutations are seen only in tumour tissues, which restricts the kinds of study in which *TP53* mutations can be used to those in which surgical or autopsy tissue specimens are available. In some cases, however, *TP53* mutations can be identified in preneoplastic tissues, and can even be amplified from serum or plasma samples by the polymerase chain reaction.

In addition to p53, other cell-growth control pathways should be included in future epidemiological studies that seek to relate exposure risk factors with specific gene targets and modes of gene inactivation. Among these additional targets is the Rb/p16 pathway. This pathway, which is important in the G_1 cell-cycle checkpoint, can be blocked by inactivation or alterations in different genes. Among these, the *CDKN2A* gene locus encodes two different proteins derived from alternate splicing: p16INK4a (exons 1α, 2, 3) is a G_1 cell-cycle regulator and p14ARF (exons 1β, 2, 3) modulates MDM2-mediated degradation of p53 (Shahnavaz *et al.*, 2001; Kresty *et al.*, 2002).

Promoter hypermethylation, a non-mutational mechanism for inactivation of *p16INK4a*, is also common in head and neck cancer. The mechanisms responsible for aberrant methylation are poorly understood. It is not yet clear whether methylation would be affected differently by viral or chemical carcinogen exposures. Another component of the Rb/p16 pathway, cyclin D1, is amplified in head and neck cancers. Amplification of cyclin D1 occurs in a high proportion of epithelial tumours and is also found in precancerous lesions. Interestingly, cyclin D1 amplification has been found in head and neck tumours that also harbour oncogenic strains of the human papillomavirus (i.e. HPV-16, HPV-18) (Cattani *et al.*, 1998; Almadori *et al.*, 2002). This observation could lead to a marker of viral carcinogenesis.

Another example of an emerging pathway is the phosphatidylinositol 3-kinase (PI-3Kinase) pathway. This pathway affects signalling invoked by cell contact and growth-promoting molecules, such as insulin, and modifies apoptotic and cell-cycle checkpoint regulation. The chromosomal region 3q2 containing PI-3Kinase subunit α is frequently amplified in head and neck squamous-cell cancer. PTEN, a lipid phosphatase, is thought to mitigate against PI-3Kinase activity by meta-bolizing the lipid second messengers produced by the enzyme. Thus, PTEN is thought to modulate the downstream effects of PI-3Kinase over-expression on such targets as Akt and p27 (Kip1). Current evidence indicates that PTEN may influence cell-cycle checkpoints through its effect on the SKP2 protein, which is involved in the pro-teolytic degradation of p27Kip1. In oral squamous-cell cancer, a striking inverse relation-ship has been observed between p27Kip and SKP2 protein expression (Gstaiger et al., 2001). Further work is needed to clarify the role of PI-3Kinase, cell cycle and apoptotic mechanisms, however, as some studies have failed to observe an influence of PI-3Kinase amplification on puta-tive downstream effectors such as Akt. Other genes in the region besides PI-3Kinase may also be involved in head and neck cancers.

Thus, it will be important in future studies to characterize multicomponent control pathways as targets of environmental exposures and genetic susceptibility. This should be approached with the idea that individual genes within a pathway can be inactivated through different mutational and epigenetic mechanisms. Additional studies aimed at relating distinct patterns of pathway inacti-vation with specific etiological exposures are needed.

3.4   Biomarkers of susceptibility
Progress in understanding the role of endogenous and exogenous xenobiotics in the pathway leading to carcinogenesis, together with the rapid advances in human genomics and molecular techniques, have enabled researchers to consider more realistically the influence of inherited genetic traits in the paradigm of cancer etiology. Genetic factors ranging from predisposing highly penetrant mutations to low-penetrance genetic polymorphisms have been shown to influence the inter-individual variation in cancer incidence

significantly. Highly penetrant mutations in genes, such as p53 in the Li–Fraumeni syndrome and Rb in familial bilateral retinoblastoma, confer a very high risk for developing cancer and are the cause of extensive morbidity and mortality in affected families. However, the prevalence of these inherited mutations is low in populations and accounts for only a small proportion of the overall incidence of cancer. In contrast, the more prevalent low-penetrance genetic polymorphisms, which are broadly defined as differences in nucleotide sequence among individuals occurring in more than 1% of the population, contribute lower levels of risk for cancer but affect a larger proportion of the population. Inherited genotypes among a number of classes of genes acting at each phase of the multistage model of carcinogenesis can potentially influence an individual's suscep-tibility to develop cancer (Rebbeck, this volume).

For example, known differences in the meta-bolism of potential carcinogens are usually detected by biochemical tests. People who are rapid oxidizers (readily activate procarcinogens), slow acetylators (poorly detoxicate certain carci-nogens) or both can be detected by urinanalysis for specific types of metabolites of caffeine following administration of a standard cup of coffee (Kadlubar et al., 1990). In a study reported by Landi et al. (1996) on the association between smoking and risk for bladder cancer, smokers were classified for their status as oxidizers and acetylators and the results were compared with the level of 4-aminobiphenyl–haemoglobin adducts present in the individuals. Rapid oxi-dizers and subjects with a combined slow acetyl-ator–rapid oxidizer phenotype had the highest levels of adducts at a low smoking dose.

As our knowledge of the human genome increases, the implementation of follow-up studies that can interpret the significance, in terms of future health effects, of the genetic poly-morphisms found becomes critical. It is not helpful to know whether individuals are fast or slow acetylators, or have any other marker of a genetic susceptibility to cancer, if we do not know (1) what the biomarker signifies in terms of pro-bability of an adverse health effect and (2) what measures can be taken to improve the probability of future health. As our ability to discover genes associated with susceptibility to disease increases, additional research must be carried out to define the degree of susceptibility to disease indicated by the polymorphism. In addition, some research should be directed towards obtaining information that will help individuals to reduce their personal risk. An example is the study reported by Mooney et al. (1997) in which the relative contributions of genetic and nutritional factors to DNA damage in heavy smokers allow some hope for intervention in the disease process in susceptible individuals.

Genetic information may have important implications for cancer detection and prevention. First, knowledge of these factors may be used to guide recommendations for modification of certain exposures (e.g. use of oral contraceptives), which may become a part of standard care in the follow-up of women who are found to carry these variants. Second, knowledge of risk-modifying factors in these individuals may lead to tailored cancer screening strategies. This could include recommendations related to the timing, intensity or organ-specific screening in subsets of people. Finally, knowledge of factors that modify cancer risk may direct research efforts to identify important carcinogenesis pathways. This may in turn lead to the novel use of existing (e.g. hormonal) agents or the development of new agents that could be applied in chemoprevention or treatment strategies specifically targeted towards individuals with a specific genetic susceptibility.

In contrast, low-penetrance genes are expected to confer a relatively low degree of risk to the individual. As a result, it is unclear how genetic information at these loci may be of value in clinical risk assessment at this time. If an array of genotypes at multiple loci (possibly in conjunction with exposure information) is identified that has a considerable effect on cancer risk, then information on low-penetrance genotype may be clinically valuable. For example, Rebbeck et al. (1997–98) evaluated the utility of using genotypes in breast cancer risk assessment, and showed that information on genotype of a low-penetrance gene (NAT2) when combined with smoking may have a similar utility in risk prediction to BRCA2 under certain conditions.

However, substantial additional information is needed on the conditions under which low-penetrance genotypes affect cancer risk.

3.4.1 Behavioural gene polymorphisms

Although exposures to lifestyle factors such as tobacco and alcohol are primarily determined by one's environment, it is possible that genes may also play an important role. For example, it has been shown that several genes may be associated with the ability to quit smoking, including the dopamine re-uptake transporter gene and dopamine D2 and D4 receptor genes (Lerman et al., 1999), as well as the cytochrome p450 2A6 gene. Individuals who are able to quit smoking reduce their risk of tobacco-related cancers substantially, and a genetic component to quitting smoking could therefore be highly relevant with respect to cancer risk. Similarly, genotypes involved in the metabolism of alcohol, including alcohol dehydrogenase and aldehyde dehydrogenase genes, may determine an individual's propensity to drink. Genotypes that influence lifestyle exposures should therefore be considered in studies of cancer susceptibility because they may elucidate mechanisms through which carcinogens act and may better define an individual's predicted pattern of exposure to relevant agents. Such studies will need to pay particular attention to the collection of the bio-behavioural data to be evaluated, including the use of appropriate data collection instruments. In addition, it may be necessary to make distinctions between the role of genes in the etiology of tumours and the role of the same genes in predicting behavioural outcomes. For example, the aldehyde dehydrogenases may influence the degree to which some individuals consume alcohol, but they may also influence relevant carcinogenic pathways directly in the etiology of disease (Brennan & Boffetta, this volume).

3.4.2 Metabolic gene polymorphisms

The literature on metabolic gene polymorphisms as cancer risk factors has demonstrated considerable heterogeneity of results, in that both weakly positive and negative findings have been reported for many variant gene alleles in association with many cancer types. Larger studies, including meta-analyses and pooled analyses, have generally found very weak or no evidence of association with cancer as the main effects. Compared with many other risk factors (both genetic and non-genetic), the degree of risk conferred by the metabolic gene variant alleles is likely to be low.

This conclusion is actually not surprising, given all we know about the biochemical functions of the enzymes coded by these genes and the complex molecular pathways that must occur for a cell to undergo malignant transformation (Rebbeck, this volume). In fact, such genes should play no role in cancer susceptibility unless the gene variant under study has a significant effect on the metabolism of the carcinogens to which people in a particular study are exposed. Furthermore, the gene in question must be expressed at an appropriate level in the target tissue. Even if these conditions are met, the metabolism of carcinogenic chemicals often proceeds by multiple pathways, only one of which might be mediated by the gene under study. Other issues are dose effects of the carcinogen, the existence of multiple molecular pathways to cancer, which might not all be affected by the relevant carcinogenic metabolite, and the existence of redundancy in many of these genes, so that lack of function of one member of the family (as in the GST family) might have no overall effect.

Since it is to be expected that no single metabolic gene variant should ever be observed to play a large role in cancer susceptibility for any general cancer type, results from recent large studies actually confirm what is known about mechanisms of environmental carcinogenesis and the role of gene–environment interactions related to metabolic susceptibility genes.

Therefore, mechanistic hypotheses should be tested, specifying that a particular gene polymorphism might affect only a particular exposure-specific, gender-specific or age-specific (etc.) metabolic pathway.

A hypothetical example illustrating how targeted hypotheses could derive a strong significant association for a gene polymorphism in a specific category of individuals, hidden in a large population for whom the risk allele has no effect, has been published (Garte et al., 1997). In this example, only 50 out of a population of 1000 cases are truly affected by the variant allele, because of their associated environmental and genetic risk factors. When these 50 people are examined, the odds ratio for having the variant allele is 9.0, whereas for the whole population it is 1.2.

There are many caveats to this approach. If it is undertaken as a form of subgroup analysis, then the problem of spurious associations due to testing multiple hypotheses could arise. This can be avoided by having strong a-priori hypotheses when designing studies of metabolic gene polymorphisms as cancer risk factors in particular groups of subjects.

Of course, targeted hypothesis testing requires large populations in order to retain adequate power to detect significant effects in small groups. The best approach to overcome the sample size and power problems is to concentrate future efforts on large studies using thousands of cases and controls, an approach that is in any case gaining favour because of the disappointing results usually obtained with smaller studies (Garte et al., 1997).

3.4.3 DNA repair gene polymorphisms

Genetic polymorphisms of DNA repair genes may also contribute to variation in DNA repair capacity (see Berwick & Vineis, 2000, for a review). For example, benzo[a]pyrene diol epoxide (BPDE)-induced DNA damage is effectively removed by the nucleotide excision repair (NER) pathway. The NER pathway alone involves at least 20 genes (Friedberg, 2001).

There have been a few studies evaluating DNA repair capacity (DRC) by the DNA repair genotype. Spitz et al. (2001) have genotyped lung cancer cases and healthy controls for two polymorphisms in the XPD/ERCC2 gene: the Lys751Gln (exon 23) locus of the XPD gene and the Asp312Asn locus. Both variant homozygous genotypes were associated with significantly poorer DNA repair capacity, as assessed by the host cell reactivation assay; cases and controls with the wild-type genotypes exhibited the most proficient DRC. These results suggest that the two XPD polymorphisms have a modulating effect on DRC. Clearly, more functional (phenotypic) studies of DNA repair in individuals with various genotypes of these polymorphisms are needed. However, it may be difficult to detect subtle differences in DNA repair capacity due to a single polymorphism of a single gene in a very complex pathway.

3.4.4 Cell-cycle control gene polymorphisms

Because carcinogenesis in most organs involves abnormalities in cell-cycle control (Scully *et al.*, 2000), polymorphisms of cell-cycle genes are good candidates for investigations of genetic susceptibility. Normal cell-cycle control ensures a rest in the cell cycle allowing DNA damage in a cell to be repaired before the cell begins the process of growth, mitosis and division. For example, the cyclin-dependent kinase inhibitor gene *TP21* (Waf1/Cip1) induces cellular growth arrest, terminal differentiation and apoptosis.

3.4.5 Immunosurveillance gene polymorphisms

An additional set of candidate genes with functional polymorphisms for consideration includes those genes involved in the immune response: encoding cytokines and their receptors, HLA and other cell-surface molecules involved in immunological recognition of infections, other (e.g. self-) antigens or in cell–cell interaction (Jepson, 1996). These genes are plausible candidates, as their functions are relevant both to infections linked to etiology and to possible responses to tumour cells. This view is endorsed by preliminary evidence suggesting that HLA alleles are involved in the etiology of childhood leukaemia (Taylor *et al.*, 1998) and Hodgkin disease (Taylor *et al.*, 1996), and tumour necrosis factor α in lymphoma (Tsukasaki *et al.*, 2001). Other candidate genes that potentially influence immune surveillance are suggested by associations between non-malignant immunological diseases and allelic variants, e.g. interleukin-12 in type 1 diabetes (Adorini, 2001).

3.4.6 Phenotypic biomarkers of susceptibility

Chromosomal damage in peripheral lymphocytes has been used to study individual sensitivity to in-vitro treatment with chemical mutagens and ionizing radiation, and as an indication of increased susceptibility to genotoxic carcinogens and increased risk for cancer. Several studies have suggested that lymphocytes from cancer patients have higher sensitivity to bleomycin, a radiomimetic genotoxin. The reasons for increased sensitivity to mutagens are not known, but it is usually considered to reflect individual differences in cellular response to DNA damage. Sensitivity to sister chromatid exchange induction by diepoxybutane *in vitro* was primarily observed to be due to the lack of erythrocytic glutathione S-transferase T1 (*GSTT1* null genotype), an enzyme that detoxifies diepoxybutane (Norppa, this volume).

Hsu and colleagues developed the mutagen sensitivity assay based on the quantification of bleomycin-induced chromatid breaks in cultured lymphocytes to measure human susceptibility to environmental carcinogens (Hsu *et al.*, 1985). Rather, it provides an integrated measure of DNA repair capacity after mutagen challenge and time for recovery. In case–control analysis, in-vitro bleomycin-induced mutagen sensitivity (either as a continuous or dichotomous variable) is an independent risk factor for head and neck cancers, after adjustment for tobacco and alcohol use, with an adjusted odds ratio of 2.5 (Spitz *et al.*, 1989; Hsu *et al.*, 1991).

A meta-analysis of three case–control studies of head and neck cancers (Cloos *et al.*, 1996) confirmed this finding, suggesting that age and use of tobacco and alcohol did not influence the mutagen sensitivity values. Heavy smoking in the absence of the hypersensitive phenotype was associated with an odds ratio of 11.5 (95% confidence interval [CI], 5.0–26.6). In heavy smokers who also exhibited mutagen hypersensitivity, the odds ratio was 44.6 (95% CI, 17.4–114).

This assay has been extended using benzo[*a*]pyrene as the challenge mutagen. In a case–control study of head and neck cancer (Wang *et al.*, 1998), BPDE-induced break/cell value was an independent risk factor for disease, with a dose–response between BPDE-induced break/cell values and risk for upper aerodigestive tract tumours. As would be expected of a phenotypic marker of genetic susceptibility, there was no significant difference among cases based on stage, site of disease or treatment status. The underlying mechanism for mutagen sensitivity associated with inclination towards cancer may reflect an altered repair process (Spitz *et al.*, 2001). However, we do not know how mutagen sensitivity as measured in lymphocytes reflects the repair capacity in the target tissue. Nor has this functional assay been validated in prospective studies. The host cell reactivation (HCR) assay measures the expression level of a damaged reporter gene as a marker of repair proficiency in the host cell (Athas *et al.*, 1991). This assay uses undamaged cells, is relatively fast and is an objective way of measuring repair. In the assay, a damaged non-replicating recombinant plasmid (pCMVcat) harbouring a chloramphenicol acetyltransferase reporter gene is introduced by transfection into primary lymphocytes. Reactivated chloramphenicol acetyltransferase enzyme activity is measured as a function of nucleotide excision repair of the damaged bacterial gene (Athas *et al.*, 1991). Both lymphocytes and skin fibroblasts from patients who have basal-cell carcinoma but not xeroderma pigmentosum have lower excision–repair rates of a reporter gene damaged with ultraviolet light (UV) than individuals without cancer (Alcalay *et al.*, 1990; Wei *et al.*, 1993). This finding suggests that the repair capacity of lymphocytes can be considered to be a reflection of an individual's overall repair capacity.

Wei *et al.* (1996) applied the HCR assay in parallel with the mutagen sensitivity assay in 16 established lymphoblastoid cell lines that included three head and neck cancer cell lines. Using UV radiation and 4-nitroquinoline oxide (4NQO) as the test mutagens, they reported that reduced cellular DNA repair capacity was significantly correlated with increased frequency of mutagen-induced chromatid breaks. The DNA repair capacity of head and neck cancer cases ($n = 55$) was significantly lower than that of the controls ($n = 61$; 8.6% versus 12.4%; $p < 0.001$).

4 Validation and application of biomarkers

Much more effort is involved in validating a biological marker as a quantitative indicator of prior exposures, of developing disease or of susceptibility to toxicant-induced disease than in the discovery of the marker itself. In most instances, we can measure many more biological phenomena than we can interpret.

For biomarkers of any kind to be useful in epidemiological studies, validation of the biomarker must be completed at several levels. First, the assay itself must be validated to indicate its accuracy, specificity and precision. Cross-laboratory comparisons help to assure the reproducibility of the assay when carried out by different groups. Assays of the same end-point by different methods must be reviewed for the influence of the methodology on the end-point of interest. Second, the association of the biomarker with the exposure or the disease process must be validated. The biomarker need not be directly on the pathway of the disease process, but the relationship to the degree of exposure or to the development of disease must be clear. Finally, validation data should be incorporated directly into the analysis of epidemiological studies of association. Using main study–validation–substudy designs with explicit modelling of measurement errors can be a powerful approach (Stram *et al.*, 1995).

The data on the amount of each marker formed and the half-life of that marker must usually be obtained in animal studies. Validation of the values for humans must come from in-vitro studies to determine whether human metabolism is similar to that in the animal model, and from limited data obtained from humans exposed to small amounts of a chemical in clinical studies or to large amounts in accidental exposures. Then, if persons with unknown exposure history are examined, one can distinguish between a person with a recent exposure to high levels of a chemical, a person who is continuously exposed to low levels of a chemical or a person who was exposed in the past but not recently. A person exposed recently to a high level of a chemical will have biomarkers that occur in large amounts and have short half-lives (e.g. urine and breath markers), but will have very little of the biomarkers that occur in small amounts but have long half-lives. A person living near a waste dump, who has been receiving low-level exposures over a long period of time, would be expected to have very little urinary or breath biomarkers, but the level of blood protein adducts should be high relative to the urinary markers. A person who was exposed to substantial amounts of a chemical in the past, but not recently, may have no biological markers in the urine but still have remnants of protein or specific DNA markers. Thus, a comparison of the levels of a series of biological markers can provide more information than a single marker (Henderson, 1995).

Finally, a biomarker can be most useful if the quantitative relationship between the biomarker and either the degree of exposure or the risk for development of a disease process is known. For example, if a certain level of a biomarker is found in a population (or an individual), it would be ideal to be able to predict the probability of subsequently developing disease in the population and the level of exposure that caused the disease (Henderson, 1995).

4.1 Development, characterization and applied transitional studies

There are many possible chemical-specific biomarkers of exposure, such as urinary metabolites, protein adducts, DNA adducts and parent compound or metabolites in exhaled breath or blood. The type of biomarker that best reflects the actual exposure can be determined in transitional studies in which external exposures are measured in the most exacting manner available and the various biomarkers of exposure are measured in the exposed population. Comparisons of the various biomarkers with the known exposure levels will indicate which biomarkers are most useful as measures of prior exposure. Such a study has been conducted in industrial plants in Czechoslovakia in which 1,3-butadiene was being produced or used in the manufacture of polymers (Albertini et al., 2001). In this case, haemoglobin adducts best reflected the exposures to butadiene and urinary metabolites were also useful.

Relating a biomarker to a disease process may be more difficult. The reactive metabolite indicated by an adducted protein or DNA base may or may not be the causative agent for the disease process of interest, but if the relationship between the adducted metabolite and the metabolic pathway leading to the primary carcinogen is known, then the adduct may be related to the disease process. For example, a biomarker such as the *HPRT* mutation is not on the pathway to disease but serves as an indicator of the mutational activity in the exposed person, and mutation can be related to the carcinogenic process (Albertini, this volume). Studies are required to determine which biomarker of effect best reflects the risk for development of disease.

Mathematical modelling of pharmacokinetic as well as pharmacodynamic processes is required to determine the quantitative relationship between the biomarker and either the degree of exposure or the risk for development of the disease. Information on the kinetics of the processes involved in dosimetry (pharmacokinetics) and the multistep responses leading to disease (pharmacodynamics) must be known. Quantitative measures of the rate constants for each step in an environmentally induced disease process and all the factors that influence those rates are difficult to obtain, particularly for the pharmacodynamic events. Physiologically based pharmacokinetic models have been developed to relate levels of metabolic biomarkers to levels of exposure, but very few attempts have been made to model biomarkers of early effects in a manner that would allow quantitative prediction of health outcome. Such pharmacodynamic modelling represents an opportunity for productive future research (Henderson, 1995).

4.2 Relevance of animal models

Animal models that reproduce the specific disease phenotype would be useful tools for mechanistic investigations and for the development and validation of biomarkers of potential use in molecular epidemiology (French, this volume). Using both random and targeted transgenic methods, mouse models may be produced that replicate the specific disease phenotype to investigate gene–environment interactions for the identification of potential etiological factors. Recent studies reported with human carcinogens using *TP53* haploinsufficiency, ras overexpression and fusion gene products of translocations have shown that lymphohaematopoietic disease may be induced.

More work is required to understand their relevance to human disease.

4.3 Criteria for selection of biomarkers for human studies

For practical reasons, biological markers for human studies must be accessible in readily available body fluids or tissues. Exhaled breath, blood, urine and buccal cells are potentially accessible, although customs in some countries may restrict use of even these samples.

Biological markers used in human studies must also be based on relatively rapid, low-cost assays. If hundreds of samples need to be tested, one cannot use a costly method that requires several days for analysis. The biological marker should be useful for determining either prior exposure levels or a developing disease process, i.e. the biomarker should be interpretable. As noted above, biological markers used in human studies must be validated as to their relationship to either exposure or the disease process, and should have a low background in non-exposed people. High backgrounds of a biomarker, from whatever source, make it difficult to interpret results from persons exposed to low levels of a chemical. The selected biomarker should be stable enough in the milieu in which it is collected to allow shipment to the point of assay. A highly unstable biomarker will subject assay results to great variability.

The completion of the human genome project provides a rich resource of genomic DNA markers for use in genetic linkage analysis and association studies. The use of genome-wide searches to identify chromosomal regions that may contain a disease-causing gene has been widely exploited in genetic linkage analyses using microsatellites and single nucleotide polymorphisms (SNPs). Choice of SNPs for linkage analysis depends on the degree of heterozygosity: the greater the heterozygosity of the SNP, the more likely the marker is to provide information on the co-segregation of a marker allele with the disease phenotype.

A crucial issue is the appropriate selection of genes and functionally significant polymorphisms in order to maximize the potential for detecting relevant effects. The general paradigm for studies of disease associations begins with the identification of genes that have ideally been characterized for relevant structural and functional characteristics. These 'candidate genes' are potentially numerous and it may be difficult to prioritize genes that are good candidates over those that are not. Thus, criteria may be used to select candidate genes and variants. For example, candidate genes are generally chosen on the basis of biological plausibility. Genes that encode enzymes with biochemical or physiological activities that have a plausible role in the pathobiology of a cancer are considered first. However, genes that lie in candidate regions with somatic changes associated with the disease (e.g. loss of constitutional heterozygosity, translocations or other somatic mutations found in tumours) may also be considered as relevant candidates.

Both functional SNPs and random (potentially non-functional) SNPs exist in the human genome, and both could be used in association studies of disease based on the concept of linkage disequilibrium in populations. Use of SNPs for genome-wide searches for association has been proposed (Risch & Merikangas, 1996), although the number of non-functional random SNPs required for a genome-wide association search could be as high as 500 000 unless population isolates are studied. Risch (2000) has argued that the use of functional SNPs is preferable because they are most likely to influence directly the traits under study and, even if they are not functionally associated with the disease of interest, they are more likely to be in linkage disequilibrium with disease-causing alleles. In either case, large sample sizes and potentially large numbers of SNPs may be required to undertake studies of genome-wide disease associations. The considerations discussed here are important, not only in the context of specifying hypotheses, but also in the context of analysis and in considering biological plausibility when making causal inferences. There is a need for a database that includes both positive and negative results and for information on the quality of studies of functional effects (De Roos *et al.*, this volume).

SNPs can be ranked according to the degree of functional significance that they are likely to have with respect to disease causation (Risch, 2000).

These rankings can therefore aid in choosing variants of greatest potential interest to disease association studies, and can be incorporated directly into the analysis using hierarchical models (Conti & Witte, 2003). The first consideration is that of the relationship between the variant and some functionally relevant phenotype. Among biologically plausible candidates, genetic polymorphisms with well-characterized relationships to biochemical or physiological traits that are known to be associated with carcinogenesis should be given first consideration. Genetic polymorphisms with well-characterized relationships to biochemical or physiological traits that have no established role in susceptibility to carcinogenesis should be given lower priority. Anonymous DNA markers (e.g. those that do not encode or regulate any known phenotype) should be considered with lowest priority. However, when the function of the gene is poorly characterized or there is reason to believe that the candidate may be in linkage disequilibrium with another gene of interest, anonymous markers may be appropriate choices. Consideration of the functionality of SNPs can therefore help to maximize the results of association studies on the genome-wide level as well as for candidate genes, as described below.

When two variants are available and are equally plausible by the criteria listed above, it may be useful to consider the more highly polymorphic marker for analysis first. A final and related consideration that is sometimes taken into account is the potential attributable risk associated with the variant of interest. This notion is related to the allele or genotype frequencies of the variants, but considers also the amount of disease in the population that may be explained by these variants. Stated differently, one may consider the potential public health impact of a variant based on the number of people that may be affected by disease as a result of having inherited a particular genotype.

5 General considerations

A number of general issues related to the design and implementation of epidemiological studies that include biomarkers have been discussed in detail elsewhere (Toniolo et al., 1997). Issues of particular importance for mechanistic studies include study design and analysis, interactions, low-dose extrapolation and ethical considerations.

5.1 Issues of study design and analysis

Epidemiological studies that use molecular techniques and specific biomarkers have the ability to test etiological hypotheses related to biological mechanisms and genetic susceptibility. Such studies are conducted in much the same way as traditional epidemiological studies, with the exception of biological sample collection and certain methodological issues, which are discussed in the following sections.

5.1.1 Case–control studies

A case–control study is a commonly used type of observational analytical design in which subjects are grouped on the basis of disease status and are assessed for certain exposures hypothesized to be related in some way to the disease. This design is particularly efficient in investigating diseases that are rare or have long latency periods, since the disease is first identified and exposures are assessed retrospectively. However, this limits the type of information that can be obtained from biological specimens. The use of biomarkers of internal dose or effective dose is appropriate only when these markers are stable over an extended period of time and reflect an accurate assessment of prior exposure that is unaffected by the disease process, diagnosis or treatment. In particular, behavioural changes following disease development might affect relevant biomarkers (e.g. dietary factors). In contrast, case–control studies are highly appropriate for studies of genetic susceptibility and those that involve end-point stratification by molecular, histological and other subtypes.

Although case–control studies have a number of advantages, including efficiency in both time and cost relative to other analytical approaches, this design is particularly susceptible to selection and information biases, since disease and exposure have already occurred. Selection bias can occur if there is differential selection of either the cases or controls into the study on the basis of their exposure status. Information bias is a result of the differential reporting of exposure information between cases and controls. However, case–control genetic association studies inherently overcome many of these limitations (Clayton & McKeigue, 2001). Mendelian genetics substantially minimize bias and residual confounding by ensuring that the allocation of individuals to specific categories defined by genotype is irrespective of other influential factors except with respect to allelic associations (linkage disequilibrium) (Davey Smith & Ebrahim, 2003).

Population stratification is a type of confounding due to population admixture that may affect genotype–disease association studies when risk allele frequencies and baseline disease risk covary between populations. It can be avoided by paying attention to the ethnic composition of the population in enrolment and analysis (Vineis *et al.*, this volume). In most instances, population stratification is likely not to be an important issue, provided that epidemiological principles of study design are rigorously applied (Thomas & Witte, 2002; Wacholder *et al.*, 2002).

5.1.2 Cohort studies
Cohort studies represent a major type of observational analytical design in which an explicitly defined cohort of individuals, classified on the basis of exposure to a suspected risk factor, is followed over a period of time to assess the occurrence of the outcome in question. The strengths and weaknesses that are characteristic of this type of study design apply to exposures in general and are not exclusive to studies employing biomarkers.

The cohort study design is recognized for its ability to assess more clearly the temporal relationship between exposure and outcome, which is critical in attempting to understand disease etiology (Hunter, 1997). Of particular importance in studies using biomarkers is the possibility for biomarker levels to be influenced by the disease. Assuming that undiagnosed or preclinical disease has not altered the level of a biomarker, exposure is generally measured before the onset of disease and one can assure that biomarker levels in cases preceded the outcome. Another strength of this study design is that biases related to the assignment of the comparison group are

minimized since they originate from the same explicitly defined source population. Finally, the nature of the follow-up period in cohort studies allows for repeated measurements of biomarkers, which can be used to test hypotheses related to different latent periods between exposure and outcome.

A major weakness of cohort studies that use biomarker data is the potential for insufficient statistical power. It may be difficult to accumulate the number of cases required for an interpretable analysis unless the cohort is large and the follow-up time is very long. However, it may be possible to overcome this by targeting a specific high-risk group for the disease. Studies using biomarkers require specimen collection, which may be an added disadvantage when recruiting participants. The opportunity for repeated biomarker measurements is considered a major strength, but there may be logistical difficulties in terms of storage space and subject consent to acquire and use the samples in a prospective manner. Furthermore, cohort studies are potentially susceptible to uncontrolled confounding, as are case–control studies.

5.1.3 Nested case–control studies
An extension of the basic cohort study design is the opportunity to conduct a case–control study using the participating cohort. In this case–control study within a cohort, or nested case–control study, controls are selected for each case accrued from the pool of participants still at risk for the disease at the time the case was diagnosed. Another variant of this idea is the case–cohort design (Prentice, 1986), in which controls are sampled at random from the entire cohort at entry. In biomarker studies, the specimens that had been collected at enrolment from this subgroup of the cohort would simply be extracted and analysed for the biomarkers in question. This design can considerably reduce the expense of data collection and analysis of the biological specimens. In addition to these reduced costs, nested case–control studies have the advantage of matching on storage duration and can be analysed together as a case–control set, which may reduce the potential for bias introduced by sample degradation and laboratory drift. Other trade-offs between the various

alternative designs are discussed by Langholz et al. (1999).

5.1.4 Case-only studies

Case–case comparisons can be useful in the study of biologically defined disease subsets when differences in the etiology of such subsets are being examined. This type of study has also been proposed to evaluate gene–environment interaction in disease etiology (Andrieu & Goldstein, 1998). A case series is defined in the same fashion as it would be in a case–control study and is grouped on the basis of the presence or absence of the susceptibility genotype in question. These two groups are compared with respect to the prevalence of the environmental exposure. An association between a genotype and exposure in this case series may suggest interaction. The main disadvantages of this study design are that (1) main effects of the genetic and environmental factors cannot be estimated; (2) the validity of the estimate of interaction is highly sensitive to the assumption of independence between genotype and exposure (Albert et al., 2001); and (3) this approach assumes that the effects of genetic and environmental factors are independent in the population at risk.

5.1.5 Family-based studies

Family studies are useful in epidemiological studies using molecular and metabolic data and can address scientific questions related to four general areas of research:

1. Does familial aggregation exist for a specific disease or characteristic?
2. Is the aggregation due to genetic factors or environmental factors or both?
3. If a genetic component exists, how many genes are involved and what is their mode of inheritance?
4. What is the physical location of these genes and what is their function?

Using linkage methods, biomarkers that characterize known DNA haplotypes have been instrumental in locating a number of cancer-related genes. Special concern must be given to ethical and counselling issues in family studies in which biomarker results for an individual may also have predictive value for other members of the family (Toniolo et al., 1997).

5.2 Interaction

The current understanding is that cancer is probably a multifactorial disease with an etiology that results from an interaction between environmental and genetic factors. This embodies the concept that genetic traits may function to modify the effects of environmental exposures in producing disease. From an analytical perspective, interaction may be inferred if the biomarker of susceptibility results in a higher disease risk in exposed susceptible groups than would be expected on the basis of relative risks in exposed non-susceptible and in non-exposed susceptible groups. The study designs that have been identified for the detection of gene–environment interactions include case-only designs, case–control study designs using unrelated controls, case–control designs using related controls, twin-study designs and combined segregation and linkage analyses (Vineis et al., this volume).

Due consideration should be given to the assessment of interaction on both additive and multiplicative scales. Interaction consistent with a multiplicative effect may imply that two exposures (either genetic and environmental, or two different genes) are involved in the same causal pathway, whereas a greater than multiplicative effect may indicate an underlying biological interaction where the effect of one exposure is enhancing the action of another. In practice, studies of gene–environment interaction rarely have sufficient power to distinguish between these two models (Clayton & McKeigue, 2001).

Of major importance in the assessment of interaction in population studies is the need for a large sample size. For example, in case–control studies, assessing interaction would require stratifying the population by the effect modifier (e.g. the genotype) and comparing the size of the odds ratios that relates the exposure to the disease. Similarly, one can consider the exposure as a modifier of the effect of genotype. The statistical power depends on the numbers of cases and controls in each of the strata rather than the case and control population as a whole. The lack of statistical power could introduce random error and make it impossible to interpret the results in a valid manner. Given the rarity of most neoplasms, large multicentre and multinational studies are encouraged.

5.3   Low-dose extrapolation

Reliable biological markers of exposure (e.g. effective dose), effect and susceptibility can be important in models used in high- to low-dose extrapolation of risk for specific health effects of chemical exposure in humans. Two types of model are essential for high- to low-dose extrapolation of health risks:

*   **dosimetry models**, which are essentially toxicokinetic models that describe quantitatively the kinetics of internal dosimetry and supply the biological effective dose (and associated uncertainty) as a function of the level of exposure to a given chemical;
*   **risk models**, which are toxicodynamic (or pharmacodynamic) models that relate effective dose (and associated uncertainty) to risk (and associated uncertainty) for a specific health effect (disease), taking into consideration the kinetics of disease induction.

Biological markers of effective dose will help reduce the uncertainty related to which value to use for effective dose for a given level of exposure to a specific chemical. Biological markers of effective dose can also be used to help decide, from a group of dosimetry models, which model is more reliable (reducing model-associated uncertainty). Similarly, biological markers of risk (e.g. risk-related DNA adducts) for a specific health effect can help decide, from a set of risk models, which model is most reliable for high- to low-dose extrapolation (reducing model-associated uncertainty). Animal studies play important roles in dosimetry and risk model selections (Henderson, 1995).

Biological markers of susceptibility can be used to identify and separate the at-risk population into different susceptibility groups (e.g. high and low) so that susceptibility-adjusted risk estimates can be developed and used in the high- to low-dose extrapolations. However, this may require different dosimetry/risk models for the different susceptibility classes.

5.4   Ethical issues in biomarker-based studies

Many aspects of the collection and long-term storage of human tissue and other biological specimens relevant in the design and implementation of molecular epidemiological studies raise ethical issues. There are potential ethical issues at each juncture of the research process, including during protocol development, when obtaining participation, and in the interpretation and notification of test and study results (Schulte *et al.*, 1997). These ethical issues arise from the possibility of abuse or misuse of biomarker data and failure to respect the rights of people participating in research. Biomarker data can be misused by failing to keep data confidential and by using them, or allowing them to be used, to stigmatize people who have been the subject of research. These people have a right to privacy, as well as a right to be told of risks of participating in biomarker studies and of any clinically important findings. Additionally, there are ethical considerations concerning the use of biological specimens collected and stored for one purpose and subsequently used for other research purposes (Toniolo *et al.*, 1997).

5.5   Guidelines for interpretation of observed associations

There are well developed and widely used guidelines for assessing causality in epidemiological studies (Hill, 1965). These can be usefully applied in the evaluation of biomarkers with disease outcome. In practice, only limited subsets of these guidelines for causal inference tend to be used. For example, in cancer epidemiology, the guidelines most often applied are consistency, strength, dose–response and biological plausibility (Weed & Gorelic, 1996). The potential applications of the guidelines for causal inference in the context of studies involving biomarkers are discussed below.

5.5.1   Guidelines for causal inference

These guidelines (modified from Surgeon General, 1964; Hill, 1965) relate to
*   consistency
*   strength
*   dose–response

- biological plausibility (including analogy)
- specificity
- temporality
- experimental support
- coherence.

Consistency: In relation to consistency, differences between studies in distributions of subjects by age and gender will be sources of heterogeneity. For example, hormonal alterations can affect ligand binding, enzyme activity, gene expression and the metabolic pathways influenced by gene expression.

In particular, some inconsistency between the results of gene–disease association studies may be secondary to variation among studies in the prevalence of interacting environmental factors that have not been assessed. It would be appropriate to test *a priori* hypotheses about differences in gene–disease associations and genotype frequencies between studies that may arise from these sources.

Heterogeneity may occur if the allele under study is associated with disease due to linkage disequilibrium with a gene that is truly causal. Such a 'marker' allele may behave differently in populations with different genetic backgrounds due to differences in the extent of the linkage disequilibrium, even if the 'causal gene' were to have the same effect in the different populations. Differences between populations in allele prevalence may result in differences between studies in the statistical power to detect both the main effects of the genotype and gene–environment interactions. Similarly, the prevalence of exposure, or variability of exposure, may influence whether an interaction is detectable.

Strength: In certain circumstances, use of biomarkers of exposure and/or effect may result in a greater magnitude of association than would be found using other measures. For example, the relationship between invasive cervical cancer and human papillomavirus is stronger than the relationship between this disease and genital warts, and this in turn is stronger than the relationship with multiple sexual partners (IARC, 1995). However, in studies of the general population, the associations between disease and biomarkers of susceptibility are not likely to be strong. In particular, many of the genetic variants so far identified as influencing susceptibility to common diseases are associated with a low relative and absolute risk (Caporaso, 1999). Therefore, exclusion of non-causal explanations for associations is crucial.

Dose–response: One of the challenges of molecular epidemiology has been the development of quantitative assays. For example, this was problematic in the initial stages of development of the ^{32}P-postlabelling and 8-oxo-7,8-dihydroguanine methods for detecting DNA adducts (Hemminki & Thilly, this volume), and in the development of biomarkers of benzene exposure (Snyder & Hong, this volume). Thus, information on the validity of biomarkers is crucial in the assessment of dose–response relationships.

In the particular instance of gene–environment interaction, even in the simplest case of a dichotomous genotype and a dichotomous exposure, there are many ways in which genotype and environment may interact (Garte *et al.*, 1997). For example, Khoury *et al.* (1993) discuss at least six different patterns of genotype–environment interaction. More patterns could be defined if more categories of exposure were introduced. For example, Taioli *et al.* (1998) have proposed a model in which an effect of the genotype is apparent at low environmental exposures, but is not apparent at high exposures. When multiple categories of dose are defined for the exposure, then many different dose–response models can be tested in the data, and, in addition, tests for interaction can be applied to the trends across strata. Similarly, more patterns of interaction could be defined if more complex classifications of genotype were considered. Even in the case of a single gene with two alleles, there needs to be a decision as to whether to combine heterozygotes with one of the two groups of homozygotes (i.e. the trait is presumed to fit either a dominant or recessive model) or to treat genotype as a trichotomous variable, i.e. treating the heterozygotes as a separate category (i.e. assuming co-dominance). Often the rarer homozygous genotype is combined with the heterozygotes because there are too few subjects for analysis in the former category. The model also will be uncertain for more common alleles for which there is limited information on co-dominance, and it will be more complex when there are multiple alleles. There is increasing emphasis on genetic pathways. In consequence, there will be a need to consider variation in multiple genes. Similarly, multiple environmental factors may be relevant.

Biological plausibility: This is a particularly important issue in the evaluation of gene–disease associations and gene–gene or gene–environment interactions. For example, in investigations of associations with genetic polymorphisms of carcinogen metabolism and DNA repair, many genotypes have been assessed without data on their functional significance. Investigations confined solely to genotypes would potentially lead to numerous false positive associations (Hemminki & Thilly, this volume). Consideration of biological plausibility involves determining: (1) whether a known function of the gene product can be linked to the observed phenotype; (2) whether the gene is expressed in the tissue of interest; and (3) temporal relationships, including the time window of gene-expression in relation to age-specific gene–disease relationships. Thus, the gene should be in the disease pathway and/or involved in the mechanism that is responsible for the development of the disease. If not, then the effect of the gene may be indirect. In studies of cancer in young people, it may also be relevant to consider maternally mediated effects of the maternal genotype and parental imprinting. Cortessis and Thomas and De Roos *et al.* (this volume) propose approaches that would integrate pharmacokinetic data in modelling gene–environment and gene–gene interactions. We do not yet know how much this will help in identifying data gaps. It is possible that carcinogen-metabolizing genes may activate carcinogens in some circumstances and detoxify them in others.

More generally, studies of biomarkers give insights into mechanisms and strengthen the evidence regarding causality (Albertini, this volume).

Specificity: Although specificity has been included as a criterion of causation, it may be inappropriate in relation to the effects of complex exposures that may influence several outcomes, e.g. tobacco smoking, or genetic variants that may influence the metabolism of a variety of exposures, e.g. cytochrome P450 gene variants.

Temporality: Although a correct time relationship is specified in many methodological texts, it seems to be seldom used in causal inference for associations of biomarkers with exposure or disease outcome (Weed & Gorelic, 1996).

In the situation of gene–disease associations, it is possible that the disease could influence the result of a phenotypic assay of the genotype under investigation. This should not be a problem with polymerase chain reaction (PCR) methods. If data were available on the time window of gene-expression, it would be relevant to consider this in relation to age-specificity of gene–disease relationships. As a perhaps extreme example, if there were an association between a type of cancer in infants and the *CYP1A1* or *CYP1A2* genotype of the index child, it is likely that this would be indirect (e.g. reflecting an effect of maternal genotype) because the enzymes coded by these genes are not expressed in the fetal liver (Cresteil, 1998; Sonnier & Cresteil, 1998).

Experimental support: Interspecies comparisons of markers of carcinogenesis, using experimental animals for which carcinogenicity data are also available, would support studies in humans of factors influencing non-cancer end-points (Albertini, this volume).

In the context of gene–disease associations, experimental support is most likely to be derived from studies of gene expression in knockout or other experimental animals, from in-vitro data on gene function or from experimental interventions based on clinical protocols aimed at normalizing the levels of a product regulated by the gene.

Coherence: This criterion has been defined as being satisfied when an association is consistent with the state of knowledge of the natural history and biology of the disease (Surgeon General,

1964). In practice, this guideline has been little used, perhaps because it has been considered to be equivalent to biological plausibility (Weed & Gorelic, 1996). Elwood (1998) defines an association as being coherent 'if it fits the general features of the distribution of both the exposure and the outcome under assessment'. He notes that the concept holds only if a high proportion of the outcome is caused by the exposure, and if the frequency of the outcome is fairly high in those exposed. An additional constraint on the use of this criterion arises when information on the distribution of the relevant exposure and outcome is inadequate. At present, information on the distribution of many biomarkers is limited. In the situation of gene–disease associations, the 'exposure' would be the genotype being investigated.

6 Conclusions

The extent to which biological markers will contribute to environmental cancer research will depend on the degree to which additional research is completed to change the markers from laboratory curiosities into useful tools for investigators. The amount of research effort and funding required to validate the usefulness of biological specimens as an indicator of prior exposure or as a predictor of disease outcome is much greater than the effort required to discover the biomarker.

Although they are still of value, some current and commonly used biomarkers have known limitations:

- Chemical-specific adducts provide evidence of exposure, but it has been difficult to establish causal relationships between adducts and cancer.
- An association has not been established between cancer risk and the frequency of sister chromatid exchange or micronuclei in peripheral lymphocytes.
- HPRT assesses mutation only in a single gene from T lymphocytes and probably preferentially in CD+ cells.

However there have been many encouraging developments in the field. For example:

- Visual assays have been enhanced by fluorescence in-situ hybridization (FISH) to include entire chromosomes.

- When specific fusion genes are involved, molecular assays can replace visual ones to assess the presence of fusion gene products of translocations, which may be used as markers of early biological effects in the classification of tumours.

Current human genome research, including SNP cataloguing, could help to identify new target genes and new metabolic/signal transduction pathways. It also opens the door for the discovery of a large number of novel genetic biomarkers. Nevertheless, it is important that the phenotype–genotype relationship be established by various experimental approaches to complement the results of population-based studies.

Large population-based studies would provide an opportunity of studying rare genetic events and gene–gene/gene–environment interactions, as well as reducing the potential of overlooking important associations that may be pertinent to specific subgroups. It is important to design hypothesis-driven studies in which mechanistic considerations involving not only target genes, but also target pathways and combinations of target pathways, may be considered. However, in the design of these types of study, one must consider the need for new statistical tools to analyse these complex associations.

6.1 *Strengths of available knowledge*

The assumption that a reporter gene used as a biomarker of effect measures a similar but unspecified response to one occurring in a cancer pathway is supported when the reporter response captures and reflects molecular mechanisms of known importance in cancer induction (Albertini et al., 1996). Large numbers of biomarkers are available for use in epidemiological studies, but only validated biomarkers are useful in predicting disease outcomes. This workshop demonstrates that, increasingly, validation data are available from both animal interspecies and human observational studies. Genotoxic changes in reporter genes have been found to be valuable not only as qualitative and quantitative measures of exposure to a carcinogen but also, by sharing the same mechanism as cancer-related genes, as surrogates for these. For instance, both the GPA and HLA mutation assays detect somatic recombinations that are the necessary events for the somatic loss of heterozygosity of many human tumours. The p53 mutational spectrum for some cancers can provide strong support for specific exogenous causation in association with cancer of a particular anatomical area. There are some reservations about using p53 mutational spectra in all instances, but they are emerging as a strong tool.

The use of susceptibility markers has increasing potential to determine relationships between the toxicant and disease. The new technology of DNA microarray for assessment of gene regulation has the potential to increase data available on gene expression. Together with data on factors affecting this variability, this information will provide important insights regarding potential confounders and effect modulators.

Polymorphisms in genes involved in metabolism, DNA repair and cell-cycle control have been shown to affect an individual's susceptibility to chemically induced cancer. Animal studies, in which homogeneity of genetic and other factors can be achieved, are less complex, but even so construction of multivariate models to incorporate etiologically important steps offers the ability to integrate the component steps and provide insight into biological pathways. Paradoxically, progress is being made in this area through recognition of the complexities of the end-points and the parameters to be included, as well as those that are missing.

6.2   Priorities for future work

Among the areas of biomarker research that were identified as priorities for future work are:
- development of models of carcinogenesis that integrate epidemiological observations;
- application of new technologies in developing biomarkers, in particular in the field of gene expression, proteomics and protein activity profiling;
- development of biomarkers of complex exposures, e.g. fruit, vegetables;
- characterization of multicomponent control pathways;
- development of mathematical models of pharmacokinetic and pharmacodynamic processes;

- integration of information on gene function, with indicators of its quality;
- availability of a database including null and negative studies of biomarker–disease associations;
- development of methods to characterize effects of multiple genes operating in pathways;
- hypothesis-driven serial tissue banking from individuals in prospective cohorts to allow comparative retrospective analyses of individuals with and without disease;
- target tissue biomarkers – microarray and proteomic studies to track induction of genes and alteration of metabolic profile;
- characterization of biomarkers in 'normal' subjects – distinction between endogenous and exogenous sources;
- use of mutations in reporter genes across species to improve risk assessment;
- development of standards for assessing evidence from studies based on genome-wide scanning;
- further research on the relevance of biomarkers in target tissues to effects in target organs.

Molecular epidemiology, and specifically the need for mechanistic information in studies of cancer etiology, has been an integrative force in bringing together the disciplines of molecular biology, toxicology and genetics with epidemiology. The successes resulting from this integration will no doubt provide the impetus for increased collaboration of these disciplines.

References

Adorini, L. (2001) Interleukin 12 and autoimmune diabetes. *Nat. Genet.*, **27**, 131–132

Albert, P.S., Ratnasinghe, D., Tangrea, J. & Wacholder, S. (2001) Limitations of the case-only design for identifying gene–environment interactions. *Am. J. Epidemiol.*, **154**, 687–693

Albertini, R.J., Nicklas, J.A. & O'Neill, J.P. (1996) Future research directions for evaluating human genetic and cancer risk from environmental exposures. *Environ. Health Perspect.* **104** (Suppl. 3), 503–510

Albertini, R.J., Sram, R.J., Vacek, P.M., Lynch, J., Wright, M., Nicklas, J.A., Boogaard, P.J., Henderson, R.F., Swenberg, J.A., Tates, A.D. &

Ward, J.B., Jr (2001) Biomarkers for assessing occupational exposures to 1,3-butadiene. *Chem.-biol. Interact.*, **135–136**, 429–453

Alcalay, J., Freeman, S.E., Goldberg, L.H. & Wolf, J.E. (1990) Excision repair of pyrimidine dimers induced by simulated solar radiation in the skin of patients with basal cell carcinoma. *J. invest. Dermatol.*, **95**, 506–509

Almadori, G., Galli, J., Cadoni, G., Bussu, F. & Maurizi, M. (2002) Human papillomavirus infection and cyclin D1 gene amplification in laryngeal squamous cell carcinoma: biologic function and clinical significance. *Head Neck*, **24**, 597–604

Andrieu, N. & Goldstein, A.M. (1998) Epidemiologic and genetic approaches in the study of gene–environment interaction: an overview of available methods. *Epidemiol. Rev.*, **20**, 137–147

Athas, W.F., Hedayati, M.A., Matanoski, G.M., Farmer, E.R. & Grossman, L. (1991) Development and field-test validation of an assay for DNA repair in circulating human lymphocytes. *Cancer Res.*, **51**, 5786–5793

Barbin, A., Laib, R.J. & Bartsch, H. (1985) Lack of miscoding properties of 7-(2-oxoethyl)guanine, the major vinyl chloride–DNA adduct. *Cancer Res.*, **45**, 2440–2444

Berwick, M. & Vineis, P (2000) Markers of DNA repair and susceptibility to cancer in humans: an epidemiologic review. *J. natl Cancer Inst.*, **92**, 874–897

Bonassi, S., Hagmar, L., Stromberg, U., Montagud, A.H., Tinnerberg, H., Forni, A., Heikkila, P., Wanders, S., Wilhardt, P., Hansteen, I.L., Knudsen, L.E. & Norppa, H. (2000) Chromosomal aberrations in lymphocytes predict human cancer independently of exposure to carcinogens. *Cancer Res.*, **60**, 1619–1625

Bond, J.A., Dahl, A.R., Henderson, R.F., Dutcher, J.S., Mauderly, J.L. & Birnbaum, L.S. (1986) Species differences in the disposition of inhaled butadiene. *Toxicol. appl. Pharmacol.*, **84**, 617–627

Bondy, M.L., Wang, L.E., El-Zein, R., de Andrade, M., Selvan, M.S., Bruner, J.M., Levin, V.A., Alfred Yung, W.K., Adatto, P. & Wei, Q. (2001) Gamma-radiation sensitivity and risk of glioma. *J. natl Cancer Inst.*, **93**, 1553–1557

Boveri, T. (1914) In: *Zur Frage der Entstehung maligner Tumoren*, Jena, Gustav Fischer

Caporaso, N. (1999) Selection of candidate genes for population studies. In: Vineis, P., Malats, N., Lang, M., d'Errico, A., Caporaso, N., Cuzick, J. & Boffetta, P., eds., *Metabolic Polymorphisms and Susceptibility to Cancer* (IARC Scientific Publications No. 148). Lyon, IARC*Press*, pp. 23–36

Cattani, P., Hohaus, S., Bellacosa, A., Genuardi, M., Cavallo, S., Rovella, V., Almadori, G., Cadoni, G., Galli, J., Maurizi, M., Fadda, G. & Neri, G. (1998) Association between cyclin D1 (CCND1) gene amplification and human papillomavirus infection in human laryngeal squamous cell carcinoma. *Clin. Cancer Res.*, **4**, 2585–2589

Chen, C.J., Wang, L.Y., Lu, S.N., Wu, M.H., You, S.L., Zhang, Y.J., Wang, L.W. & Santella, R.M. (1996) Elevated aflatoxin exposure and increased risk of hepatocellular carcinoma. *Hepatology*, **24**, 38–42

Ciroussel, F., Barbin, A., Eberle, G. & Bartsch, H (1990) Investigations on the relationship between DNA ethenobase adduct levels in several organs of vinyl chloride-exposed rats and cancer susceptibility. *Biochem. Pharmacol.*, **39**, 1109–1113

Clayton, D. & McKeigue, P.M. (2001) Epidemiological methods for studying genes and environmental factors in complex diseases. *Lancet*, **358**, 1356–1360

Cloos, J., Spitz, M.R., Schantz, S.P., Hsu, T.C., Zhang, Z.F., Tobi, H., Braakhuis, B.J. & Snow, G.B. (1996) Genetic susceptibility to head and neck squamous cell carcinoma. *J. natl Cancer Inst.*, **88**, 530–535

Conti, D.V. & Witte, J.S. (2003) Hierarchical modeling of linkage disequilibrium: genetic structure and spatial relations. *Am. J. hum. Genet.*, **72**, 351–363

Cresteil, T. (1998) Onset of xenobiotic metabolism in children: toxicological implications. *Food Addit. Contam.*, **15** (Suppl.), 45–51

Davey Smith, G. & Ebrahim, S (2003) 'Mendelian randomization': can genetic epidemiology contribute to understanding environmental determinants of disease? *Int. J. Epidemiol.*, **32**, 1–22

Elwood, M. (1998) *Critical Appraisal of Epidemiological Studies and Clinical Trials*, Oxford, Oxford University Press

Fedtke, N., Boucheron, J.A., Walker, V.E. & Swenberg, J.A. (1990) Vinyl chloride-induced DNA adducts. II: Formation and persistence of 7-(2'-oxoethyl)-guanine and N2,3-ethenoguanine in rat tissue DNA. *Carcinogenesis*, **11**,1287–1292

Friedberg, E.C. (2001) How nucleotide excision repair protects against cancer. *Nat. Rev. Cancer*, **1**, 22–33

Garte, S., Zocchetti, C. & Taioli, E. (1997) Gene–environment interactions in the application of biomarkers of cancer susceptibility in epidemiology. In: Toniolo, P., Boffetta, P., Shuker, D.E.G., Rothman, N., Hulka, B. & Pearce, N., eds, *Application of Biomarkers in Cancer Epidemiology* (IARC Scientific Publications No. 142), Lyon, IARC*Press*, pp. 251–264

Groopman, J.D., Wang, J.S. & Scholl, P. (1996) Molecular biomarkers for aflatoxins: from adducts to gene mutations to human liver cancer. *Can. J. Physiol. Pharmacol.*, **74**, 203–209

Gstaiger, M., Jordan, R., Lim, M., Catzavelos, C., Mestan, J., Slingerland, J. & Krek, W. (2001) Skp2 is oncogenic and overexpressed in human cancers. *Proc. natl Acad. Sci. USA*, **98**, 5043–5048

Hall, J.A., Saffhill, R., Green, T. & Hathway, D.E. (1981) The induction of errors during in vitro DNA synthesis following chloroacetaldehyde-treatment of poly(dA-dT) and poly (dC-dG) templates. *Carcinogenesis*, **2**, 141–146

Henderson, R.F. (1995) Strategies for use of biological markers of exposure. *Toxicol. Lett.*, **82–83**, 379–383

Hernandez, T.M. & Hainaut, P. (1999) A specific spectrum of p53 mutations in lung cancer from smokers: review of mutations compiled in the IARC p53 database. *Environ. Health Perspect.*, **106**, 385–391

Hill, A.B. (1965) The environment and disease: association or causation? *Proc. R. Soc. Med.*, **58**, 295–300

Hsu, T.C., Cherry, L.M. & Samaan, N.A. (1985) Differential mutagen susceptibility in cultured lymphocytes of normal individuals and cancer patients. *Cancer Genet. Cytogenet.*, **17**, 307–313

Hsu, T.C., Spitz, M.R. & Schantz, S.P. (1991) Mutagen sensitivity: a biological marker of cancer susceptibility. *Cancer Epidemiol. Biomarkers Prev.*, **1**, 83–89

Hunter, D.J. (1997) Methodological issues in the use of biological markers in cancer epidemiology: cohort studies. In: Toniolo, P., Boffetta, P., Shuker, D.E.G., Rothman, N., Hulka, B. & Pearce, N., eds, *Application of Biomarkers in Cancer Epidemiology* (IARC Scientific Publications No. 142), Lyon, IARC*Press*, pp. 39–46

IARC (1993) *IARC Monographs on the Evaluation of Carcinogenic Risks to Humans*, Vol. 56, *Some Naturally Occurring Substances: Food Items and Constituents, Heterocyclic Aromatic Amines and Mycotoxins*, Lyon, IARC*Press*, pp. 245–395

IARC (1994) Ethylene oxide. In: *IARC Monographs on the Evaluation of Carcinogenic Risks to Humans*, Vol. 60, *Some Industrial Chemicals*, Lyon, IARC*Press*, pp. 73–159

IARC (1995) *IARC Monographs on the Evaluation of Carcinogenic Risks to Humans*, Vol. 64, *Human Papillomaviruses*, Lyon, IARC*Press*

Jepson, A.P. (1996) Infection . . . by the new genetics. *J. Infect.*, **33**, 1–5

Kadlubar, F.F., Talaska, G., Butler, M.A., Teitel, C.H., Massengill, J.P. & Lang, N.P. (1990) Determination of carcinogenic arylamine N-oxidation phenotype in humans by analysis of caffeine urinary metabolites. *Prog. clin. biol. Res.*, **340B**, 107–114

Khoury, M., Beaty, T.H. & Cohen, B.L. (1993) *Fundamentals of Genetic Epidemiology*, New York, Oxford University Press

Kresty, L.A., Mallery, S.R., Knobloch, T.J., Song, H., Lloyd, M., Casto, B.C. & Weghorst, C.M. (2002) Alterations of p16(INK4a) and p14(ARF) in patients with severe oral epithelial dysplasia. *Cancer Res.*, **62**, 5295–5300

Landi, M.T., Zocchetti, C., Bernucci, I., Kadlubar, F.F., Tannenbaum, S., Skipper, P., Bartsch, H., Malaveille, C., Shields, P., Caporaso, N.E. & Vineis, P. (1996) Cytochrome P4501A2: enzyme induction and genetic control in determining 4-aminobiphenyl–hemoglobin adduct levels. *Cancer Epidemiol. Biomarkers Prev.*, **5**, 693–698

Langholz, B., Rothman, N., Wacholder, S. & Thomas, D.C. (1999) Cohort studies for characterizing measured genes. *Natl Cancer Inst. Monogr.*, **26**, 39–42

Lerman, C., Caporaso, N.E., Audrain, J., Main, D., Bowman, E.D., Lockshin, B., Boyd, N.R. & Shields, P.G. (1999) Evidence suggesting the role of specific genetic factors in cigarette smoking. *Health Psychol.*, **18**, 14–20

Lohmueller, K.E., Pearce, C.L., Pike, M., Lander, E.S. & Hirschhorn, J.N. (2003) Meta-analysis of genetic association studies supports a contribution of common variants to susceptibility to common disease. *Nat. Genet.*, **33**, 177–182

Miller, A.B., Bartsch, H., Boffetta, P., Dragsted, L. & Vainio, H., eds. (2001) *Biomarkers in Cancer Chemoprevention* (IARC Scientific Publications No. 154). Lyon, IARC*Press*

Moolgavkar, S.H. & Knudson, A.G., Jr (1981) Mutation and cancer: a model for human carcinogenesis. *J. natl Cancer Inst.*, **66**, 1037–1052

Mooney, L.A., Bell, D.A., Santella, R.M., Van Bennekum, A.M., Ottman, R., Paik, M., Blaner, W.S., Lucier, G.W., Covey, L., Young, T.L., Cooper, T.B., Glassman, A.H. & Perera, F.P. (1997) Contribution of genetic and nutritional factors to DNA damage in heavy smokers. *Carcinogenesis*, **18**, 503–509

Mori, H., Colman, S.M., Xiao, Z., Ford, A.M., Healy, L.E., Donaldson, C., Hows, J.M., Navarrete, C. & Greaves, M. (2002) Chromosome translocations and covert leukemic clones are generated during normal fetal development. *Proc. natl Acad. Sci. USA*, **99**, 8242–8247

Perera, F.P. & Weinstein, I.B. (1982) Molecular epidemiology and carcinogen–DNA adduct detection: new approaches to studies of human cancer causation. *J. chronic Dis.*, **35**, 581–600

Peto, J. (2001) Cancer epidemiology in the last century and the next decade. *Nature*, **411**, 390–395

Prentice, R.L. (1986) A case–cohort design for epidemiologic studies and disease prevention trials. *Biometrika*, **73**, 1–11

Ramsey, J.C. & Andersen, M.E. (1984) A physiologically based description of the inhalation pharmacokinetics of styrene in rats and humans. *Toxicol. appl. Pharmacol.*, **73**, 159–175

Rebbeck, T.R., Rogatko, A. & Viana, M.A. (1997–98) Evaluation of genotype data in clinical risk assessment: methods and application to BRCA1, BRCA2, and N-acetyl transferase-2 genotypes in breast cancer. *Genet. Test.*, **1**, 157–164

Risch, N.J. (2000) Searching for genetic determinants in the new millennium. *Nature*, **405**, 847–856

Risch, N. & Merikangas, K (1996) The future of genetic studies of complex human diseases. *Science*, **273**, 1516–1517

Ross, R.K., Yuan, J.M., Yu, M.C., Wogan, G.N., Qian, G.S., Tu, J.T., Groopman, J.D., Gao, Y.T. & Henderson, B.E. (1992) Urinary aflatoxin bio-

markers and risk of hepatocellular carcinoma. *Lancet*, **339**, 943–946

Rowley, J.D. (2001) Chromosome translocations: dangerous liaisons revisited. *Nat. Rev. Cancer*, **1**, 245–250

Sabourin, P.J., Chen, B.T., Lucier, G., Birnbaum, L.S., Fisher, E. & Henderson, R.F. (1987) Effect of dose on the absorption and excretion of [14C]benzene administered orally or by inhalation in rats and mice. *Toxicol. appl. Pharmacol.*, **87**, 325–336

Scully, C., Field, J.K. & Tanzawa, H. (2000) Genetic aberrations in oral or head and neck squamous cell carcinoma (SCCHN): 1. Carcinogen metabolism, DNA repair and cell cycle control. *Oral Oncol.*, **36**, 256–263

Schulte, P.A., Hunter, D. & Rothman, N. (1997) Ethical and social issues in the use of biomarkers in epidemiological research. In: Toniolo, P., Boffetta, P., Shuker, D.E.G., Rothman, N., Hulka, B. & Pearce, N., eds, *Application of Biomarkers in Cancer Epidemiology* (IARC Scientific Publications No. 142), Lyon, IARC*Press*, pp. 313–318

Shahnavez, S.A., Bradley, G., Regezi, J.A., Thakker, N., Gao, L., Hogg, D. & Jordan, R.C. (2001) Patterns of CDKN2A gene loss in sequential oral epithelial dysplasias and carcinomas. *Cancer Res.*, **61**, 2371–2375

Singer, B., Spengler, S.J., Chavez, F. & Kusmierek, J.T. (1987) The vinyl chloride-derived nucleoside, N2,3-ethenoguanosine, is a highly efficient mutagen in transcription. *Carcinogenesis*, **8**, 745–747

Smith, M.T., Zhang, L., Wang, Y., Hayes, R.B., Li, G., Wiemels, J., Dosemeci, M., Titenko-Holland, N., Xi, L., Kolachana, P., Yin, S. & Rothman, N (1998) Increased translocations and aneusomy in chromosomes 8 and 21 among workers exposed to benzene. *Cancer Res.*, **58**, 2176–2181

Snijders, A.M., Nowak, N., Segraves, R., Blackwood, S., Brown, N., Conroy, J., Hamilton, G., Hindle, A.K., Huey, B., Kimura, K., Law, S., Myambo, K., Palmer, J., Ylstra, B., Yue, J.P., Gray, J.W., Jain, A.N., Pinkel, D. & Albertson, D.G. (2001) Assembly of microarrays for genome-wide measurement of DNA copy number. *Nat. Genet.*, **29**, 263–264

Sonnier, M. & Cresteil, T. (1998) Delayed ontogenesis of CYP1A2 in the human liver. *Eur. J. Biochem.*, **251**, 893–898

Spitz, M.R., Fueger, J.J., Beddingfield, N.A., Annegers, J.F., Hsu, T.C., Newell, G.R. & Schantz, S.P. (1989) Chromosome sensitivity to bleomycin-induced mutagenesis, an independent risk factor for upper aerodigestive tract cancers. *Cancer Res.*, **49**, 4626–4628

Spitz, M.R., Wu, X., Wang, Y., Wang, L.E., Shete, S., Amos, C.I., Guo, Z., Lei, L., Mohrenweiser, H. & Wei, Q. (2001) Modulation of nucleotide excision repair capacity by XPD polymorphisms in lung cancer patients. *Cancer Res.*, **61**, 1354–1357

Stram, D.O., Longnecker, M.P., Shames, L., Kolonel, L.N., Wilkens, L.R., Pike, M.C. & Henderson, B.E. (1995) Cost-efficient design of a diet validation study. *Am. J. Epidemiol.*, **142**, 353–362

Surgeon General (1964) (Advisory Committee) *Smoking and Health*, Washington DC, US Department of Health, Education and Welfare

Swenberg, J.A., Fedtke, N., Fennel, T.R. & Walker, V.E. (1990) Relationships between carcinogen exposure, DNA adducts and carcinogenesis. In: Clayson, D.B., Munro, I.C., Shubik, P. & Swenberg, J.A., eds, *Progress in Predictive Toxicology*. Amsterdam, Elsevier Science, pp. 161–184

Taioli, E., Zocchetti, C. & Garte, S. (1998) Models of interaction between metabolic genes and environmental exposure in cancer susceptibility. *Environ. Health Perspect.*, **106**, 67–70

Tang, D.L., Rundle, A., Warburton, D., Santella, R.M., Tsai, W.Y., Chiamprasert, S., Hsu, Y.Z. & Perera, F.P. (1998) Associations between both genetic and environmental biomarkers and lung cancer: evidence of a greater risk of lung cancer in women smokers. *Carcinogenesis*, **19**, 1949–1953

Taylor, G.M., Gokhale, D.A., Crowther, D., Woll, P., Harris, M., Alexander, F., Jarrett, R. & Cartwright, R.A. (1996) Increased frequency of HLA-DPB1*0301 in Hodgkin's disease suggests that susceptibility is HVR-sequence and subtype-associated. *Leukemia*, **10**, 854–859

Taylor, G.M., Dearden, S., Payne, N., Ayres, M., Gokhale, D.A., Birch, J.M., Blair, V., Stevens, R.F., Will, A.M. & Eden, O.B. (1998) Evidence that an HLA-DQA1-DQB1 haplotype influences susceptibility to childhood common acute lymphoblastic leukaemia in boys provides further support for an infection-related aetiology. *Br. J. Cancer*, **78**, 561–565

Thomas, D.C. & Witte, J.S. (2002) Point: population stratification: a problem for case–control studies of candidate–gene associations? *Cancer Epidemiol. Biomarkers Prev.*, **11**, 505–512

Toniolo, P., Boffetta, P., Shuker, D.E.G., Rothman, N., Hulka, B. & Pearce, N., eds (1997) *Application of Biomarkers in Cancer Epidemiology* (IARC Scientific Publications No. 142), Lyon, IARC*Press*

Tsao, J.L., Yatabe, Y., Salovaara, R., Jarvinen, H.J., Mecklin, J.P., Aaltonen, L.A., Tavaré, S., & Shibata, D. (2000) Genetic reconstruction of individual colorectal tumor histories. *Proc. natl Acad. Sci. USA*, **97**, 1236–1241

Tsukasaki, K., Miller, C.W., Kubota, T., Takeuchi, S., Fujimoto, T., Ikeda, S., Tomonaga, M. & Koeffler, H.P. (2001) Tumor necrosis factor α polymorphism associated with increased susceptibility to development of adult T-cell leukemia/lymphoma in human T-lymphotropic virus type I carriers. *Cancer Res.*, **61**, 3770–3774

Vainio, H., Magee, P.N., McGregor, D.B. & McMichael, A.J. (1992) *Mechanisms of Carcinogenesis in Risk Identification* (IARC Scientific Publication No. 116), Lyon, IARC*Press*

Vineis, P., Malats, N., Lang, M., d'Errico, A., Caporaso, N., Cuzick, J. & Boffetta, P., eds (1999) *Metabolic Polymorphisms and Susceptibility to Cancer* (IARC Scientific Publications No. 148), Lyon, IARC*Press*

Wacholder, S., Rothman, N. & Caporaso, N (2002) Counterpoint: bias from population stratification is not a major threat to the validity of conclusions from epidemiological studies of common polymorphisms and cancer. *Cancer Epidemiol. Biomarkers Prev.*, **11**, 513–520

Wang, L.E., Sturgis, E.M., Eicher, S.A., Spitz, M.R., Hong, W.K. & Wei, Q (1998) Mutagen sensitivity to benzo(a)pyrene diol epoxide and the risk of squamous cell carcinoma of the head and neck. *Clin. Cancer Res.*, **4**, 1773–1778

Ward, J.B., Jr & Henderson, R.E. (1996) Identification of needs in biomarker research. *Environ. Health Perspect.*, **104** (Suppl.), 895–900

Waters, M.D., Stack, H.F. & Jackson, M.A. (1999) Genetic toxicology data in the evaluation of potential human environmental carcinogens. *Mutat. Res.*, **437**, 21–49

Weed, D.L. & Gorelic, L.S. (1996) The practice of causal inference in cancer epidemiology. *Cancer Epidemiol. Biomarkers Prev.*, **5**, 303–311

Wei, Q., Matanoski, G.M., Farmer, E.R., Hedayati, M.A. & Grossman, L (1993) DNA repair and aging in basal cell carcinoma: a molecular epidemiology study. *Proc. natl Acad. Sci. USA*, **90**, 1614–1618

Wei, Q., Spitz, M.R., Gu, J., Cheng, L., Xu, X., Strom, S.S., Kripke, M.L. & Hsu, T.C. (1996) DNA repair capacity correlates with mutagen sensitivity in lymphoblastoid cell lines. *Cancer Epidemiol. Biomarkers Prev.*, **5**, 199–204

Wiemels, J.L., Smith, R.N., Taylor, G.M., Eden, O.B., Alexander, F.E. & Greaves, M.F. (2001) Methylene-tetrahydrofolate reductase (MTHFR) polymorphisms and risk of molecularly defined subtypes of childhood acute leukemia. *Proc. natl Acad. Sci. USA*, **98**, 4004–4009

Xiong, P., Bondy, M.L., Li, D., Shen, H., Wang, L.E., Singletary, S.E., Spitz, M.R. & Wei, Q. (2001) Sensitivity to benzo(a)pyrene diol-epoxide associated with risk of breast cancer in young women and modulation by glutathione S-transferase polymorphisms: a case–control study. *Cancer Res.*, **61**, 8465–8469

Mechanisms of Carcinogenesis: Contributions of Molecular Epidemiology
Patricia Buffler, Jerry Rice, Robert Baan, Michael Bird and Paolo Boffetta, eds
IARC Scientific Publications No. 157
International Agency for Research on Cancer, Lyon, 2004

Subgroup Report: Stomach Cancer

Robert Newton, Jerry Rice and Patricia Buffler

Background

In the 1990s, about 800 000 deaths were attributable to gastric cancer each year, making it the 14th leading cause of death in the world and the second leading cause of death from cancer (Murray & Lopez, 1997; Plummer *et al.*, this volume). Despite rapidly declining incidence rates in developed countries, gastric cancer will remain a major cause of death for many years as a result of population ageing, population growth in developing countries and poor prognosis. The incidence of gastric cancer varies approximately 15–20-fold worldwide, with the highest rates being recorded in Japan and East Asia, and the lowest rates in North America. Patterns of mortality reflect those of incidence, largely because the fatality rate from gastric cancer is high. The tumour is about two to three times more common in men than in women and the incidence increases markedly with age in both sexes.

Known and suspected risk factors

Data, primarily from prospective sero-epidemiological studies, suggest that infection with the gastric bacterium, *Helicobacter pylori*, is a leading cause of gastric cancer (IARC, 1994), with estimates of attributable risk ranging from about 40 to 70% (Forman *et al.*, 1994; Danesh, 1999). Both gastric carcinoma (of all histological subtypes) and gastric non-Hodgkin lymphoma (which comprises about 3% of stomach tumours) have been associated with *H. pylori* infection, although the mechanism of carcinogenesis and other risk factors for disease may differ. However, epidemiological evidence indicates that the etiology of gastric carcinoma differs according to site within the stomach (Plummer *et al.*, this volume). Tumours of the cardia, which are relatively rare, do not appear to be related to infection with *H. pylori* and differ in a number of other important ways from non-cardia cancers. It is therefore important to distinguish between cardia and non-cardia tumours in epidemiological or molecular studies of gastric cancer.

H. pylori is a spiral, flagellated, gram-negative bacterium that colonizes the human gastrointestinal tract and lives beneath the mucus overlaying the gastric epithelium. It causes gastritis in all infected people and, although many cases remain asymptomatic, some result in gastric or duodenal ulceration. In a very small proportion of infected individuals, *H. pylori* may be involved in the etiology of gastric adenocarcinomas and the much rarer primary gastric non-Hodgkin lymphoma. It is estimated that about 50% of the world's population is chronically infected with *H. pylori*. The prevalence of infection is highest in developing countries and increases rapidly during the first two decades of life, such that 80–90% of the population may be infected by early adulthood. In most developed countries, the prevalence of infection is substantially lower at all ages, particularly in childhood. Everywhere, the prevalence of *H. pylori* is strongly correlated with markers of poverty and, indeed, has been decreasing in developing countries for decades, presumably because of improvements in living conditions. Transmission occurs from person to person, probably from mouth to mouth or faecally–orally, or both.

Drug therapy consisting of two antibiotics in combination with either a bismuth preparation or an acid inhibitor for 14 days is effective in eradicating *H. pylori* in about 80% of cases. Given the high incidence of stomach cancer, the availability of screening tests and eradication regimens, but the relatively low progression rates to cancer in people with *H. pylori* infection, very large randomized trials are needed to establish the value of eradication for the prevention of gastric cancer. However, the large-scale use of antimicrobial treatment is potentially problematic — eradication might be difficult to achieve and re-infection can occur. Furthermore, extensive use of antibiotics may lead to the development of resistant strains (Coursaget & Muñoz, 1999). Nevertheless, it is essential to bear in mind, when considering further research on carcinogenesis in relation to gastric cancer, that primary prevention of the tumour might be possible on the basis of information already available. However, a better understanding of mechanisms is potentially useful for secondary prevention of gastric cancer, for example, by allowing identification of high-risk individuals.

In the future, immunization may be a better strategy for the prevention of *H. pylori*-associated diseases, particularly in developing countries. It has been demonstrated in mouse models that *H. pylori* vaccines can not only protect against infection, but may also induce regression of associated lesions. However, in models more relevant to humans, such as monkeys, results have been disappointing. In phase I trials of a recombinant vaccine in humans, no adverse events were observed, but neither were there any changes in gastric bacterial density. Further work is required to identify appropriate target antigens and delivery systems and to understand the mechanism of protective immunity. Therefore, there is currently little realistic prospect of a cheap and effective vaccine becoming available in the foreseeable future.

Relatively less is known about other risk factors for gastric cancer. A consistent finding in many studies is that a diet rich in fresh fruits and vegetables appears to be protective against the disease. The role of other dietary factors remains unclear, although high salt consumption may be associated with an increased risk. Familial aggregation of cases might suggest a genetic component and several candidate genes have been studied as potential risk factors.

Stages in tumour development

The mechanisms by which gastric tumours develop are unclear and may differ for different types. In particular, the way in which *H. pylori* might increase the risk for gastric cancer is unknown. The bacteria cause lifelong inflammation, possibly leading to oxidative damage, with the production of mutagenic compounds, as well as loss of gastric acidity and epithelial cell proliferation. Any or all of the above might contribute to carcinogenesis. There is evidence that the development of cancer is preceded by progressive changes to the stomach mucosa — from inflammation to atrophy and cellular proliferation, a process that is thought to be related to infection with *H. pylori* (Correa, this volume). This may be particularly true of the pro-inflammatory strains of *H. pylori* — those that possess the cytotoxin associated gene A (*CagA*) — because they markedly affect gastric cytokine levels and promote cell turnover, without inducing a corresponding increase in apoptosis. Therefore, *CagA* strains of *H. pylori* might be expected to show a stronger association with gastric cancer, but the evidence for this remains scant.

The Mongolian gerbil is currently the best available animal model of gastric cancer in relation to infection with *H. pylori* and perhaps also other risk factors, but is currently relatively underdeveloped. Furthermore, the presence of a gastric cancer lesion (or the precancerous lesions that precede it) in the stomach may influence the measurement of factors associated with disease. Therefore, prospective studies are likely to be more informative than retrospective ones. This has significant practical implications, as the collection of biological material on large numbers of healthy individuals is expensive and difficult. It also places limitations on the type of biological material that can be collected (gastric biopsies are probably not feasible) and draws attention to the need to develop relatively non-invasive methods of obtaining samples from the stomach (perhaps via saliva or faecal material).

Available biomarkers

Markers of H. pylori infection
Almost all sero-epidemiological studies of *H. pylori* and gastric cancer have classified subjects as 'positive' or 'negative', and it may be useful to consider anti-*H. pylori* antibody titres as a quantitative measure of risk for the tumour. Such a strategy has proved useful in studies of viruses and cancer in which high titres of viral antibodies are associated with the subsequent development of

malignancy (de Thé et al., 1978). Information on anti-H. pylori antibody titres might allow discrimination of high-risk individuals in populations with a high prevalence of infection, and the presence of a dose–response would be further evidence of causality. It could also be useful in epidemiological studies to investigate the role of duration and timing of infection — the determinants of chronic infection — in relation to cancer risk, and in studies of the transmission of H. pylori.

A classification of H. pylori strains has been proposed based on the presence (type I) or absence (type II) of a 40-kb pathogenicity island which makes type I strains more virulent. Since only type I strains have the CagA gene, antibodies to CagA can be used as a marker of infection with type I strains. The role of CagA-positive strains in the pathogenesis of gastric cancer requires further investigation and could be achieved using the newly developed anti-CagA antibody assays.

Markers of Epstein–Barr virus (EBV) infection
Epstein–Barr virus (EBV) DNA is clonally present in all tumour cells of approximately 10% of gastric adenocarcinomas worldwide. However, the role of EBV in the etiology of gastric carcinoma is unclear and warrants further investigation. Anti-EBV antibodies could be measured in cases and controls using sera from prospective studies — this might be particularly informative if the subset of cases with evidence of EBV DNA in malignant tissue could be selected.

Markers of inflammation and oxidative damage
Inflammation and oxidative damage precede the development of gastric carcinoma and gastric

non-Hodgkin lymphoma, but the relative importance of these two processes is unclear. The epidemiological finding that a diet rich in fresh fruits and vegetables is protective against gastric carcinoma has led to the hypothesis that this effect is mediated through anti-oxidant vitamins. In prospective studies, intake of anti-oxidant vitamins (A, C and E) could be estimated using dietary questionnaires or measured directly in serum. Furthermore, in a randomized trial of the chemoprevention of gastric dysplasia, anti-oxidant supplements (vitamins A and C) were as effective as H. pylori eradication in causing the regression of existing premalignant lesions. This suggests that oxidative damage may be of particular mechanistic importance for carcinomas, although the number of subjects in the trial was relatively small (Correa et al., 2000). Conversely, the development of extranodal non-Hodgkin lymphoma is sometimes preceded by site-specific inflammation, which may be more relevant than oxidative damage in this instance.

Non-specific biomarkers of inflammation, oxidative damage and gastric tissue damage are available (see Table 1) and could be used in prospective studies of gastric cancer. Certain markers of inflammation and gastric tissue damage can be measured in blood. Most markers of oxidative damage require biopsy material.

Markers of genetic susceptibility
It is established that individuals with blood group A have a slightly increased risk for gastric cancer. The role of other susceptibility genes is less certain. Genes affecting susceptibility to gastric cancer may act at any stage of the carcinogenic process from infection with H. pylori through to invasive malignancy. Of particular interest are

---

Table 1. Non-specific biomarkers

Inflammation	Oxidative damage	Gastric tissue damage
C-reactive protein	Hydrogen peroxide	Gastrin
Lymphocyte counts	Nitric oxide radicals	Pepsinogen I & II
Cytokines	Nitrotyrosine	
Interleukins	Malondialdehyde	

those genes, such as *IL-1β*, which are polymorphic and linked to the process of gastric acid secretion. A more extensive list of candidate genes is presented in the chapter by Correa (this volume).

Mutational spectra

An extensive range of genetic mutations associated with gastric cancer or premalignant lesions has been characterized (Tahara, this volume). These include alterations to tumour suppressor genes, cell-cycle regulators, oncogenes and adhesion molecules, as well as microsatellite instability.

DNA adducts

It has been hypothesized that endogenous nitrosamine formation may influence risk for gastric carcinoma. Exposure to nitrosamines should give rise to alkylation of gastric DNA and could be measured as DNA adducts such as O^6-methylguanine.

Dietary markers

The role of dietary factors (in addition to antioxidant vitamins) is being studied in the EPIC (European Prospective Investigation of Cancer — International Agency for Research on Cancer) and other studies. Intake of dietary components is estimated using questionnaires and diet diaries, and serum is collected for measurement of dietary biomarkers. The role of salt consumption — another putative risk factor for gastric cancer — is difficult to assess, although it could be estimated in nested case–control studies using urine samples collected over a 24-h period.

Conclusions

Although gastric cancer remains the second most common cause of cancer death worldwide, incidence and mortality rates have been steadily declining over the last 50 years, in both former high- and low-incidence countries. For example, in Japan, gastric cancer mortality rates have declined by more than half since the 1950s, with an average reduction of 1% per year, although rates remain the highest in the world. Mortality rates have also declined in other high-incidence countries, as well as in low-incidence countries

such as the USA. These reductions are thought to be largely due to changes in dietary patterns and methods of preserving foods, together with a reduction in the prevalence of infection with *H. pylori*. Perhaps the best hope for increasing the rate of decline in the incidence and mortality from gastric cancer lies with interventions against *H. pylori*, ideally through vaccination or perhaps mass treatment of infection.

References

Correa, P., Fontham, E.T., Bravo, J.C., Bravo, L.E., Ruiz, B., Zarama, G., Realpe, J.L., Malcom, G.T., Li, D., Johnson, W.D. & Mera, R. (2000) Chemoprevention of gastric dysplasia: randomized trial of antioxidant supplements and anti-Helicobacter pylori therapy. *J. natl Cancer Inst.*, **92**, 1881–1888

Coursaget, P. & Muñoz, N. (1999) Vaccination against infectious agents associated with human cancer. In: Newton, R., Beral, V. & Weiss, R.A., eds, *Infections and Human Cancer* (Cancer Surveys Vol. 33), New York, Cold Spring Harbor Laboratory Press, pp. 355–381

Danesh, J. (1999) *Helicobacter pylori* infection and gastric cancer: systematic review of the epidemiological studies. *Aliment. Pharmacol. Ther.*, **13**, 851–856

de Thé, G., Geser, A., Day, N.E., Tukei, P.M., Williams, E.H., Beri, D.P., Smith, P.G., Dean, A.G., Bornkamm, G.W., Feorino, P. & Henle, W. (1978) Epidemiological evidence for causal relationship between Epstein-Barr virus and Burkitt's lymphoma from Ugandan prospective study. *Nature*, **274**, 756–761

Forman, D., Webb, P. & Parsonnet, J. (1994) *H. pylori* and gastric cancer. *Lancet*, **343**, 243–244

IARC (1994) *IARC Monographs on the Evaluation of Carcinogenic Risks to Humans*, Vol. 64, *Schistosomes, Liver Flukes and* Helicobacter Pylori, Lyon, IARC*Press*, pp. 177–240

Murray, C.J. & Lopez, A.D. (1997) Global mortality, disability, and the contribution of risk factors: Global Burden of Disease Study. *Lancet*, **349**, 1436–1442

Mechanisms of Carcinogenesis: Contributions of Molecular Epidemiology
Patricia Buffler, Jerry Rice, Robert Baan, Michael Bird and Paolo Boffetta, eds
IARC Scientific Publications No. 157
International Agency for Research on Cancer, Lyon, 2004

Subgroup Report: Lymphohaematopoietic Neoplasms

Julian Little, Michael Bird and Patricia Buffler

Background

Target tissue

In contrast to other types of cancer, the target tissues (blood and bone marrow) for investigation of the etiology and pathogenesis of lympho-haematopoietic neoplasms are relatively easily accessible. From studies of cord blood, it is known that only a fraction (approximately 1%) of preleukaemic clones present at birth go on to develop leukaemia. In consequence, it has been possible to characterize the biology of the various diseases relatively better than has been the case for epithelial tumours.

Lymphomas and lymphoid leukaemias versus myeloid leukaemias

Lymphoma and leukaemia are diverse diseases with multiple subtypes that probably have different etiologies. However, a distinction between two general types of these diseases is useful: (1) lymphoid and (2) myeloid.

Current evidence suggests that lymphoma and lymphoid leukaemias may have an immunogenic etiology. Autoimmunity, immunosuppression and chronic infection have been associated with various forms of lymphoma. For example, chronic *Helicobacter pylori* infection appears to cause gastric mucosa-associated lymphoid tissue lymphoma, whereas infection with the Epstein–Barr virus in certain regions is associated with Burkitt's lymphoma (Smith *et al.*, this volume). Acute lymphoblastic leukaemia in children may be associated with an abnormal immune response to a common infectious agent (Greaves, 1997) or exposure to a specific viral agent (Kinlen, 1995).

One of the best-documented environmental agents is in-utero exposure to ionizing radiation (X-rays and γ-radiation). No cases of childhood leukaemia were observed in the study of atomic bomb survivors who were exposed *in utero*, whereas a 40% increase in risk for leukaemia was noted for children medically exposed just before birth (IARC, 2000).

Myeloid leukaemia, in contrast, may result from chemical or dietary exposures. Treatment with topoisomerase II inhibitors and alkylating agents has been shown to produce treatment-related acute myeloid leukaemia with distinctive chromosomal aberrations. Acute myeloid leukaemia arising in elderly patients exhibits some of the same chromosomal abnormalities, suggesting a possible chemical etiology (Smith *et al.*, this volume). Occupational exposure to benzene has also been conclusively linked with development of leukaemia, mostly of the acute myeloid type (NTP, 2002).

Myeloid leukaemias and metabolism of chemicals

Some types of acute myelogenous leukaemia have been shown to be induced by chemicals. The specific chemicals involved are benzene, an industrial chemical, and two forms of cancer chemotherapeutic agent, i.e. alkylating agents and topoisomerase II inhibitors. It is thought that these chemicals, or their metabolites, can damage DNA, either by covalent binding to DNA, by the generation of reactive oxygen species or by interfering with DNA repair. The results of the DNA damage are most likely to be chromosomal aberrations or translocations, which in themselves are biomarkers of effect. To fill a gap in our knowledge of the role of these chemicals in leukemogenesis, a fuller appreciation of the intermediate steps that lead to DNA damage is needed. Thus, it is known that benzene must undergo hepatic metabolism, the products of which enter the bone marrow and probably undergo further metabolism, ending in a process, as yet not fully understood, which results in DNA damage. DNA adduct formation may play a role. Alternatively, benzene metabolites may be auto-oxidizable and yield reactive oxygen species that may cause DNA damage. Some alkylating agents, such as melphalan, may react directly with DNA. Others, such as cyclophosphamide, may require metabolic activation both for their anti-cancer activity and for covalent binding to DNA. Topoisomerase II inhibitors may act by preventing the DNA repair function of the enzyme or may function by some other mechanism, as yet not identified. The role played by the metabolism of each of these types of compound and the ultimate chemical species that produce the DNA damage require further study. It is possible that studies of this type may uncover additional, previously unrecognized biomarkers.

Research strategies

Molecular epidemiological studies of leukaemia and lymphoma in high-risk populations should provide insights relevant to the design and evaluation of general population studies that seek to identify causal factors which have appreciable population attributable risks. In particular, such research can provide a basis to bridge results from toxicological studies to studies of exposed human populations or for generating hypotheses for general population research. In the interim, biomarkers should be developed that will facilitate the conduct of improved general population studies. Perhaps most important is the development of biomarkers of exposure which, given the skewed nature of exposure distributions for many environmental factors, seems necessary to minimize exposure misclassification and to provide a basis to judge potential human risk where epidemiological studies are unlikely to be feasible.

One way in which biomarkers may be used is to compare changes that arise at different stages of evolution of clonal lineages with each other. For example, assuming that clonal populations can be developed for sequentially evolving lineages, technologies such as comparative genomic hybridization between representatives of steps in evolution may reveal the importance of each step and

its place in the sequence of overall changes that arise. The general principle is to apply methods that are currently used to compare the overall genome between malignant and normal tissue in a comparison of intermediate changes at different steps in the evolution of clonal lineages. We propose that the validation of currently available biomarkers, and development and validation of new ones, would proceed by an iterative process. Thus, new biomarkers might be developed on the basis of the results of ongoing case–control studies and animal models, validated in studies of individuals at high risk, and then tested in studies of individuals at lower risk. Those validated would then be investigated in population-based studies (mainly nested case–control studies). This would be expected to generate new leads and the process of development and validation would then be implemented once again.

Validation in cohorts of individuals at high risk

Biomarkers might be best validated in the context of cohort studies of individuals at risk. Examples include cancer patients treated with genotoxic chemotherapy or radiotherapy, patients suffering from autoimmune conditions, immunosuppressed patients (notably as a result of acquired immunodeficiency syndrome or organ transplant), human T-lymphotropic virus type 1-infected individuals and patients with myelodysplastic syndromes. There is no evidence that the cancers experienced by immunosuppressed individuals are different from those occurring in the general population, but there are several important considerations in study design. As a malignant outcome in most of the situations is relatively rare (~ 1%), a practical approach would be to organize systematic banking of appropriate serial blood and bone-marrow cell samples from the cohort. This hypothesis-driven tissue banking is a strategy that allows the testing of specific hypotheses regarding the type, numbers and sequencing of biological changes revealed by biomarkers involved in leukaemogenesis/lymphomagenesis.

Once individuals with leukaemia/lymphoma are identified, their samples could be analysed retrospectively in comparison with a set without disease. This would enable identification of bio-marker assays that are informative. Moreover, with this approach, genetic markers of DNA damage or repair could be quantified along side measurements of genetic change directly involved in the causal pathway, e.g. chromosome trans-locations identified by real-time polymerase chain reaction (PCR) methods (Taqman), genomic PCR (using fusion gene sequence) and fluorescence in-situ hybridization (with gene-specific probes).

Given the rarity of these patients, large multi-centre (probably multinational) studies are essen-tial. The initial design of such studies (prior to funding applications) should be conducted in close collaboration with the appropriate clinical working groups (i.e. as active participants in the study).

Large-scale molecular epidemiological studies to identify and validate biomarkers for biological processes involved in leukaemogenesis/lympho-magenesis are not practical given the current state of understanding. Rather, nested case–control studies of a subset of cases and controls of high-risk individuals may be a methodologically sound alternative for identifying important processes. The purpose of these nested studies is to allow for focused subsequent prospective studies in the general population. One high-risk group will be cancer patients receiving chemotherapy or radio-therapy for a primary malignancy for whom the risk for subsequent treatment-related acute mye-loid leukaemia is substantial. Biological samples will consist of target tissues for treatment-related acute myeloid leukaemia, i.e. blood and bone marrow. Samples should be obtained before and at intervals during and following treatments, providing material for longitudinal observations. Samples should be cryopreserved to allow for functional analyses of certain biomarkers. Ethical issues involved in the conduct of such studies have been previously reviewed (Schulte et al., 1997).

Available biomarkers
The only validated biomarkers of early effect for haematological malignancies are classical chro-mosomal aberrations (Bonassi et al., 2001). This classic assay is, however, time-consuming and expensive, and scoring may be subjective; thus

new methods are needed. An automated quanti-tative molecular version of this assay would be highly desirable, but it will be important to deve-lop this in the context of clonality.

Several ongoing case–control studies are exa-mining the relationship between childhood and lymphohaematopoietic neoplasms, a variety of exposures, genetic factors that may modulate these exposures, such as metabolic polymor-phisms including glutathione S-transferase variants, NAD(P)H:quinone oxidoreductase, and gene fusions. Information from these studies may provide useful information to guide the future selection of putative biomarkers of susceptibility and effect for study. There is therefore a need to develop approaches for a critical appraisal and synthesis of the data from these studies, e.g. following the Human Genome Epidemiology Network (Little et al., 2003).

Novel biomarkers
There is a need to develop additional biomarkers for assessing biological processes involved in leukaemogenesis/lymphomagenesis. These will be biomarkers of exposure, effect and susceptibi-lity. In nested case–control studies of high-risk subjects, the biomarkers of exposure would be those that measure internal and target doses of the agents used in the therapy of primary tumours. Biomarkers of susceptibility will be in part geno-typic markers. Additional susceptibility bio-markers will be those that detect specific infec-tions (lymphomagenesis) or immunodeficiencies. For the latter, specific rather than global immuno-deficiencies are likely to be most informative. Biomarkers of effect will include non-specific and, more importantly in this context, specific genetic events (i.e. chromosomal rearrangements, mutations). Furthermore, it is likely that several rather than single genetic events will characterize the process of leukaemogenesis/lymphoma-genesis. These several processes will probably occur sequentially and they must occur in clonal lineages. Therefore, it is important that additional biomarkers of clonality be developed to allow longitudinal observations of clonal evolutions. These specific biomarkers of effect must be assessed in target tissues.

Genomic DNA translocation biomarkers

At present, work is being conducted on the development of genomic DNA translocation biomarkers. Chromosomal translocations are a frequent hallmark of leukaemias and lymphomas. In many cases, these can be identified as early events in the pathogenesis of disease with close temporal association with the causal agents or processes. Biomarker assays that focus on measuring translocations in healthy individuals (early effect) or leukaemia patients (disease) or indirect measures of the processes that form translocations should prove to be useful biomarkers that could link exposure/etiology to disease.

Current translocation biomarker assay development is based on real-time PCR scanning for functional translocations (Greaves, Smith *et al.*, this volume). Such assays rely on the consistent structure of translocations at the RNA level and are highly useful for diagnostic classification of disease. These have also been used as an early disease event or exposure effect biomarker in apparently normal subjects. Such assays are dependent on uniform quality of RNA among samples, and minimization of potential laboratory cross-contamination. Therefore, in banking specimens, consideration needs to be given to the fact that translocation detection requires high-quality RNA to be isolated and stored appropriately. In addition, the ability to quantify the effect depends on the assay used. It is a difficult challenge to develop a molecular assay that is quantitative and uses DNA stored mainly as frozen buffy coats. However, any novel assay could be readily validated by comparing it with the classic chromosomal aberration test. Other novel biomarkers that use serum for immunological assays or proteomics would also be highly desirable. Recently, the structures of several types of leukaemia translocations have been elucidated on the DNA scale, revealing that each individual translocation event in each patient clone has specific break-points on the genes involved in the fusion. One characteristic feature of the translocations is the clustering of break-points within specific defined regions (Wiemels *et al.*, 2000; Xiao *et al.*, 2001). This clustering will allow the

design of genomic DNA translocation biomarker assays that will be highly specific to each translocation event. Such assays might, however, be less sensitive but resistant to confounding from clonal outgrowths. More quantifiable assays of risk of translocations could be developed that assess DNA breakage and rejoining processes. Increased double-strand break formation and altered rejoining could be utilized as susceptibility markers, perhaps in conjunction with assessment of genetic susceptibility conferred by variability on DNA double-strand break repair.

Subtypes of non-Hodgkin lymphoma are associated with specific oncogene-associated translocations with immunoglobulin (IGH) genes. In addition, these neoplastic clones also harbour clonally rearranged functional IGH genes. Both of these genetic rearrangements are biomarkers of the origin of the disease. First, the oncogenic translocation (IGH-BCL2, IGH-BCL1, etc.) can provide clues to the developmental window of the cell and its physical and locational context at the time of transformation. These oncogenic translocations leave vestigial remnants of their timing and mechanism of origin, much more specifically than those found in the leukaemias noted above. Similar information can be gleaned from the functional IGH rearrangement. For instance, B-cell chronic lymphocytic leukaemias/lymphomas can be divided into two categories based on IGH mutation status (Damle *et al.*, 2000). One class derives from non-mutated naive B-cells and the other from mutated postgerminal centre cells. Similar clues are evident from IGH genes at all stages of B-cell differentiation, allowing the ascertainment of the exact location and functional context of the cell at the time of transformation (Hummel & Stein, 2000). This information may provide direct clues to the etiology of the cancer or at least provide more meaningful classification of lymphomas in epidemiological studies (Damle *et al.*, 2000). Second, the IGH fusion itself provides information about the etiological agent that induced proliferation of the clone. This gene encodes an antibody that should recognize an epitope, the most concise piece of information required by the T cell to generate an immune response, on the antigen associated with the initial expansion of the B-cell clone in normal processes. This gene could be cloned, expressed and screened against antigens produced by putative infectious causes of the lymphoma. High-throughput methods using this approach could be used in population studies. Epitopes of these antibodies may be directly relevant to the environmental causes of the lymphoma.

Functional effects of germ-line polymorphic variants

Germ-line genetic variants (alleles and haplotypes) that confer susceptibility to neoplastic disease have been studied in the context of cancer risk factors. Results of such studies, using genes involved in carcinogen metabolism, DNA repair and various other processes related to carcinogenesis have been mixed with respect to strength and consistency of association. An important issue to consider in such studies is the functional consequence of the allelic variant under study. Some such variants lead to a complete or partial loss of activity of a particular enzyme (e.g. homozygous deletion of a gene such as *GSTM1*), whereas others produce increased activity. Certain polymorphic genetic variants may have statistically significant but functionally irrelevant effects on the risk for disease (or other end-points) because they are in linkage disequilibrium with a true causative locus. Before initiating studies on any specific allele, it is critical to have some knowledge about the phenotype (broadly defined) of the genetic variant. Association studies using alleles, SNPs or other genetic markers whose functional relevance is unknown run the risk of being non-informative and/or non-reproducible if different populations with different disequilibrium patterns are studied, especially if further research determines such variants to be in fact devoid of any phenotypic effect. It is possible to observe a significant and consistent association due to linkage disequilibrium; but the problem is that this would not explain the underlying biology.

Information on gene function is important both in the context of specifying hypotheses, but also in the context of analysis (Cortessis & Thomas, this volume), and in considering biological plausibility when making causal inferences. There is a need for a database that includes information on the quality of studies of functional effects (De Roos *et al.*, this volume). In relation to lymphohaematopoietic neoplasms, so far, the main use of this information has been in the selection of candidate genes. For example, in the case of benzene-induced leukaemia, metabolic genes that have allelic variants with well-established phenotypic effects (such as *NQO1* C609T) on metabolism, conjugation and elimination of benzene intermediary metabolites have been specifically selected for study (Smith *et al.*, this volume).

Genome-wide association scans, and even massive explorations for gene–environment and gene–gene interactions, perhaps using such machine-learning techniques as artificial neural networks, will soon be technically feasible, but problems of interpretation will still persist after the formidable laboratory and bioinformatics challenges are overcome. In data sets with many more predictors than subjects, one can expect that combinations of variables will usually be found that almost perfectly predict the outcome in the data used to fit the model. However, these will have little or no predictive value when using new data. Use of highly conservative significance criteria, cross-validation techniques and especially independent replication will help overcome the problem of false positives, but formal guidelines for interpreting results from genome-wide scans remain to be developed.

Conclusions

Leukaemia and lymphoma are distinct but heterogeneous diseases characterized by well-defined morphological and molecular subtypes (Jaffe *et al.*, 2001; Greaves, Smith *et al.*, this volume) and are likely to be associated with a number of different etiological factors. The extent of this heterogeneity and the lack of known causes of disease warrant the need for large, multicentre, international studies so that these relatively small subgroups are no longer analysed together, but can be examined individually. These larger studies would provide the opportunity to study rare genetic events and gene–gene/gene–environment interactions, as well as reduce the potential of overlooking important associations that may be pertinent to specific subgroups.

New technologies in molecular genetics have made it possible to screen a large fraction of the genome (thousands of genes) in a single association study. The use of such genome-wide screening for biomarkers of susceptibility and/or effect has been proposed, but it should be noted that currently there are severe technical computational and conceptual problems with the analyses and interpretation of such large data-generating experiments. These include problems such as low signal-to-noise ratios. Therefore, it is recommended that a mechanistic pathway-driven method be applied, using a number of genetic loci that can be managed appropriately with respect to data interpretation, as a more rational approach to the use of this technology for biomarker development. The number of genetic loci that can be managed is expected to rise with time as improvements in data handling and other associated methodologies become available and may eventually approach the scale of genome-wide screening.

Priorities for future work include:

- Development of international multicentre consortia to implement large studies of the well-defined morphological and molecular subtypes of the lymphohaematopoietic neoplasms, initially in subjects at high risk;
- Development of models of leukaemogenesis/lymphomagenesis that are informed by coordinated work in different branches of biology;
- Exploitation of new technologies in developing biomarkers, e.g. development of translocation detection methods applied to DNA rather than RNA, and use of serum-based immunological or proteomic assays;
- Validation of biomarkers in high-risk individuals;
- In developing quality standards for this work (cf. MIAME [minimum information about a microarray experiment], Brazma *et al.*, 2001), it is important to take account of epidemiological issues (which are not really addressed by MIAME);
- Integration of gene function information, with indication of quality;
- Need for database including null as well as positive studies of biomarker–disease associations.

References

Bonassi, S., Neri, M. & Puntoni, R. (2001) Validation of biomarkers as early predictors of disease. *Mutat. Res.*, **480–481**, 349–358

Brazma, A., Hingamp, P., Quackenbush, J., Sherlock, G., Spellman, P., Stoeckert, C., Aach, J., Ansorge, W., Ball, C.A., Causton, H.C., Gaasterland, T., Glenisson, P., Holstege, F.C., Kim, I.F., Markowitz, V., Matese, J.C., Parkinson, H., Robinson, A., Sarkans, U., Schulze-Kremer, S., Stewart, J., Taylor, R., Vilo, J. & Vingron, M. (2001) Minimum information about a microarray experiment (MIAME) – toward standards for microarray data. *Nat. Genet.*, **29**, 365–371

Damle, R.N., Fais, F., Ghiotto, F., Valetto, A., Albesiano, E., Wasil, T., Batliwalla, F.M., Allen, S.L., Schulman, P., Vinciguerra, V.P., Rai, K.R., Gregersen, P.K., Ferrarini, M. & Chiorazzi, N. (2000) Chronic lymphocytic leukemia: a proliferation of B cells at two distinct stages of differentiation. *Curr. Top. Microbiol. Immunol.*, **252**, 285–292

Greaves, M.F. (1997) Aetiology of acute leukaemia. *Lancet*, **349**, 344–349

Hummel, M. & Stein, H. (2000) Clinical relevance of immunoglobulin mutation analysis. *Curr. Opin. Oncol.*, **12**, 395–402

IARC (2000) *IARC Monographs on the Evaluation of Carcinogenic Risks to Humans*, Vol. 75, *Ionizing Radiation, Part 1: X- and Gamma-Radiation, and Neutrons*, Lyon, IARCPress

Jaffe, E.S., Lee Harris, N., Stein, H. & Vardiman, J.W. (2001) *WHO Classification of Tumours: Pathology and Genetics of Tumours of Haematopoietic and Lymphoid Tissues*, Lyon, IARCPress

Kinlen, L.J. (1995) Epidemiological evidence for an infective basis in childhood leukaemia. *Br. J. Cancer*, **71**, 1–5

Little, J., Khoury, M.J., Bradley, L., Clyne, M., Gwinn, M., Lin, B., Lindegren, M.L. & Yoon, P. (2003) The human genome project is complete. How do we develop a handle for the pump? *Am. J. Epidemiol.*, **157**, 667–673

NTP (2002) *Report on Carcinogens*, 10th Ed., Research Triangle Park, National Toxicology Program

Schulte, P.A., Hunter, D. & Rothman, N. (1997) Ethical and social issues in the use of biomarkers in epidemiological research. In: Toniolo, P., Boffetta, P.,

Shuker, D.E.G., Rothman, N., Hulka, B. & Pearce, N., eds, *Application of Biomarkers in Cancer Epidemiology* (IARC Scientific Publications No. 142), Lyon, IARC*Press*, pp. 313–318

Wiemels, J.L., Alexander, F.E., Cazzaniga, G., Biondi, A., Mayer, S.P. & Greaves, M. (2000) Micro-clustering of TEL-AML1 translocation breakpoints in childhood acute lymphoblastic leukemia. *Genes Chromosomes Cancer*, **29**, 219–228

Xiao, Z., Greaves, M.F., Buffler, P., Smith, M.T., Segal, M.R., Dicks, B.M., Wiencke, J.K. & Wiemels, J.L. (2001) Molecular characterization of genomic AML1-ETO fusions in childhood acute leukemia. *Leukemia*, **15**, 1906–1913

Mechanisms of Carcinogenesis: Contributions of Molecular Epidemiology
Patricia Buffler, Jerry Rice, Robert Baan, Michael Bird and Paolo Boffetta, eds
IARC Scientific Publications No. 157
International Agency for Research on Cancer, Lyon, 2004

Subgroup Report: Head and Neck Cancer

Margaret R. Spitz, Regina M. Santella, Paolo Boffetta and
Patricia Buffler

Background

The incidence of head and neck cancer (cancers of the oral cavity, pharynx and larynx) varies widely throughout the world, with little discernable pattern. Worldwide, the established etiological factors for head and neck cancer include tobacco smoking and heavy alcohol drinking, chewing of betel nut and tobacco, and infection with human papillomavirus (HPV). The model of head and neck cancer provides many advantages for evaluating and validating biomarkers of risk, early detection and response. The lesions are histologically homogeneous (originating from the squamous cell) and the two major risk factors — alcohol and tobacco — are well known. The accessibility of oral cavity tissue as a target or a potentially close surrogate for the target tissue facilitates these studies. Premalignant lesions are readily accessible and lend themselves to biomarker studies. Finally, the well-documented risk these patients incur for second primary cancers may be used to validate markers of risk and early detection.

Tobacco and alcohol consumption account for 75–90% of cases of head and neck cancer, but cannot explain the strong variation in incidence between countries. The risk increases rapidly with increasing tobacco and alcohol consumption, with evidence of a multiplicative effect of these two exposures. Few studies have had sufficient power to assess whether the contribution of alcohol and tobacco may differ by subsite within the upper aerodigestive tract. Moreover, because only a fraction of exposed individuals will develop neoplastic lesions, the role of genetic susceptibility and its interaction with these and other exposures (including diet) must be considered. Epidemiological evidence from studies using traditional case–control study designs suggests that a diet high in animal fat and low in fruit and vegetables may also be a risk factor for these cancers.

The combined effects of alcohol and tobacco highlight the importance of interactions in the study of head and neck cancer. However, the mechanism of this interaction is not understood. Alcohol itself is not a proven carcinogen. The possibility has been raised that dietary deficiency of folate, which is common in heavy drinkers, may play a role, but this has not been studied. Alcohol may potentiate the carcinogenic effect of tobacco at every level of tobacco use. However, this effect is most striking at the highest levels of tobacco consumption, and its magnitude is at least additive but may be multiplicative, dependent on the subsite of head and neck cancer and level of exposure.

The clastogenic effect of acetaldehyde, a metabolite of alcohol, is well established, and local carcinogenic effects of acetaldehyde have been related to this type of genotoxicity.

Polymorphisms exist in the many genes involved in addictive behaviours, in metabolism of tobacco carcinogens and alcohol, in DNA repair and in cell-cycle control, and these may contribute to interindividual variation in risk. These genes are logical candidates for the examination of interactions with environmental factors. Given the multiple interactions that can be considered, the use of mechanistic modelling methods such as those discussed by Cortessis and Thomas (this volume) could be fruitfully applied to investigate this disease. This type of analysis, as well as traditional logistic regression models for evaluating multi-pathway interactions, will require very large sample sizes. Given the rarity of head and neck cancers, multicentre collaborative studies or pooling of individual studies will be necessary to provide sufficient power to examine these interacting factors.

The role of HPV-16 infection, as a primary or interacting factor, has not been explored in detail. To investigate further the role of HPV, reliable methods to examine the prevalence of infection are needed. For example, good serological and molecular methods are required to conduct valid case–control studies. Clearly, studies need to evaluate multiple interactions between environmental factors.

The timing of these exposures may also be important. The pathogenic processes may be augmented by exposure to carcinogens during periods of organ growth and development. Consequently, further studies related to age at starting smoking, alcohol drinking and HPV infection should be undertaken.

Stages in tumour development and progression

Slaughter's concept of field cancerization (Slaughter et al., 1953) suggests that multiple neoplastic lesions of independent origin that occur within an epithelial field result from repeated exposure to carcinogens of a whole field, in combination with endogenous processes such as carcinogen metabolism, repair capability and inherent genetic instability. This process places whole tissue fields at increased cancer risk. Sustained exposure to carcinogens leads to the accumulation of genetic damage throughout the tissue. When cell proliferation occurs, particularly in association with wound healing, DNA damage may be transformed into permanent genetic changes (e.g. mutations, deletions, rearrangements, loss and gain of chromosome regions, gene amplification). When specific gene regions that are functionally important for selection (i.e. render cells resistant to apoptosis or differentiation, give proliferative/survival advantage) are altered, clonal outgrowths occur throughout the field and may be clinically evident as premalignant lesions. Continued genomic change in the outgrowing clones increases their neoplastic potential. This process explains both the existence of well-defined premalignant lesions and the well-documented risk for second cancers in the exposed epithelial tract.

Premalignant lesions of the upper aerodigestive tract are an excellent system for studying carcinogenesis and testing chemopreventive agents in humans. Oral premalignant lesions are white (leukoplakia) and/or red (erythroplasia) mucosal patches in the oral cavity or oropharynx that are easily monitored (visually and by biopsy). Individuals with these lesions are at increased risk for cancer, and the degree of risk can exceed 40% if severe dysplasia is present. Advanced premalignant lesions of the larynx, defined as mild to severe dysplasia (and carcinoma in situ), are ultimately destined to develop into invasive carcinoma (45–60% after 3–5 years). The variability in these rates of progression may be due to age, gender, histology, and site and duration of the lesions. These lesions serve as an excellent, accessible system for studying carcinogenesis of the head and neck in humans.

Another unique characteristic of upper aerodigestive tract cancers is their high predilection for the development of second primary tumours. Patients with cancer of the upper aerodigestive tract face an annual risk of 4–7% for developing a potentially fatal second primary tumour. The development of these second primary cancers is also a consequence of field cancerization, and risks are higher with continuing carcinogenic exposures. Knowledge of the genetic mechanisms underlying the development of head and neck cancer has greatly increased in the last decade, and it has been estimated that 5–10 genetic events are required. The main alterations found in head and neck cancer are cyclin D1 amplification and loss, mutation or methylation of p16 (an early event), TP53 and FHIT (or other genes present on chromosome 3p). Models have been proposed for the accumulation of these and other alterations. This area of research is extremely promising with respect to the elucidation of mechanisms of head and neck carcinogenesis and its relationship with environmental exposures and host factors. However, the available information on the interplay between exposure to environmental carcinogens (tobacco, betel nuts, alcoholic beverages, HPV), host-susceptibility factors and acquired alterations is still limited. Most of the available data refer to the prevalence and pattern of *TP53* mutations, which show a clear increase in prevalence of G–T transversions in tobacco-related cancers. Future studies should clarify the role of genetic alterations in head and neck cancer by incorporating valid information on exposure to environmental factors and by measuring susceptibility markers.

Available biomarkers
Genetic polymorphisms

The study of germ-line polymorphisms in head and neck cancer etiology can help identify high-risk subgroups as well as elucidate mechanisms of carcinogenesis. Issues of bias and confounding are not unique to head and neck cancer. Population stratification is a type of confounding due to population admixture that may affect studies of genotype–disease association when risk allele frequencies and baseline disease risk co-vary between populations. This can be avoided by paying attention to the ethnic composition of the population at enrolment and in analysis. Reliable data on lifetime alcohol and tobacco consumption are important for testing interactions as covariates in the analysis. It goes without saying that representative control groups need to be selected. Also crucial is the appropriate selection of candidate genes and functionally significant polymorphisms to maximize the potential for detecting relevant effects. Finally, appropriate study design and power considerations need to be made to allow the detection of potentially subtle effects as well as interactions among various bio-behavioural factors and genotypes.

Biobehavioural factors: Exposures to tobacco and alcohol may be dictated by genotypes that determine bio-behavioural propensity to drink or smoke. For example, inherited genotypes that regulate dopamine or serotonin metabolism have been associated with propensity to be a smoker and determine risk-taking behaviours and nicotine dependence (Lerman *et al.*, 1999). Similarly, genotypes involved in the metabolism of alcohol, including the alcohol dehydrogenases and aldehyde dehydrogenases, may determine an individual's propensity to drink. Genotypes that predict a propensity to smoke tobacco or drink alcohol should therefore be considered in studies of susceptibility to head and neck cancers because they may define better an individual's predicted pattern of exposure to these agents. This information may be used to tailor chemical and behavioural interventions related to avoidance of exposure, cessation of the habit or chemoprevention, relevant to the individual's genotype.

Although the literature suggests that genotypes that predict exposure patterns may exist, there are a number of caveats. First, careful consideration must be given of the bio-behavioural data to be evaluated. Appropriate data collection instruments include detailed assessment of personality type and other behavioural factors. These data may be used not only as end-points to be predicted by genotype data, but also as stratification variables to define relevant population subsets. Second, it may be necessary to make distinctions between the role of genes in the etiology of tumours and the role of the same genes in predicting bio-behavioural outcomes such as propensity to smoke or drink. For example, the aldehyde dehydrogenases may influence the degree to which some individuals consume alcohol, but they may also influence relevant carcinogenic pathways directly implicated in the etiology of disease. Similarly, variants of the *CYP2A6* gene may determine not only the degree of nicotine dependence (and thereby the amount of tobacco carcinogen exposure), but also the individual's ability to metabolize carcinogenic nitrosamines in the cigarettes, and therefore to modulate the risk for tobacco-induced cancer.

Metabolism: Many published studies on the impact of human polymorphisms of xenobiotic metabolizing enzymes in the development of head and neck cancer, in relation to tobacco and alcohol consumption, have suggested gene–environment interactions (Olshan *et al.*, 2000; Brennan & Boffetta, this volume). In general, larger studies to evaluate such interactions fully are needed.

DNA repair: Genetic polymorphisms of DNA repair genes may contribute to variation in DNA repair capacity. Benzo[*a*]pyrene diolepoxide

(BPDE)-induced DNA damage is effectively removed by the nucleotide excision repair (NER) pathway. The NER pathway alone involves at least 20 genes. Acetaldehyde adducts are removed through base-excision repair. There is a need to conduct larger, well-designed, well-powered studies to investigate the etiological significance of these polymorphisms, with comprehensive evaluation of genes in specific repair pathways. Clearly, functional (phenotypic) studies of DNA repair in individuals with various genotypes of these polymorphisms are needed. However, it will be difficult to detect subtle differences in DNA repair capacity due to a single polymorphism of a single gene in a very complex pathway.

Additional polymorphisms: Because carcinogenesis of the head and neck also involves abnormalities in cell-cycle control (Scully *et al.*, 2000), polymorphisms of cell-cycle control genes are good candidates for investigations of genetic susceptibility. An additional set of candidate genes for consideration includes those involved in immune surveillance. Appropriate candidates among these genes include the cytokines because they may influence response to HPV infection as well as indicating the presence of a tumour. The effect of these genotypes should be considered in combination with characteristics of HPV infection.

Surrogate tissue biomarkers

Cytogenetic: In-vitro chromosomal analysis has been used to study individual sensitivity to genotoxicity and cancer risk, and the technique is gaining wider approval in formal hypothesis testing using classic epidemiological methodology. The value of using chromosomal aberrations in peripheral lymphocytes as markers of risk for head and neck cancer has yet to be shown.

A number of functional assays using lymphocytes treated *in vitro* have been developed to look at the sensitivity of cells to DNA damage and their capacity to repair this damage. The mutagen sensitivity assay is a functional assay that measures chromatid breaks in response to in-vitro exposure to carcinogens in short-term cultures of peripheral blood lymphocytes. The challenge

mutagens selected include bleomycin (a radiomimetic agent) and BPDE, the activated form of the tobacco carcinogen, benzo[*a*]pyrene. The host cell reactivation assay measures the level of expression of a damaged reporter gene as a marker of repair proficiency in the host cell. It is another relevant assay that uses undamaged cells, is relatively fast and is an objective method of measuring DNA repair capacity. None of these functional assays has been validated prospectively. Nor do we know how well these markers of DNA repair capacity correlate with genotype and with measures of genomic instability in the target tissue. There have been only a few small studies evaluating DNA repair capacity by genotype.

Adducts: Acetaldehyde yields a number of unstable and stable adducts with proteins and DNA, the major ones resulting from Schiff base formation. One of the most promising biomarkers for alcohol consumption is the presence of acetaldehyde adducts in peripheral blood proteins. Several groups have used specific antibodies to detect acetaldehyde–protein epitopes in blood from heavy drinkers. Recently, antibodies against very low-density lipoprotein/acetaldehyde have been claimed to provide the most effective detection of acetaldehyde adducts in blood *in vivo* (Latvala *et al.*, 2001). There is a need to evaluate the specificity and sensitivity of these immunochemical methods further before their application in epidemiological studies.

Experimental studies in rodents fed ethanol also demonstrated the formation of acetaldehyde–protein adducts in various tissues. In humans, such adducts have been investigated in liver and bone marrow but not yet in tissues from the oral cavity. An ELISA assay for measuring keratin–acetaldehyde adducts in hair has also been reported. It could be a useful non-invasive method for use in humans, but it has only been tested in mice (Watson *et al.*, 1998). Another promising approach is the use of methods based on mass spectrometry, for example to analyse a stable imidazoline–protein adduct (Conduah Birt *et al.*, 1998).

Although several adducts of acetaldehyde with DNA have been characterized *in vitro*, there is a lack of sensitive and specific methods for their detection *in vivo*, with only the ^{32}P-postlabelling technique reported in the literature so far. Using this method, Fang and Vaca (1997) measured elevated levels of an acetaldehyde–DNA adduct in granulocyte and lymphocyte DNA from alcoholic patients, as compared with control subjects. Subsequently, the same DNA adduct was detected in untreated and acetaldehyde-treated human buccal epithelial cells in culture (Vaca *et al.*, 1998). The detection of other types of DNA adducts in blood samples of cases and controls may also be of interest since these methods have been of use in lung and other cancers.

Target tissue biomarkers

The metabolism of alcohol, tobacco components, especially aromatic amines, polycyclic aromatic hydrocarbons (PAHs) and NNK-related compounds has been studied extensively; however, additional work could be carried out to characterize the metabolism of these compounds in the target tissues, i.e. head and neck tissues (Vondracek *et al.*, 2001). Metabolic studies in humans, large enough to permit an exploration of these metabolic characteristics among a population, should be performed. In particular, the ability of these compounds and metabolites to induce various genes that, in turn, alter metabolic profiles could also be studied. Microarray and proteomic studies may ultimately be the ideal means by which this issue can be examined in the future.

In contrast to many other cancers, studies of DNA adducts in target tissue of cases and controls are quite feasible in head and neck cancer because of the ready availability of the appropriate tissues. Most studies to date have used immunohistochemical methods to investigate oral cell damage, although there are also ^{32}P-postlabelling data. Adducts measured include those of PAH, 4-aminobiphenyl and malondialdehyde as well as 1,N2-propanodeoxyguanosine and 8-hydroxydeoxyguanosine. N7-Alkylguanine has also been measured in laryngeal tissue. Much more work is needed in this area to determine the adducts of alcohol and tobacco carcinogens as well as damage related to oxidative stress.

Studies on the spectrum of genetic changes in tumours may also provide much useful informa-tion. In addition to *TP53* mutation, other targets within the p53 pathway, as well as other cell-growth control pathways, should be included in future epidemiological studies to relate exposure risk factors to specific gene targets and modes of gene inactivation. For example, among these targets is the Rb/p16 pathway which is important in the G_1 cell-cycle checkpoint and can be blocked by inactivation of different genes. Further, individual genes can be inactivated through different mutational and epigenetic mechanisms. Inactivation of tumour-suppressor genes by methylation of CpG-rich promoter regions is another area of active investigation. Additional studies with the goal of relating distinct patterns of pathway inactivation with specific etiological exposures are needed.

Recent studies have demonstrated that tumour DNA released into the bloodstream can be detected in cancer patients. Only a subset of cases has any one specific genetic alteration in their tumour, with an even lower frequency of this same alteration found in tumour DNA in blood. However, these methods have potential as early markers of disease in high-risk populations and to monitor recurrence in patients.

Future biomarkers

The detection of multiple susceptibility factors will probably reveal the true dimensions of gene–environment interactions. The most should be made of technological advances in high-through-put, automated approaches for rapid, large-scale genotyping in order to identify and evaluate biological markers that are more selectively predictive of individual risk, disease behaviour and response to intervention. Identification of protein patterns in serum using high-throughput proteomics linked to novel bioinformatics approaches has provided interesting data that suggest that information on predisposition to disease, early diagnosis and evaluation of response to therapy can be obtained from sera. Tumour DNA can also be isolated from serum or plasma; it is a useful source for screening specific transcripts or mutations in mitochondria or nuclear DNA sequences and may have a potential role in early detection. Pharmacogenetic profiles could be used to individualize therapy and to understand the functional consequences of response to chemoprevention, chemotherapy or radiotherapy. Increased emphasis will also be placed on correlating biomarker data derived from surrogate tissues (peripheral lymphocytes, serum) with molecular changes in the target tissue. The techniques and technologies of molecular epidemiology are highly applicable to these pursuits. Linking of tissue repositories with well-characterized epidemiological, clinical and follow-up data enhances the value of these resources. There will be a concomitant need for state-of-the-art archiving laboratories for long-term storage and tracking of human samples using individualized bar coding and tracking systems, a cryogenic repository of blood components and a room temperature-based, automated storage system for acquiring large DNA libraries. The ethical, educational, social and informatics considerations that will result are challenging.

The ability to identify smokers with the highest risks for developing cancer has substantial preventive implications. These subgroups could be targeted for the most intensive smoking cessation interventions, could be enrolled into chemoprevention trials and might be suitable for more aggressive screening programmes that are not appropriate for the general population. Finally, studying susceptibility to common cancers and widely prevalent exposures may provide further insight into the basic mechanisms of carcinogenesis. This knowledge is essential for the design of future epidemiological and intervention studies.

Public health implications

A better understanding of the pathogenesis and mechanistic pathways of head and neck cancers has public health importance. If HPV-16 infection is important in etiology, immunization of young adults, which is currently being evaluated for cervical cancer prevention, may also prevent some head and neck cancers. This is especially important given that there is some evidence that smoking and alcohol are less strongly associated with HPV-16-positive tumours. Although avoiding smoking and heavy drinking is clearly

important to reduce overall mortality, the reduction of mortality from head and neck cancer among moderate drinkers due to alcohol cessation would probably be outweighed by an increase in overall mortality. This would mainly be due to an increase in cardiovascular risk, which is higher in non-drinkers than in moderate drinkers. The overall negative effects of alcohol cessation may even be more important among nonsmokers.

The understanding of dietary cofactors, such as folate deficiency or other nutritional deficiencies, could enable chemopreventive interventions for high-risk groups, including those who have smoked and drunk heavily, as well as survivors of head and neck cancer who have a high rate of development of new tumours.

References

Conduah Birt, J.E., Shuker, D.E. & Farmer, P.B. (1998) Stable acetaldehyde–protein adducts as biomarkers of alcohol exposure. *Chem. Res. Toxicol.*, **11**, 136–142

Fang, J.L. & Vaca, C.E. (1997) Detection of DNA adducts of acetaldehyde in peripheral white blood cells of alcohol abusers. *Carcinogenesis*, **18**, 627–632

Latvala, J., Melkko, J., Parkkila, S., Jarvi, K., Makkonen, K. & Niemela, O. (2001) Assays for acetaldehyde-derived adducts in blood proteins based on antibodies against acetaldehyde/lipoprotein condensates. *Alcohol clin. exp. Res.*, **25**, 1648–1653

Lerman, C., Caporaso, N.E., Audrain, J., Main, D., Bowman, E.D., Lockshin, B., Boyd, N.R. & Shields, P.G. (1999) Evidence suggesting the role of specific genetic factors in cigarette smoking. *Health Psychol.*, **18**, 14–20

Olshan, A.F., Weissler, M.C., Watson, M.A. & Bell, D.A. (2000) GSTM1, GSTT1, GSTP1, CYP1A1, and NAT1 polymorphisms, tobacco use, and the risk of head and neck cancer. *Cancer Epidemiol. Biomarkers Prev.*, **9**, 185–191

Scully, C., Field, J.K. & Tanzawa, H. (2000) Genetic aberrations in oral or head and neck squamous cell carcinoma (SCCHN): 1. Carcinogen metabolism, DNA repair and cell cycle control. *Oral Oncol.*, **36**, 256–263

Slaughter, D.P., Southwick, H.W. & Smejkal, W. (1953) Field cancerization in oral stratified squamous epithelium. *Cancer*, **6**, 963–968

Vaca, C.E., Nilsson, J.A., Fang, J.L. & Grafstrom, R.C. (1998) Formation of DNA adducts in human buccal epithelial cells exposed to acetaldehyde and methylglyoxal in vitro. *Chem.-biol. Interact.*, **108**, 197–208

Vondracek, M., Xi, Z., Larsson, P., Baker, V., Mace, K., Pfeifer, A., Tjalve, H., Donato, M.T., Gomez-Lechon, M.J. & Grafstrom, R.C. (2001) Cytochrome P450 expression and related metabolism in human buccal mucosa. *Carcinogenesis*, **22**, 481–488

Watson, R.R., Solkoff, D., Wang, J.Y. & Seeto, K. (1998) Detection of ethanol consumption by ELISA assay measurement of acetaldehyde adducts in murine hair. *Alcohol*, **16**, 279–284

General Considerations

Mechanisms of Carcinogenesis: Contributions of Molecular Epidemiology
Patricia Buffler, Jerry Rice, Robert Baan, Michael Bird and Paolo Boffetta, eds
IARC Scientific Publications No. 157
International Agency for Research on Cancer, Lyon, 2004

Metabolic and Biochemical Issues in the Molecular Epidemiology of Cancer

Robert Snyder and Jun-Yan Hong

Summary
In this chapter, we highlight the significance of some metabolic and biochemical issues in molecular epidemiology. We discuss biomarkers and biologically reactive intermediates and describe the significance of polymorphisms in xenobiotic metabolizing enzymes, with emphasis on the role of some of these enzymes in the generation of reactive metabolites and on the related issue of susceptibility biomarkers. In the final section, we have selected an example of a specific compound, benzene, for which a variety of different biomarkers have been studied.

Introduction
Human responses to xenobiotic chemicals are in many instances genetically controlled. Extensive descriptions of genetically controlled variations in drug metabolism were reviewed by Kalow (1992). Some of the more convincing arguments for the genetic control of drug metabolism have come from studies of fraternal and identical twins in which it was shown that in identical twins the pharmacokinetics for a given chemical were essentially identical, whereas the differences between fraternal twins approached those seen in the general population (Vesell, 1973). Although transient changes in xenobiotic metabolism, as in the case of enzyme induction, may be environmentally mediated, basal levels appear to be genetically determined and within a given population may display enzymatic polymorphisms.

The development of newer methodologies to explore polymorphisms has led to studies both of the aberrant proteins that result from xenobiotic insult and of the underlying damage to DNA itself. The field has come to be called molecular epidemiology, and its success depends heavily on the observation and interpretation of so-called **biomarkers**. Some types of biomarkers are biological, such as the qualitative or quantitative examination of specific cells. The purpose of this chapter is to discuss biomarker formation from a biochemical perspective as a genetically determined event. Biomarkers can provide information on:

- exposure to a chemical,
- the extent to which a chemical has had a health impact or
- relative individual susceptibility to the effects of a chemical or family of chemicals.

Thus, we refer to biomarkers of exposure, effect and susceptibility.

Biomarkers have been used for years as indicators of exposure to many chemicals. Table 1 lists a number of chemicals, the exposure to which can be studied on the basis of the chemical or a metabolite in blood, urine or exhaled air (Gil & Pla, 2001). Studies of soluble or volatile chemicals and their metabolites can provide valuable information for detecting enzymatic polymorphisms. However, biochemical or metabolic issues underpinning biomarkers frequently arise from the non-enzymatic reactions of reactive chemicals with cellular macromolecules, such as nucleic acids or proteins. Drugs or chemicals may enter the body by a variety of routes. Although oral intake is the most common, inhalation of gases, vapours or aerosols or administration of drugs parenterally, either for a therapeutic purpose or during drug abuse, are alternative routes of exposure. The chemicals themselves may be chemically reactive or they may be activated enzymatically. For example, when mechlorethamine, an early

Table 1. Some examples of biomarkers measured in urine, blood or exhaled air (Gil & Pla, 2001)

Chemical	Biomarker	Measured in
Cadmium	Cadmium	Urine, blood
Mercury	Mercury	Urine, blood
Zinc	Zinc	Urine, blood
n-Hexane	2-Hexanol	Urine
	2,5-Hexanedione	Urine
Styrene	Styrene	Blood, exhaled air
	Mandelic acid	Urine
	Phenylglyoxilic acid	Urine
Aniline	Aniline	Urine
	para-Aminophenol	Urine
	Methaemoglobin	Blood, exhaled air
Ethylene glycol	Oxalic acid	Urine

nitrogen mustard, anticancer alkylating drug comes into contact with water, it loses a chlorine atom and assumes the structure of an ethylenimonium ion which can react with nucleophilic sites on cellular macromolecules such as DNA. No enzyme is required to generate the reactive species. More frequently, xenobiotic chemicals require metabolic activation via one of a series of reactions. The result is the conversion of an otherwise inert chemical to a biologically reactive intermediate (BRI) (Jollow et al., 1975; Snyder et al., 1982; Kocsis et al., 1986; Witmer et al., 1991; Snyder et al., 1996; Dansette et al., 2001) which can then react non-enzymatically at nucleophilic sites on proteins or nucleic acids. The significance of these reactions with respect to cancer is that BRI-directed formation of DNA adducts may be an initiating event in carcinogenesis.

The usefulness of a biochemical biomarker can be defined by several characteristics. Ideally the biomarker should be unique to the exposure under consideration. It should be either the chemical itself or a metabolite produced by that chemical and no other. For use in human studies it should be measurable using relatively non-invasive procedures such as urine collection or a blood sample, as opposed to an organ biopsy. Chemical analysis of the biomarker should be accurate and precise. If possible, the biomarker should be indi-

cative of the degree of exposure. Another important feature is that, to provide an early warning of impending toxicity, it should be measurable before development of overt toxicity.

Enzymes that mediate the activation of carcinogens are termed xenobiotic metabolizing enzymes (XMEs). Differential responses to chemicals among individuals within a population may be related to interindividual differences in enzyme activity due to enzyme inhibition or induction. Alternatively, the polymorphic distribution of XMEs could serve as the basis of a molecular epidemiological study. Hong and Yang (1997) reviewed molecular epidemiological studies on genetic polymorphism of XMEs in human susceptibility to environmental cancers. With the large number of novel XME genetic polymorphisms that can be expected to be identified in projects related to the human genome and the availability of various high through-put genotyping technologies, research interest in this area is expected to increase. However, selection of suitable XMEs and their relevant genetic polymorphisms for cancer molecular epidemiological studies remains a challenge. In the following discussions, we emphasize some specific metabolic and biochemical issues in the molecular epidemiology of cancer. We believe these mechanistic considerations should be helpful in the design and interpretation of molecular epidemiological studies.

Metabolism of most, if not all, environmental carcinogens clearly involves multiple pathways and is controlled by the rate-limiting XME in each pathway. The concentrations of reactive metabolites that can attack DNA and other macromolecules to initiate mutagenic or carcinogenic events will be determined by the final balance between the production of BRI by activation pathways and their elimination by inactivation pathways. Therefore, it would be ideal to combine the XMEs responsible for different metabolic pathways in the design of molecular epidemiological studies. If possible, non-XME enzymes or proteins that play important roles in the post-activation stages of carcinogenesis, such as DNA repair enzymes, should also be included in the experimental design.

Human cancers may result from exposure to a variety of chemical carcinogens. For example, heterocyclic amines such as 2-amino-1-methyl-6-phenylimidazo[4,5-b]pyridine (PhIP) in over-cooked meat have been associated with the risk of breast and colon cancer; nitrosamines in tobacco such as 4-(methylnitrosamino)-1-(3-pyridyl)-1-butanone (NNK) have been implicated in the etiology of human lung cancer. Therefore, the selection of XMEs for studies of cancer risk depends first on knowledge of the most relevant or suspected carcinogen exposure in the study population. In some early molecular epidemiological studies, there was no careful consideration linking the candidate XME with the existence of specific environmental carcinogens. The candidate XMEs were chosen simply on the basis of their general roles in carcinogen activation or inactivation. These studies usually provided little information on the roles of XMEs and their genetic polymorphisms in human cancer risk.

If a specific carcinogen to which the study population is exposed can be identified, the next critical issue is to choose the most relevant XME for the study. It is well known that XMEs such as cytochrome P450 (CYP) enzymes have overlapping substrate specificities. Very often, a specific chemical carcinogen can be metabolized by more than one XME. For example, the activation of PhIP to its carcinogenic product N-OH PhIP can be catalysed by human CYP1A1, CYP1A2 and CYP1B1 (Crofts et al., 1998). Assessment of the relative contribution of each XME to the activation or inactivation of the relevant carcinogen is, therefore, very important in the study design. There are two major considerations in the assessment of the relative contributions of more than one XME to a metabolic reaction. First, although several different XMEs may be involved in a single step in the metabolism of a specific carcinogen, the affinities of the substrate for the different enzymes (measured as K_m) and the catalytic efficiencies of each reaction (V_{max}/K_m) could be significantly different. Since levels of carcinogen exposures in daily life are expected to be low, the XME with the highest substrate affinity (i.e. the lowest K_m) and high catalytic efficiency is believed to be the most relevant to carcinogen metabolic activation *in vivo*. A panel of heterogeneously expressed XMEs can be used to obtain the required information on enzyme kinetics. The second important consideration is the expression profile of the relevant XME in different human tissues. Because the ultimate carcinogenic BRI species formed during metabolic activation of a chemical usually has a very short half-life, production of these highly reactive metabolites within the target tissues for carcinogenesis (in-situ activation) could be an important factor in determining the organ or tissue specificity of a specific carcinogen. Obviously, for a XME that is known to catalyse carcinogen activation, it would be relevant if the XME were expressed to a significant level in the cancer target tissue.

An example is the metabolic activation of the tobacco-specific carcinogen NNK. Of the human CYP enzymes examined previously, CYP1A1, 1A2, 2A6, 2B6, 2D6, 2E1, 2F1 and 3A4 all displayed activity in the formation of carcinogenic metabolites of NNK (Smith et al., 1992; Penman et al., 1993; Smith et al., 1995; Patten et al., 1996; Smith et al., 1996). However, when the kinetic properties of these CYP enzymes are considered, CYP2A6 and 1A2 have the lowest K_m (120 and 300 µmol/L, respectively) and relatively high V_{max} values for the formation of the carcinogenic metabolites of NNK (Smith et al., 1992; Patten et al., 1996; Smith et al., 1996). Therefore, CYP2A6 and 1A2 are more likely than other CYP enzymes to metabolize NNK under normal exposure conditions. Su et al. (2000) found that CYP2A13 has an even higher substrate affinity for NNK, with a K_m value of approximately 10 µmol/L. CYP2A13 also has a relatively higher V_{max} than that of CYP2A6 (Table 2). The catalytic efficiency of CYP2A13 for the formation of a keto aldehyde, which is produced in one of the NNK activation pathways, was much higher than that of CYP2A6 (0.36 versus 0.008). Furthermore, although the CYP2A13 mRNA expression level was almost 2000-fold lower than the level of CYP2A6 in human liver, its expression level is higher than CYP2A6 in human respiratory tract tissues such as lung and trachea. All these findings suggest that CYP2A13 may be more important than CYP2A6 in the metabolic activation of NNK

Table 2. Comparison of *CYP2A6* and *CYP2A13* in enzyme kinetics of NNK metabolism and human tissue expression (Su *et al.*, 2000)

	CYP2A6	CYP2A13
Enzyme kinetics		
Keto aldehyde formation		
K_m (μM)	118	11.3 ± 3.5
V_{max}/K_m	0.008	0.36
Keto alcohol formation		
K_m (μM)	141	13.1 ± 5.1
V_{max}/K_m	0.003	0.09
mRNA expression		
(amol/mg total RNA)		
Liver	13000	7
Nasal mucosa	160	750
Lung	9	78
Trachea	76	130

NNK is a tobacco-specific carcinogen. Keto aldehyde and keto alcohol are the metabolites formed in the metabolic activation of NNK. a = atto = 10^{-18}

in human respiratory tract tissues such as lung and trachea (Su *et al.*, 2000) and may play an important role in tobacco-related carcinogenesis in these tissues.

The enzymatic generation of biologically reactive intermediates

When xenobiotic chemicals enter the body by the oral route they must be sufficiently lipid-soluble to permit passive diffusion across the lipoprotein membranes of the gastrointestinal tract. They are transported via the portal circulation to the liver where, for the most part, they are converted metabolically to more polar compounds to enhance their ultimate excretion via the kidney. Indeed, when Williams (1959) first described the enzymatic metabolism of xenobiotics as phase I and phase II reactions, he termed them 'detoxication mechanisms'. Nevertheless he realized that in many instances the products of these reactions could be more toxic than the original substrate of the enzyme, but that synthetic conjugation reactions could provide ultimate detoxication. It is

now understood that cleavage enzymes, whose substrates are the phase II conjugation products, may also produce reactive metabolites, as can other pathways. This phenomenon was not appreciated by earlier investigators.

Reactions mediated by cytochrome P450

CYP is a general designation for a large group of mixed-function oxidases encountered throughout the animal and plant kingdoms which can activate oxygen for the purpose of hydroxylating or otherwise oxidizing aliphatic, alicyclic or aromatic hydrocarbon compounds, or organic compounds containing oxygen, nitrogen or sulfur. CYP enzymes dealkylate compounds containing nitrogen, sulfur or phosphorus that have alkyl groups at these heteroatoms, and also mediate desulfuration, dehalogenation and deamination reactions. They may also reduce nitro or azo compounds. In higher animals, they are found primarily in the endoplasmic reticulum of the liver, but can also be observed in lesser quantities in many other organs. The expression of each type of CYP depends upon the organ in which it is found and on the possibility of enzyme induction. The expression of each type of CYP can be increased by administration of specific inducers.

CYPs are oxygen-activating enzymes similar to mitochondrial cytochrome oxidase. Indeed the same approach, the photochemical action spectrum technique, was used to identify each CYP as the terminal oxygen acceptor in an electron transport chain (Snyder, 2000a). Figure 1 shows the scheme for the series of reactions mediated by CYP using benzene as the substrate. The active site of CYP utilizes a haem–iron complex to bind oxygen close to the protein site at which the substrate binds. Since only reduced iron (Fe^{2+}) binds oxygen, a flavoprotein (NADPH-CYP reductase) passes electrons from NADPH to CYP. The specificity of each CYP is dependent on the structure of the apoprotein. One of the potential BRIs derived from benzene, benzene oxide, is the end-product of these reactions.

The potential role of CYP in the metabolic activation of environmental chemicals to BRIs may be to catalyse an attack by oxygen on a carbon–carbon bond to yield an epoxide in the form of a

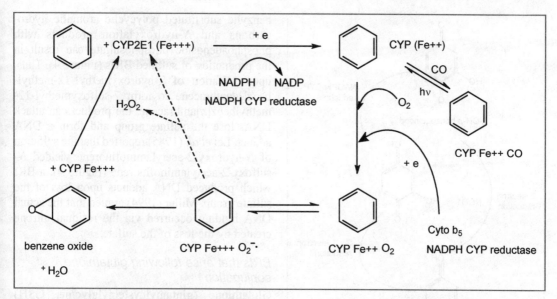

Figure 1. CYP cycle with benzene as substrate.

highly strained, very reactive, three-membered oxirane ring (Figure 1). Subsequent electrophilic attack by epoxides on nucleophilic centres can result in the formation of covalently bound adducts to proteins or nucleic acids. Whether or not binding occurs depends upon whether the BRI rearranges to form phenolic compounds, which are not binding species, before the covalent bond is established. Alternatively, the epoxide may be de-activated by the enzyme epoxide hydrolase to yield a dihydrodiol. The dihydrodiol may be oxidized to a catechol-like structure by dihydrodiol dehydrogenase, which is a step in the course of benzene metabolism, or a second epoxidation may occur on an adjacent carbon–carbon bond to yield a dihydrodiol epoxide, which is a step in the metabolism of benzo[a]pyrene and other polycyclic aromatic hydrocarbons. These reactions result in the formation of BRIs. The extent to which BRIs are formed in any individual is a function of the distributions of the various polymorphic CYP enzymes.

NAD(P)H:quinone oxidoreductase

NAD(P)H:quinone oxidoreductase (NQO1, DT-diaphorase) is a polymorphic flavin-containing enzyme which carries out a two-electron reduc-

tion of quinones to hydroquinones (Ross, 1997). Quinones may also be reduced via two one-electron steps (Figure 2). NQO1 is present in various cell types at different levels of expression. In some cases no NQO1 protein can be detected, but the enzyme may be induced by one of two mechanisms:

• Dioxin and aromatic hydrocarbons induce NQO1 by a so-called **bifunctional** mechanism in which they form a complex with the Ah receptor, which reacts with the ARNT protein and traverses the cell to the nucleus where it binds to the xenobiotic responsive element (XRE), resulting in transcriptional activation of NQO1;

• The **monofunctional** mechanism involves a variety of agents such as phenolic antioxidants, hydrogen peroxide and β-naphthoflavone, which act via a pathway involving the antioxidant response element, and the fos and jun proteins.

NQO1 has been thought of as a means of detoxifying reactive quinones to the level of unreactive hydroquinones. Thus, the reduction of para-benzoquinone to hydroquinone by NQO1 is thought to protect against benzene toxicity (Rothman et al., 1997; Moran et al., 1999). The

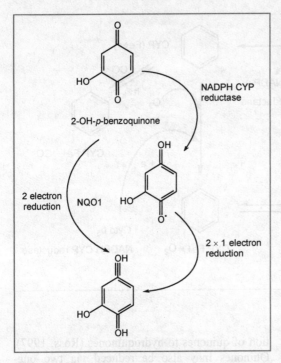

Figure 2. Quinone reductases (Ross, 1997).

data indicate a more complex view of this enzyme (Smith, 1999). Cadenas (1995) suggested that the chemical reactivity of the product of quinone reduction, i.e. the resulting hydroquinone, depends on the non-quinone functional group chemistry of the initial substrate (Figure 3). Thus, the products of the reduction may be hydroquinones which are (1) redox stable and susceptible to conjugation, the products of which are sulfates or glucuronides, (2) alkylating agents capable of covalent binding to DNA or (3) redox-labile products which may undergo auto-oxidation to yield superoxide anion radical. In the presence of superoxide dismutase, the product may be converted to a redox-stable hydroquinone and then conjugated, or the process may give rise to oxygen radicals capable of causing DNA damage.

BRIs arising as a result of sulfate conjugation

Although the formation of sulfate conjugates has generally been thought to result in detoxication, Miller *et al.* (1991) suggested that the reaction of

benzylic substituted polycyclic aromatic hydrocarbons and *N*-hydroxylation products with phosphoadenosine phosphosulfate can result in the production of sulfated BRIs (Figure 4). Thus, upon sulfation of 7-hydroxymethyl-12-methylbenz[*a*]anthracene to form 7-sulfoxymethyl-12-methylbenz[*a*]anthracene, the product can attack DNA, lose the sulfate group and form a DNA adduct. Lai *et al.* (1985) reported that the sulfation of *N*-hydroxy-2-acetylaminofluorene yielded *N*-sulfoxy-2-acetylaminofluorene (Figure 4), a BRI which produced DNA adducts upon loss of the sulfate group. Miller (1994) argued that the actual DNA binding occurred via the residual nitrone created by the loss of the sulfate.

BRIs that arise following glutathione conjugation

Glutathione (glutamylcysteinylglycine, GSH) transferases are a series of microsomal and cytoplasmic enzymes that bind GSH to electrophilic species in liver and other organs. The conjugates are then transported to the kidney, the glutamate and glycine residues are removed and the amino group of cysteine is acetylated before the resulting mercapturic acid is excreted in the urine (Figure 5). GSH conjugates may, however, form BRIs by four different mechanisms (Stevens & Wallin, 1990):

- The GSH conjugate with ethylene chloride leads to the formation of a sulfur half mustard, i.e. *S*-(2-chloroethyl)-*N*-acetyl-L-cysteine. Both *S*-(2-choloroethyl)-*N*-acetyl-L-cysteine and *S*-(2-choloroethyl)-cysteine form guanine adducts.
- Wefers and Sies (1983) and Brunmark and Cadenas (1988) suggest that GSH conjugates with hydroquinones, such as menadione, result in the formation of auto-oxidizable species which give rise to superoxide anion radicals. GSH conjugates of hydroquinones have also been demonstrated to be toxic and carcinogenic to the kidney with toxicity increasing as more GSH molecules are added to the ring. Weber *et al.* (2001) suggest that 2,3,5-tris(glutathionyl)hydroquinone imposes oxidative stress on kidney cells.
- Another mode of formation of BRIs due to GSH conjugation occurs from the action of

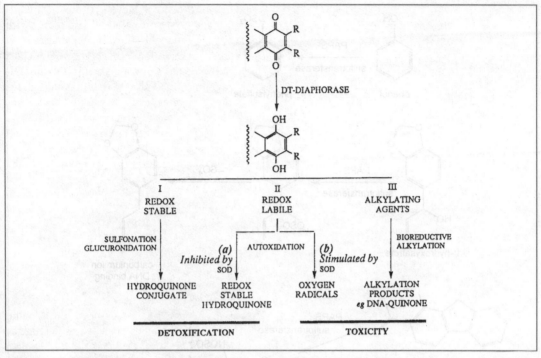

Figure 3. Anti-oxidant and prooxidant functions of DT-diaphorase in quinone metabolism. The reactivity of the hydroquinone formed during DT-diaphorase catalysis, (I) redox stable, (II) redox labile, or (III) alkylating agents, is a function of the substitution pattern (R) of the quinone. SOD, superoxide dismutase. From Cadenas (1995)

cysteine conjugate β-lyases (Vamvakas & Anders, 1991). An example is shown in Figure 6 where hexachlorobutadiene is shown to be converted to either an inactive mercapturic acid or a reactive thioketene (Dekant *et al.*, 1988). Another example is the fate of the trichloroethylene conjugate of GSH in which binding occurs by displacement of one chlorine atom to yield either S-1,2-dichlorovinyl-L-cysteine or S-2,2-dichlorovinyl-L-cysteine after removal of glutamate and glycine. Cysteine conjugate β-lyase cleaves the molecule between the sulfur and carbon-3 atoms of cysteine (β elimination) leading to the formation of another reactive thioketene species.

- GSH adducts may release the original active metabolite, providing a mechanism for transferring a BRI from one organ to another (Armstrong, 1997).

Susceptibility biomarkers related to polymorphisms among xenobiotic metabolizing enzymes

XMEs play a critical role in the metabolic activation or inactivation of most environmental carcinogens. In carcinogenesis induced by chemical carcinogens in experimental animals, it has been demonstrated that either inhibition of XME-catalysed carcinogen activation or induction of XME-catalysed carcinogen inactivation results in a reduction of tumour occurrence. The existence of functional genetic polymorphisms of XME that have a significant impact on the expression and catalytic activity of the enzymes has also been well documented. All of these provide strong support for the notion that genetic polymorphisms of XME may serve as appropriate susceptibility biomarkers of environmental carcinogenesis in humans. In addition, genetic polymorphisms of XME, by affecting carcinogen

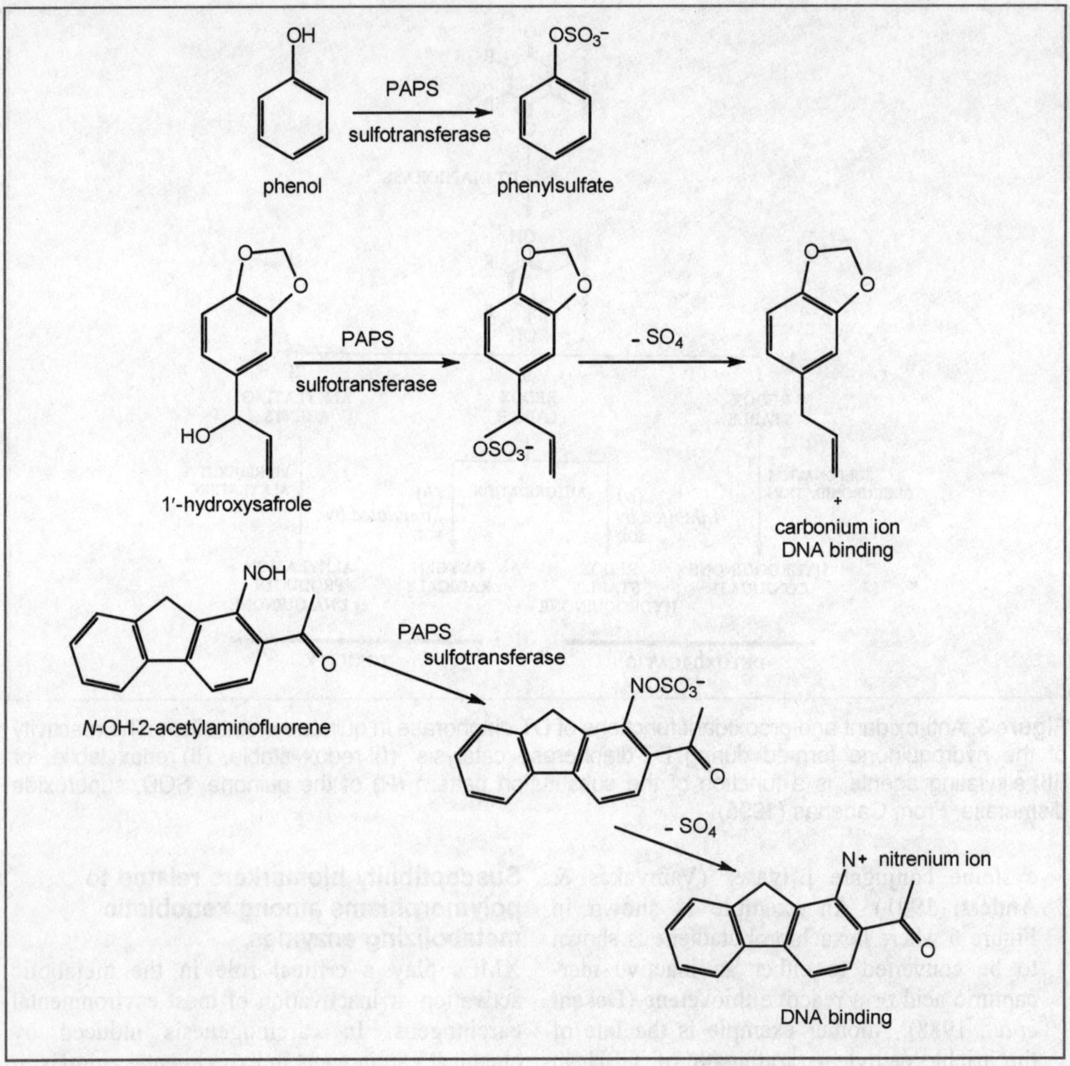

Figure 4. Examples of sulfo-conjugation leading to metabolic activation. PAPS, 3'-phosphoadenosine 5'-phosphosulfate synthase.

metabolism, could have profound effects on the level of carcinogen-derived DNA adducts, which are generally accepted as an intrinsic biomarker of exposure.

Genetic polymorphisms of xenobiotic metabolizing enzymes

Because of the power of the available technology, single nucleotide polymorphisms (SNPs, the most common form of DNA sequence variation) are readily detected. Overall, it can be estimated that there is approximately 1 SNP in every 100–500 bases in human DNA (Collins *et al.*, 1998). On the basis of this estimation, every human gene, including those that code for XMEs, is expected to have at least several polymorphic sequence variations. One should always bear in mind that most of these polymorphic variations do not have functional significance, even though they may occur in the most important cancer-related genes.

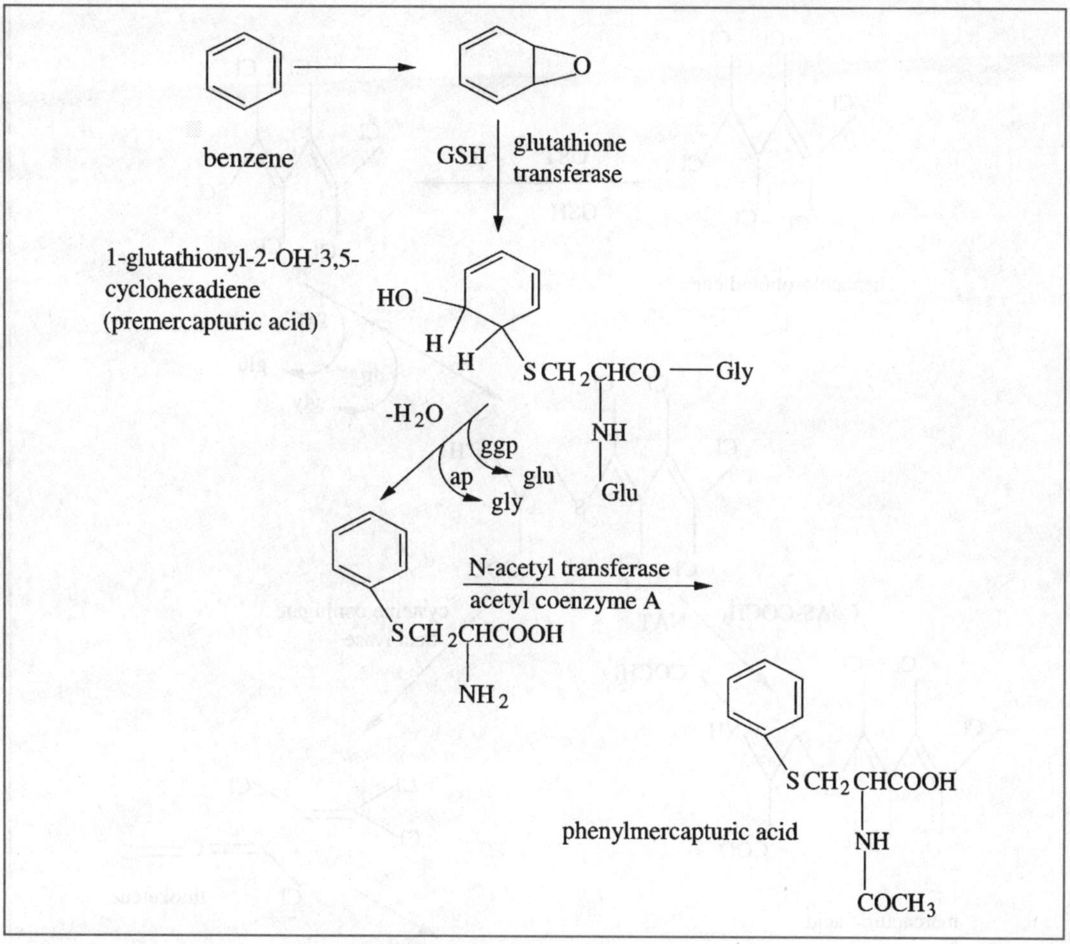

Figure 5. Formation of a non-toxic mercapturic acid derived from benzene.

Localization of polymorphic variations in the regulatory region of a gene and in the protein coding region which results in amino acid sequence variation (missense variation) may also not necessarily cause any alterations in the expression of that gene or the biological activity of its encoded protein. Therefore, when designing molecular epidemiological studies on the relationship between XME genetic polymorphisms and human cancer risk, it is important to realize that genetic polymorphisms may be detected that lack functional significance.

Table 3 summarizes the reported molecular epidemiological studies on XME genetic polymorphisms and the risk for human stomach cancer,

leukaemia/lymphoma and aerodigestive cancer. This summary was based on a PubMed search for publications from 1991 to October 2001. Although the functional significance issue did not appear to be a major concern in some early molecular epidemiological studies, more and more epidemiologists have recently recognized the importance of this issue in designing their studies. As biochemists and toxicologists, we strongly believe that establishing the significance of XME genetic polymorphisms, before attempting to assess their roles in human susceptibility to cancer by large population-based studies, would be a more meaningful and more cost-effective approach. For deletion-related XME genetic polymorphisms

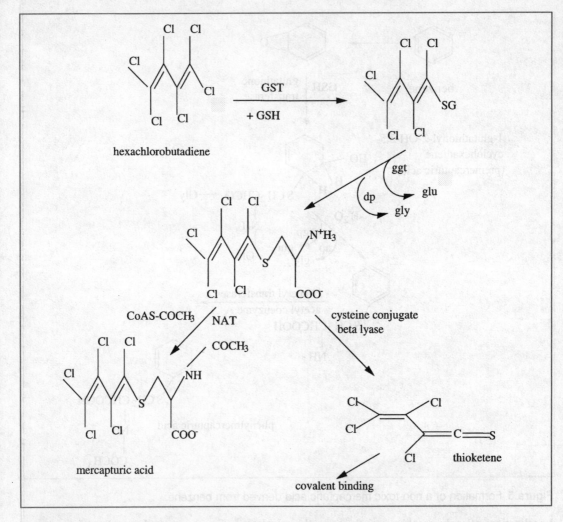

Figure 6. Glutathione conjugation with hexachlorobutadiene resulting in either a non-toxic mercapturic acid or a biological reactive intermediate.

such as GSTM1 and GSTT1 'null' polymorphisms, the functional consequences could be easily predicted. However, for XME genetic polymorphisms that involve sequence variations at the single nucleotide level, the functional characterization represents a challenging task.

Various molecular and biochemical approaches have been applied to characterization studies. In general, if a SNP is localized in a non-coding regulatory region such as the promoter, a reporter gene assay could be used to determine whether the SNP affects gene transcription. On the other hand,

if the SNP is within the protein coding region and results in a missense alteration of the DNA nucleotide sequence, the corresponding variant protein can be produced by site-directed mutagenesis or heterologous expression to study its biochemical properties. In combination with computer modelling, knowledge of the protein structure–activity relationship may also be useful in predicting the functional consequences of certain missense polymorphisms. In addition, use of human microsomes or of cells from donors with known XME genetic polymorphisms for in-vitro metabolism studies, or

Table 3. Molecular epidemiological studies on XME genetic polymorphism and the risk of human aerodigestive cancer, leukaemia/lymphoma and stomach cancer

	Aerodigestive cancer	Leukaemia/lymphoma	Stomach cancer
Cytochrome P450 (CYP)			
CYP1A1	Jahnke et al. (1996); Lucas et al. (1996); Matthias et al. (1998)	Hengstler et al. (1998); Krajinovic et al. (1999); Sassai et al. (1999); Garte et al. (2000); Infante-Rivard et al. (2000); Krajinovic et al. (2000); Sarmanova et al. (2001)	Kato et al. (1995); Nishimoto et al. (2000); Shimada et al. (2001); Zhang & Bian (2001)
CYP2D6	Jahnke et al. (1996); Matthias et al. (1998)		
CYP 2E1	Jahnke et al. (1996); Lucas et al. (1996); Matthias et al. (1998); Bouchardy et al. (2000)	Garte et al. (2000); Sarmanova et al. (2001)	Katoh et al. (1996, 1999); Saadat & Saadat (2001)
CYP3A4		Wundrack et al. (1994); Krajinovic et al. (1999); Naoe et al. (2000)	
Glutathione S-transferase (GST)			
GSTM1	Jahnke et al. (1996); Matthias et al. (1998)	Hengstler et al. (1998); Krajinovic et al. (1999); Sassai et al. (1999); Anderer et al. (2000); Davies et al. (2000); Garte et al. (2000); Krajinovic et al. (2000); Naoe et al. (2000); Rollinson et al. (2000); Saadat & Saadat (2000); Allan et al. (2001); Sarmanova et al. (2001)	Katoh et al. (1996, 1999); Saadat & Saadat (2001)
GSTM3	Jahnke et al. (1996); Matthias et al. (1998)	Hengstler et al. (1998); Krajinovic et al. (1999)	
GSTP1	Jahnke et al. (1996)	Hengstler et al. (1998); Rollinson et al. (1999); Allan et al. (2000); Sarmanova et al. (2001)	Katoh et al. (1999); Alves et al. (2000)
GSTT1	Jahnke et al. (1996); Matthias et al. (1998); Garte et al. (2000)	Hengstler et al. (1998); Krajinovic et al. (1999); Sassai et al. (1999); Anderer et al. (2000); Davies et al. (2000); Naoe et al. (2000); Rollinson et al. (2000); Allan et al. (2001); Sarmanova et al. (2001)	Katoh et al. (1996,1999); Saadat & Saadat (2001); Zhang & Bian (2001)
N-Acetyltransferases (NAT)			
NAT1		Hengstler et al. (1998); Krajinovic et al. (1999)	Boissy et al. (2000); Katoh et al. (2000)
NAT2		Hengstler et al. (1998); Krajinovic et al. (1999)	Boissy et al. (2000); Katoh et al. (2000)
NAD(P)H:quinone oxidoreductase (NQOl)		Naoe et al. (2000)	
Alcohol and aldehyde dehydrogenases	Tanabe et al. (1999); Bouchardy et al. (2000); Muto et al. (2000)		Zhang & Bian (2001)

the use of genotyped human subjects for in-vivo metabolism studies, could be a reasonable approach. However, it should be noted that the throughput of currently available technologies for functional characterization of XME genetic polymorphisms is relatively low, which significantly limits our capability in this extremely important research area.

The impact of functional genetic polymorphisms can be determined at various phenotypic levels *in vitro* and *in vivo*. These include the expression of mRNA and protein, the enzyme catalytic properties and the toxicokinetics. For example, Kitagawa *et al.* (1999) and Oscarson *et al.* (1998) reported that, in test subjects carrying homozygous CYP2A6 deletion alleles, urinary levels of cotinine (a major metabolite of nicotine) and 7-hydroxycoumarin (a major metabolite of coumarin) were much lower than in subjects carrying homozygous CYP2A6 wild-type alleles who received the same doses of nicotine or coumarin. These results demonstrate a significant effect of CYP2A6 'null' alleles on the toxicokinetics *in vivo* and are consistent with the predominant role of CYP2A6 in metabolizing nicotine and coumarin. Selection of such XME genetic polymorphisms that have great impact on toxicokinetics would provide us a better chance to elucidate the relationship between XME genetic polymorphisms and human susceptibilities to environmental carcinogens in molecular epidemiological studies. Whenever possible, this type of validation of the in-vitro results should always be encouraged.

Example of multiple biomarkers for a single chemical (benzene)

Desirable characteristics of biochemical biomarkers were discussed above. The best biomarkers are not always chemicals. Benzene is a chemical to which large numbers of people have been, and continue to be, exposed. In this section we discuss potential biomarkers for benzene.

Metabolite biomarkers of exposure

Selection of biomarkers of exposure presupposes that the biomarker is uniquely related to the chemical in question. Thus, measurement of

benzene in the breath, blood, urine or tissues of an exposed person would be the best biomarker for benzene since its presence would most likely be the result of exposure to benzene. A series of methods have been proposed for measuring benzene in humans (ATSDR, 1997). Because of inconsistencies in quantifying unchanged benzene, quantification of metabolites of benzene, usually in urine, has been preferred. Inoue *et al.* (1986) collected urine from men and women at the end of a 7-hour shift in workplaces where exposure to benzene was reported. The workers wore passive dosimeters for the assessment of exposure to benzene and phenol was measured in urine. Exposure to 10 mg/kg (parts per million) benzene resulted in urinary phenol levels of 47.5 mg/L (57.9 mg/g creatinine; 46.6 mg/L when corrected to a specific gravity of 1.016). Further studies were directed to the measurement of catechol and hydroquinone (quinol) in urine after exposure to benzene (Inoue *et al.*, 1988). The data suggested that when workers were exposed to 100 mg/kg of benzene about 25% of the dose could be found in the urine as phenol (13.2%), catechol (1.6%) and hydroquinone (10.2%). It is significant that earlier studies of benzene metabolism in rabbits by Parke and Williams (1953) gave similar results. Studies on urinary excretion of 1,2,4-benzenetriol (Inoue *et al.*, 1989a) suggested that it is derived from phenol and hydroquinone, but not from catechol, and does not offer an approach to direct measurement of exposure to benzene. Nevertheless, the measurement of phenolic metabolites in the urine has not gained universal acceptance because of the likelihood that they may also arise from dietary components.

The search for urinary metabolites uniquely derived from benzene has focused on *trans, trans* (*t,t*)-muconic acid and phenylmercapturic acid. Methods for determining *t,t*-muconic acid concentrations in urine of benzene-exposed workers were reported by Inoue *et al.* (1989b), Ducos *et al.* (1992) and Marrubini *et al.* (2001). Boogaard and van Sittert (1995) found *t,t*-muconic acid in the urine of non-exposed people at a level of 710 μg/g creatinine. Goba *et al.* (1997) found that, among 80 bus drivers exposed to benzene over a range of 10–1000 μg/m³, the mean value for *t,t*-muconic acid in urine was 297 µg/g creatinine, but the range of values varied from 20 to 1295 µg/g. The authors attributed this to inter-individual variability of benzene metabolism. Sanguinetti *et al.* (2001) suggested that urinary *t,t*-muconic acid was not a good marker for attempting to determine exposure to benzene in the µg/kg (parts per billion) range of exposures. Nevertheless, *t,t*-muconic acid is relatively easy to measure compared to other metabolites.

Certain problems arise when *t,t*-muconic acid is used as a measure of exposure to benzene. One difficulty is that an enzyme called pyrocatechase, which is present in several microorganisms, can open the catechol ring to yield *cis,cis*-muconic acid (Knox, 1961). If dietary catechol is attacked by enzymes of the gastrointestinal flora, muconic acid may appear in urine but unrelated to exposure to benzene. It is also clear that benzene in cigarette smoke is a significant contributor to urinary *t,t*-muconic acid (Ruppert *et al.*, 1997). Furthermore, Ruppert *et al.* (1997) and Weaver *et al.* (2000) reported that sorbic acid, a commonly used food preservative that is metabolized to *t,t*-muconic acid, might interfere with the measurement of the metabolite after exposure to benzene. It should be noted, however, that Renner *et al.* (1999) offered a method for determining the proportion of *t,t*-muconic acid in urine that is derived from sorbic acid as distinct from that derived from benzene.

As an alternative, it has been suggested that *S*-phenylmercapturic acid in urine would be a valuable marker of exposure. Boogaard and van Sittert (1995, 1996) suggested that the measurement of *S*-phenylmercapturic acid in urine is superior to that of *t,t*-muconic acid because it has a longer half-life, is more specific for benzene and detects exposure to lower levels, i.e. 0.3 mg/kg of benzene. Taken together, the data suggest that at high exposure levels either *t,t*-muconic acid or *S*-phenylmercapturic acid can detect exposure but at lower levels the mercapturate may have an advantage.

The major problem with all of these methods has been the difficulty of relating accurately any of the potential biomarkers to specific levels of benzene exposure. Thus, we may conclude that observation of these biomarkers suggests exposure to environmental benzene, provided that one can account for possible co-exposures to sorbic acid or cigarette smoke.

Other metabolites of benzene have been identified in urine but not evaluated as quantitative biomarkers of exposure. These include *N*-acetyl-*S*-(2,5-dihydroxyphenyl)-L-cysteine, a presumed metabolite of hydroquinone (Nerland & Pierce, 1990) and *N*7-phenylguanine, which was identified in the urine of rats treated with radiolabelled benzene (Norpoth *et al.*, 1988).

It is known that exposure to benzene can result in covalent binding of reactive metabolites to proteins throughout the body (Snyder *et al.*, 1978). Covalent binding to blood proteins has been suggested as a biomarker of exposure to benzene. Thus, Melikian *et al.* (1992) exposed rats to labelled benzene and recovered *S*-(2,5-dihydroxyphenyl)cysteine and *S*-phenylcysteine from hydrolysed haemoglobin. Bechtold *et al.* (1992a) and Bechtold and Henderson (1993) identified *S*-phenylcysteine in the haemoglobin of both rats and mice exposed to benzene. Bechtold *et al.* (1992b) and Bechtold and Strunk (1996) studied the production of *S*-phenylcysteine in albumin of benzene-exposed rats. Rappaport and Yeowell-O'Connor (1999) examined haemoglobin and albumin adducts in the blood of 88 Chinese workers exposed to benzene over a range of doses estimated at 0–138 mg/kg and detected *S*-phenylcysteine. It is significant that these adducts were observed in the exposed workers, in control subjects and in commercial human proteins.

Biomarkers of effect

The earliest biomarkers of effect of benzene are not measurements of metabolism. The earliest biomarkers of effect are decreased levels of circulating erythrocytes, leukocytes or platelets as a function of exposure to benzene (Snyder *et al.*, 1993). As benzene toxicity progresses it may lead to bone marrow aplasia or to dysplasia which may then progress to acute myelogenous leukaemia. Benzene-induced chromosomal damage is another biomarker of effect, which is discussed in another chapter (Smith *et al.*, this volume).

Biomarkers of susceptibility

It has long been recognized that benzene toxicity is mediated by benzene metabolites. The activity of enzymes involved in benzene metabolism can determine the susceptibility of an individual to benzene-induced bone marrow disease. It has been postulated that hydroquinone is a key metabolite in the initiation of benzene toxicity. Hydroquinone is thought to function via its oxidation to *para*-benzoquinone, presumably via myeloperoxidase (Smith *et al.*, 1989). *para*-Benzoquinone is highly reactive and can bind covalently to macromolecules but it is inactivated by reduction to hydroquinone via NQO1 (Ross, 1996). Rothman *et al.* (1997) studied a group of Chinese workers who had been exposed to benzene and exhibited benzene toxicity. They suggested that risk factors for increased susceptibility to benzene included the activity of CYP2E1 coupled with a mutation, which decreased the activity of NQO1. Indeed, it has been suggested (Snyder, 2000b) that polymorphisms in hepatic CYP2E1 and GST and myeloperoxidase and NQO1 in bone marrow may help to define an individual's susceptibility to benzene toxicity.

In summary, many chemicals exhibit their carcinogenicity only after metabolic activation by XMEs. We have summarized the role of phase I enzymes such as the CYP family of enzymes as well as phase II enzymes such as NQO1, GSTs and sulfotransferase in the generation of BRIs. These phase I and phase II enzymes are expressed polymorphically among individuals and specifically among organs. Variability in susceptibility to the carcinogenic effects of a chemical within a given population may be determined by the polymorphic distribution of specific XMEs. To assign an etiological role of an XME to a specific cancer requires both genetic and kinetic analysis of the enzyme. We emphasize that the interactions among epidemiologists, molecular biologists and toxicologists are critically important for successful cancer molecular epidemiological studies. Finally, we have used benzene as an example to discuss the application of several different biomarkers to study exposure, effect and susceptibility to a specific chemical.

References

Allan, J.M., Wild, C.P., Rollinson, S., Willett, E.V., Moorman, A.V., Dovey, G.J., Roddam, P.L., Roman, E., Cartwright, R.A. & Morgan, G.J. (2001) Polymorphism in glutathione *S*-transferase P1 is associated with susceptibility to chemotherapy-induced leukemia. *Proc. natl Acad. Sci. USA*, **98**, 11592–11597

Alves, C., Silva, F., Gusmao, L., Seruca, R., Soares, P., Reis, R.M. & Amorim, A. (2000) Extended structural variation of a pentanucleotide repeat in the GSTP1 gene: characterisation in a normal population and in thyroid and gastric tumors. *Eur. J. hum. Genet.*, **8**, 540–544

Anderer, G., Schrappe, M., Brechlin, A.M., Lauten, M., Muti, P., Welte, K. & Stanulla, M. (2000) Polymorphisms within glutathione *S*-transferase genes and initial response to glucocorticoids in childhood acute lymphoblastic leukaemia. *Pharmacogenetics*, **10**, 715–726

Armstrong, R.N. (1997) Glutathione transferases. In: Sipes, I.G., McQueen, C.A. & Gandolfi, A.J., eds (Guengerich, F.P., volume ed.), *Comprehensive Toxicology*, New York, Pergamon, Vol. 3, pp. 307–327

ATSDR (Agency for Toxic Substances and Disease Registry) (1997) *Toxicological Profile for Benzene*, US Department of Health and Human Services, Public Health Service, pp. 309–313

Bechtold, W.E. & Henderson, R.F. (1993) Biomarkers of human exposure to benzene. *J. Toxicol. environ. Health*, **40**, 377–386

Bechtold, W.E. & Strunk, M.R. (1996) *S*-Phenylcysteine in albumin as a benzene biomarker. *Environ. Health Perspect.*, **104** (Suppl. 6), 1147–1149

Bechtold, W.E., Willis, J.K., Sun, J.D., Griffith, W.C. & Reddy, T.V. (1992a) Biological markers of exposure to benzene: S-phenylcysteine in albumin. *Carcinogenesis*, **13**, 1217–1220

Bechtold, W.E., Sun, J.D., Birnbaum, L.S., Yin, S.N., Li, G.L., Kasicki, S., Lucier, G. & Henderson, R.F. (1992b) *S*-Phenylcysteine formation in hemoglobin as a biological exposure index to benzene. *Arch. Toxicol.*, **66**, 303–309

Boissy, R.J., Watson, M.A., Umbach, D.M., Deakin, M., Elder, J., Strange, R.C. & Bell, D.A. (2000) A pilot study investigating the role of NAT1 and

NAT2 polymorphisms in gastric adenocarcinoma. *Int. J. Cancer*, **87**, 507–511

Boogaard, P.J. & van Sittert, N.J. (1995) Biological monitoring of exposure to benzene: a comparison between *S*-phenylmercapturic acid, *trans,trans*-muconic acid and phenol. *Occup. environ. Med.*, **52**, 611–620

Boogaard, P.J. & van Sittert, N.J. (1996) Suitability of *S*-phenylmercapturic acid and *trans,trans*-muconic acid as biomarkers for exposure to low concentrations of benzene. *Environ. Health Perspect.*, **104** (Suppl 6), 1151–1157

Bouchardy, C., Hirvonen, A., Coutelle, C., Ward, P.J., Dayer, P. & Benhamou, S. (2000) Role of alcohol dehydrogenase 3 and cytochrome P-4502E1 genotypes in susceptibility to cancers of the upper aerodigestive tract. *Int. J. Cancer*, **87**, 734–740

Brunmark, A. & Cadenas, E. (1988) Reductive addition of glutathione to *p*-benzoquinone, 2-hydroxy-*p*-benzoquinone, and *p*-benzoquinone epoxides. Effect of the hydroxy- and glutathionyl substitutents on *p*-benzohydroquinone autooxidation. *Chem.-biol. Interact.*, **68**, 273–298

Cadenas, E. (1995) Antioxidant and prooxidant functions of DT-diaphorase in quinone metabolism. *Biochem. Pharmacol.*, **49**, 127–140

Collins, F.S., Brooks, L.D. & Chakravarti, A. (1998) A DNA polymorphism discovery resource for research on human genetic variation. *Genome Res.*, **8**, 1229–1231

Crofts, F.G., Sutter, T.R. & Strickland, P.T. (1998) Metabolism of 2-amino-1-methyl-6-phenylimidazo[4,5-b]pyridine by human cytochrome P4501A1, P4501A2 and P4501B1. *Carcinogenesis*, **19**, 1969–1973

Dansette, P.M., Snyder, R., Delaforge, M., Monks, T.J., Gibson, G.G., Jollow, D.J., Greim, H. & Glenn Sipes, I., eds (2001) *Biological Reactive Intermediates VI: Chemical and Biological Mechanisms in Susceptibility to and Prevention of Environmental Diseases*, New York, Plenum Press

Davies, S.M., Robison, L.L., Buckley, J.D., Radloff, G.A., Ross, J.A. & Perentesis, J.P. (2000) Glutathione *S*-transferase polymorphisms in children with myeloid leukemia: a Children's Cancer Group study. *Cancer Epidemiol. Biomarkers Prev.*, **9**, 563–566

Dekant, W., Schrenk, D., Vamvakas, S. & Henschler, D. (1988) Metabolism of hexachloro-1,3-butadiene in mice: in vivo and in vitro evidence for activation by glutathione conjugation. *Xenobiotica*, **18**, 803–816

Ducos, P., Gaudin, R., Bel, J., Maire, C., Francin, J.M., Robert, A. & Wild, P. (1992) *trans,trans*-Muconic acid, a reliable biological indicator for the detection of individual benzene exposure down to the ppm level. *Int. Arch. environ. Health*, **64**, 309–313

Garte, S., Taioli, E., Crosti, F., Sainati, L., Barisone, E., Luciani, M., Jankovic, M. & Biondi, A.G (2000) Deletion of parental GST genes as a possible susceptibility factor in the etiology of infant leukemia. *Leukemia Res.*, **24**, 971–974

Gil, F. & Pla, A. (2001) Biomarkers as biological indicators of xenobiotic exposure. *J. appl. Toxicol.*, **21**, 245–255

Goba, F., Rovesti, S., Borella, P., Vivoli, R., Casegrandi. E. & Viovoli, G. (1997) Inter-individual variability of benzene metabolism to *trans,trans*-muconic acid and its implications in the biological monitoring of occupational exposure. *Sci. total Environ.*, **199**, 41–48

Hengstler, J.G., Arand, M., Herrero, M.E. & Oesch, F. (1998) Polymorphisms of *N*-acetyltransferases, glutathione *S*-transferases, microsomal epoxide hydrolase and sulfotransferases: influence on cancer susceptibility. *Recent Results Cancer Res.*, **154**, 47–85

Hong, J.Y. & Yang, C.S. (1997) Genetic polymorphism of cytochrome P450 as a biomarker of susceptibility to environmental toxicity. *Environ. Health Perspect.*, **105** (Suppl. 4), 759–762

Infante-Rivard, C., Krajinovic, M., Labuda, D. & Sinnett, D. (2000) Parental smoking, CYP1A1 genetic polymorphisms and childhood leukemia (Quebec, Canada). *Cancer Causes Control*, **11**, 547–553

Inoue, O., Seiji, K., Kasahara, M., Nakatsuka, H., Watanabe, T., Yin, S.G., Li, G.L., Jin, C., Cai, S.X., Wang, X.Z. & Ikeda, M. (1986) Quantitative relation of urinary phenol levels to breath zone benzene concentrations: a factory survey. *Br. J. ind. Med.*, **43**, 692–697

Inoue, O., Seiji, K., Kasahara, M., Nakatsuka, H., Watanabe, T., Yin, S., Li, G.L., Cai, S.X., Jin, C. & Ikeda, M. (1988) Determination of catechol and quinol in the urine of workers exposed to benzene. *Br. J. ind. Med.*, **45**, 487–492

Inoue, O., Seiji, K., Nakatsuka, H., Watanabe, T., Yin, S., Li, G.L., Cai, S.X., Jin, C. & Ikeda, M. (1989a) Excretion of 1,2,4-benzenetriol in urine of workers exposed to benzene. *Br. J. ind. Med.*, **46**, 559–565

Inoue, O., Seiji, K., Nakatsuka, H., Watanabe, T., Yin, S.N., Li, G.L., Cai, S.X., Jin, C. & Ikeda, M. (1989b) Urinary t,t-muconic acid as an indicator of exposure to benzene. *Br. J. ind. Med.*, **46**, 122–127

Jahnke, V., Matthias, C., Fryer, A. & Strange, R. (1996) Glutathione *S*-transferase and cytochrome-P-450 polymorphism as risk factors for squamous cell carcinoma of the larynx. *Am. J. Surg.*, **172**, 671–673

Jollow, D.J., Kocsis, J.J., Snyder, R. & Vainio, H. (1975) *Biological Reactive Intermediates: Formation, Toxicity and Inactivation*, New York, Plenum Press

Kalow, W., ed. (1992) Pharmacogenetics of drug metabolism. In: *International Encyclopedia of Pharmacology and Therapeutics*, New York, Pergamon Press

Kato, S., Onda, M., Matsukura, N., Tokunaga, A., Tajiri, T., Kim, D.Y., Tsuruta, H., Matsuda, N., Yamashita, K. & Shields, P.G. (1995) Cytochrome P4502E1 (CYP2E1) genetic polymorphism in a case–control study of gastric cancer and liver disease. *Pharmacogenetics*, **5**, S141–S144

Katoh, T., Nagata, N., Kuroda, Y., Itoh, H., Kawahara, A., Kuroki, N., Ookuma, R. & Bell, D.A. (1996) Glutathione *S*-transferase M1 (GSTM1) and T1 (GSTT1) genetic polymorphism and susceptibility to gastric and colorectal adenocarcinoma. *Carcinogenesis*, **17**, 1855–1859

Katoh, T., Kaneko, S., Takasawa, S., Nagata, N., Inatomi, H., Ikemura, K., Itoh, H., Matsumoto, T., Kawamoto, T. & Bell, D.A. (1999) Human glutathione *S*-transferase P1 polymorphism and susceptibility to smoking related epithelial cancer; oral, lung, gastric, colorectal and urothelial cancer. *Pharmacogenetics*, **9**, 165–169

Katoh, T., Boissy, R., Nagata, N., Kitagawa, K., Kuroda, Y., Itoh, H., Kawamoto, T. & Bell, D.A. (2000) Inherited polymorphism in the N-acetyltransferase 1 (*NAT1*) and 2 (*NAT2*) genes and susceptibility to gastric and colorectal adenocarcinoma. *Int. J. Cancer*, **85**, 46–49

Kitagawa, K., Kunugita, N., Katoh, T., Yang, M. & Kawamoto, T. (1999) The significance of the homozygous CYP2A6 deletion on nicotine metabolism: a new genotyping method of CYP2A6 using a single PCR-RFLP. *Biochem. biophys. Res. Commun.*, **262**, 146–151

Knox, W.E. (1961) Pyrocatechase. In: Long, C., Kong, E.J. & Sperry, W.M., eds, *Biochemist's Handbook*, Princeton, NJ, Van Nostrand

Kocsis, J.J., Jollow, D., Witmer, C.M., Nelson, J.O. & Snyder, R., eds (1986) *Biological Reactive Intermediates III: Mechanisms of Action in Animal Models and Human Disease*, New York, Plenum Press

Krajinovic, M., Labuda, D., Richer, C., Karimi, S. & Sinnett, D. (1999) Susceptibility to childhood acute lymphoblastic leukemia: influence of CYP1A1, CYP2D6, GSTM1, and GSTT1 genetic polymorphisms. *Blood*, **93**, 1496–1501

Krajinovic, M., Richer, C., Sinnett, H., Labuda, D. & Sinnett, D. (2000) Genetic polymorphisms of *N*-acetyltransferases 1 and 2 and gene–gene interaction in the susceptibility to childhood acute lymphoblastic leukemia. *Cancer Epidemiol. Biomarkers Prev.*, **9**, 557–562

Lai, C.C., Miller, J.A., Miller, E.C. & Liem, A. (1985) *N*-sulfooxy-2-aminofluorene is the major ultimate electrophilic and carcinogenic metabolite of *N*-hydroxy-2-acetylaminofluorene in the liver of infant male (C57BL/6J × C3H/HeJ)F$_1$ (B6C3F1) mice. *Carcinogenesis*, **6**, 1037–1045

Lucas, D., Menez, C., Floch, F., Gourlaouen, Y., Sparfel, O., Joannet, I., Bodenez, P., Jezequel, J., Gouerou, H., Berthou, F., Bardou, L.G. & Menez, J.F. (1996) Cytochromes P4502E1 and P4501A1 genotypes and susceptibility to cirrhosis or upper aerodigestive tract cancer in alcoholic Caucasians. *Alcohol clin. exp. Res.*, **20**, 1033–1037

Marrubini, G., Hogendoorn, E.A., Coccini, T. & Manzo, L. (2001) Improved coupled column liquid chromatographic method for high-speed direct analysis of urinary *trans,trans*-muconic acid, as a biomarker of exposure to benzene. *J. Chromatogr. B Biomed. Sci. Appl.*, **751**, 331–339

Matthias, C., Bockmuhl, U., Jahnke, V., Jones, P.W., Hayes, J.D., Alldersea, J., Gilford, J., Bailey, L., Bath, J., Worrall, S.F., Hand, P., Fryer, A.A. & Strange, R.C. (1998) Polymorphism in cytochrome

P450 CYP2D6, CYP1A1, CYP2E1 and glutathione S-transferase, GSTM1, GSTM3, GSTT1 and susceptibility to tobacco-related cancers: studies in upper aerodigestive tract cancers. *Pharmacogenetics*, **8**, 91–100

Melikian, A.A., Prahalad, A.K. & Coleman, S. (1992) Isolation and characterization of two benzene-derived hemoglobin adducts *in vivo* in rats. *Cancer Epidemiol. Biomarkers Prev.*, **1**, 307–313

Miller, J.A. (1994) Research in chemical carcinogenesis with Elizabeth Miller – A trail of discovery with our associates. *Drug Metab. Rev.*, **26**, 1–36

Miller, J.A., Surh, Y.-J., Liem, A. & Miller, E.C. (1991) Electrophilic sulfuric acid ester metabolites of hydroxy-methyl aromatic hydrocarbons as precursors of hepatic benzylic DNA adducts. In: Witmer, C.M., Snyder, R., Jollow, D.J., Kalf, G.F., Kocsis, J.J. & Sipes, I.G., eds, *Biological Reactive Intermediates IV: Molecular and Cellular Effects and Their Impact on Human Health*, New York, Plenum Press, pp. 555–567

Moran, J.L., Siegel, D. & Ross, D. (1999) A potential mechanism underlying the increased susceptibility of individuals with a polymorphism in NAD(P)H: quinone oxidoreductase 1 (NQO1) to benzene toxicity. *Proc. natl Acad. Sci. USA*, **96**, 8150–8155

Muto, M., Hitomi, Y., Ohtsu, A., Ebihara, S., Yoshida, S. & Esumi, H. (2000) Association of aldehyde dehydrogenase 2 gene polymorphism with multiple esophageal dysplasia in head and neck cancer patients. *Gut*, **47**, 256–261

Naoe, T., Takeyama, K., Yokozawa, T., Kiyoi, H., Seto, M., Uike, N., Ino, T., Utsunomiya, A., Maruta, A., Jin-nai, I., Kamada, N., Kubota, Y., Nakamura, H., Shimazaki, C., Horiike, S., Kodera, Y., Saito, H., Ueda, R., Wiemels, J. & Ohno, R. (2000) Analysis of genetic polymorphism in NQO1, GST-M1, GST-T1, and CYP3A4 in 469 Japanese patients with therapy-related leukemia/myelodysplastic syndrome and de novo acute myeloid leukemia. *Clin. Cancer Res.*, **6**, 4091–4095

Nerland, D.E. & Pierce, W.M. (1990) Identification of N-acetyl-S-(2,5-dihydroxyphenyl)-L-cysteine as a urinary metabolite of benzene, phenol and hydroquinone. *Drug Metab. Dispos.*, **18**, 958–961

Nishimoto, I.N., Hanaoka, T., Sugimura, H., Nagura, K., Ihara, M., Li, X.J., Arai, T., Hamada, G.S., Kowalski, L.P. & Tsugane, S. (2000) Cytochrome P450 2E1 polymorphism in gastric cancer in Brazil: case–control studies of Japanese Brazilians and non-Japanese Brazilians. *Cancer Epidemiol. Biomarkers Prev.*, **9**, 675–680

Norpoth, K., Stucker, W., Krewet, E. & Muller, G. (1988) Biomonitoring of benzene exposure by trace analyses of phenylguanine. *Int. Arch. occup. environ. Health*, **60**, 163–168

Oscarson, M., Gullsten, H., Rautio, A., Bernal, M.L., Sinues, B., Dahl, M.L., Stengard, J.H., Pelkonen, O., Raunio, H. & Ingelman-Sundberg, M. (1998) Genotyping of human cytochrome P450 2A6 (CYP2A6), a nicotine C-oxidase. *FEBS Lett.*, **438**, 201–205

Parke, D.V. & Williams, R.T. (1953) Studies in detoxication 49. The metabolism of benzene containing $^{14}C_1$ benzene. *Biochem. J.*, **54**, 231

Patten, C.J., Smith, T.J., Murphy, S.E., Wang, M.H., Lee, J., Tynes, R.E., Koch, P. & Yang, C.S. (1996) Kinetic analysis of the activation of 4-(methylnitrosamino)-1-(3-pyridyl)-1-butanone by heterologously expressed human P450 enzymes and the effect of P450-specific chemical inhibitors on this activation in human liver microsomes. *Arch. Biochem. Biophys.*, **333**, 127–138

Penman, B.W., Reece, J., Smith, T., Yang, C.S., Gelboin, H.V., Gonzalez, F.J. & Crespi, C.L. (1993) Characterization of a human cell line expressing high levels of cDNA-derived CYP2D6. *Pharmacogenetics*, **3**, 28–39

Rappaport, S.M. & Yeowell-O'Connell, K. (1999) Protein adducts as dosimeters of human exposure to styrene, styrene-7,8-oxide and benzene. *Toxicol. Lett.*, **108**, 117–126

Renner, T., Baer-Koetzle, M. & Scherer, G. (1999) Determination of sorbic acid in urine by gas chromatography-mass spectrometry. *J. Chromatogr. A*, **847**, 127–133

Rollinson, S., Roddam, P., Kane, E., Roman, E., Cartwright, R., Jack, A. & Morgan, G.J. (2000) Polymorphic variation within the glutathione S-transferase genes and risk of adult acute leukaemia. *Carcinogenesis*, **21**, 43–47

Ross, D. (1996) Metabolic basis of benzene toxicity. *Eur. J. Hematol.*, **60** (Suppl.), 111–118

Ross, D. (1997) Quinone reductases. In: Sipes, I.G., McQueen, C.A. & Gandolfi, A.J., eds (Guengerich,

F.P., volume ed.), *Comprehensive Toxicology*, New York, Pergamon, Vol. 3, pp. 179–197

Rothman, N., Smith, M.T., Hayes, R.B., Traver, R.D., Hoener, B., Campleman, S., Li, G., Dosemeci, M., Linet, M., Zhang, L., Xi, L., Wacholder, S., Lu, W., Meyer, K.B., Titenko-Holland, N., Stewart, J.T., Yin, S. & Ross, D. (1997) Benzene poisoning, a risk factor for hematological malignancy, is associated with the NQO1 609 C→T mutation and rapid fractional excretion of chlorzoxazone. *Cancer Res.*, **57**, 2839–2842

Ruppert, T., Scherer, G., Tricker, A.R. & Adlkofer, F. (1997) *trans,trans*-Muconic acid as a biomarker of non-occupational environmental exposure to benzene. *Int. Arch. occup. environ. Health.*, **69**, 247–251

Saadat, I. & Saadat, M. (2000) The glutathione *S*-transferase mu polymorphism and susceptibility to acute lymphocytic leukemia. *Cancer Lett.*, **158**, 43–45

Saadat, I. & Saadat, M. (2001) Glutathione *S*-transferase M1 and T1 null genotypes and the risk of gastric and colorectal cancers. *Cancer Lett.*, **169**, 21–26

Sanguinetti, G., Accorsi, A., Barbieri, A., Raffi, G.B. & Violante, F.S. (2001) Failure of urinary *trans,trans*-muconic acid as a biomarker for indoor environmental benzene exposure at ppb levels. *J. Toxicol. environ. Health A.*, **63**, 599–604

Sarmanova, J., Benesova, K., Gut, I., Nedelcheva-Kristensen, V., Tynkova, L. & Soucek, P. (2001) Genetic polymorphisms of biotransformation enzymes in patients with Hodgkin's and non-Hodgkin's lymphomas. *Hum. mol. Genet.*, **10**, 1265–1273

Sasai, Y., Horiike, S., Misawa, S., Kaneko, H., Kobayashi, M., Fujii, H., Kashima, K. & Taniwaki, M. (1999) Genotype of glutathione *S*-transferase and other genetic configurations in myelodysplasia. *Leukemia Res.*, **23**, 975–981

Shimada, K., Matsukawa, M., Kurihara, M., Nishimura, Y. & Kurata, N. (2001) [Molecular mechanism of carcinogenesis in human stomach cancer: Genetic polymorphism of cytochrome P4502E1]. *Nippon Rinsho*, **59** (Suppl. 4), 48–52 (in Japanese)

Smith, M.T. (1999) Benzene, NQO1, and genetic susceptibility to cancer. *Proc. natl Acad. Sci. USA*, **96**, 7624–7626

Smith, M.T., Yager, J.W., Steinmetz, K.L. & Eastmond, D.A. (1989) Peroxidase-dependent metabolism of benzene's phenolic metabolites and its potential role in benzene toxicity and carcinogenicity. *Environ. Health Perspect.*, **82**, 23-29

Smith, T.J., Guo, Z., Gonzalez, F.J., Guengerich, F.P., Stoner, G.D. & Yang, C.S. (1992) Metabolism of 4-(methylnitrosamino)-1-(3-pyridyl)-1-butanone in human lung and liver microsomes and cytochromes P-450 expressed in hepatoma cells. *Cancer Res.*, **52**, 1757–1763

Smith, T.J., Stoner, G.D. & Yang, C.S. (1995) Activation of 4-(methylnitrosamino)-1-(3-pyridyl)-1-butanone (NNK) in human lung microsomes by cytochromes P450, lipoxygenase, and hydroperoxides. *Cancer Res.*, **55**, 5566–5573

Smith, T.J., Guo, Z., Guengerich, F.P. & Yang, C.S. (1996) Metabolism of 4-(methylnitrosamino)-1-(3-pyridyl)-1-butanone (NNK) by human cytochrome P450 1A2 and its inhibition by phenethyl isothiocyanate. *Carcinogenesis*, **17**, 809–813

Snyder, R. (2000a) Cytochrome P450, the oxygen activating enzyme in xenobiotic metabolism. *Toxicol. Sci.*, **58**, 3–4

Snyder, R. (2000b) Overview of the toxicology of benzene. *J. Toxicol. environ. Health A*, **61**, 339–346

Snyder, R., Lee, E.W. & Kocsis, J.J. (1978) Binding of labeled benzene metabolites to mouse liver and bone marrow. *Res. Commun. chem. Pathol. Pharmacol.*, **20**, 191–194

Snyder, R., Park, D.V., Kocsis, J.J., Jollow, D.V., Gibson, G.G. & Witmer, C.M., eds (1982) *Biological Reactive Intermediates II: Chemical Mechanisms and Biological Effects*, New York, Plenum Press

Snyder, R., Witz, G. & Goldstein, B.D. (1993) The toxicology of benzene. *Environ. Health Perspect.*, **100**, 293–306

Snyder, R., Kocsis, J.J., Sipes, I.G., Kalf, G.F., Jollow, D.J., Greim, H., Monks, T.J. & Witmer, C.M., eds (1996) *Biological Reactive Intermediates V: Basic Mechanistic Research in Toxicology and Human Risk Assessment*, New York, Plenum Press

Stevens, J.L. & Wallin, A. (1990) Is the toxicity of cysteine conjugates formed during mercapturic acid synthesis relevant to the toxicity of covalently bound drug residues? *Drug Metab. Rev.*, **22**, 617–635

Su, T., Bao, Z., Zhang, Q.-Y., Smith, T.J., Hong, J.-Y. & Ding, X. (2000) Human cytochrome P450 CYP2A13: predominant expression in the respiratory tract and its high efficiency metabolic activation of a tobacco-specific carcinogen, 4-(methylnitrosamino)-1-(3-pyridyl)-1-butanone. *Cancer Res.*, **60**, 5074–5079

Tanabe, H., Ohhira, M., Ohtsubo, T., Watari, J., Yokota, K. & Kohgo, Y. (1999) Genetic polymorphism of aldehyde dehydrogenase 2 in patients with upper aerodigestive tract cancer. *Alcohol clin. exp. Res.*, **23** (Suppl 4), 17S–20S

Vamvakas, S. & Anders, M.W. (1991) Formation of reactive intermediates by phase II enzymes: glutathione-dependent bioactivation reactions. *Adv. exp. Med. Biol.*, **283**, 13–24

Vesell, E.S. (1973) Advances in pharmacogenetics. *Prog. med. Genet.*, **9**, 291–367

Weaver, V.M., Buckley, T. & Groopman, J.D. (2000) Lack of specificity of *trans,trans*-muconic acid as a benzene biomarker after ingestion of sorbic acid-preserved foods. *Cancer Epidemiol. Biomarkers Prev.*, **9**, 749–755

Weber, T.J., Huang, Q., Monks, T.J. & Lau, S.S. (2001) Differential regulation of redox responsive transcription factors by the nephrocarcinogen 2.3.5-tris(glutathion-*S*-yl)hydroquinone. *Chem. Res. Toxicol.*, **14**, 814–821

Wefers, H. & Sies, H. (1983) Hepatic low-level chemiluminescence during redox cycling of menadione and the menadione-glutathione conjugate: relation to glutathione and NAD(P)H:quinone reductase (DT-diaphorase) activity. *Arch. Biochem. Biophys.*, **224**, 568–578

Williams, R.T. (1959) *Detoxication Mechanisms: The Metabolism and Detoxication of Drugs, Toxic Substances and Other Organic Compounds*, New York, John Wiley & Sons, pp. 734–739

Witmer, C.M., Snyder, R., Jollow, D.J., Kalf, G.F., Kocsis, J.J. & Sipes, I.G., eds (1991) *Biological Reactive Intermediates IV: Molecular and Cellular Effects and Their Impact on Human Health*, New York, Plenum Press

Wundrack, I., Meese, E., Mullenbach, R. & Blin, N. (1994) Debrisoquine hydroxylase gene polymorphism in meningioma. *Acta neuropathol.*, **88**, 472–474

Zhang, Z. & Bian, J. (2001) [Progress in researches on the relationship between genetic polymorphisms of alcohol-metabolizing enzymes and cancers]. *Zhonghua Yi Xue Yi Chuan Xue Za Zhi*, **18**, 62–65 (in Chinese)

Corresponding author:

Robert Snyder
Professor of Toxicology,
EOHSI, Rutgers University,
170 Frelinghuysen Road,
Piscataway, NJ 08854, USA
rsnyder@eohsi.rutgers.edu

Mechanisms of Carcinogenesis: Contributions of Molecular Epidemiology
Patricia Buffler, Jerry Rice, Robert Baan, Michael Bird and Paolo Boffetta, eds
IARC Scientific Publications No. 157
International Agency for Research on Cancer, Lyon, 2004

Exposure Biomarkers for the Study of Toxicological Impact on Carcinogenic Processes

Peter B. Farmer

Summary

Exposure biomarkers for carcinogens in humans include the measurement of the genotoxin or its active metabolite in blood, urine or other tissues, and the determination of the interaction products (adducts) of the carcinogen with protein or DNA. The latter approach may indicate the amount of genotoxically active material that has reached the tissue under study and provides invaluable information for molecular epidemiological studies. Protein adducts are not repaired and are considered primarily as exposure monitors, but DNA adducts may give further information about the mutagenic significance of the exposure. The techniques available for measurement of protein and DNA adducts include mass spectrometry, immunoassay, high performance liquid chromatography with UV, fluorescence or electrochemical detection, ^{32}P-postlabelling (for DNA only) and accelerator mass spectrometry. The lowest limits of sensitivity of the protein adduct measurements is less than 1 pmol adduct/g protein, and the procedures for DNA adduct determination have sensitivities ranging from of 1 adduct in 10^8 to 1 in 10^{11} nucleotides. All these techniques are capable of measuring environmental, occupational and dietary exposures to a variety of genotoxic compounds, as exemplified in this review.

Introduction

This chapter assesses the applicability for molecular epidemiological purposes of available exposure biomarkers for carcinogens, with special reference to the biomarkers that are relevant to the toxicological impact of these exposures. In particular, it considers the analytical approaches that have been used, the compounds to which they have been applied and the ongoing problems that are related to this area. The value of exposure biomarkers to epidemiologists is without doubt. They give improved measures of dose of carcinogens, and are of particular value if they are on an individual person basis, i.e. they take into account interindividual differences in uptake of carcinogens and their active metabolites.

It should be stressed that the detection of exposure to a carcinogen is only the first stage in assessing possible risk derived from an exposure. The interpretation of exposure monitoring data is highly complex because of the variability in biological response to carcinogen exposure between human individuals. Additionally many carcinogen exposure biomarkers also show 'background' levels of exposure, for example due to endogenous production of carcinogenic species, which must be considered in any risk assessment procedures. Such factors will be considered in later chapters in this volume.

Human exposure to carcinogens may be determined using three different sources of material for analysis:

• external monitors
• human blood, urine and other tissues for determining the concentration of carcinogen or metabolites
• cellular macromolecules containing covalently bound interaction products of the carcinogens.

The value of these measurements differs. The measurement of external sources is clearly important for those involved in public health and environmental protection, whereas the measurement of carcinogen interaction products is the most valuable if one wishes to consider the biological significance of the exposure. It is this latter approach to which most attention will be paid in this chapter.

The procedures for measuring the biologically relevant dose of a carcinogen are more highly advanced for organic genotoxic carcinogens than for non-genotoxic carcinogens, because of our greater understanding of the mechanism for the former. Thus organic genotoxic carcinogens are known to be electrophilic species (or metabolized to these) and interact with nucleophilic sites within DNA and other cellular molecules. Consequently it has been possible to develop highly specific analytical approaches for detecting circulating carcinogenically active species by measuring their interaction products with biological target sites.

In contrast, the mechanisms for non-genotoxic carcinogens are varied and not all fully understood, and biomarkers of exposure for these carcinogens are more limited. The compounds themselves or their active metabolites may be measured, but there are no direct interaction products with DNA for determination. Secondary effects, such as radical damage to DNA, may also be produced and can be used as indirect exposure biomarkers to non-genotoxic carcinogens.

Exposure biomarkers for inorganic carcinogens depend largely on determination of the toxic elements in blood or urine, for example by atomic absorption spectrometry (AAS) or inductively complex plasma mass spectrometry (ICP-MS). Exposure to some metals may also be detected in readily available tissues — such as fingernails, toenails and hair — which gives the potential for longer-term and retrospective monitoring of exposure.

Monitoring of exogenous carcinogens

Monitoring of external concentrations of carcinogens in air, diet and occupational environment has played an important role in epidemiological studies, but does not affect directly the toxicological impact of such exposures to individuals. A summary of some representative carcinogens whose exposure is currently being monitored in this way is given in Table 1. The analytical procedures include high-performance liquid chromatography (HPLC) with fluorescence detection

(LC-FL) or UV detection (LC-UV), gas chromatography (GC) with flame ionization detection (FID), electron capture detection (ECD), photoionization detection (PID) or mass spectral detection (MS).

Internal dose of carcinogens and metabolites

Internal doses of carcinogens and their metabolites have mostly been measured in blood or urine, although fatty tissues have been analysed for some lipophilic compounds, such as dibenzo-para-dioxins and polychlorinated dibenzofurans (IARC, 1997; Schuhmacher et al., 1999; Arfi et al., 2001). These procedures are extensively used in the occupational setting, although dietary and environmental intakes have also been measured. In some cases the parent carcinogen molecule may be analysed, but often the compound is extensively metabolized. Three examples of compounds where metabolites have been especially useful to monitor exposure (styrene, benzene and polycyclic aromatic hydrocarbons) are summarized below, and a more complete listing of a selection of carcinogens and complex mixtures is given in Table 2.

Styrene
For styrene the determination of metabolites gives a fairly unique representation of how much of the compound has passed through the pathway leading to the active carcinogenic metabolite. Styrene is metabolized to styrene oxide, which is electrophilic and may interact with DNA. The major detoxification of styrene oxide is by hydrolysis to styrene glycol, which is oxidized to mandelic acid and subsequently to phenylglyoxylic acid, which are excreted in the urine (Sumner & Fennel, 1994). Analysis of these by HPLC has been extensively used in occupational studies (e.g. Vodicka et al., 1999; Symanski et al., 2001, for reinforced plastics workers; and Ong et al., 1994; Triebig et al., 2001, for boat builders).

Benzene
The relevance of a metabolite measurement to toxicological impact depends greatly on its structure. This may be demonstrated using

Table 1. Monitoring of exogenous carcinogens

Biomarker	Source	Method	Reference
Benzene	Air, water, diet, dermal	GC-FID, GC-MS, GC-PID, GC-ECD	Institute for Environment and Health (1999); Skov et al. (2001)
1,3-Butadiene	Air	GC-FID	Fajen et al. (1993)
Styrene	Air, food, water	GC-FID, GC-MS	Miller et al. (1994); Ong et al. (1994)
PAHs (from particulate matter)	Air	LC-FL, silica gel chromatography, GC-MS	Topinka et al. (2000); Binkova et al. (1995, 1999); Georgiadis et al. (2001)
Chromium	Various	AAS, ICP, XRF, etc.	IARC (1990)
Dioxins	Air, food	GC-MS	IARC (1997)
Aflatoxin B$_1$	Food	ELISA, TLC, LC-UV, LC-FL	IARC (1993)
Chloroform	Air, food, water	GC-FID, GC-ECD, GC-MS	IARC (1999)

LC, liquid chromatography; FL, fluorescence; UV, ultraviolet; MS, mass spectrometry; GC, gas chromatography; FID, flame ionization detection; ECD, electron capture detection; PID, photoionization detection; TLC, thin-layer chromatography; AAS, atomic absorption spectrometry; ICP, inductively couple plasma; XRF, X-ray fluorescence; ELISA, enzyme linked immunosorbent assay; PAHs, polycyclic aromatic hydrocarbons

benzene as an example, for which biomarkers that are of possibly different toxicological relevance may be obtained by selecting different metabolites for analysis (see chapter by Snyder & Hong, this volume). After exposure, it is possible to determine unchanged benzene in expired air, blood or urine as a marker of exposure (Crebelli et al., 2001; Waidyanatha et al., 2001), but benzene is also metabolized by a complex series of pathways, and the critical carcinogenic metabolite is not known with certainty. Benzene is epoxidized to benzene oxide, a genotoxic compound, and this results in the formation of phenol. The determination of phenol in urine was originally proposed to monitor exposure to benzene (Van Haaften & Sie, 1965), but phenol concentrations are not specific for exposure to benzene. Further metabolites on this pathway are catechol and hydroquinone, which may be involved in the mutagenic or toxic effects resulting from exposure to benzene, and monitoring of these is possible in urine (Ong et al., 1995). Alternatively the initial epoxide metabolite, benzene oxide, reacts with cellular nucleophiles (see also

'Carcinogen adducts' below), including both macromolecules and some small molecules. One of the sites of attack is the sulfydryl group of glutathione and further metabolism of this yields S-phenylmercapturic acid which is excreted in urine. This may be detected by GC-MS (Boogaard & van Sittert, 1995), LC-UV (Inoue et al., 2000), LC-FL (Crebelli et al., 2001) and LC-MS-MS (Melikian et al., 1999a) as a very specific marker of exposure to benzene and the subsequent formation of benzene oxide. Immunoaffinity purification coupled with HPLC has also been used for this determination (Ball et al., 1997). A further pathway for benzene metabolism is ring opening, which results in the formation of trans,trans-muconaldehyde and trans,trans-muconic acid, which again may be possible contributors to the carcinogenic pathway of benzene. Trans,trans-muconic acid may be measured in urine using GC-MS (Bechtold et al., 1991), LC-UV (Boogaard & van Sittert, 1995) or LC-MS (Melikian et al., 1999a) and is a reasonably specific marker of exposure to benzene and its metabolism through this pathway. Thus the meta-

Table 2. Monitoring of internal doses of carcinogens and metabolites

Compound	Biomarker	Source	Method	Reference
Styrene	Mandelic acid, phenyl-glyoxylic acid	Urine	HPLC	Ong et al. (1994); Vodicka et al. (1999); Symanski et al. (2001); Triebig et al. (2001)
Benzene	Benzene	Blood, urine, breath	GC-FID, GC-MS	Crebelli et al. (2001); Waidyanatha et al. (2001)
Benzene	Trans, trans-muconic acid	Urine	GC-MS, LC-MS-MS, LC-UV	Bechtold et al. (1991); Boogaard & van Sittert (1995); Melikian et al. (1999a); Fang et al. (2000); Crebelli et al. (2001)
Benzene	S-Phenylmercapturic acid	Urine	GC-MS, LC-UV, LC-FL, LC-MS-MS	Boogaard & van Sittert (1995); Ball et al. (1997); Melikian et al. (1999a); Inoue et al. (2000, 2001); Crebelli et al. (2001)
Benzene	Catechol, hydroquinone	Urine	LC-FL	Ong et al. (1995)
Chloroform	Chloroform	Breath, blood	GC	Aggazzotti et al. (1993); Cammann & Hubner (1995)
Dioxins	Dioxins	Blood, fat	GC-MS	Schuhmacher et al. (1999); Arfi et al. (2001)
PAHs	1-Hydroxypyrene	Urine	LC-FL	Jongeneelen (1994); Ovrebo et al. (1995); Nielsen et al. (1996); Schoket al. (1999); Scherer et al. (2000); van Delft et al. (2001)
Heterocyclic aromatic amines	Parent compounds and metabolites	Urine	GC-NICI-MS, LC-FL	Stilwell et al. (1999); Friesen et al. (2001); Murray et al. (2001); Strickland et al. (2001)

LC, liquid chromatography; FL, fluorescence; UV, ultraviolet; MS, mass spectrometry; GC, gas chromatography; FID, flame ionization detection; PAH, polycyclic aromatic hydrocarbon; HPLC, high-performance liquid chromatography; NICI, negative in chemical ionization bolite markers of exposure to benzene vary greatly in their specificity for exposure to benzene and may hold different significances as regards the toxicological effects of the exposure. A variety of exposures to benzene have been assessed by measurements of the metabolites above. As a recent example, in a study of traffic police in Rome, smoking was shown to increase S-phenyl-mercapturic acid and *trans,trans*-muconic acid in both occupationally exposed and control groups (Crebelli *et al.*, 2001).

Polycyclic aromatic hydrocarbons

Exposure to polycyclic aromatic hydrocarbons (PAHs) is normally as part of a complex mixture, such as urban air pollution. In this mixture, there is a range of possibly carcinogenic aromatic components, and a widely used procedure is to analyse a marker of the exposure rather than carry out a complete analysis of all components. In the case of PAHs, urinary 1-hydroxypyrene may be measured as a marker of overall exposure to PAH (Jongeneelen, 1994). This is normally carried out using LC-FL. Occupational exposure, for example in coke oven workers (Ovrebo *et al.*, 1995; Van Delft *et al.*, 2001), garage mechanics (Schoket *et al.*, 1999) and diesel exhaust (Nielsen *et al.*, 1996), has been well documented. 1-Hydroxypyrene has also been used as a bio-marker of exposure to PAHs in non-occupationally exposed people where an effect of smoking is observed (Scherer *et al.*, 2000).

Carcinogen adducts

The chemical process for formation of adducts from genotoxic carcinogens involves a reaction of the compound or its active metabolite with a nucleophilic group in a cellular molecule. The sites of adduct formation are summarized in Table 3.

The most abundant nucleophile within the cell is water and reaction of the carcinogen with this (hydrolysis) normally results in production of a detoxified metabolite (which may also be measured as a biomarker of exposure). The most relevant adducts for carcinogenic risk assessment are those formed at the target site in DNA, i.e. on the nucleotides critically involved in a mutational

lesion in a target tissue. Tissues are available for a number of important neoplasms and specific mutational effects in these have been associated with adduct formation with carcinogens, for example PAHs (Denissenko *et al.*, 1996) and afla-toxin B_1 (Hsu *et al.*, 1991). However, the carci-nogen adducts originally present in these tissues at the time of cancer initiation may no longer be present in the tumour tissue, and the analysis of these adducts at the target site at the time of exposure is difficult. Other sites of relevance as useful biomarkers are glutathione, protein and non-target DNA, summarized below.

Glutathione

The sulfydryl group of glutathione is powerfully nucleophilic and is a site of attack for many geno-toxic carcinogens. Metabolism of the product yields mercapturic acids, which are excreted in the urine. This process occurs with a relatively short time scale, so that urinary mercapturic acids reflect recent exposure to genotoxic species (half-lives 1.5–9 h; Van Welie *et al.*, 1992; De Rooij *et al.*, 1998). Analysis is by a variety of tech-niques, including GC with MS and other detection systems, HPLC (including LC-MS), immuno-assay and spectrophotometry, and over 20 com-pounds have been monitored in human urine (De Rooij *et al.*, 1998). Application to S-phenylmer-capturic acid, derived from benzene, is described in the section above.

Proteins

Nucleophilic side-chains of amino acids in proteins are sites of reaction of carcinogens, and the adducts formed here normally have no toxicological effect and may be considered simply as a measure of exposure to the genotoxic species. The amino acids involved include cysteine, histidine, aspartic acid, glutamic acid, lysine and the N-terminal amino acid. Protein adducts are generally stable and are not enzymatically repaired, and for exposure monitoring they are normally used with globin or albumin, because of the long lifetime and ready availability of these proteins in blood. Because of the 4-month lifetime of globin in humans, retrospective exposure monitoring can be carried out after several weeks.

Table 3. Sites of carcinogen adduct formation

Site of interaction	Significance	Lifetime of adduct
Target DNA	Most relevant for risk assessment, but not readily available from human subjects	Hours to weeks
Non-target DNA	May be used as a quantitative marker of target site DNA reactions	Hours to weeks
Protein	May be used as a quantitative marker of DNA interactions, and also represents a (generally) stable exposure monitor	Normally same lifetime as protein, e.g. 120 days for globin
Glutathione	Normally a detoxification process. May be used as a short term exposure monitor	< 1 day

Hair has been used on rare occasions and holds some potential for tracking exposures over an extended time period. Protein adducts have now been determined as a biomarker of exposure to more than 30 compounds (examples taken from the period 1998–2001 in Table 4; for earlier reviews see Farmer, 1994; Farmer & Sweetman, 1995; Sweetman *et al.*, 1998). However, unlike the situation for DNA, there are no screening systems for detection of a wide variety of protein adducts in one analysis.

N-Terminal amino acid adducts: In globin, the amino group of the N-terminal amino acid valine forms adducts with a variety of electrophilic compounds of low molecular weight, such as methylating agents, epoxides of ethylene, propylene, 1,3-butadiene and styrene, acrylonitrile and acrylamide, and isocyanates (see Sweetman *et al.*, 1998 and Table 4). These adducts are analysed by a modified Edman degradation procedure, devised by Tornqvist *et al.* (1986), followed by GC-MS or LC-MS. For quantitation, adducts of the genotoxin with globin or a model peptide (e.g. valine–leucine–serine, the N-terminal peptide of the α-chain of globin; Tavares *et al.*, 1996) are used as calibration standards. Stable isotopically labelled analogues of these adducts are also synthesized to be used as MS internal standards.

Levels of adducts as low as 1 pmol/g globin can be determined, allowing environmental exposure to many carcinogens to be measured. The procedure is designed to be used for specific (and predetermined) chemicals, i.e. one needs to know in advance what adduct one is analysing, as selective ion monitoring of adducts that have been separated chromatographically is used. Thus synthesis of the analytes is needed in every case, to act as standards.

Cysteine adducts: For some carcinogens, cysteine adducts are the predominant interaction products in proteins. Because the cysteine residues are present within the polypeptide chain in both globin and albumin, it is necessary to carry out a complete protein hydrolysis if one wishes to analyse the adducted amino acid. This approach may result in severe chromatographic problems. Alternative methods have been developed for removal of the adducted group from the cysteine adduct before its analysis, for example by reaction with trifluoroacetic anhydride and methane sulfonic acid (Yeowell-O'Connell *et al.*, 1998), which simplifies the analysis of the adduct, although assumptions need to be made about the original source of the adducted group within the protein. In the case of aromatic amines, the reactive metabolite reacts with the sulfydryl

Table 4. Occupational, environmental, and experimental exposures detected from protein adducts. Representative examples from the period 1998–2001

Class	Compound	Exposure	Adduct	Method	Reference
Epoxides	Ethylene oxide	Occupation, rat model	N-terminal valine in globin	GC-MS(-MS)	Van Sittert et al. (2000)
	Propylene oxide	Occupation			Boogaard et al. (1999)
	Epoxides of butadiene	Occupation			Begemann et al. (2001)
	Styrene oxide	Occupation			Vodicka et al. (1999)
	Epichlorohydrin	Rat model			Landin et al. (1999)
PAHs	Benzo[a]pyrene	Environment and occupation	COOH of globin COOH of albumin	GC-MS	Melikian et al. (1999a) Pastorelli et al. (2000)
Aromatic amines	Methylene-4,4'-dianiline	Mice, rat models	N-terminal valine in globin	MS	Kautiainen et al. (1998)
Monocyclic aromatic hydrocarbons	Benzene	Occupation and environment	SH of globin SH of albumin	GC-MS	Hanway et al. (2000) Yeowell-O'Connell et al. (1998)
Isocyanates	4,4'-Methylenediphenyl diisocyanate	Rat model	N-terminal valine in globin	LC-MS-MS, GC-MS	Sabbioni et al. (2000)
α,β–Unsaturated compounds	Acrylamide Acrylonitrile	Occupation Smoking Rat model	N-terminal valine in globin N-terminal valine in globin	GC-MS(-MS), immunoassay	Hagmar et al. (2001); Perez et al. (1999); Wong et al. (1998)
Mycotoxins	Aflatoxin B$_1$	Diet	Lys in albumin	Immunoassay	Ahsan et al. (2001)
Methylating agents		Smoking	N-terminal valine in globin	GC-MS	Thier et al. (2001)
Amides	Dimethylformamide	Occupation	N-terminal valine in globin	GC-MS	Kafferlein & Angerer (2001); Angerer et al. (1998)
Heterocyclic amines	PhIP	Human volunteers	Acid hydrolysable adducts	GC-NICI-MS	Magagnotti et al. (2000)
Aldehydes	Acetaldehyde	In vitro	N-terminal valine in globin	LC-MS	Birt et al. (1998)

LC, liquid chromatography; MS, mass spectrometry; GC, gas chromatography; PAH, polycyclic aromatic hydrocarbon; NICI, negative ion chemical ionization group of cysteine to produce a sulfinamide residue. This may be hydrolysed under mild alkaline conditions to yield the parent amine, which is analysed by GC-MS after derivatization.

Other protein adducts: The adducts formed with aspartic acid and glutamic acid are esters, and are readily hydrolysed by mild acid or alkali. This hydrolytic reaction is the basis of the analytical approach for these adducts. Thus for the tobacco-specific nitrosamine adducts, mild hydrolysis of the protein with alkali results in for example 4-hydroxy-1-(3-pyridyl)-1-butanone (HPB), which is analysed by GC-MS (Hecht *et al.*, 1993). Benzo[*a*]pyrene adducts may similarly be analysed by GC-MS after acid hydrolysis (Melikian *et al.*, 1999b; Pastorelli *et al.*, 2000). Histidine adducts with ethylene oxide have been monitored as an exposure biomarker for ethylene oxide, but the procedure for this was complex and has been replaced with the Edman procedure for the N-terminal adduct. Aflatoxin–lysine in albumin continues to be monitored, using an immunochemical approach, to detect exposure to this mycotoxin.

DNA

DNA is not as readily available as proteins from exposed subjects and consequently the methodology for adduct detection needs to be extremely sensitive. The main analytical procedures currently used for DNA adducts are summarized in Table 5, and include chemically specific procedures such as LC-MS and less specific, but more sensitive procedures such as ^{32}P-post-labelling and accelerator mass spectrometry (AMS).

The source of the DNA is normally lymphocytes (or white blood cells) although buccal smears, placenta, bladder epithelial cells, lung, cervix and sperm have also been used. DNA repair products are excreted in urine and may also be used as an exposure biomarker (see below). Unlike the situation in protein adduct analysis, the lifetime of the adduct is not always clear. Repair processes remove with different efficiencies many adducts, although some (e.g. phosphotriesters) are apparently not subject to repair in eukaryotic

Table 5. Analytical procedures for DNA adducts

	Sensitivity (approximate)	Amount of DNA needed for analysis (µg)
Immunoassay	$1/10^8$	1–100
Mass spectrometry	$1/10^7$–$1/10^8$	100
HPLC/ECD or fluorescence	$1/10^8$	1–100
^{32}P-Postlabelling	$1/10^9$–$1/10^{10}$	1–10
Accelerator mass spectrometry	$1/10^{11}$	1–1000

HPLC/ECD, high-performance liquid chromatography/electron capture detection

systems. Also the lifetime of the DNA *in vivo* is variable according to the tissue from which it was derived. It is not possible to give a comprehensive review of DNA adduct determinations for carcinogens, because of the large number that have been carried out. However, representative examples of recent studies, over the period 1998–2001, are given in Table 6, and summaries of some successes and limitations of the analytical approaches are given below. Earlier reviews summarize previously successful uses of DNA adducts for carcinogen exposure determination (Farmer, 1994; Hemminki *et al.*, 1994; Schoket, 1999; Shuker, 1999).

GC- and LC-MS: The improving sensitivity of LC-MS suggests that it may become the method of choice for analysing carcinogen–DNA adducts in the future. To date it has been successfully applied for example to adducts from amines, nitrosamines, olefins and etheno adducts. It has the advantage that it confirms with certainty the chemical nature of the adduct being studied, and that, with the appropriate internal standard, very accurate quantitation can be carried out. At present, however, it requires amounts of DNA that may not always be available from the sampling procedures carried out in normal human studies.

Table 6. Occupational, environmental and experimental exposures detected from DNA adducts. Representative examples from the period 1998–2001

Method	Compound	Exposure	Tissue	Reference
32P-Postlabelling	PAHs	Environment	Lymphocytes	Kyrtopoulos et al. (2001)
		Occupation	WBC, lymphocytes	Binkova et al. (1998)
		Environment, diet	Varied	Schoket et al. (1999)
		Environment	WBC	Whyatt et al. (2001)
		Oil-well fires	Placenta	Marafie et al. (2000)
		Environment	WBC, granulocytes	Butkiewitz et al. (1998)
		Human controls, cancer patients	Breast	Pfau et al. (1998)
	Styrene	Occupation	Lymphocytes	Vodicka et al. (1999)
	4-Aminobiphenyl	Smoking	Lymphocytes	Dallinga et al. (1998)
	Malondialdehyde	Control humans	Liver, lung, pancreas	Yi et al. (1998)
	Aristocholic acid	Chinese herbs nephropathy patients	Urinary tract	Arlt et al. (2001)
	Methylating agents	Occupation	Lymphocytes	Reh et al. (2000)
	Acrolein	Acrolein (cockerels)	Aorta	Penn et al. (2001)
	Acrolein, crotonaldehyde	Smoking	Oral tissue	Nath et al. (1998)
	Etheno adducts	Familial adenomatous polyposis	Colon polyps	Schmid et al. (2000)
	trans-4-Hydroxy-2-nonenal	Control humans, rats	Colon, brain	Wacker et al. (2000)
		Control humans, rats (CCl$_4$)	Liver, colon	Chung et al. (2000)
Immunoassay	PAHs	Oil-well fires	WBC	Poirier et al. (1998)
	Aflatoxin B$_1$	Varied	Varied	Kriek et al. (1998)
		Diet	Urine	Nayak et al. (2001)
		Diet	Albumin	Turner et al. (1998)
Immunoslot blot	Malondialdehyde	Control humans	WBC, gastric tissue	Leuratti et al. (1998)
		Helicobacter pylori	Gastric mucosa	Everett et al. (2001)
	Methylating agents	Cancer chemotherapy	Blood, colon	Harrison et al. (2001)
	Ethylating agents	N-Nitrosodiethylamine (mice)	Varied	Oreffo et al. (2000)

Table 6 (contd)

Method	Compound	Exposure	Tissue	Reference
Mass spectrometry	Heterocyclic amines	IQ (rats)	Liver	Soglia et al. (2001)
	Aromatic amines	4-Aminobiphenyl (mice)	Liver	Doerge et al. (1999)
	1,3-Butadiene	1,3-Butadiene (rats, mice)	Liver, lung	Tretyakova et al. (1998)
	Etheno adducts	Control humans	Placenta	Chen et al. (1999)
		Control rats	Urine	Yen et al. (1998)
		Vinyl chloride (rats)	Liver	Morinello et al. (2001)
	Tobacco-specific nitrosamines	Smoking	Lung	Hecht (1999)
Accelerator mass spectrometry	Heterocyclic aromatic amines	14C-Labelled compounds administered to human volunteers	Colon, tumour	Mauthe et al. (1999)
			Colon	Turteltaub et al. (1999)
	Benzo[a]pyrene		Breast, tumour	Lightfoot et al. (2000)
			Breast, tumour	Lightfoot et al. (2000)

PAHs, polycyclic aromatic hydrocarbons; WBC white blood cells; IQ, 2-Amino-3-methylimidazo[4,5-f]quinoline

Immunoassays: Immunoassays can have about the same sensitivity for DNA adduct analysis as the best MS techniques, but again relatively large amounts of DNA may be needed for analysis by standard immunochemical procedures. Innovations such as the immunoslot blot assay now allow highly sensitive analyses to be carried out with much smaller DNA samples (see review by Shuker, 1999). One very useful application of the antibodies that have been made to DNA adducts is in the preparation of immunoaffinity columns that enable the specific purification of these adducts as a preliminary step before analysis by any of the techniques discussed here.

32P-Postlabelling: 32P-Postlabelling remains the most versatile and sensitive procedure for analysis of carcinogen–DNA adducts (Figure 1). The original problems of irreproducibility between laboratories have been partially removed by the production of standard protocols (Phillips & Castegnaro, 1999). However, the degree of enrichment and labelling varies according to the adduct being analysed, meaning that preliminary studies with standard compounds are very important for accurate quantitation. The advantage of 32P-postlabelling is that mixtures can be studied, although one disadvantage is that the structures of the postlabelled products detected are not known with certainty and can normally only be postulated on the basis of chromatographic comparison with standards. Again MS may hold the solution to this, although attempts to use it for structure characterization of 32P-postlabelled products from in-vivo experiments have so far not been extensive.

Accelerator mass spectrometry: AMS detects specific isotopes with great sensitivity. One such isotope is 14C, and experiments have been established in which the fate of trace levels of 14C-labelled carcinogens have been studied in humans. For example, both metabolites and adducts have been detected for heterocyclic amines after administration of the 14C-labelled species. The particular advantage of AMS is its sensitivity, which is at least an order of magnitude greater than 32P-postlabelling and which allows

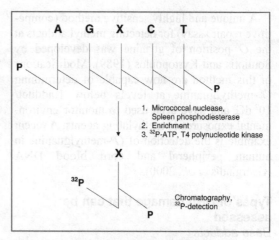

Figure 1. 32P-Postlabelling of DNA adducts.

1. Micrococcal nuclease, Spleen phosphodiesterase
2. Enrichment
3. 32P-ATP, T4 polynucleotide kinase

Chromatography, 32P-detection

the detection of 1 adduct per 10^11 nucleotides. The disadvantages are that the experiments at present require the deliberate administration of the isotopically labelled species, which is unsuitable for routine monitoring, and that the structural characterization of the adduct is hard to achieve as the molecule is destroyed before the AMS analysis. One possible solution to this is to develop a 14C-postlabelling technique, so that unlabelled compounds could be studied in humans, but with the superior sensitivity of AMS.

Other techniques: HPLC has the sensitivity to detect adducts, but only when combined with highly sensitive detectors, such as fluorescence (FL) or electrochemical detection (EC). For example, some alkylated nucleic acid bases are fluorescent, and some oxidative DNA lesions are particularly suitable for EC detection. Synchronous fluorescence spectroscopy has been used for the detection of PAH adducts with DNA, by detection of benzo[*a*]pyrene tetrol released by hydrolysis of the adduct (Weston *et al.*, 1989). The recent use of a laser-induced fluorescent detector by Ozbal *et al.* (2000) for detecting protein adducts derived from the active metabolite from benzo[*a*]pyrene has demonstrated the potential of this highly sensitive detection mechanism, and application to DNA adducts seems appropriate.

A unique and highly sensitive method (competitive repair assay) for detecting methyl adducts at the O^6-position of guanine was developed by Souliotis and Kyrtopoulos (1989). Modifications of this method are now capable of determining O^6-methylguanine at levels below 1 adduct/10^7 dG, and have been used to monitor environmental exposures to methylating agents. A recent example is the detection of O^6-methylguanine in human peripheral and cord blood DNA (Georgiadis et al., 2000).

Types of DNA damage that can be assessed

Base adducts

Carcinogen adducts are formed at all the nucleophilic sites on the DNA bases, with different specificities according to the nature of the genotoxic compound. Thus for alkylating agents of low molecular weight, the major site of adduct formation is guanine N7. Adenine N3 and guanine O^6 are sites for more minor adducts. Adducts from polycyclic aromatic hydrocarbons include guanine N7 and N^2 and those from aromatic amines, guanine C8. All of these lesions can be detected by the techniques described above, although adducts at N7 of guanine and N3 of adenine are unstable to chemical and enzymic hydrolysis of the glycolytic bond. Such adducts are readily lost from the DNA, which may make their quantitative determination in the nucleic acid difficult (but see 'Repair products from DNA adducts', below). Repair processes vary in their efficiency towards the other adducts, and the kinetics of these should be considered before choosing the timing of the human sample collections.

Phosphotriesters

In addition to reacting with the nucleophilic sites on the DNA bases, many carcinogens also react with the oxygen of the internucleotidic phosphodiester linkages to form phosphotriesters. The biological significance (if any) of these lesions is not known. Although bacterial repair of phosphotriesters occurs (Ada protein), repair mechanisms in eukaryotic systems are not known and long lifetimes of phosphotriesters have been demonstrated in vivo and in human cell lines.

Thus these lesions, which are relatively abundant for some alkylating carcinogens, may serve as ideal biomarkers with which to assess cumulative genotoxic exposure. Methods for assessing amounts of phosphotriesters include:

- transalkylation of a nucleophile, such as cob(1)alamin, followed by HPLC of the product (Haglund et al., 1997, 2000)
- digestion of the DNA to dinucleoside phosphotriesters, hydrolysis to dinucleotides and ^{32}P-postlabelling analysis using chromatography (Saris et al., 1995) or polyacrylamide gel electrophoresis (Guichard et al., 2000) to separate the products.

Repair products from DNA adducts

Both N7 adducts of guanine and N3 adducts of adenine are removed from the DNA by glycosylases and some have been shown to be excreted unchanged in the urine during the next few days (Shuker & Farmer, 1992). Analysis of these repair products offers an attractive non-invasive way to detect the amount of nucleic acid damage that has occurred. The analytical methods employed include LC-UV, LC-FL, GC-MS and immunoassay. The most important study in this area with regard to human carcinogenic risk assessment was of a population from the People's Republic of China, where urinary excretion of the N7-guanine adduct of aflatoxin B_1 was found to be correlated with the incidence of hepatocellular carcinoma (Ross et al., 1992; Qian et al., 1994). Other examples of the use of this technique include the excretion of 3-methyladenine after treatment of cancer patients with dacarbazine (Shuker et al., 1997) or N-methyl-N-nitrosourea (Prevost et al., 1996) and an investigation of the possibility that bromhexine was nitrosated to a methylating product by studying the excretion of N7-methylguanine (Farmer et al., 1988). The disadvantage of the approach of measuring excretion products is that the source of the adduct is not known. Conceivably some of it could arise from RNA as well as from DNA, although mechanistic arguments contest this (Shuker & Farmer, 1992).

Oxidatively damaged DNA bases

Most DNA damage arises not from electrophilic alkylating organic carcinogens, but from radical attack. In particular the hydroxyl radical, which is produced by a variety of exogenous sources and also through endogenous metabolism, reacts with many DNA bases, the major product being 8-hydroxyguanine. Oxidized DNA bases may be measured by GC-MS, LC-MS, LC-EC and immunoassay, and there is continuing confusion regarding the precision of some of these assays. Oxidation of bases may occur during DNA preparation or during the analytical procedure (e.g. derivatization for GC-MS) which might cause an error to the determination of the original oxidative damage in the DNA. These oxidative lesions, although potentially of mutagenic importance, are generally not suitable for determining exposure to a carcinogen.

Indirect sources of DNA damage

In some cases, the agent responsible for DNA damage is not itself an electrophilic alkylating agent, but generates this compound by secondary processes in the body. Thus nitrite may generate N-nitrosamines, which are then metabolized to alkylating agents. Radical attack affects DNA bases directly (see 'Oxidatively damaged DNA bases', above), but can also generate DNA-reacting species from other molecules. Thus, during lipid peroxidation, electrophilic molecules such as malondialdehyde and 4-hydroxy-2-nonenal are formed and may subsequently form DNA adducts. The methods of analyses for malondialdehyde–DNA adducts are immuno-assay (particularly immunoslot blot assay) and ^{32}P-postlabelling; for 4-hydroxynonenal–DNA adducts, ^{32}P-postlabelling has also been used (see Table 6).

Conclusion

As illustrated above, internal exposure to carcinogens in humans may be monitored either by measurement of the carcinogen or its metabolites in a body fluid or tissue, or by determining the interaction products of the carcinogen with cellular macromolecules. The technology for the latter procedure has developed rapidly over the last decade and is now capable of measuring DNA adducts at levels as low as 1 adduct/10^{11} nucleotides. As the sensitivity of these analyses has increased, the confirmation of the structure of the adduct being analysed is not always as easy to achieve. Thus, for example, the most sensitive techniques of ^{32}P-postlabelling and AMS depend on co-chromatography for characterization of the adducts being determined. Ultimately other mass spectrometric techniques may be able to play a greater role in increasing the chemical specificity of the analyses. Thus, technology such as the use of nanospray interfaces and capillary liquid chromatography, combined with tandem MS, hold great potential for future adduct analyses.

Protein adducts are particularly useful for exposure determination, but DNA adducts may be of more value with regard to the risk associated with the exposure. However, although mutational effects produced by DNA adducts may be detected in in-vitro systems, the current measuring techniques for mutations are not sensitive enough to inform us about the mutational significance of the very low levels of adducts that can be determined by ^{32}P-postlabelling and AMS. Thus it is difficult to confirm that there is no threshold for the relationship between mutational effects and adduct measurements, although this is often assumed in regulatory assessments. Another fact that should also be considered if risk assessments are to be made on the basis of adduct measurements is that many adducts are produced from endogenous sources, and the significance of this damage in comparison with that caused by exogenous genotoxins is as yet not understood.

References

Aggazzotti, G., Fantuzzi, G., Righi, E., Tartoni, P., Cassinadri, T. & Predieri, G. (1993) Chloroform in alveolar air of individuals attending indoor swimming pools. *Arch. environ. Health*, **48**, 250–254

Ahsan, H., Wang, L.Y., Chen, C.J., Tsai, W.Y. & Santella, R.M. (2001) Variability in aflatoxin-albumin adduct levels and effects of hepatitis B and C virus infection and glutathione S-transferase M1 and T1 genotype. *Environ. Health Perspect.*, **109**, 833–837

Angerer, J., Goen, T., Kramer, A. & Kafferlein, H.U. (1998) N-Methylcarbamoyl adducts at the N-terminal valine of globin in workers exposed to N,N-dimethylformamide. *Arch. Toxicol.*, **72**, 309–313

Arfi, C., Seta, N., Fraisse, D., Revel, A., Escande, J.P. & Momas, I. (2001) Dioxins in adipose tissue of non-occupationally exposed persons in France; correlation with individual food exposure. *Chemosphere*, **44**, 1347–1352

Arlt, V.M., Pfohl-Leszkowicz, A., Cosyns, J. & Schmeiser, H.H. (2001) Analyses of DNA adducts formed by ochratoxin A and aristolochic acid in patients with Chinese herbs nephropathy. *Mutat. Res.*, **494**, 143–150

Ball, L., Wright, A.S., Van Sittert, N.J. & Aston, P. (1997) Immunoenrichment of urinary S-phenylmercapturic acid. *Biomarkers*, **2**, 29–33

Bechtold, W.E., Lucier, G., Birnbaum, L.S., Yin, S.N., Li, G.L. & Henderson, R.F. (1991) Muconic acid determinations in urine as a biological exposure index for workers occupationally exposed to benzene. *Am. ind. Hyg. Assoc. J.*, **52**, 473–478

Begemann, P., Sram, R.J. & Neumann, H.G. (2001) Hemoglobin adducts of epoxybutene in workers occupationally exposed to 1,3-butadiene. *Arch. Toxicol.*, **74**, 680–687

Binkova, B., Lewtas, J., Miskova, I., Lenicek, J. & Šrám, R.J. (1995) DNA adducts and personal air monitoring of carcinogenic polycyclic aromatic hydrocarbons in an environmentally exposed population. *Carcinogenesis*, **16**, 1037–1046

Binkova, B., Topinka, J., Mrackova, G., Gajdosova, D., Vidova, P., Stavkova, Z., Peterka, V., Pilcik, T., Rimar, V., Dobias, L., Farmer, P.B. & Šrám, R.J. (1998) Coke oven workers study: the effect of exposure and GSTM1 and NAT2 genotypes on DNA adduct levels in white blood cells and lymphocytes as determined by P-32-postlabelling. *Mutat. Res.*, **416**, 67–84

Binkova, B., Vesely, D., Vesela, D., Jelinek, R. & Šrám, R.J. (1999) Genotoxicity and embryotoxicity of urban air particulate matter collected during winter and summer period in two different districts of the Czech Republic. *Mutat. Res.*, **440**, 45–58

Birt, J.E.E.C., Shuker, D.E.G. & Farmer, P.B. (1998) Stable acetaldehyde–protein adducts as biomarkers of alcohol exposure. *Chem. Res. Toxicol.*, **11**, 136–142

Boogaard, P.J. & Van Sittert, N.J. (1995) Biological monitoring of exposure to benzene: a comparison between S-phenylmercapturic acid, trans,trans-muconic acid, and phenol. *Occup. environ. Med.*, **52**, 611–620

Boogaard, P.J., Rocchi, P.S.J. & Van Sittert, N.J. (1999) Biomonitoring of exposure to ethylene oxide and propylene oxide by determination of hemoglobin adducts: correlation between airborne exposure and adduct levels. *Int. Arch. occup. environ. Health*, **72**, 142–150

Butkiewicz, D., Grzybowska, E., Hemminki, K., Ovrebo, S., Haugen, A., Motykiewicz, G. & Chorazy, M. (1998) Modulation of DNA adduct levels in human mononuclear white blood cells and granulocytes by CYP1A1, CYP2D6 and GSTM1 genetic polymorphisms. *Mutat. Res.*, **415**, 97–108

Cammann, K. & Hubner, K. (1995) Trihalomethane concentrations in swimmers' and bath attendants' blood and urine after swimming or working in indoor swimming pools. *Arch. environ. Health*, **50**, 61–65

Chen, H.J.C., Chiang, L.C., Tseng, M.C., Zhang, L.L., Ni, J.S. & Chung, F.L. (1999) Detection and quantification of 1,N(6)-ethenoadenine in human placental DNA by mass spectrometry. *Chem. Res. Toxicol.*, **12**, 1119–1126

Chung, F.L., Nath, R.G., Ocando, J., Nishkawa, A. & Zhang, L. (2000) Deoxyguanosine adducts of t-4-hydroxy-2-nonenal are endogenous DNA lesions in rodents and humans: detection and potential sources. *Cancer Res.*, **60**, 1507–1511

Crebelli, R., Tomei, F., Zijno, A., Ghittori, S., Imbriani, M., Gamberale, D., Martini, A. & Carere, A. (2001) Exposure to benzene in urban workers: environmental and biological monitoring of traffic police in Rome. *Occup. environ. Med.*, **58**, 165–171

Dallinga, J.W., Pachen, D.M.F.A., Wijnhoven, S.W.P., Breedijk, A., van't Veer, L., Wigbout, G., van Zandwijk, N., Maas, L.M., van Agen, E., Kleinjans, J.C.S. & van Schooten, F.J. (1998) The use of 4-aminobiphenyl hemoglobin adducts and aromatic DNA adducts in lymphocytes of smokers as biomarkers of exposure. *Cancer Epidemiol. Biomarkers Prev.*, **7**, 571–577

van Delft, J.H.M., Steenwinkel, M.S., van Asten, J.G., De Vogel, N., Bruijntjes-Rozier, T.C.D.M., Schouten, T., Cramers, P., Maas, L., van Herwijnen,

M.H., van Schooten, F.J. & Hopmans, P.M.J. (2001) Biological monitoring of the exposure to polycyclic aromatic hydrocarbons of coke oven workers in relation to smoking and genetic polymorphisms for GSTM1 and GSTT1. *Ann. occup. Hyg.*, **45**, 395–408

De Rooij, B.M., Commandeur, J.N.M. & Vermeulen, N.P.E. (1998) Mercapturic acids as biomarkers of exposure to electrophilic chemicals: applications to environmental and industrial chemicals. *Biomarkers*, **3**, 239–303

Denissenko, M.F., Pao, A., Tang, M. & Pfeifer, G.P. (1996) Preferential formation of benzo(*a*)pyrene adducts at lung cancer mutational hotspots in P53. *Science*, **274**, 430–432

Doerge, D.R., Churchwell, M.I., Marques, M.M. & Beland, F.A. (1999) Quantitative analysis of 4-aminobiphenyl-C8-deoxyguanosyl DNA adducts produced in vitro and in vivo using HPLC-ES-MS. *Carcinogenesis*, **20**, 1055–1061

Everett, S.M., Singh, R., Leuratti, C., White, K.L.M., Neville, P., Greenwood, D., Marnett, L.J., Schorah, C.J., Forman, D., Shuker, D. & Axon, A.T.R. (2001) Levels of malondialdehyde–deoxyguanosine in the gastric mucosa: relationship with lipid peroxidation, ascorbic acid, and *Helicobacter pylori*. *Cancer Epidemiol. Biomarkers Prev.*, **10**, 369–376

Fajen, J.M., Lunsford, R.A. & Roberts, D.R. (1993) Industrial exposure to 1,3-butadiene in monomer, polymer and end-user industries. In: Sorsa, M., Peltonen, K., Vainio, H. & Hemminki, K., eds, *Butadiene and Styrene: Assessment of Health Hazards* (IARC Scientific Publications No. 127), Lyon, IARC*Press*, pp. 3–13

Fang, M.Z., Shin, M.K., Park, K.W., Kim, Y.S., Lee, J.W. & Cho, M.H. (2000) Analysis of urinary S-phenylmercapturic acid and *trans,trans*-muconic acid as exposure biomarkers of benzene in petrochemical and industrial areas of Korea. *Scand. J. Work Environ. Health*, **26**, 62–66

Farmer, P.B. (1994) Carcinogen adducts: use in diagnosis and risk assessment. *Clin. Chem.*, **40**, 1438–1443

Farmer, P.B. & Sweetman, G.M.A. (1995) Mass spectrometry detection of carcinogen adducts. *J. mass Spect.*, **30**, 1369–1379

Farmer, P.B., Parry, A., Franke, H. & Schmid, J. (1988) Lack of detectable DNA alkylation for bromhexine in man. *Arzneimittelforschung*, **38**, 1351–1354

Friesen, M.D., Rothman, N. & Strickland, P.T. (2001) Concentration of 2-amino-1-methyl-6-phenyl-imidazo(4,5-b)pyridine (PhIP) in urine and alkali-hydrolyzed urine after consumption of charbroiled beef. *Cancer Lett.*, **173**, 43–51

Georgiadis, P., Samoli, E., Kaila, S., Katsouyanni, K. & Kyrtopoulos, S.A. (2000) Ubiquitous presence of O⁶-methylguanine in human peripheral and cord blood DNA. *Cancer Epidemiol. Biomarkers Prev.*, **9**, 299–305

Georgiadis, P., Topinka, J., Stoikidou, M., Kaila, S., Gioka, M., Katsouyanni, K., Šrám, R.J., Autrup, H. & Kyrtopoulos, S.A. (2001) Biomarkers of genotoxicity of air pollution (the AULIS project): bulky DNA adducts in subjects with moderate to low exposures to airborne polycyclic aromatic hydrocarbons and their relationship to environmental tobacco smoke and other parameters. *Carcinogenesis*, **22**, 1447–1457

Guichard, Y., Jones, G.D.D. & Farmer, P.B. (2000) Detection of DNA alkylphosphotriesters by ³²P-postlabeling: evidence for the nonrandom manifestation of phosphotriester lesions *in vivo*. *Cancer Res.*, **60**, 1276–1282

van Haaften, A.B. & Sie, S.T. (1965) The measurement of phenol in urine by gas chromatography as a check on benzene exposure. *Am. ind. Hyg. Assoc. J.*, **26**, 52–58

Haglund, J., Ehrenberg, L. & Törnqvist, M. (1997) Studies of transalkylation of phosphotriesters in DNA: reaction conditions and requirements on nucleophiles for determination of DNA adducts. *Chem.-biol. Interact.*, **108**, 119–133

Haglund, J., Rafiq, A., Ehrenberg, L., Golding, B.T. & Tornqvist, M. (2000) Transalkylation of phosphotriesters using Cob(I)alamin: toward specific determination of DNA-phosphate adducts. *Chem. Res. Toxicol.*, **13**, 253–256

Hagmar, L., Tornqvist, M., Nordander, C., Rosen, I., Bruze, M., Kautianinen, A., Magnusson, A.L. Malmberg, B., Aprea, P., Granath, F. & Axmon, A. (2001) Health effects of occupational exposure to acrylamide using hemoglobin adducts as biomarkers of internal dose. *Scand. J. Work Environ. Health*, **27**, 219–226

Hanway, R., Cavicchioli, A., Kaur, B., Parsons, J., Lamb, J.H., Buckberry, L.D. & Farmer, P.B. (2000) Analysis of S-phenyl-L-cysteine in globin as a marker of benzene exposure. *Biomarkers*, **5**, 252–262

Harrison, K.L., Wood, M., Lees, N.P., Hall, C.N., Margison, G.P. & Povey, A.C. (2001) Development and application of a sensitive and rapid immunoassay for the quantitation of N7-methyldeoxyguanosine in DNA samples. *Chem. Res. Toxicol.*, **14**, 295–301

Hecht, S.S. (1999) DNA adduct formation from tobacco-specific *N*-nitrosamines. *Mutat. Res.*, **424**, 127–142

Hecht, S.S., Carmella, S.G., Foiles, P.G., Murphy, S.E. & Peterson, L.A. (1993) Tobacco-specific nitrosamine adducts: studies in laboratory animals and humans. *Environ. Health Perspect.*, **99**, 57–63

Hemminki, K., Bartsch, H., Shuker, D.E.G., Segerback, D., Kadlubar, F. & Dipple, A., eds (1994) *DNA Adducts: Identification and Biological Significance* (IARC Scientific Publications No. 125), Lyon, IARC*Press*

Hsu, I.C., Metcalf, R.A., Sun, T., Welsh, J.A., Wang, N.J. & Harris, C.C. (1991) Mutational hotspot in the p53 gene in human hepatocellular carcinomas. *Nature*, **350**, 427–428

IARC (1990) *IARC Monographs on the Evaluation of Carcinogenic Risks to Humans*, Vol. 49, *Chromium, Nickel and Welding*, Lyon, IARC*Press*, pp. 49–256

IARC (1993) *IARC Monographs on the Evaluation of Carcinogenic Risks to Humans*, Vol. 56, *Some Naturally Occurring Substances: Food Items and Constituents, Heterocyclic Aromatic Amines and Mycotoxins*, Lyon, IARC*Press*, pp. 245–395

IARC (1997) *IARC Monographs on the Evaluation of Carcinogenic Risks to Humans*, Vol. 69, *Polychlorinated Dibenzo-para-dioxins and Polychlorinated Dibenzofurans*, Lyon, IARC*Press*

IARC (1999) *IARC Monographs on the Evaluation of Carcinogenic Risks to Humans*, Vol. 73, *Some Chemicals that Cause Tumours of the Kidney or Urinary Bladder in Rodents and Some Other Substances*, Lyon, IARC*Press*, pp. 131–182

Inoue, O., Kanno, E., Kakizaki, M., Watanabe, T., Higashikawa, K. & Ikeda, M. (2000) Urinary phenylmercapturic acid as a marker of occupational exposure to benzene. *Ind. Health*, **38**, 195–204

Inoue, O., Kanno, E., Yusa, T., Kakizaki, M., Watanabe, T., Higashikawa, K. & Ikeda, M. (2001)

A simple HPLC method to determine urinary phenylmercapturic acid and its application to gasoline station attendants to biomonitor occupational exposure to benzene at less than 1 ppm. *Biomarkers*, **6**, 190–203

Institute for Environment and Health (1999) *Benzene in the Environment: An Evaluation of Exposure of the UK General Population and Possible Adverse Health Effects* (Report R12), London, Medical Research Council, pp. 20–59

Jongeneelen, F.J. (1994) Biological monitoring of environmental exposure to polycyclic aromatic hydrocarbons; 1-hydroxypyrene in urine of people. *Toxicol. Lett.*, **72**, 205–211

Kafferlein, H.U. & Angerer, J. (2001) *N*-Methylcarbamoylated valine of hemoglobin in humans after exposure to *N,N*-dimethylformamide: evidence for the formation of methyl isocyanate? *Chem. Res. Toxicol.*, **14**, 833–840

Kautiainen, A., Wachtmeister, C.A. & Ehrenberg, L. (1998) Characterization of hemoglobin adducts from a 4,4′-methylenedianiline metabolite evidently produced by peroxidative oxidation in vivo. *Chem. Res. Toxicol.*, **11**, 614–621

Kriek, E., Rojas, M., Alexandrov, K. & Bartsch, H. (1998) Polycyclic aromatic hydrocarbon–DNA adducts in humans: relevance as biomarkers for exposure and cancer risk. *Mutat. Res.*, **400**, 215–231

Kyrtopoulos. S.A., Georgiadis, P., Autrup, H., Demopoulos, N.A., Farmer, P., Haugen, A., Katsouyanni, K., Lambert, B., Ovrebo, S., Šram, R., Stefanou, G.S., Topinka, J., Stefanou, G. & Demopoulos, N. (2001) Biomarkers of genotoxicity of urban air pollution — Overview and descriptive data from a molecular epidemiology study on populations exposed to moderate-to-low levels of polycyclic aromatic hydrocarbons: the AULIS project. *Mutat. Res.*, **496**, 207–228

Landin, H.H., Segerback, D., Damberg, C. & Osterman-Golkar, S. (1999) Adducts with haemoglobin and with DNA in epichlorohydrin-exposed rats. *Chem.-biol. Interact.*, **117**, 49–64

Leuratti, C., Singh, R., Lagneau, C., Farmer, P.B., Plastaras, J.P., Marnett, L.J. & Shuker, D.E.G. (1998) Determination of malondialdehyde-induced DNA damage in human tissues using an immunoslot blot assay. *Carcinogenesis*, **19**, 1919–1924

Lightfoot, T.J., Coxhead, J.M., Cupid, B.C., Nicholson, S. & Garner, R.C. (2000) Analysis of DNA adducts by accelerator mass spectrometry in human breast tissue after administration of 2-amino-1-methyl-6-phenylimidazo[4,5-b]pyridine and benzo[a]pyrene. *Mutat. Res.*, **472**, 119–127

Magagnotti, C., Orsi, F., Bagnati, R., Celli, N., Rotilio, D., Fanelli, R. & Airoldi, L. (2000) Effect of diet on serum albumin and hemoglobin adducts of 2-amino-1-methyl-6-phenylimidazo[4,5-b]pyridine (PhIP) in humans. *Int. J. Cancer*, **88**, 1–6

Marafie, E.M., Marafie, I., Emery, S.J., Waters, R. & Jones, N.J. (2000) Biomonitoring the human population exposed to pollution from the oil fires in Kuwait: analysis of placental tissue using ^{32}P-postlabeling. *Environ. mol. Mutag.*, **36**, 274–282

Mauthe, R.J., Dingley, K.H., Leveson, S.H., Freeman, S.P.H.T., Turesky, R.J., Garner, R.C. & Turteltaub, K.W. (1999) Comparison of DNA-adduct and tissue-available dose levels of MeIQx in human and rodent colon following administration of a very low dose. *Int. J. Cancer*, **80**, 539–545

Melikian, A.A., O'Connor, R., Prahalad, A.K., Hu, P., Li, H., Kagan, M. & Thompson, S. (1999a) Determination of the urinary benzene metabolites S-phenylmercapturic acid and *trans,trans*-muconic acid by liquid chromatography-tandem mass spectrometry. *Carcinogenesis*, **20**, 719–726

Melikian, A.A., Malpure, S., John, A., Meng, M., Schoket, B., Mayer, G., Vinze, I., Kolozsi-Ringelhann, A. & Hecht, S.S. (1999b) Determination of hemoglobin and serum albumin adducts of benzo[a]pyrene by gas chromatography-mass spectrometry in humans and their relation to exposure and to other biological markers. *Polycyclic Arom. Comp.*, **17**, 125–134

Miller, R.R., Newhook, R. & Poole, A. (1994) Styrene production, use and human exposure. *Crit. Rev. Toxicol.*, **24** (Suppl) S1–S10

Morinello, E.J., Ham, A.J.L., Ranasinghe, A., Sangaiah, R. & Swenberg, J.A. (2001) Simultaneous quantitation of N(2),3-ethenoguanine and 1,N(2)-ethenoguanine with an immunoaffinity/gas chromatography/high-resolution mass spectrometry assay. *Chem. Res. Toxicol.*, **14**, 327–334

Murray, S., Lake, B.G., Gray, S., Edwards, A.J., Springall, C., Bowey, E.A., Williamson, G., Boobis, A.R. & Gooderham, N.J. (2001) Effect of cruciferous vegetable consumption on heterocyclic aromatic amine metabolism in man. *Carcinogenesis*, **22**, 1413–1420

Nath, R.G., Ocando, J.E., Guttenplan, J.B. & Chung, F.L. (1998) 1,N(2)-propanodeoxyguanosine adducts: potential new biomarkers of smoking-induced DNA damage in human oral tissue. *Cancer Res.*, **58**, 581–584

Nayak, S., Sashidhar, R.B. & Bhat, R.V. (2001) Quantification and validation of enzyme immunoassay for urinary aflatoxin B1–N(7)-guanine adduct for biological monitoring of aflatoxins. *Analyst*, **126**, 179–183

Nielsen, P.S., Andreassen, A., Farmer, P.B., Ovrebo, S. & Autrup, H. (1996) Biomonitoring of diesel exhaust-exposed workers. DNA and hemoglobin adducts and urinary 1-hydroxpyrene as markers of exposure. *Toxicol. Lett.*, **86**, 27–37

Ong, C.N., Shi, C.Y., Chia, S.E., Chua, S.C., Ong, H.Y., Lee, B.L., Ng, T.P. & Teramoto, K. (1994) Biological monitoring of exposure to low concentrations of styrene. *Am. J. ind. Med.*, **25**, 719–730

Ong, C.N., Kok, P.W., Lee, B.L., Shi, C.Y., Ong, H.Y., Chia, K.S., Lee, C.S & Luo, X.W. (1995) Evaluation of biomarkers for occupational exposure to benzene. *Occup. environ. Med.*, **52**, 528–533

Oreffo, V., Singh, R., Rich, K.J., Shuker, D.E.G., Carthew, P., Cordero, R., Van Delft, J.H.M. & Farmer, P.B. (2000) DNA adducts in relation to lung tumour outcome are not markers of susceptibility following a single dose treatment of SWR, BALB/c and C57BL/6J mice with N-nitrosodiethylamine. *Biomarkers*, **5**, 323–340

Ovrebo, S., Haugen, A., Farmer, P.B. & Anderson, D. (1995) Evaluation of biomarkers in plasma, blood, and urine samples from coke oven workers: significance of exposure to polycyclic aromatic hydrocarbons. *Occup. environ. Med.*, **52**, 750–756

Ozbal, C.C., Skipper, P.L., Yu, M.C., London, S.J., Dasari, R.R. & Tannenbaum, S.R. (2000) Quantification of (7S,8R)-dihydroxy-(9R,10S)-epoxy-7,8,9,10-tetrahydrobenzo(a)pyrene adducts in human serum albumin by laser-induced fluorescence: implications for the in vivo metabolism of benzo(a)pyrene. *Cancer Epidemiol. Biomarkers Prev.*, **9**, 733–739

Pastorelli, R., Guanci, M., Cerri, A., Minoa, C., Carrer, P., Negri, E., Fanelli, R. & Airoldi, L. (2000)

Benzo(*a*)pyrene diolepoxide haemoglobin and albumin adducts at low levels of benzo[*a*]pyrene exposure. *Biomarkers*, **5**, 245–251

Penn, A., Nath, R., Pan, J., Chen, L., Widmer, K., Henk, W. & Chung, F.L. (2001) 1,N(2)-propanodeoxyguanosine adduct formation in aortic DNA following inhalation of acrolein. *Environ. Health Perspect.*, **109**, 219–224

Perez, H.L., Segerback, D. & Osterman-Golkar, S. (1999) Adducts of acrylonitrile with hemoglobin in nonsmokers and in participants in a smoking cessation program. *Chem. Res. Toxicol.*, **12**, 869–873

Pfau, W., Stone, E.M., Brockstedt, U., Carmichael, P.L., Marquardt, H. & Phillips, D.H. (1998) DNA adducts in human breast tissue: association with N-acetyltransferase-2 (*NAT2*) and *NAT1* genotypes. *Cancer Epidemiol. Biomarkers Prev.*, **7**, 1019–1025

Phillips, D.H. & Castegnaro, M. (1999) Standardization and validation of DNA adduct postlabelling methods: report of interlaboratory trials and production of recommended protocols. *Mutagenesis*, **14**, 301–315

Poirier, M.C., Weston, A., Schoket, B., Shamkhani, H., Pan, C.F., McDiarmid, M.A., Scott, B.G., Deeter, D.P., Heller, J.M., Jacobson-Kram, D. & Rothman, N. (1998) Biomonitoring of United States army soldiers serving in Kuwait in 1991. *Cancer Epidemiol. Biomarkers Prev.*, **7**, 545–551

Prevost, V., Likhachev, A.J., Loktionova, N.A., Bartsch, H., Wild, C.P., Kazanova, O.I., Arkhipov, A.I., Gershanovich, M.L. & Shuker, D.E.G. (1996) DNA base adducts in urine and white blood cells of cancer patients receiving combination chemotherapies which include N-methyl-N-nitrosourea. *Biomarkers*, **1**, 244–251

Qian, G.S., Ross, R.K., Yu, M.C., Yuan, J.M. Gao, Y.T., Henderson, B.E., Wogan, G.N. & Groopman, J.D. (1994) A follow-up study of urinary markers of aflatoxin exposure and liver cancer risk in Shanghai, People's Republic of China. *Cancer Epidemiol. Biomarkers Prev.*, **3**, 3–10

Reh, B.D., DeBord, D.G., Butler, M.A., Reid, T.M., Mueller, C. & Fajen, J.M. (2000) O[6]-Methylguanine DNA adducts associated with occupational nitrosamine exposure. *Carcinogenesis*, **21**, 29–33

Ross, R.K., Yuan, J.M., Yu, M.C., Wogan, G.N., Qian, G.S., Tu, J.T., Groopman, J.D., Gao, Y.T. & Henderson, B.E. (1992) Urinary aflatoxin biomarkers and risk of hepatocelullar carcinoma. *Lancet*, **339**, 943–946

Sabbioni, G., Hartley, R., Henschler, D., Hollrigl-Rosta, A., Koeber, R. & Schneider, S. (2000) Isocyanate-specific hemoglobin adduct in rats exposed to 4,4′-methylenediphenyl diisocyanate. *Chem. Res. Toxicol.*, **13**, 82–89

Saris, C.P., Damman, S.J., van den Ende, A.M.C., Westra, J.G. & den Engelse, L. (1995) A ^{32}P-postlabeling assay for the detection of alkylphosphotriesters in DNA. *Carcinogenesis*, **16**, 1543–1548

Scherer, G., Frank, S., Riedel, K., Meger-Kossien, I. & Renner, T. (2000) Biomonitoring of exposure to polycyclic aromatic hydrocarbons of nonoccupationally exposed persons. *Cancer Epidemiol. Biomarkers Prev.*, **9**, 373–380

Schmid, K., Nair, J., Winde, G., Velic, I. & Bartsch, H. (2000) Increased levels of promutagenic etheno-DNA adducts in colonic polyps of FAP patients. *Int. J. Cancer*, **87**, 1–4

Schoket, B. (1999) DNA damage in humans exposed to environmental and dietary polycyclic aromatic hydrocarbons. *Mutat. Res.*, **424**, 143–153

Schoket, B., Poirer, M.C., Mayer, G., Torok, G., Kolozsi-Ringelhann, A., Bognar, G., Bigbee, W.L. & Vincze, I. (1999) Biomonitoring of human genotoxicity induced by complex occupational exposures. *Mutat. Res.*, **445**, 193–203

Schuhmacher, M., Domingo, J.L., Llobet, J.M., Lindstrom, G. & Wingfors, H. (1999) Dioxin and dibenzofuran concentrations in adipose tissue of a general population from Tarragona, Spain. *Chemosphere*, **38**, 2475–2487

Shuker, D.E.G. (1999) DNA adducts in mammalian cells as indicators of exposure to carcinogens. In: McGregor, D.B., Rice, J.M. & Venitt, S., eds, *The Use of Short- and Medium-term Tests for Carcinogens and Data on Genetic Effects in Carcinogenic Hazard Evaluation* (IARC Scientific Publications No. 146), Lyon, IARC*Press*, pp. 287–307

Shuker, D.E.G. & Farmer, P.B. (1992) Relevance of urinary DNA adducts as markers of carcinogen exposure. *Chem. Res. Toxicol.*, **5**, 450–460

Shuker, D.E.G., Braybrooke, J., Crawley, J.E., Flanagan, E. & Harris, A.L. (1997) 3-Methyladenine excretion in patients with malignant melanoma receiving dacarbazine. *Br. J. Cancer*, **75**, 44 van Sittert, N.J., Boogaard, P.J., Natarajan, A.T., Tates, A.D., Ehrenberg, L.G. & Tornqvist, M.A. (2000) Formation of DNA adducts and induction of mutagenic effects in rats following 4 weeks inhalation exposure to ethylene oxide as a basis for cancer risk assessment. *Mutat. Res.*, **447**, 27–48

Skov, H., Lindskog, A., Palmgren, F. & Christensen, C.S. (2001) An overview of commonly used methods for measuring benzene in ambient air. *Atmos. Environ.*, **35**, S141–S148

Soglia, J.R., Turesky, R.J., Paehler, A. & Vouros, P. (2001) Quantification of the heterocyclic aromatic amine DNA adduct N-(deoxyguanosin-8-yl)-2-amino-3-methylimidazo[4,5-*f*]quinoline in livers of rats using capillary liquid chromatography/microelectrospray mass spectrometry: a dose–response study. *Anal. Chem.*, **73**, 2819–2827

Souliotis, V.L. & Kyrtopoulos, S.A. (1989) A novel, sensitive assay for O^6-methyl- and O^6-ethylguanine in DNA based on repair by the enzyme O^6-alkylguanine DNA alkyltransferase in competition with an oligonucleotide containing O^6-methylguanine. *Cancer Res.*, **49**, 6997–7001

Stillwell, W.G., Turesky, R.J., Sinha, R., Skipper, P.L. & Tannenbaum, S.R. (1999) Biomonitoring of heterocyclic aromatic amine metabolites in human urine. *Cancer Lett.*, **143**, 145–148

Strickland, P.T., Qian, Z., Friesen, M.D., Rothman, N. & Sinha, R. (2001) Measurement of 2-amino-1-6-phenylimidazo(4,5-b)pyridine (PhIP) in acid-hydrolyzed urine by high-performance liquid chromatography with fluorescence detection. *Biomarkers*, **6**, 313–325

Sumner, S.J. & Fennell, T.R. (1994) Review of the metabolic fate of styrene. *Crit. Rev. Toxicol.*, **24**, S11–S33

Sweetman, G.M.A., Shuker, D.E.G., Glover, R.P. & Farmer, P.B. (1998) Mass spectrometry in carcinogenesis research. *Adv. mass Spect.*, **14**, 343–376

Symanski, E., Bergamaschi, E. & Mutti, A. (2001) Inter-and intra-individual sources of variation in levels of urinary styrene metabolites. *Int. Arch. occup. environ. Health*, **74**, 336–344

Tavares, R., Borba, H., Monteiro, M., Proenca, M.J., Lynce, N., Rueff, J., Bailey, E., Sweetman, G.M.A., Lawrence, R.M. & Farmer, P.B. (1996) Monitoring of exposure to acrylonitrile by determination of

N-(2-cyanoethyl)valine at the N-terminal position of haemoglobin. *Carcinogenesis*, **17**, 2655–2660

Thier, R., Lewalter, J. Selinski, S. & Bolt, H.M. (2001) Re-evaluation of the effect of smoking on the methylation of N-terminal valine in haemoglobin. *Arch. Toxicol.*, **75**, 270–273

Topinka, J., Schwarz, L.R., Wiebel, F.J., Cerna, M. & Wolff, T. (2000) Genotoxicity of urban air pollutants in the Czech Republic. Part II. DNA adduct formation in mammalian cells by extractable organic matter. *Mutat. Res.*, **469**, 83–93

Tornqvist, M., Mowrer, J., Jensen, S. & Ehrenberg, L. (1986) Monitoring of environmental cancer initiators through hemoglobin adducts by a modified Edman degradation method. *Anal. Biochem.*, **154**, 255–266

Tretyakova, N.Y., Chiang, S.Y., Walker, V.E. & Swenberg, J.A. (1998) Quantitative analysis of 1,3-butadiene-induced DNA adducts *in vivo* and *in vitro* using liquid chromatography electrospray ionization tandem mass spectrometry. *J. mass Spect.*, **33**, 363–376

Triebig, G., Stark, T., Ihrig, A. & Diez, M.C. (2001) Intervention study on acquired color vision deficiencies in styrene-exposed workers. *J. occup. environ. Med.*, **43**, 494–500

Turner, P.C., Dingley, K.H., Coxhead, J., Russell, S. & Garner, R.C. (1998) Detectable levels of serum aflatoxin B1–albumin adducts in the United Kingdom population: implications for aflatoxin B1 exposure in the United Kingdom. *Cancer Epidemiol. Biomarkers Prev.*, **7**, 441–447

Turteltaub, K.W., Dingley, K.H., Curtis, K.D., Malfatti, M.A., Turesky, R.J., Garner, R.C., Felton, J.S. & Lang, N.P. (1999) Macromolecular adduct formation and metabolism of heterocyclic amines in humans and rodents at low doses. *Cancer Lett.*, **143**, 149–155

Vodicka, P., Tvrdik, T., Osterman-Golkar, S., Vodickova, L., Peterkova, K., Soucek, P., Sarmanova, J., Farmer, P.B., Granath, F., Lambert, B. & Hemminki, K. (1999) An evaluation of styrene genotoxicity using several biomarkers in a 3-year follow-up study of hand-lamination workers. *Mutat. Res.*, **445**, 205–224

Wacker, M., Schuler, D., Wanek, P. & Eder, E. (2000) Development of a ^{32}P-postlabeling method for the detection of 1,N(2)-propanodeoxyguanosine adducts of trans-4-hydroxy-2-nonenal *in vivo*. *Chem. Res. Toxicol.*, **13**, 1165–1173

Waidyanatha, S., Rothman, N., Fustinoni, S., Smith, M.T., Hayes, R.B., Bechtold, W., Dosemeci, M., Guilan, L., Yin, S.N. & Rappaport, S.M. (2001) Urinary benzene as a biomarker of exposure among occupationally exposed and unexposed subjects. *Carcinogenesis*, **22**, 279–286

van Welie, R.T.H., van Dijck, R.G.J.M., Vermeulen, N.P.E. & van Sittert, N.J. (1992) Mercapturic acids, protein adducts, and DNA adducts as biomarkers of electrophilic chemicals. *Crit. Rev. Toxicol.*, **22**, 271–306

Weston, A., Rowe, M.L., Manchester, D.K., Farmer, P.B., Mann, D.L. & Harris, C.C. (1989) Fluorescence and mass spectral evidence for the formation of benzo[a]pyrene anti-diolepoxide–DNA and –hemoglobin adducts in humans. *Carcinogenesis*, **10**, 251–257

Whyatt, R.M., Jedrychowski, W., Hemminki, K., Santella, R.M., Tsai, W.Y., Yang, K. & Perera, F.P. (2001) Biomarkers of polycyclic aromatic hydrocarbon-DNA damage and cigarette smoke exposures in paired maternal and newborn blood samples as a measure of differential susceptibility. *Cancer Epidemiol. Biomarkers Prev.*, **10**, 581–588

Wong, J.L., Zheng, Y.T., Li, J.Y., Tamburrow, C.H. & Benz, F.W. (1998) Immunoassay of haemoglobin–acrylonitrile adduct in rat as a biomarker of exposure. *Biomarkers*, **3**, 317–326

Yen, T.Y., Holt, S., Sangaiah, R., Gold, A. & Swenberg, J.A. (1998) Quantitation of 1,N⁶-ethenoadenine in rat urine by immunoaffinity extraction combined with liquid chromatography/electrospray ionization mass spectrometry. *Chem. Res. Toxicol.*, **11**, 810–815

Yeowell-O'Connell, K., Rothman, N., Smith, M.T., Hayes, R.B., Li, G., Waidyanatha, S., Dosemeci, M., Zhang, L., Yin, S., Titenko-Holland, N. & Rappaport, S.M. (1998) Hemoglobin and albumin adducts of benzene oxide among workers exposed to high levels of benzene. *Carcinogenesis*, **19**, 1565–1571

Yi, P., Sun, X., Doerge, D.R. & Fu, P.P. (1998) An improved ³²P-postlabeling/high-performance liquid chromatography method for the analysis of the malondialdehyde-derived 1,N(2)-propanodeoxyguanosine DNA adduct in animal and human tissues. *Chem. Res. Toxicol.*, **11**, 1032–1041

Corresponding author

Peter B. Farmer
MRC Toxicology Unit, Hodgkin Building,
University of Leicester, Lancaster Road,
PO Box 138, Leicester LE1 9HN, UK
pbf1@le.ac.uk

Mechanisms of Carcinogenesis: Contributions of Molecular Epidemiology
Patricia Buffler, Jerry Rice, Robert Baan, Michael Bird and Paolo Boffetta, eds
IARC Scientific Publications No. 157
International Agency for Research on Cancer, Lyon, 2004

Biomarkers of Inherited Susceptibility and Cancer

Timothy R. Rebbeck

Summary

The etiology of cancer is likely to involve the effects of inherited genotypes at various points in the multistage process of carcinogenesis. For example, inherited genotypes could influence propensity to be exposed to carcinogens, generation of somatic mutations that initiate tumours, determination of a tumour's natural history or clinical prognosis and response to chemoprevention and treatment. Classes of inherited genotypes involved in multistage carcinogenesis are defined here to help focus the role inherited genotypes may have in the etiology and prevention of cancer. Knowledge of inherited genotype may assist in elucidating the nature and timing of specific genetic events in carcinogenesis, identify exposures that correlate with specific steps in carcinogenesis, lead to the development of risk assessment models and target relevant biochemical pathways for the development of preventive or therapeutic interventions.

Introduction: Inherited genotypes and multistage carcinogenesis

The characterization of the human genome has provided a large amount of information about human germline genetic variation. A major challenge facing the scientific community is how to relate these variants to functionally and clinically meaningful end-points. Central to this process are basic science investigations that characterize the effects of germline variation on gene expression, regulation, and function on a molecular, biochemical or tissue level. A complementary approach is that of molecular epidemiology, which provides evidence for statistical associations between inherited genetic variation and end-points relevant to human disease on a population level.

The multistage model of carcinogenesis in the context of molecular epidemiology studies (Perera & Weinstein, 1982) describes biomarkers that characterize the progression of normal cells to initiated and preneoplastic cells, and finally to malignant disease. This model further considers the consequences of malignancy to the morbidity and mortality of the affected individual. These biomarkers include measures of internal and biologically effective exposure doses, early biological effect, altered structure or function, disease and prognosis (Schulte & Perera, 1993). Although biomarkers measured in somatic tissues play a central role in these models, inherited genotypes also play a prominent role as susceptibility factors that in part determine the course of multistage carcinogenesis.

In this context, inherited genotype information can be thought of as acting to affect exposure, disease susceptibility and outcome. A number of classes of genes acting at each phase of this multistage model can be identified, as shown in Figure 1. In this presentation, G denotes genotypes at a single locus. Subscripts to G are used to distinguish different classes of genes that may act at different points in the development and progress of a tumour. First, G_E comprises those genes involved in metabolic pathways that determine propensity to be exposed to endogenous or exogenous carcinogens. Chemoprevention is the active administration of agents with the goal of reducing the incidence of cancer. G_P, the genes involved in the metabolism of chemopreventive agents, can determine the degree to which an individual's cancer risk may be modified, or the degree to which an individual will suffer adverse side-effects from exposure to the agent. G_D comprises those genes that are directly involved in the

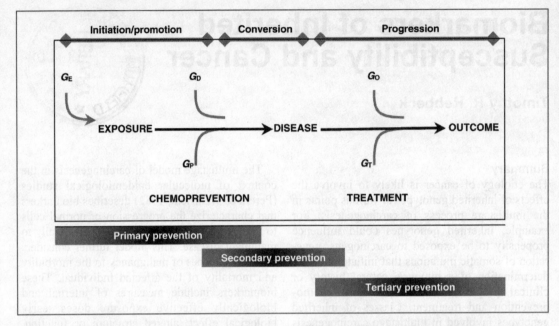

Figure 1. Inherited susceptibility genes on the continuum from exposure to disease outcome

etiology of a tumour, and include those typically considered in studies addressing disease susceptibility (e.g. *BRCA1*, *TP53*, *APC*). G_T are therefore those genes involved in the determination of drug dissemination and metabolism (e.g. of chemotherapies used in cancer treatment). As with G_P, G_T in part determine an agent's efficacy and toxicity. G_O can be distinguished from G_T and G_D because they are associated with the course of an individual's disease at or after the time of diagnosis. G_O are therefore determinants of the natural history of a tumour, as it progresses from a more benign to a more progressive stage.

Defining these classes of genes could assist in understanding the point in carcinogenesis at which a particular gene may be acting. This may elucidate specific carcinogenic events controlled by a gene, including relevant biochemical pathways or exposures. It may also help to identify genes and related pathways for the development of preventive or therapeutic interventions. For example, it seems likely that G_E and G_P play a substantial role in studies involving cancer prevention, whereas G_D are more likely to contribute to studies of etiology. By understanding that the same gene works during different phases of carcinogenesis, a better understanding of a gene's role in cancer may be gained. Implicit in this model is the role that inherited genotypes may play in cancer prevention by better defining modifiable aspects of carcinogenesis.

In this chapter, each of these classes of genes is defined and examples are provided that illustrate how inherited genotype information can be used to understand better the multistep carcinogenesis process and potentially to improve cancer prevention and treatment.

G_E: Inherited genetic determinants of carcinogenic exposures

G_E are involved in metabolic pathways that determine propensity to be exposed to endogenous or exogenous carcinogens. For example, a number of investigators have related G_E in genes related to neurotransmitter metabolism including *DRD4*, *SLCA3* and *5-HTTLPR* with propensity to smoke, early age at smoking initiation, ability to stop smoking and nicotine dependence (Shields *et al.*, 1998; Lerman *et al.*, 1999; Sabol *et al.*, 1999; Lerman *et al.*, 2000). Similarly, genotypes that are involved in steroid hormone metabolism may also in part explain interindividual variability in hormone-related risk factors, and therefore in propensity to be exposed to these factors. For example, *CYP17* is a member of the cytochrome P450 multigene family that is responsible for conversion of progesterone to androstenedione in the biosynthesis of estrone. A number of authors have evaluated the relationship of a 5′-untranslated region polymorphism with age at menarche (Feigelson *et al.*, 1997a; Helzlsouer *et al.*, 1998; Weston *et al.*, 1998; Haiman *et al.*, 1999), use of hormone replacement therapy (HRT; Feigelson *et al.*, 1997b) or circulating hormone levels (Haiman *et al.*, 1999). The relationship of *CYP17* genotype with age at menarche was not consistent in all studies, and there have not been independent confirmations of the reported associations of HRT use or circulating hormone levels. However, this example points to the possibility that G_E may influence propensity to be exposed to 'traditional' cancer risk factors, elucidate biologically relevant prevention pathways and identify people who should be targeted for prevention.

G_P: Inherited genetic determinants of chemoprevention response and toxicity

G_P include those genes that are most likely to predict an individual's response to a chemopreventive agent, and in addition may define those individuals who may suffer increased toxicities when exposed to these agents. There are few examples of the use of G_P in cancer chemoprevention studies. A potential example is that of tamoxifen, an antiestrogenic drug used for the prevention of breast cancer. Tamoxifen is metabolized to the antiestrogenic 4-hydroxytamoxifen (4-OHT) by SULT1A1 and to *N*-desmethyl tamoxifen by CYP3A4. The *N*-desmethyl form is quantitatively the major antiestrogenic metabolite, although the 4-OHT form is 100-fold more antiestrogenic than the *N*-desmethyl form. Therefore, *SULT1A1* and *CYP3A4* may be considered candidate G_P, since variants that affect the metabolism of tamoxifen to 4-OHT or *N*-desmethyl tamoxifen may predict which individuals have either an optimal chemopreventive response or the potential for increased toxicity after

administration of tamoxifen. For example, individuals with a specific G_P genotype may be at highest risk for adverse reactions. For tamoxifen chemoprevention, these reactions can include hot flashes, which may affect a woman's long-term compliance with the preventive regimen. Although SULT1A1 and CYP3A4 are key enzymes in the metabolism of tamoxifen, a number of others, including CYP2D6 and CYP2C9, are also involved in tamoxifen metabolism. Furthermore, sulfate conjugation of 4-OHT by *SULT1A1* can reduce the antiestrogenic properties of tamoxifen metabolites. Therefore, as with most complex metabolic systems, multiple G_P may need to be considered before we can fully evaluate the pharmacogenetics of cancer chemoprevention. However, knowledge of G_P could help us to understand better whether the chemopreventive regimen is effective, and in what individuals.

Knowledge of G_P may have important implications for study design and analysis in cancer chemoprevention. First, studies that attempt to identify chemopreventive agents may not identify protective effects if only a subset of individuals with a specific G_P genotype are likely to respond with a decreased cancer incidence. Consequently, sample size requirements will be dictated not only by the proposed reduction in cancer incidence in the treatment arm, but also by the proportion of individuals in the population who carry a particular G_P. Furthermore, fairly detailed knowledge about the pharmacogenetics of the G_P under study may be required in order to model optimally the effect of a G_P. These considerations, although potentially resulting in a more informative result, could make the design and execution of chemopreventive studies considerably more difficult to achieve than if G_P were not considered.

G_D: Inherited genetic determinants of cancer etiology

Two classes of G_D have been inferred or found to be associated with cancer aetiology and risk. First, there are a few genes with allelic variants that confer a high degree of risk to the individual. These genes will be referred to here as **high-penetrance** genes. Relatively few individuals in the population are predicted to carry risk-increasing genotypes at these loci. Therefore, the population attributable risk (e.g. the proportion of prostate cancer in the population that may be explained by these genotypes) is low. Because of the large magnitude of effects these genotypes have on cancer risk, one hallmark of high-penetrance genes is the creation of a Mendelian (often auto-somal dominant) pattern of cancer. Examples of these genes include *BRCA1* and *BRCA2* in breast and ovarian cancer, *CDKN2a* in melanoma and *APC* in colorectal cancer.

Second, it is hypothesized that genes exist that confer a small-to-moderate degree of prostate cancer risk to the individual. These **low-pene-trance** genes may not be associated with Mende-lian patterns of cancer occurrence in families, but may rather be associated with sporadic cancer. In addition, it is expected that allelic variability at these genes may be relatively common, and thus may explain a relatively larger proportion of certain cancers in the population.

High-penetrance G_D

The hereditary pattern of many cancers conferred by high-penetrance genes makes it possible to use principles of Mendelian genetics to identify the DNA sequence responsible for the etiology of these tumours by using a positional cloning approach. This approach involves a wide variety of genetic epidemiological methods using pedi-gree data, including both ad-hoc and formal quan-titative methods. Identification of effects of high-penetrance G_D on cancer risk may begin by eva-luating whether the cancer aggregates in families (i.e. whether cancer incidences in some families are higher than expected). Quantitative methods using twin, sib-pair, nuclear family, extended pedigree and other family-based data can be used for more formal quantitation of the degree of familial aggregation. Simple familial aggregation analyses may not be able to distinguish shared environmental effects from the effects of genes, but more sophisticated methods of familial aggre-gation analysis may provide insight into genetic etiologies. These approaches include comparing cancer aggregation in biological relatives and non-biologically related family members.

If there is no evidence for familial aggregation of a disease, then it is highly unlikely that subse-quent family-based methods will identify a high-penetrance G_D that explains cancer etiology; epi-demiological methods, possibly using measured biomarkers, may then be employed to identify cancer risk factors (see below for discussion of low-penetrance G_D). However, evidence of fami-lial aggregation can lead to evaluation of Mende-lian or more complex patterns of segregation of cancer in families. The goal of these methods is to determine whether the pattern of cancer in a family is consistent with inheritance of a suscep-tibility gene. These methods are often highly quantitative, requiring sophisticated model fitting and intensive computational analysis. If a pattern of inheritance consistent with a single-gene effect is observed (even if reduced penetrance, genetic heterogeneity, interaction with environmental factors, etc., are observed), identifying the DNA sequence responsible for the observed pattern of cancer can then be accomplished by using genetic linkage analysis. The goal of genetic linkage ana-lysis is to identify the co-segregation of poly-morphic DNA markers that have a known location in the human genome with the inheritance of disease in families. Again, these methods may be computationally intense, and use affected pairs of relatives in a family, nuclear families or large extended pedigrees. Successful linkage analyses culminate in the molecular cloning of the DNA sequence responsible for the hereditary disease pattern.

Prostate cancer represents a particularly complex example of high-penetrance G_D. It has long been known that an excess of prostate cancer occurs in some families (Morganti *et al.*, 1956). Since the time that prostate cancer was recognized as a familial disease, complex segregation ana-lyses have been undertaken (Carter *et al.* 1992; Grönberg *et al.*, 1997a,b; Schaid *et al.*, 1998) which indicated that a rare, autosomal dominant gene segregated in some families to explain patterns of hereditary prostate cancer. This puta-tive gene or genes confers a relatively high lifetime prostate cancer penetrance (e.g. 63–89%, depending on the data set and model applied). However, the frequency of disease-causing alleles in the populations studied was inferred to be 0.3–0.6% in the USA and 1.7% in Scandinavia. These figures, and the estimates emanating from these analyses, suggest that only a small proportion (perhaps no more than 10%) of all prostate cancer may occur in men who carry a single-gene mutation with an autosomal dominant pattern of inheritance. A number of loci have been identified which explain these hereditary patterns of prostate cancer (reviewed by Ostrander & Stanford, 2000). Only one cloned gene that may confer prostate cancer risk has been identified, *HPC2/ELAC2* (Rebbeck *et al.*, 2000; Tavtigian *et al.*, 2001), although the role of this gene in prostate cancer etiology has not been observed in all studies (Xu *et al.*, 2001a,b,c). Although it has not yet been cloned, the strongest evidence to date for a high-penetrance prostate cancer G_D is for *HPC1* on chromosome 1q24–25 (Smith *et al.*, 1996). However, this gene is likely to explain only a small proportion of hereditary prostate cancers. Additional linkage analyses have identified putative hereditary prostate cancer loci on chromosomes 1p36 (*CAPB*), 20q13 (*HPC20*), Xq27–28 (*HPCX*) and 1q42.2–q43 (*PCAP*), although few of the reports of linkage at these loci have been confirmed in an independent report. Therefore, the genetics of hereditary prostate cancer involving G_D remains unresolved.

Low-penetrance G_D

As implied above, the search for genotype–disease associations for genes that do not confer high risk of disease cannot rely on the use of hereditary patterns of disease in families. Instead, the search for G_D that confer a relatively low degree of risk usually relies on knowledge about biochemical or physiological pathways that are thought to be involved in carcinogenesis. Because the genes involved in these processes are too numerous to consider in any single study of cancer susceptibility, a number of criteria can be used to define one or more candidate genes that have the most promise as cancer susceptibility genes. Criteria for candidate gene selection include biological plausibility, whether there is a known functional relationship between genotype

and phenotypes relevant to cancer risk and the degree of polymorphism.

When one or more candidate genes have been selected, a series of steps can be taken to establish the relationship of G_D with cancer. First, optimization and validation of genotyping methods should be undertaken that take into account the type of biosamples from which genotypes will be obtained. These and related investigations are often referred to as 'transitional studies' (Schulte & Perera, 1993). For the genotype–disease associations themselves, a number of study designs are available (see Schulte & Perera, 1993 for a complete discussion of these approaches). These designs include traditional epidemiological methods of case–case, case–control and cohort studies. In addition to these more traditional epidemiological methods, modified family study designs are also available to identify important genotype–disease associations. These include the transmission-disequilibrium (TDT) and haplotype relative risk (HRR) methods. A comprehensive review of these approaches is presented by Goldstein and Andrieu (1999). These designs provide efficient means of using genotype data in small families, and have the advantage of controlling for background genotype, ethnicity and possibly other unmeasured confounders.

Again using prostate cancer as an example, molecular epidemiological studies have yet to provide consistent inferences about the role of low penetrance G_D in prostate cancer etiology. There are a number of examples of low-penetrance genes in the etiology of prostate cancer (reviewed by Rebbeck, 2001). These include genes involved in the metabolism of environmental carcinogens (e.g. *CYP2D6*, *CYP2C19*, *GSTM1*, *GSTP1*, *GSTT1*, *NAT1* and *NAT2*), those involved in androgen metabolism (*AR*, *CYP17* and *SRD5A2*) and the vitamin D receptor (*VDR*). In addition, *HPC2* has been inferred by some (Rebbeck *et al.*, 2000) but not all (Vesprini *et al.*, 2001) studies to confer hereditary prostate cancer risk outside the context of hereditary cancer families. Despite the many potential candidate genes, few consistent associations between these genes and prostate cancer risk have been identified. The majority of these studies have been undertaken in small sample sets, and rarely have there been confirmatory analyses using independent samples. Therefore, it is difficult to assess whether consistent and strong associations exist.

The *AR* (androgen receptor) *CYP17*, *SRD5A2* (5α-reductase type II) and *VDR* genes have been the most widely studied of those reported to date. Length of the *AR-CAG* and *AR-GGN* repeat polymorphisms has been reported to be associated with risk for prostate cancer in a number of studies (Giovannucci *et al.*, 1997; Ingles *et al.*, 1997; Platz *et al.*, 1998; Hsing *et al.*, 2000) but not in all studies (Bratt *et al.*, 1999; Edwards *et al.*, 1999). Similarly, associations of *SRD5A2* have been reported by some groups (Makridakis *et al.*, 1999; Nam *et al.*, 2001) but not others (Febbo *et al.*, 1999; Lunn *et al.*, 1999). *CYP17* has been consistently reported to be associated with risk for prostate cancer by a number of groups. However, the direction of the genotypic association for the same polymorphism has been reported to be positive in some studies (Lunn *et al.*, 1999; Wadelius *et al.*, 1999; Gsur *et al.*, 2000) and inverse in one other (Habuchi *et al.*, 2000). Finally, a number of polymorphisms in *VDR* exist and have been studied in association with risk for prostate cancer. Some studies have shown no association of any *VDR* polymorphism and risk for prostate cancer (Ma *et al.*, 1998; Blazer *et al.*, 2000). Others have reported an association with one of many polymorphisms studied (Taylor *et al.*, 1996; Ingles *et al.*, 1997; Habuchi *et al.*, 2000), without consistent replication of findings regarding the same polymorphic variant in different studies. Therefore, although many of these genes may play a role in the etiology of prostate cancer, there remains relatively little information about which genes, which polymorphisms and in which populations these genes will exert their effects on prostate cancer risk.

This type of inconsistency is typical for candidate gene association investigations for most cancer sites studied to date. Obtaining consistent inferences, or explaining the sources of this inconsistency, remains a major challenge for molecular epidemiology. In part, limited statistical power may play a role in these inconsistent inferences. In addition, differences in the definition and distribution of tumour stages and grades among studies may affect the inferences made. For example, screening practices at the time of case ascertainment may result in inconsistencies in the nature of the case sample studied, and affect the results of a study of this type. This information is often not available or not presented, and thus inconsistencies among studies that could be explained by very different study populations may be perceived as inconsistent results. Future studies in this area should report and evaluate the distribution of screening and tumour stage or grade in studies that evaluate inherited genotype and tumour characteristics, natural history or prognosis. Similarly, differences among study populations with respect to ethnicity or geography could affect the inferences of a study. Population substructure has been hypothesized to affect inferences from association studies, but there is mounting evidence that it may be possible to assess and correct for confounding by ethnicity (population stratification) using relatively straightforward means (Wacholder *et al.*, 2000). These approaches include standard methods of adjustment for confounding, family-based studies that inherently 'match' analyses for ethnicity (e.g. Spielman *et al.*, 1993) or formal evaluations of population substructure using random molecular markers (Devlin & Roeder, 1999; Pritchard & Rosenberg, 1999). However, it cannot be discounted that etiological differences by ethnicity may reflect real differences across populations, and not a failure of the methodology to detect (or reject) these effects.

A final aspect should be the consideration of multiple factors simultaneously, to determine whether inherited genotype provides additional information about natural history, prognosis or treatment response independent of that found in traits that are more easily obtained, including histopathological characteristics. It will be increasingly valuable to consider haplotype data and make use of linkage disequilibrium among variants to better understand the role of multi-allelic variability at a locus or among loci on disease risk (e.g. Cargill *et al.*, 1999). The effects of low-penetrance genes are also likely to involve interactions with other genes and with environmental exposures. A critical aspect of research that evaluates these genes is the ability to determine the specific environmental context in which these genes exert their effects. For example, in the absence of exposure, it is possible that a gene may have no meaningful effect on cancer etiology. In the presence of one exposure (e.g. cigarette smoke), the gene may result in an increase in cancer risk, whereas in the presence of a second exposure (e.g. diet), the gene may be associated with a reduction in cancer risk. The cumulative balance of these effects across a multitude of such genes and exposures is likely to be involved in the etiology of a particular cancer. Therefore, a hallmark of this class of gene will be the generation of a complex multifactorial etiological pattern of cancer.

G_T: Inherited genetic determinants of treatment response and toxicity

G_T are conceptually similar to G_P, because they are involved in the dissemination and metabolism of a pharmacological agent, and thereby contribute to an agent's efficacy and toxicity. Response to cancer treatment is determined in part by drug pharmacokinetics, which control levels of the absorption and dissemination of the drug in the bloodstream as well as in target tissues. In addition to pharmacodynamic determinants, the metabolic activation and excretion of drugs may also determine the amount and type of drug at the target tissue. G_T may influence the structure or amount of these agents and thereby influence drug pharmacodynamics and metabolism, and therefore may predict interindividual variability in response to or toxicity of a drug. A paradigm for the role of G_T dictating choice of treatment regimen is the use of thiopurine-containing drugs that are metabolized by thiopurine methyltransferase (TPMT; reviewed by Krynetski & Evans, 2000). Approximately 1 in 300 white Americans carries a TPMT genotype that results in the inability to methylate thiopurine drugs, which can produce potentially fatal myelosuppression (Krynetski et al., 1996). Therefore, knowledge of an individual's TPMT genotype and phenotype has become part of standard clinical practice when treatments involve thiopurines (Krynetski et al., 1996; Otterness et al., 1997). Other classes of enzymes, including dihydropyrimidine dehydrogenase, aldehyde dehydrogenases, glutathione S-transferases, uridine diphosphate glucuronosyl-transferases and cytochromes P450 used in cancer therapy may also have pharmacogenetic significance in determining cancer chemotherapy regimens (reviewed by Iyer & Ratain, 1998).

There are also data suggesting that specific treatments for commonly occurring cancers may be influenced by G_T, based not on detailed knowledge of specific genes and their regulation of well-characterized metabolic pathways, but rather on epidemiological association studies of candidate genes. For the example of prostate cancer, Bratt et al. (1999) reported that response to endocrine therapy (orchiectomy, gonadotropin-releasing hormone or bicalutamide monotherapy) improved by 25% for each increase in triplet repeat length, or a fourfold better prognosis for men with 25 CAG repeats compared to those with only 19. Despite a relatively small sample size ($n = 73$), this relationship remained marginally significant even after adjusting for pretreatment level of prostate-specific antigen (PSA) and tumour grade and stage. These results exemplify the type of relationship inherited genotype may have with prognosis in response to therapy. However, Bratt et al. (1999) also reported that longer AR-CAG repeat length was also associated with tumour stage. Thus, a difficulty in assessing this type of data is to tease apart the value of the inherited genotype to predict natural history of disease (G_O, see below) rather than response to treatment, or whether both phenomena contribute to outcome. Thus, studies designed to address this problem must be able to distinguish specifically the effects of genotypes on natural history from those of treatment response.

The use of G_T also has implications for epidemiological and clinical study design and analysis. For the most part, the studies reporting genotype–tumour trait effects have not been designed specifically to study these relationships, but instead were reported in the context of case–control or cohort studies. Often, case inclusion–exclusion criteria are not adequately defined or are some-times inappropriately collected for the evaluation of natural history and prognosis. Studies are often not specifically designed to have adequate statistical power for the evaluation of these questions. Prospective follow-up of a well-defined cohort of patients may be inadequate or incomplete. Evidence for the sample size limitation of many studies is clear from the many reports in which genotype was inferred to have no effect when the associated p-values fell in the 0.05–0.10 range with some moderately large effect sizes.

G_O: Inherited genetic determinants of clinical outcome

G_O may influence the natural history of disease if they are involved in tumour progression. For example, genotype may influence tumour histopathology including the stage or grade of disease, the rate of disease progression or the propensity for metastasis. These events include regulation of somatic DNA damage or repair directly or via the metabolism of compounds that induce DNA damage and the metabolism of steroid hormones that induce the growth of tumours. Therefore, some of the genes that may be considered candidate G_D may also be candidates for tumour progression and prognosis. G_O can be distinguished from G_T because they are associated with the course of an individual's disease even before treatment initiation. Because some genes may affect both natural history (i.e. G_O) and treatment response (i.e. G_T), it is also important to design studies that can tease apart these potentially separate effects. In contrast to the study of inherited genetic variants and clinical outcome, there is a large body of research that evaluates biochemical (e.g. levels of PSA), histopathological (e.g. tumour grade, stage) or somatic genetic measures in relation to cancer progression or prognosis. The role of somatic genetic mutations, including loss or amplification of specific genes in tumours, has been correlated with the natural history of cancer progression and therefore clinical prognosis (reviewed by Latil & Lidereau, 1998; Ozen & Pathak, 2000).

Prostate cancer again represents a useful example of G_O predicting clinical outcome.

Unlike most cancers, a sizeable proportion of prostate tumours may exist without producing symptoms (Baron & Angrist, 1941; Edwards *et al.*, 1953; Franks, 1954; Halpert & Schmalhorst, 1966; Lundberg & Berge, 1970). The prevalence of prostate cancer in these studies among men who were studied at autopsy but had no clinical evidence of the disease is high, with estimates ranging from 27% in men in their 30s to 34% of men in their 40s (Sakr *et al.*, 1993). Although most prostate cancers that are detected by PSA screening and are treated surgically have clinical significance to the patient (Epstein *et al.*, 1994; Ohori *et al.*, 1994), even tumours with a potentially poor prognosis may not lead to significant morbidity or mortality, particularly in older men. There is therefore controversy about what kind of treatment (if any) should be pursued in these cases (reviewed by Hoff & Pow-Sang, 2001). Furthermore, unnecessary treatments may result in morbidity that could be avoided if tumours that are destined to take an indolent course could be identified. Factors, including inherited genotype, that could predict who will have a poorer clinical outcome could therefore be of particular value in prostate cancer.

For example, Grönberg *et al.* (1997b) undertook a genetic linkage analysis of 74 hereditary prostate cancer families from North America, and compared prostate cancer characteristics in the linked and unlinked families. Linked families had a significantly earlier mean age at prostate cancer diagnosis than unlinked families. Tumours in the linked families were of higher grade and more advanced stage than in the unlinked families. Goddard *et al.* (2001) also found that detection of linkage to *HPC1* was enhanced when Gleason score was considered in the linkage model. These results suggest that *HPC1* confers not only susceptibility to develop prostate cancer, but also a propensity for more aggressive disease. Thus, *HPC1*-associated prostate cancers may have a different natural history from non-*HPC1* cancers.

Witte *et al.* (2000) undertook a genome-wide linkage analysis to identify genes associated with aggressiveness of prostate tumours. Using a sample of 513 brothers with prostate cancer, they undertook a genome-wide scan for genes associated with Gleason score. Those authors identified regions on chromosomes 5q, 7q and 19q as containing putative prostate cancer 'aggressiveness' genes. Although no gene has been isolated in these regions that could explain these results, the findings represent an approach to identify G_O that may confer clinically significant disease in some families.

There is limited evidence to date about the role of other G_O as modulators of the natural history or clinical outcome of prostate cancer. It is biologically plausible that G_O at a variety of loci may be associated with clinical outcome. For example, genes involved in androgen metabolism could modulate the bioavailability of androgens to prostate tumours, thus giving differential growth potential to some tumours. Despite reports that shorter polyglutamine repeat variants in AR are associated with tumour stage, grade or survival (Giovannucci et al., 1997; Ingles et al., 1997; Stanford et al., 1997; Nam et al., 2000), a relationship between AR alleles and prostate tumour characteristics has not been seen in all studies. Three studies reported no strong relationship of AR polymorphism with higher tumour stage or grade (Bratt et al., 1999; Edwards et al., 1999; Hsing et al., 2000). Nam et al. (2000) reported no overall association of short AR-CAG repeat length with survival, but they found that in low-grade and -stage cancers (i.e. those with generally favourable prognosis), the risk of recurrence was eightfold higher in men with shorter AR-CAG repeats than in men with longer repeats. Although there is some evidence that AR alleles are associated with differential stage, grade or survival, the inconsistencies among studies could be due to low power in some samples studied to detect effects when stratified by tumour characteristics.

Conclusions

Knowledge of the human genome provides a wealth of information about germline genetic variation. A challenge of molecular and genetic epidemiology is to relate these genotypes to biologically and clinically meaningful end-points. A series of classes of germline genotypes has been defined here to help focus the role that genotype data may have in the complex, multistage etiology and prevention of cancer. Defining these gene classes could elucidate the nature and timing of specific carcinogenic events, and may identify exposures that correlate with specific steps in carcinogenesis. Knowledge of these genotypes could also identify individuals for targeted risk evaluation, chemoprevention or treatment.

References

Baron, E. & Angrist, A. (1941) Incidence of occult adenocarcinoma of the prostate after 50 years of age. Arch. Pathol., 32, 787–793

Blazer, D.G., III, Umbach, D.M., Bostick, R.M. & Taylor J.A. (2000) Vitamin D receptor polymorphisms and prostate cancer. Mol. Carcinog., 27, 18–23

Bratt, O., Borg, A., Kristoffersson, U., Lundgren, R., Zhang, Q.X. & Olsson, H. (1999) CAG repeat length in the androgen receptor gene is related to age at diagnosis of prostate cancer and response to endocrine therapy, but not to prostate cancer risk. Br. J. Cancer, 81, 672–676

Cargill, M., Altshuler, D., Ireland, J., Sklar, P., Ardlie, K., Patil, N., Shaw, N., Lane, C.R., Lim, E.P., Kalyanaraman, N., Nemesh, J., Ziaugra, L., Friedland, L., Rolfe, A., Warrington, J., Lipshutz, R., Daley, G.Q. & Lander, E.S. (1999) Characterization of single-nucleotide polymorphisms in coding regions of human genes. Nat. Genet., 22, 231–238

Carter, B.S., Beaty, T.H., Steinberg, G.D., Childs, B. & Walsh P.C. (1992) Mendelian inheritance of familial prostate cancer. Proc. natl Acad. Sci. USA, 89, 3367–3371

Devlin, B. & Roeder, K. (1999) Genomic control for association studies. Biometrics, 55, 997–1004

Edwards, C., Steinthorsson, N. & Nicholson, D. (1953) An autopsy study of latent prostatic cancer. Cancer, 6, 531–554

Edwards, S.M., Badzioch, M.D., Minter, R., Hamoudi, R., Collins, N., Ardern-Jones, A., Dowe, A., Osborne, S., Kelly, J., Shearer, R., Easton, D.F., Saunders, G.F., Dearnaley, D.P. & Eeles, R.A. (1999) Androgen receptor polymorphisms: association with prostate cancer risk, relapse, and overall survival. Int. J. Cancer, 84, 458–465

Epstein, J.I., Carmichael, M.J., Partin, A.W. & Walsh, P.C. (1994) Small high grade adenocarcinoma of the prostate in radical prostatectomy specimens performed for nonpalpable disease: pathogenetic and clinical implications. *J. Urol.*, **151**, 1587–1592

Febbo, P.G., Kantoff, P.W., Platz, E.A., Casey, D., Batter, S., Giovannucci, E., Hennekens, C.H. & Stampfer, M.J. (1999) The V89L polymorphism in the 5alpha-reductase type 2 gene and risk of prostate cancer. *Cancer Res.*, **59**, 5878–5881

Feigelson, H.S., Coetzee, G.A., Kolonel, L.N., Ross, R.K. & Henderson, B.E. (1997a) A polymorphism in the *CYP17* gene increases the risk of prostate cancer. *Cancer Res.*, **57**, 1063–1065

Feigelson, H.S., Henderson, B.E. & Pike, M.C. (1997b) Re: Recent trends in U.S. breast cancer incidence, survival, and mortality rates. *J. natl Cancer Inst.*, **89**, 1810–1812

Franks, L.M. (1954) Latent carcinoma of the prostate. *J. Pathol. Bacteriol.*, **68**, 603–616

Giovannucci, E., Stampfer, M.J., Krithivas, K., Brown, M., Dahl, D., Brufsky, A., Talcott, J., Hennekens, C.H. & Kantoff, P.W. (1997) The CAG repeat within the androgen receptor gene and its relationship to prostate cancer. *Proc. natl Acad. Sci. USA*, **94**, 3320–3323

Goddard, K.A., Witte, J.S., Suarez, B.K., Catalona, W.J. & Olson, J.M. (2001) Model-free linkage analysis with covariates confirms linkage of prostate cancer to chromosomes 1 and 4. *Am. J. hum. Genet.*, **68**, 1197–1206

Goldstein, A.M. & Andrieu, N. (1999) Detection of interaction involving identified genes: available study designs. *Natl Cancer Inst. Monograph*, **26**, 49–54

Grönberg, H., Damber, L., Damber, J.E. & Iselius, L. (1997a) Segregation analysis of prostate cancer in Sweden: support for dominant inheritance. *Am. J. Epidemiol.*, **146**, 552–557

Grönberg, H., Xu, J., Smith, J.R., Carpten, J.D., Isaacs, S.D., Freije, D., Bova, G.S., Damber, J.E., Bergh, A., Walsh, P.C., Collins, F.S., Trent, J.M., Meyers, D.A. & Isaacs, W.B. (1997b) Early age at diagnosis in families providing evidence of linkage to the hereditary prostate cancer locus (*HPC1*) on chromosome 1. *Cancer Res.*, **57**, 4707–4709

Gsur, A., Bernhofer, G., Hinteregger, S., Haidinger, G., Schatzl, G., Madersbacher, S., Marberger, M.,

Vutuc, C. & Micksche, M. (2000) A polymorphism in the *CYP17* gene is associated with prostate cancer risk. *Int. J. Cancer*, **87**, 434–437

Habuchi, T., Liqing, Z., Suzuki, T., Sasaki, R., Tsuchiya, N., Tachiki, H., Shimoda, N., Satoh, S., Sato, K., Kakehi, Y., Kamoto, T., Ogawa, O. & Kato, T. (2000) Increased risk of prostate cancer and benign prostatic hyperplasia associated with a *CYP17* gene polymorphism with a gene dosage effect. *Cancer Res.*, **60**, 5710–5713

Haiman, C.A., Hankinson, S.E., Spiegelman, D., Colditz, G.A., Willett, W.C., Speizer, F.E., Kelsey, K.T. & Hunter, D.J. (1999) The relationship between a polymorphism in CYP17 with plasma hormone levels and breast cancer. *Cancer Res.*, **59**, 1015–1020

Halpert, B. & Schmalhorst, W.R. (1966) Carcinoma of the prostate in patients 70 to 79 years old. *Cancer*, **19**, 695–698

Helzlsouer, K.J., Huang, H.Y., Strickland, P.T., Hoffman, S., Alberg, A.J., Comstock, G.W. & Bell, D.A. (1998) Association between CYP17 polymorphisms and the development of breast cancer. *Cancer Epidemiol. Biomarkers Prev.*, **7**, 945–949

Hoff, B. & Pow-Sang, J.M. (2001) Observation in the management of localized prostate cancer. *Cancer Control*, **8**, 151–154

Hsing, A.W., Gao, Y.T., Wu, G., Wang, X., Deng, J., Chen, Y.L., Sesterhenn, I.A., Mostofi, F.K., Benichou, J. & Chang, C. (2000) Polymorphic *CAG* and *GGN* repeat lengths in the androgen receptor gene and prostate cancer risk: a population-based case–control study in China. *Cancer Res.*, **60**, 5111–5116

Ingles, S.A., Ross, R.K., Yu, M.C., Irvine, R.A., La Pera, G., Haile, R.W. & Coetzee, G.A. (1997) Association of prostate cancer risk with genetic polymorphisms in vitamin D receptor and androgen receptor. *J. natl Cancer Inst.*, **89**, 166–170

Iyer, L. & Ratain, M.J. (1998) Pharmacogenetics and cancer chemotherapy. *Eur. J. Cancer*, **34**, 1493–1499

Krynetski, E.Y. & Evans, W.E. (2000) Genetic polymorphism of thiopurine *S*-methyl-transferase: molecular mechanisms and clinical importance. *Pharmacology*, **61**, 136–146

Krynetski, E.Y., Tai, H.L., Yates, C.R., Fessing, M.Y., Loennechen, T., Schuetz, J.D., Relling, M.V. &

Evans, W.E. (1996) Genetic polymorphism of thiopurine *S*-methyltransferase: clinical importance and molecular mechanisms. *Pharmacogenetics*, **6**, 279–290

Latil, A. & Lidereau, R. (1998) Genetic aspects of prostate cancer. *Virchows Arch.*, **432**, 389–406

Lerman, C., Caporaso, N.E., Audrain, J., Main, D., Bowman, E.D., Lockshin, B., Boyd, N.R. & Shields, P.G. (1999) Evidence suggesting the role of specific genetic factors in cigarette smoking. *Health Psychol.*, **18**, 14–20

Lerman, C., Caporaso, N.E., Audrain, J., Main, D., Boyd, N.R. & Shields, P.G. (2000) Interacting effects of the serotonin transporter gene and neuroticism in smoking practices and nicotine dependence. *Mol. Psychiatr.*, **5**, 189–192

Lundberg, S. & Berge, T. (1970) Prostatic carcinoma. An autopsy study. *Scand. J. Urol. Nephrol.*, **4**, 93–97

Lunn, R.M., Bell, D.A., Mohler, J.L. & Taylor, J.A. (1999) Prostate cancer risk and polymorphism in 17 hydroxylase (*CYP17*) and steroid reductase (SRD5A2). *Carcinogenesis*, **20**, 1727–1731

Ma, J., Stampfer, M.J., Gann, P.H., Hough, H.L., Giovannucci, E., Kelsey, K.T., Hennekens, C.H. & Hunter, D.J. (1998) Vitamin D receptor polymorphisms, circulating vitamin D metabolites, and risk of prostate cancer in United States physicians. *Cancer Epidemiol. Biomarkers Prev.*, **7**, 385–390

Makridakis, N.M., Ross, R.K., Pike, M.C., Crocitto, L.E., Kolonel, L.N., Pearce, C.L., Henderson, B.E. & Reichardt, J.K. (1999) Association of missense substitution in SRD5A2 gene with prostate cancer in African-American and Hispanic men in Los Angeles, USA. *Lancet*, **354**, 975–978

Morganti, G., Gianferrari, L. & Cresseri, A. (1956) [Clinicostatistical and genetic studies of prostatic neoplasias.] *Acta gen. med. gem.*, **6**, 304–305 (in French)

Nam, R.K., Elhaji, Y., Krahn, M.D., Hakimi, J., Ho, M., Chu, W., Sweet, J., Trachtenberg, J., Jewett, M.A. & Narod, S.A. (2000) Significance of the CAG repeat polymorphism of the androgen receptor gene in prostate cancer progression. *J. Urol.*, **164**, 567–572

Nam, R.K., Toi, A., Vesprini, D., Ho, M., Chu, W., Harvie, S., Sweet, J., Trachtenberg, J., Jewett, M.A. & Narod, S.A. (2001) V89L polymorphism of type-2,5-alpha reductase enzyme gene predicts prostate cancer presence and progression. *Urology*, **57**, 199–204

Ohori, M., Goad, J.R., Wheeler, T.M., Eastham, J.A., Thompson, T.C. & Scardino, P.T. (1994) Can radical prostatectomy alter the progression of poorly differentiated prostate cancer? *J. Urol.*, **152**, 1843–1849

Ostrander, E.A. & Stanford, J.L. (2000) Genetics of prostate cancer: too many loci, too few genes. *Am. J. hum. Genet.*, **67**, 1367–1375

Otterness, D., Szumlanski, C., Lennard, L., Klemetsdal, B., Aarbakke, J., Park-Hah, J.O., Iven, H., Schmiegelow, K., Branum, E., O'Brien, J. & Weinshilboum, R. (1997) Human thiopurine methyltransferase pharmacogenetics: gene sequence polymorphisms. *Clin. Pharmacol. Ther.*, **62**, 60–73

Ozen, M. & Pathak, S. (2000) Genetic alterations in human prostate cancer: a review of current literature. *Anticancer Res.*, **20**, 1905–1912

Perera, F.P. & Weinstein, I.B. (1982) Molecular epidemiology and carcinogen–DNA adduct detection: new approaches to studies of human cancer causation. *J. chron. Dis.*, **35**, 581–600

Platz, E.A., Giovannucci, E., Dahl, D.M., Krithivas, K., Hennekens, C.H., Brown, M., Stampfer, M.J. & Kantoff, P.W. (1998) The androgen receptor gene GGN microsatellite and prostate cancer risk. *Cancer Epidemiol. Biomarkers Prev.*, **7**, 379–384

Pritchard, J.K. & Rosenberg, N.A. (1999) Use of unlinked genetic markers to detect population stratification in association studies. *Am. J. hum. Genet.*, **65**, 220–228

Rebbeck, T.R. (2001) Molecular epidemiology of prostate cancer. In: Greenlee, W.F., Samson, L. & Vanden Heuvel, J.P., eds, *Cellular and Molecular Toxicology*, New York, Elsevier

Rebbeck, T.R., Walker, A.H., Zeigler-Johnson, C., Weisburg, S., Martin, A.M., Nathanson, K.L., Wein, A.J. & Malkowicz, S. B. (2000) Association of *HPC2*/ELAC2 genotypes and prostate cancer. *Am. J. hum. Genet.*, **67**, 1014–1019

Sabol, S.Z., Nelson, M.L., Fisher, C., Gunzerath, L. Brody, C.L., Hu, S., Sirota, L.A., Marcus, S.E., Greenberg, B.D., Lucas, F.R., IV, Benjamin, J., Murphy, D.L. & Hamer, D.H. (1999) A genetic association for cigarette smoking behavior. *Health Psychol.*, **18**, 7–13

Sakr, W.A., Haas, G.P., Cassin, B.F., Pontes, J.E. & Crissman, J.D. (1993) The frequency of carcinoma and intraepithelial neoplasia of the prostate in young male patients. *J. Urol.*, **150**, 379–385

Schaid, D.J., McDonnell, S.K., Blute, M.L. & Thibodeau, S.N. (1998) Evidence for autosomal dominant inheritance of prostate cancer. *Am. J. hum. Genet.*, **62**, 1425–1438

Schulte, P.A. & Perera, F.P. (1993) *Molecular Epidemiology: Principles and Practices*, San Diego, Academic Press

Shields, P.G., Lerman, C., Audrain, J., Bowman, E.D., Main, D., Boyd, N.R. & Caporaso, N.E. (1998) Dopamine D4 receptors and the risk of cigarette smoking in African-Americans and Caucasians. *Cancer Epidemiol. Biomarkers Prev.*, **7**, 453–458

Smith, J.R., Freije, D., Carpten, J.D., Gronberg, H., Xu, J., Isaacs, S.D., Brownstein, M.J., Bova, G.S., Guo, H., Bujnovszky, P., Nusskern, D.R., Damber, J.E., Bergh, A., Emanuelsson, M., Kallioniemi, O.P., Walker-Daniels, J., Bailey-Wilson, J.E., Beaty, T.H., Meyers, D.A., Walsh, P.C., Collins, F.S., Trent, J.M. & Isaacs, W.B. (1996) Major susceptibility locus for prostate cancer on chromosome 1 suggested by a genome-wide search. *Science*, **274**, 1371–1374

Stanford, J.L., Just, J.J., Gibbs, M., Wicklund, K.G., Neal, C.L., Blumenstein, B.A. & Ostrander, E.A. (1997) Polymorphic repeats in the androgen receptor gene: molecular markers of prostate cancer risk. *Cancer Res.*, **57**, 1194–1198

Tavtigian, S.V., Simard, J., Teng, D.H., Abtin, V., Baumgard, M., Beck, A., Camp, N.J., Carillo, A.R., Chen, Y., Dayananth, P., Desrochers, M., Dumont, M., Farnham, J.M., Frank, D., Frye, C., Ghaffari, S., Gupte, J.S., Hu, R., Iliev, D., Janecki, T., Kort, E.N., Laity, K.E., Leavitt, A., Leblanc, G., McArthur-Morrison, J., Pederson, A., Penn, B., Peterson, K.T., Reid, J.E., Richards, S., Schroeder, M., Smith, R., Snyder, S.C., Swedlund, B., Swensen, J., Thomas, A., Tranchant, M., Woodland, A.M., Labrie, F., Skolnick, M.H., Neuhausen, S., Rommens, J. & Cannon-Albright, L.A. (2001) A candidate prostate cancer susceptibility gene at chromosome 17p. *Nat. Genet.*, **27**, 172–180

Taylor, J.A., Hirvonen, A., Watson, M., Pittman, G., Mohler, J.L. & Bell, D.A. (1996) Association of prostate cancer with vitamin D receptor gene polymorphism. *Cancer Res.*, **56**, 4108–4110

Vesprini, D., Nam, R.K., Trachtenberg, J., Jewett, M.A., Tavtigian, S.V., Emami, M., Ho, M., Toi, A. & Narod, S.A. (2001) HPC2 variants and screen-detected prostate cancer. *Am. J. hum. Genet.*, **68**, 912–917

Wacholder, S., Rothman, N. & Caporaso, N. (2000) Population stratification in epidemiologic studies of common genetic variants and cancer: quantification of bias. *J. natl Cancer Inst.*, **92**, 1151–1158

Wadelius, M., Andersson, A.O., Johansson, J. E., Wadelius, C. & Rane, E. (1999) Prostate cancer associated with *CYP17* genotype. *Pharmacogenetics*, **9**, 635–639

Weston, A., Pan, C.F., Bleiweiss, I.J., Ksieski, H.B., Roy, N., Maloney, N. & Wolff, M.S. (1998) CYP17 genotype and breast cancer risk. *Cancer Epidemiol. Biomarkers Prev.*, **7**, 941–944

Witte, J.S., Goddard, K.A., Conti, D.V., Elston, R.C., Lin, J., Suarez, B.K., Broman, K.W., Burmester, J.K., Weber, J.L. & Catalona, W.J. (2000) Genome-wide scan for prostate cancer-aggressiveness loci. *Am. J. hum. Genet.*, **67**, 92–99

Xu, J., Zheng, S.L., Chang, B., Smith, J.R., Carpten, J.D., Stine, O.C., Isaacs, S.D., Wiley, K.E., Henning, L., Ewing, C., Bujnovszky, P., Bleeker, E.R., Walsh, P.C., Trent, J.M., Meyers, D.A. & Isaacs, W.B. (2001a) Linkage of prostate cancer susceptibility loci to chromosome 1. *Hum. Genet.*, **108**, 335–345

Xu, J., Zheng, S.L., Hawkins, G.A., Faith, D.A., Kelly, B., Isaacs, S.D., Wiley, K.E., Chang, B., Ewing, C.M., Bujnovszky, P., Carpten, J.D., Bleeker, E.R., Walsh, P.C., Trent, J.M., Meyers, D.A. & Isaacs, W.B. (2001b) Linkage and association studies of prostate cancer susceptibility: evidence for linkage at 8p22–23. *Am. J. hum. Genet.*, **69**, 341–350

Xu, J., Zheng, S.L., Carpten, J.D., Nupponen, N.N., Robbins, C.M., Mestre, J., Moses, T.Y., Faith, D.A., Kelly, B.D., Isaacs, S.D., Wiley, K.E., Ewing, C.M., Bujnovszky, P., Chang, B., Bailey-Wilson, J., Bleeker, E.R., Walsh, P.C., Trent, J.M., Meyers, D.A. & Isaacs, W.B. (2001c) Evaluation of linkage and association of HPC2/ELAC2 in patients with familial or sporadic prostate cancer. *Am. J. hum. Genet.*, **68**, 901–911

Corresponding author:

Timothy R. Rebbeck
Department of Biostatistics and Epidemiology,
Center for Clinical Epidemiology and Biostatistics,
and Cancer Center, University of Pennsylvania
School of Medicine, 904 Blockley Hall,
423 Guardian Drive, Philadelphia, PA 19104-6021,
USA
trebbeck@cceb.med.upenn.edu

Mechanisms of Carcinogenesis: Contributions of Molecular Epidemiology
Patricia Buffler, Jerry Rice, Robert Baan, Michael Bird and Paolo Boffetta, eds
IARC Scientific Publications No. 157
International Agency for Research on Cancer, Lyon, 2004

Toxicological Considerations in the Application and Interpretation of Susceptibility Biomarkers in Epidemiological Studies

Anneclaire J. De Roos, Martyn T. Smith, Stephen Chanock
and Nathaniel Rothman

Summary

With major advances in genotyping technology, it has become practical and affordable to screen biological samples for multiple polymorphisms for which there is more or less knowledge about their functional relevance in relation to toxicological agents or disease. This situation creates some unique epidemiological challenges in which careful consideration of the mechanisms underlying genotype–disease and genotype–exposure–disease relationships, or the lack of knowledge thereof, may help to prevent false-positive results or misinterpretation of data that could mislead future research. Coordination and linkage of data resources on toxicological exposures, genes and disease would be useful as an integrated source of information to devise study design, analysis and interpretation. Such a database could be useful in collating information from which to determine relevant exposures for the disease and to guide the selection of susceptibility markers for study. Further information on toxicological mechanisms and functional relevance of gene variants in relation to disease could be accounted for in statistical analyses and interpretation. Statistical methods that can incorporate this prior information on mechanism, such as hierarchical regression modelling, may help to mitigate some of the problems inherent to these studies by adjusting estimates and confidence limits according to this prior information. Even in the situation where little information on etiological mechanisms is available, application of a less informed prior can be beneficial in improving the accuracy and
precision for an ensemble of estimates. The changing paradigm of epidemiological research with regard to increasing detail of underlying mechanisms and the sheer amount of data being evaluated necessitates access to sources of information and analytic methods that can integrate this complexity.

Introduction

Application of susceptibility biomarkers in epidemiological studies holds some potential for elucidating underlying toxicological mechanisms. Conversely, knowledge about toxicological mechanisms can aid in planning and interpretation of studies using susceptibility markers. These studies have allowed scientists to start asking new types of questions about toxicological effects. There is a hope that exposure–disease associations, which may be controversial because of small magnitude of the relative risks, will be clarified by discerning susceptible subpopulations. The annotation of the genome, which, so far, has focused on the discovery and validation of the single-nucleotide polymorphism (SNP), has resulted in an exponential increase in SNPs; it is estimated that there are between 2 and 11 million common SNPs (i.e. with a frequency of greater than 1%). With major advances in genotyping technology, it has become practical and affordable to analyse multiple polymorphisms in DNA from biological samples of various types and qualities (e.g. blood, buccal cells). No longer restricted to analysis of a single polymorphism of interest that is thought to interact with a toxicological agent, these new genotyping capabilities allow investigators to screen multiple gene variants for which there may be more or less knowledge about their relevance in relation to toxicological agents and disease. Given that most chronic diseases probably arise from a complex and often poorly understood combination of multiple genetic and environmental factors, a broad-based approach in which multiple associations are screened could be beneficial in building more realistic models of disease.

Within this new paradigm lie some unique epidemiological challenges. New considerations must be applied to study design, analysis and interpretation of epidemiological studies that are becoming more complicated with such an unprecedented amount of data. It is particularly important to overcome these challenges in the situation where genotypes are evaluated on the basis of little prior information of functional significance in relation to toxicological agents or disease. Presumably, scientists will look toward results of such preliminary studies for guidance in focusing future research. False-positive results due to chance will unavoidably occur, leading investigators astray. Although improved genotyping capabilities make rapid replication of study results possible in order to negate false positives, the limiting factor will be attaining access to epidemiological study populations with biological samples. Careful consideration of the toxicological mechanisms underlying genotype–disease and genotype–exposure–disease relationships, or consideration of the lack of knowledge, may help to prevent false-positive results or misinterpretation of data, leading to thoughtful pursuit of refined hypotheses in subsequent studies.

Data resources

Currently, the fields of genetics and toxicology are both undergoing substantial change, primarily as a consequence of the first draft sequence of the human genome. There is a strong research need for a database incorporating the various types of data that are available separately and which could be brought to bear on the selection of genes and pathways in the study of toxicological agents and disease. Attempts to organize integrated databases

have lagged significantly behind the generation of data. An ideal database could guide investigators in the design, analysis and interpretation of epidemiological studies incorporating susceptibility markers. Specifically, it would be useful to guide researchers through the process of identifying important genes for a specific toxicological agent and disease of interest. In doing so, it could present reliable information on gene function, SNPs and other variants in those genes, and functional consequences of the variants. Furthermore, the database could include information on toxicological mechanisms and toxicokinetics for the main exposure of interest and for other exposures that are important because of their associations with disease or gene function. These data would be useful for consideration in the study design phase, and could be accounted for in statistical analyses. The database could thus be designed to provide cutting edge information on the paradigm of exposure–gene–disease (E-G-D database). For example, in planning a study on exposure to benzene as a risk factor for leukaemia, a search of the proposed E-G-D database could result in the type of information listed in Table 1. In addition to text and tables containing such information, contributions from leading toxicologists could include diagrams depicting metabolic pathways for toxicological agents such as benzene (Figure 1). In addition to metabolic pathways, downstream pathways through which the toxicological agent is thought to affect the disease process would also be described in the database, including processes such as DNA repair, immune function and cell-cycle control, with database links to aid in identification of variants in relevant genes involved in those pathways.

Before creating a new database, it is essential to take stock of those that are currently publicly available, primarily for the purpose of connecting reliable resources (database links are provided in Table 2). There are several toxicology databases containing detailed information on biological effects of toxicological agents. Useful examples include the National Library of Medicine's (NLM) Toxline, the National Institute for Occupational Safety and Health's (NIOSH) Registry of Toxic Effects of Chemical Substances (RTECS),

Table 1. Types of information to be obtained from a search on 'benzene and leukaemia' in the proposed E-G-D database

Feature	Result	Other lists or links
Benzene	(search item)	Toxicokinetic data on general distribution and metabolism of benzene in the human body and mechanism of action
Leukaemia	(search item)	Known or suspected risk factors for leukaemia to consider in study design
Genes	Genes affecting or affected by benzene exposure, e.g. *CYP2E1*, *NQO1*	Other genes potentially relevant for leukaemia (not necessarily relevant for benzene)
Gene function	Function of gene in relation to toxicological agent of interest, e.g.: *CYP2E1*: phase I metabolism; converts benzene to phenol *NQO1*: converts toxic benzoquinones to less toxic polyphenols Factors which affect gene expression, e.g. *CYP2E1*: alcohol, obesity (McCarver *et al.*, 1998)	Toxicokinetic data on relevant metabolic reactions Data on expression in key organs Exposures affecting gene function and exposures involved in same pathway as benzene
Polymorphisms	Identified polymorphisms for genes of interest, e.g.: *CYP2E1*: *RsaI*, *Ins96* *NQO1*: ^{609}C→T mutation	Genomic information necessary to perform genotyping assays
Effect of polymorphism on gene function	Information on effect of polymorphisms on gene function, e.g.: *CYP2E1*: unknown functional significance of polymorphisms — phenotype may be more relevant for epidemiological studies *NQO1*: complete loss of enzyme activity among homozygous variants	Expression and proteomic data Toxicokinetic data for a given genotype and substrate

the Agency for Toxic Substances and Disease Registry's (ATSDR) Toxicological Profiles and the US National Toxicology Program (NTP) databases. Currently, these resources do not provide a comprehensive overview of the functional pathways of genes thought to be involved in disease processes relevant for a specific toxicological agent; nor do the databases contain information on the effects of exposures on expression of genetic pathways.

Similarly, none of the SNP databases contains comprehensive information addressing the functional significance of SNPs, especially in relation to toxicological agents, or the effects of exposures on the function of variant genotypes. From the

National Center for Biotechnology (NCBI) website, one can access the public version of the draft of the genome as well as many analytical sites for genetic analyses. LocusLink, curated by NCBI, is a central public database for genes that provide links to gene structure, location, known sequence and common variants. Also linked to the NCBI site is the international database, db-SNP, a central repository for putative SNPs that is fed by a series of public databases which include sequence data, either directly generated in re-sequencing projects or derived from computer algorithms that examine public databases in search of possible SNPs. Several public efforts within the National Cancer Institute (NCI) have

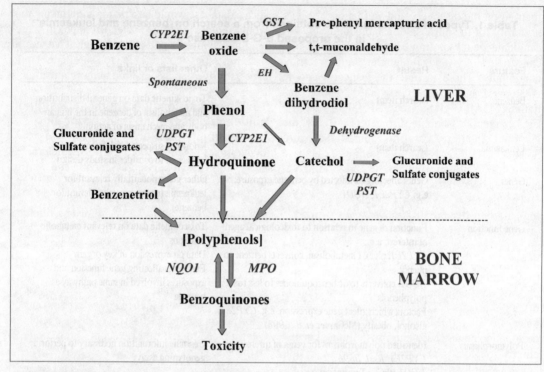

Figure 1. Pathways of benzene metabolism in the human body

Table 2. Existing databases containing information on toxicology and genes

Toxicology

National Toxicology Program (NTP) databases (http://ntp-server.niehs.nih.gov) including the Report on Carcinogens (RoC) and Chemical Health & Safety Information

Agency for Toxic Substances and Disease Registry's Toxicological Profiles (http://www.atsdr.cdc.gov/toxpro2.html)

National Library of Medicine's Toxnet databases (http://toxnet.nlm.nih.gov) including Toxline and Gene-Tox

National Institute for Occupational Safety and Health's (NIOSH) Registry of Toxic Effects of Chemical Substances (RTECS) (http://www.cdc.gov/niosh/rtecs.html)

Genes

National Center for Biotechnology Information (NCBI) databases (http://www.ncbi.nlm.nih.gov) including LocusLink, RefSeq, and dbSNP

Environmental Genome Project (EGP) of the National Institute for Environmental Health Sciences (NIEHS) (http://www.niehs.nih.gov/envgenom/home.htm)

Cancer Genome Anatomy Project - Genetic Annotation Initiative (CGAP-GAI) (http://lpg.nci.nih.gov/GAI/)

Online Mendelian Inheritance in Man (OMIM) (http://www3.ncbi.nlm.nih.gov/Omim/searchomim.html)

Human Genome Epidemiology Network (HuGENet) (http://www.cdc.gov/genetics/hugenet/)

The SNP Consortium Ltd (http://snp.cshl.org/)

focused on the discovery and validation of SNPs primarily for the purpose of establishing SNPs in candidate genes of immediate relevance to the cancer biology and molecular epidemiology community. These include the Cancer Genome Anatomy Project – the Genetic Annotation Initiative (CGAP-GAI) and the SNP500 project. The Environmental Genome Project (EGP) of the National Institute for Environmental Health Sciences (NIEHS) is also developing a database cataloguing polymorphisms in environmental response genes, based on resequencing efforts.

The next step is to attach functional or biological significance to known gene variants. Several ongoing projects, such as NIEHS's EGP and Microarray Center, are focused on evaluating the function of genes and gene variants in relation to toxicological agents. The most comprehensive database containing information on the function of gene variants is the Online Mendelian Inheritance in Man (OMIM™) database. OMIM is designed to conduct searches by individual genes, clinical outcomes or exposures. Search results contain summarized text about gene function, gene variants and epidemiological studies pertaining to the gene, with links to the published literature via PubMed (http://www4.ncbi.nlm.nih.gov/entrez/query.fcgi). A similar resource is being developed by the Centers for Disease Control (CDC) Human Genome Epidemiology Network (HuGENet). The emphasis of these databases is on compiling comprehensive information about genetic associations with disease; toxicological exposures are represented, but not as a primary organizing principle for the databases.

The proposed E-G-D database could be a useful resource for epidemiologists in providing information to consider when designing studies and for interpreting data on susceptibility markers and disease. Although many parts of such a database already exist, the three major axes — exposures, genes, and disease — are not at present linked together in a useful way. The creation of such a database could provide a valuable framework for organizing information generated from ongoing projects researching toxicology, gene variants and their functional significance in relation to disease. However, development of

such a database would be a major undertaking that would require continued scientific input in screening and synthesizing data, although advances in bioinformatics could help to automate some aspects of the data acquisition and organization.

Toxicological considerations in design of epidemiological studies incorporating susceptibility markers

In addition to the typical concerns of epidemiological study design (e.g. unbiased case and control selection), there are some important considerations inherent to studies incorporating susceptibility markers. New considerations include choosing which susceptibility markers to study. In addition, factors such as exposure measurement take on new importance when a major focus of studies is to examine genotype–exposure interactions. However, the level of detail for such considerations will depend on existing prior information on the mechanism of disease etiology relating to toxicological agents and genetic pathways.

Studies with little prior information on toxicological mechanism

There are diseases for which no specific toxicological agent is suspected as a cause. In some instances clues from the occupational epidemiology literature indicate that certain occupations are at high risk of a disease (e.g. farm work as a risk factor for adult brain cancer (Inskip et al., 1995), but no specific exposure within the job has been identified as a probable risk factor. In such a situation, examination of a wide range of susceptibility markers can be usefully applied to home in on relevant etiological pathways (e.g. phase I or phase II metabolic pathways, DNA repair, cell-cycle control). In this way, if associations are observed with gene variants in a certain pathway, new hypotheses concerning groups of compounds that are known to affect, or be affected by, those pathways could be further investigated.

The proposed E-G-D database could be used in such a situation by simply conducting a search on the disease to be studied (e.g. glioma). The database could retrieve potentially relevant gene families for study, on the basis of observations from mechanistic studies of disease. For example, observations that lymphocytes from patients with glioma have a higher sensitivity to a mutagenic dose of ionizing radiation (Bondy et al., 2001) may prompt investigation into the relevance of genes involved in DNA repair. Furthermore, genes involved in the metabolism of exogenous compounds (phase I and phase II) could be important upstream of the DNA repair pathway, and would also warrant study in this situation. In this way, the E-G-D database could provide a forum for synthesis of such mechanistic information to help researchers identify potentially relevant gene families for a specific disease. It would thus differ from existing databases which catalogue existing literature on already observed associations between genotype and disease, but do not include input from studies of potential mechanisms.

Studies with strong hypotheses of underlying toxicological mechanisms

Choosing susceptibility markers: Benzene has been declared a known human leukaemogen (IARC, 1982; McMichael, 1988), and incorporation of susceptibility markers into future studies on benzene and leukaemia will probably help to elucidate further the underlying toxicological mechanism. In this type of situation, where a specific agent is already known or suspected to be a risk factor for disease, it is critical to consider existing knowledge about the underlying toxicology, such as that provided by the proposed E-G-D database (in Table 1 and Figure 1), when choosing susceptibility markers for study. A visual representation of the metabolic pathways of benzene (Figure 1) makes it clear that it is important to study not only genes involved in the initial metabolic step (*CYP2E1*), but also those genes that play a role later in the metabolic pathway (*GSTs, EH, PST, UDPGT, NQO1* and *MPO*). Other pathways downstream from benzene metabolism but relevant to toxicity may be critical in the disease process, including DNA repair, immune function and cell-cycle control, and it would also be important to consider genes in these pathways. After important genes and their functions have been identified, the E-G-D database could provide links to catalogues of poly-

morphisms in those genes and functional information about variants, in order to judge their relevance for the exposure–disease hypothesis under study. For example, the *CYP2E1 Rsa*1 and *Ins*96 polymorphisms, which may decrease (Marchand et al., 1999) or increase (McCarver et al., 1998) CYP2E1 activity, respectively, would each be valid candidates to study since this phase I step is crucial to benzene metabolism. In addition, the *NQO1* [609]C→T mutation, which results in a complete loss of enzyme activity among homozygotes, would be an important variant to study in order to characterize the crucial metabolic step of conversion of toxic benzoquinones back to less toxic polyphenols (Rothman et al., 1997). After candidate gene variants are identified, further links in the E-G-D database could lead the researcher to sites in which bioinformatics information necessary for conducting the genotyping assays would be located.

Exposure measurement: Choosing relevant susceptibility markers for study is important, but equally careful consideration must be given to exposure measurement. It is crucial to obtain a high-quality exposure measure of any toxicological agent for which genotype–exposure interaction is of primary interest. Although physical or biological measures of exposure may be useful in characterizing a subject's exposure status at one point in time, it should be recognized that studies of diseases with a long latency period, such as cancer, should ideally integrate different types of exposure information including questionnaire data, historical records and geographically linked databases. Thoughtful modelling of biological exposure measures should recognize that such measures already reflect some of the genotypic variability in metabolism between individuals; therefore, assessment of genotype–exposure interaction may not be appropriate in some instances.

In the design phase of studies incorporating susceptibility markers, it is critical to consider certain exposures other than the main toxicological agent of interest. It is important to collect information on factors that may act through the same genetic pathway as the main exposure. For example, in addition to benzene, other industrial solvents such as styrene and carbon tetrachloride are metabolized via the CYP2E1 pathway (Stubbins & Wolf, 1999). Therefore, studies of genotype–exposure interaction of benzene and variants in CYP2E1 should ideally include measurement of other solvents suspected to be common in the population, particularly those exposures which frequently occur together with benzene in occupational settings, in order to consider potential confounding or to create an integrated exposure measure. Other exposures may not act through the same pathway as the main toxicological agent of interest, but may affect, or be affected by, the pathway. It is important to consider factors that may affect the phenotypic response of interest, either through induction of gene expression or by affecting post-transcriptional- or post-translational processing. For example, CYP2E1 activity appears to be induced by alcohol consumption and obesity (McCarver et al., 1998; Marchand et al., 1999), and studies of CYP2E1 polymorphisms should take these factors into account as potential effect modifiers of genotype effects. It is critically important to consider all such extraneous factors in the study design phase, so that adequate information can be collected to allow evaluation of potential confounding or effect modification in the analysis phase. The proposed E-G-D database could be used to improve exposure measurement planning by listing, for a given disease and gene of interest, exposures potentially relevant to the disease that are known to affect, or be affected by, the gene's expression.

Using toxicological information in analysing and interpreting epidemiological studies incorporating susceptibility markers

Epidemiological studies incorporating susceptibility markers will have a wide range of analytic aims. The proposed E-G-D database could be useful in addressing these aims by providing information relevant for statistical analysis and interpretation of specific genotype or genotype–exposure effects.

Estimating genotype-specific effects without prior information on toxicological mechanism
If no specific toxicological agent is known or suspected to be a risk factor for a disease, association of gene variants with the disease can provide some clues about underlying disease mechanisms and groups of compounds that could be important in the etiological pathway. However, because the number of toxicological agents affected by or affecting a certain pathway is generally large, this strategy is likely to be of limited utility for identifying specific exposures as etiological agents. For example, because of the low degree of substrate specificity of genes such as *GSTP1*, observed associations between polymorphisms in *GSTP1* and a certain disease could indicate any of a variety of potential toxicological risk factors, including solvents, pesticides or components present in cigarette smoke (Strange & Fryer, 1999). Another consideration relates to the fact that an observed association between one variant and disease may actually result from its linkage disequilibrium with another polymorphism located nearby on the same chromosome. Statistical methods aimed at analysing haplotype instead of genotype may overcome some of this difficulty, since haplotypes may be more specific markers of common inherited genetic variation than any single polymorphism (Johnson et al., 2001). Although the inherent uncertainty of haplotype assignments for unrelated individuals may somewhat dilute their possibly greater information content, there have recently been some promising reports concerning the accuracy and predictive value of estimated haplotype frequencies (Fallin & Schork, 2000; Fallin et al., 2001).

Screening large numbers of genotypes or haplotypes for their associations with disease is likely to pose problems of false-positive findings and sparse data resulting in imprecise estimates. Without any context of a hypothesized underlying etiological mechanism, results from such studies will be difficult to interpret. Statistical methods in which this lack of specific prior information is taken into account offer some potential as an alternative to unstructured modelling of multiple variables (see 'Integrating prior toxicological information into analyses of multiple exposures', below).

Genotype–exposure interaction

Studies of genotype–exposure interaction can provide clues about susceptible subpopulations and toxicological mechanisms of disease. Because of increasing feasibility and affordability of genotyping and the fact that larger epidemiological studies are supporting more intensive statistical analyses, epidemiologists are evaluating potential interactions more than ever, even when there are no prior hypotheses about interaction. Some important analytical issues have recently re-emerged.

Exposure assessment and definition: Examination of genotype–exposure interaction places a new importance on defining relevant exposures, and this is a topic that should be revisited with serious consideration of the underlying toxicological mechanism. Improving exposure assessment should focus on decreasing misclassification, since even small amounts of exposure misclassification can not only bias the effect estimate for exposure, but can also substantially bias the estimate of the joint genotype–exposure effect (Rothman *et al.*, 1999). Efforts to decrease misclassification should take the prevalence of the exposure of interest into consideration. In studies where the prevalence of exposures is low (< 15%), a true positive association of the exposure can be substantially attenuated by even small numbers of individuals incorrectly non-differentially classified as exposed, whereas an equal proportion of individuals incorrectly classified as unexposed will contribute little bias to the estimate; in this scenario the focus should be on increasing specificity of exposure measures, whereas increasing sensitivity of exposure measures may be more important in situations where the prevalence of exposure is high (Flegal *et al.*, 1986; Dosemeci & Stewart, 1996).

Exposures of interest should be defined in such a way as to represent the most relevant exposure to the disease end-point of interest. Refinement of the definition of exposure should focus on the type, duration, intensity and timing of exposure.

The type of exposure refers to the specificity of the exposure measure. For example, because many solvents have different toxicological properties, a crudely defined categorical exposure to solvents is likely to cause reduced power to detect a genotype–exposure effect if only a few specific types of solvents are truly associated with the disease. For most toxicological agents thought to cause cancer, the longest and most intense exposures are likely to be of importance, although this cannot always be assumed to be the case. The relevant timing of exposure will vary depending on the hypothesized mechanism; early- versus late-stage carcinogenesis should be considered. A putative biochemical mechanism by which toxicological agents exert their effects is related to the actual dose of the active carcinogenic metabolite that reaches the genome in the target cell, so toxicokinetic data relating the external exposure level to a dose at the target site may be useful in defining estimates of dose rather than simply exposure. For example, because the phase I reaction by CYP2E1 converting benzene to its metabolic by-products occurs in the liver, a more refined measure of benzene exposure could take toxicokinetic data on uptake, elimination and transport through the body into account in order to estimate a relevant dose of benzene in liver tissue. Factors relating to variability in toxicokinetics (e.g. body mass index, age) could be useful in incorporating some measures of interindividual variability into dose estimates. Because the internal dose at the target site is also related to the activity of multiple genes involved in metabolic pathways, more sophisticated toxicokinetic modelling takes genotypes at critical loci into account. With a well-described toxicokinetic model, an estimate of each individual's internal dose that integrates their constellation of exposures and metabolic activities specific to their genotypes could obviate the need to assess genotype–exposure interaction, instead allowing direct modelling of an integrated measure of metabolic product at the target site. Cortessis and Thomas (this volume) describe such a physiologically based pharmacokinetic (PBPK) modelling approach. In most cases, however, the detailed toxicokinetic data required for such modelling will not be available, and a simple assessment of genotype and external exposure will be the logical analytical approach.

Estimating and interpreting interaction: A simple question that scientists want to answer in studies of toxicological agents and genotypes is 'Does the effect of exposure differ between persons with different genotypes?' Presentation of the absolute risk of exposure within people of each genotype is a straightforward way to conceive the comparison that is being made when testing statistical interaction. Since the absolute risk cannot be calculated directly using case–control data, the relative effects of exposure in each stratum of genotype are often presented; however, because the magnitude of the relative effects is dependent on the underlying incidence of the disease in each stratum, a direct comparison between relative effect measures can sometimes be misleading (Thompson, 1991). Thus, comparison of the joint and individual effects of the gene variant and exposure using a common referent becomes essential for evaluating interaction.

There is a recurring debate and some misunderstanding of whether statistical interaction should be tested using an additive or multiplicative joint effect as the null hypothesis. Because of the ease of testing for interaction on the multiplicative scale by including product terms in logistic regression models, it has become the standard. However, the choice of either scale as the null is based on underlying assumptions, and simply noting the p-value from a test of interaction may cause the scientist to miss valuable information. For example, a joint effect that is exactly multiplicative (therefore indicating no statistical interaction on the multiplicative scale) is likely to be considerably more than additive, and may be of biological or public health importance. Emphasis on detecting interaction may also inhibit useful description of relationships that fit well using an additive or multiplicative model. Issues and guidelines for testing and reporting of statistical interactions have been discussed in detail elsewhere (Botto & Khoury, 2001), and are not extensively reviewed here. Despite the choice of whether or not to conduct a formal statistical test, or whether to declare an additive or multiplicative

joint effect as the null hypothesis, it is useful to present the results of individual and joint effects in a 2×4 table, as described by Botto and Khoury (2001), since this straightforward presentation highlights important aspects of the data, and allows other measures of interest to be calculated from it. This presentation, however, applies to the situation in which dichotomization of exposure is appropriate; another format would be necessary if a toxicological exposure had a linear relationship with disease. Nevertheless, a simple presentation of effects is important because most of the existing studies are underpowered on either scale to test for interactions of probably modest effects; therefore, the estimated effects are all that remains to inform scientists about the direction for future research.

After careful consideration of exposure definition and assessment of joint and individual effects, researchers are left with the challenge of interpreting results. Some scientists have postulated different underlying biological mechanisms for interpretation of joint effects that are observed to fall anywhere along the spectrum relative to additivity or multiplicativity; others have pointed out that data fitting any specific statistical model could potentially have multiple explanations because of the unknown nature of underlying pathological processes and unmeasured intervening variables (Thompson, 1991). Therefore, although such models can be useful in providing clues about underlying toxicological mechanisms, they offer no means for obtaining definitive information. Interpretation may seem clear in an extreme case for which the effect of one factor appears to be entirely dependent on the presence of the other factor, or when 'cross-over effects' are observed in which the direction of an association is reversed across different levels of one factor. But even in such extreme cases, nothing more than hypotheses about underlying mechanisms can be derived from estimated effects (Thompson, 1991). The role of chance and error inherent to epidemiological studies also cannot be ruled out as an explanation of observed statistical interaction. Replication thus becomes extremely important in providing a basis for developing hypotheses about results indicating subtle interactive effects. Replication in different study populations can offer valuable insight into associations within the context of differing exposure scenarios and co-factors. In addition, pooling of studies, where appropriate, can offer greater statistical power to detect interaction. Epidemiological findings of interactive effects, once established, can then provide some direction for toxicological research, where hypotheses about underlying toxicological mechanisms of genotype–exposure effects can be tested in animal or in-vitro systems.

Integrating prior toxicological information into analyses of multiple exposures

Because genotyping has become more accessible and affordable, many researchers will pursue the objective of screening multiple 'exposures' (e.g. genotypes, haplotypes or genotype–exposure combinations) as potential risk factors for cancer. Since each person is exposed to a combination of genotypes and toxicological agents that may be associated with each other in the population, multiple exposures should in many cases be modelled simultaneously to account for their probable correlation. Although conventional methods of estimating effects (such as maximum likelihood estimation) are informative in providing clues about the direction of effects, the accuracy and precision of estimates calculated using these methods may be inadequate. Where data are sparse, as is often the case when studying low-frequency genotypes, imprecision of estimates can hinder interpretation. In addition, some estimates will be very inaccurate, as a result of either chance or systematic error. Small datasets will also limit the number of parameters that can be fitted using conventional statistical methods. Since the results of preliminary studies will probably be used to define a focus for further research, it is important to minimize the total error in estimating associations of multiple genotypes or genotype–exposure combinations with disease.

Hierarchical regression using empirical or semi-Bayes methods provides some advantage over frequentist methods when modelling multiple exposures, by using prior information on the similarities between exposure effects to adjust estimates (Greenland, 1994; Greenland & Poole,

1994; Witte *et al.*, 1994). In theory, frequentist regression models objective functional relations among measured variables, whereas Bayesian regression brings subjectivity into the modelling process by incorporating data that may be informative in explaining the variation between exposures and the outcome (Greenland, 1997). These methods allow the researcher to specify prior distributions for the true effects, or distributions from which the true effect parameters are assumed to arise (Dunson, 2001). For example, in a study of the effects of multiple gene variants on disease, the researcher may assume *a priori* that the true effects of the gene variants arise from a distribution that is more constrained than the set of observed effects (i.e. the estimated beta coefficients) (Figure 2); separate prior distributions could alternatively be defined for the true effects of individual gene variants. In empirical Bayes and semi-Bayes analyses, prior information about factors that are hypothesized to determine or explain the magnitude of the true effect parameters can be used to specify the form of the prior distributions, whose magnitudes are then estimated. Such prior information could include various factors such as results from previous studies or characteristics of the genotypes or genotype–exposure combinations that are postulated to relate to the underlying etiological mechanisms. Effect estimates and confidence limits are then adjusted according to the prior distributions, generally resulting in improved accuracy and precision for an ensemble of estimates (Greenland 1994, 2000a; Steenland *et al.*, 2000). Hierarchical regression, also called multilevel, multistage or random coefficient modelling, has been described extensively (Greenland, 1994, 2000a,b), but has not been applied frequently in studies of susceptibility markers and disease. Use of these methods has been hindered in part by the lack of simple software for hierarchical regression modelling; however, S-Plus or SAS Proc GLIMMIX can be adapted to this purpose (Steenland *et al.*, 2000; Witte *et al.*, 2000).

The method can be conceptualized as a multilevel model (see Figure 3) (Witte *et al.*, 1994), although different levels of the model can be solved simultaneously using iterative procedures

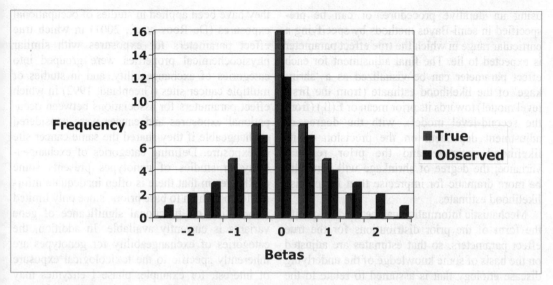

Figure 2. Example of prior and observed distributions of betas from a study of the effects of multiple gene variants on disease

- **First-level model: log (p / 1-p) = Xβ + Wγ**

- **Second-level model: β = Zπ + 0**
  - **Model predicts E(β_j) for any combination of prior covariates**

- **Posterior estimates:**
  - **Adjustment of first-level estimate toward E(β), with degree of shrinkage determined by variance of first-level estimate and prior residual variance**

Where: **p = risk of disease in the population, X = matrix of exposures, β = vector of logistic coefficients for exposures, W = matrix of covariates, γ = vector of logistic coefficients for covariates, Z = matrix of prior covariates, π = vector of coefficients for prior covariates, 0 = vector of residual variation terms, E(β_j) = expected value of beta for each exposure.**

Figure 3. Multilevel models in hierarchical regression analysis

such as penalized likelihood (Witte *et al.*, 2000). In the first-level model, disease outcome is regressed on multiple exposures (*X*; e.g. geno-types, haplotypes or genotype–exposure combinations) and any potential confounders (*W*; e.g. age, sex) to calculate maximum likelihood estimates for the exposures of interest. The beta coefficients from the first level (β_j, for each exposure) are then modelled as values of an outcome variable in a second-level linear regression model, as a function of second-level or 'prior' covariates (*Z*) that

are thought to determine the magnitude of the true effect parameters. A prior distribution for each true effect parameter is inferred from this second-level model by calculation of an expected value of beta, E(β_j), or prior mean, for each exposure, based on its values for the prior covariates. The prior distribution also includes a value for the prior residual variance, which represents effects of the exposures above and beyond effects accounted for by the second-level prior covariates; it is estimated in empirical Bayes methods using an iterative procedure, or can be pre-specified in semi-Bayes methods by specifying a particular range in which the true effect parameter is expected to lie. The final adjustment for each effect parameter can be visualized as a 'shrinkage' of the likelihood estimate (from the first-level model) towards its prior mean or $E(\beta_j)$ (from the second-level model), with the degree of adjustment dependent on the precision of its likelihood estimate and the prior residual variance; the degree of shrinkage will generally be more dramatic for imprecise than for precise likelihood estimates.

Mechanistic information can be used to specify the form of the prior distributions for the true effect parameters, so that estimates are adjusted on the basis of some knowledge of the underlying disease etiology that is assumed to relate to the magnitude of effects. In the simple case, indicator variables can be used to represent subsets of true effect parameters within which parameters can be regarded as 'exchangeable' or as drawn from a common prior distribution (Greenland, 1994, 2000a). This definition could conceivably be applied to groups of gene variants that are hypothesized to result in similar function with the same direction of effect on disease (e.g. groups of variants in phase I, phase II or DNA repair genes). Such categories of exchangeability could also be applied in a situation in which multiple genotype–exposure interaction terms are evaluated, and terms incorporating a common exposure (e.g. polycyclic aromatic hydrocarbons (PAHs)) are considered exchangeable (e.g. parameters for effects of interaction terms for variants in *GSTM1* and *GSTP1* with exposure to PAH would be considered exchangeable). In the final adjustment for each effect parameter, estimates for exposures included in the same category of exchangeability would be shrunk towards a common prior mean, while those in another category would be shrunk towards the mean of their group. It is important to note, however, that the quantitative magnitude of the similarities between parameters need not be specified absolutely, but can rather be estimated from the data. Such categories of exchangeability have not often been applied to studies of genotypes or genotype–exposure combinations, but

they have been applied in studies of occupational exposures (De Roos *et al.*, 2001) in which true effect parameters for exposures with similar physicochemical properties were grouped into categories of exchangeability, and in studies of multiple cancer sites (Greenland, 1992) in which effect parameters for associations between occupational exposures and cancer were considered exchangeable if they shared the same cancer site or exposure. Defining categories of exchangeability in studies of genotypes presents some challenges in that there is often inadequate information on which to base priors, since only limited information on functional significance of gene variants is currently available. In addition, the categories of exchangeability for genotypes are inherently specific to the toxicological exposure of interest; for example, phase I enzymes may have a common effect in relation to one substrate, but may have little in common in relation to another substrate for which some phase I enzymes may act more like phase II enzymes. In many studies in which main effects of genotypes are estimated, defined categories of exchangeability should relate to the functional activity of the gene variant in the context of background exposures. When screening multiple exposures for which little prior information is available, it may alternatively be appropriate to specify prior distributions in which a certain proportion of exposures are expected to have no effect. For example, in a simulation study of the effect of multiple HLA genotypes on insulin-dependent diabetes mellitus, Thomas *et al.* (1992) postulated a 'mixture prior' by which the proportion of null haplotype effects and the prior distribution of non-null effects were estimated from the data.

Rather than, or in addition to, categories of exchangeability, prior covariates can be based on quantitative characteristics which provide an indication of the degree of similarity between exposures on factors that are thought to underlie the effects of exposures on disease. For example, in a study of the effects of foods on breast cancer incidence, Witte *et al.* (1994) defined prior covariates representing nutrient content in foods. Thus, estimates for foods with similar nutrient content were shrunk closer to each other. In analyses of multiple haplotypes, prior covariates could be defined as a set of weights indicating the degree of similarity between haplotypes, based on the number of shared alleles or the length of the longest segment in common (Thomas *et al.*, 1992, 2001). The observed pattern of correlations could thus be used to adjust the effect of each haplotype, while borrowing information from estimates for similar haplotypes.

Much more sophisticated prior distributions can be constructed that integrate very specific toxicological data, but there are few such examples in the epidemiological literature. Aragaki *et al.* (1997) used multilevel modelling in a study of 45 joint effects of *NAT2* genotypes with different types of meat food items on the incidence of colorectal adenomas. The hypothesized toxicological mechanism behind *NAT2* genotype–meat effects was that cooked meat contains heterocyclic amines (HCAs) which are activated to a carcinogenic form by *NAT2*-produced enzymes. Different types of meat contain different concentrations of specific HCAs, and different *NAT2* genotypes confer different rates of HCA metabolism. In this analysis, the authors defined a prior distribution for each of the true *NAT2* genotype–meat effects comprised of toxicokinetic data on the genotype–meat-specific rates of metabolism for each of four different HCAs. In this way, the effect estimates for *NAT2* genotype–meat combinations that had similar rates of metabolism for the four HCAs were shrunk closer to each other, compared with the estimate for a *NAT2* genotype–meat combination with a very different toxicokinetic profile. Whereas the estimates calculated using maximum likelihood estimation indicated that eating one serving of bacon per day was associated with increased incidence of colorectal adenomas among persons with certain *NAT2* genotypes but not others, the results from hierarchical regression indicated increased risk associated with bacon consumption that was common to all the *NAT2* genotypes, after adjusting estimates based on the toxicokinetic data. Thus, integration of prior information on toxicological mechanism can result in qualitatively different interpretation of genotype–exposure effects.

The analysis by Aragaki *et al.* (1997) provides an interesting example of how prior toxicological data can be used to adjust effect estimates, which also underlines the fact that the specificity of toxicological information integrated into the prior should be supported by the strength of the hypothesis of the underlying mechanism. Such a prior integrating specific toxicological information is appropriate for studies in which the underlying hypothesis is well defined. The hypothesis that HCAs may increase the risk of colorectal adenomas or colon cancer has been supported by several studies in animals and humans (Lang *et al.*, 1994; Roberts-Thompson *et al.*, 1996; Toyota *et al.*, 1996; Sinha *et al.*, 2001). In addition, the role of NAT2 in HCA activation is well described (Vatsis *et al.*, 1995), as are the differing concentrations of HCAs in different types of cooked meat (Layton *et al.*, 1995; Sinha *et al.*, 2001). Many studies of genotype–exposure interactions will be more exploratory by nature. In this type of situation, it would be inappropriate to define a prior integrating specific toxicological data, because an incorrectly specified prior distribution will result in incorrectly adjusted estimates. Even where some knowledge of mechanism exists, the available toxicological data may be of limited quality or their applicability may be uncertain. Nevertheless, in a situation where there is little available data on which to base a prior distribution, empirical Bayes and semi-Bayes methods can be used to improve estimates using a vague prior, such as a prior in which all true effect parameters are considered exchangeable and likelihood estimates are shrunk towards one common prior mean, or a prior in which loose categories, or multiple overlapping categories of exchangeability, are defined. Simulation studies have indicated that even where only crude prior information exists (as in the form of categories of exchangeability), a hierarchical model with a simplified prior can outperform maximum likelihood estimation in enhancing the accuracy and precision of an ensemble of estimates (Witte & Greenland, 1996).

The sensitivity of the model to the selected prior covariates can and should be assessed in the light of uncertain data, but this should not be used as a strategy to select prior covariates. It is also possible to determine the relative importance of the different prior covariates using the fitted second-level regression coefficients. The ability to estimate parameters at the second level, however, depends on the richness of the data structure; this ability is enhanced by a large number of effects being estimated at the first level to inform the second-level model. In this sense, evaluation of multiple exposures could be viewed as an advantage to analysis, rather than the more typical view of multiple comparisons as a problem related to a greater probability of false-positive findings (Goodman, 1998). There are certain trade-offs in the modelling strategy, however, in terms of the choice of prior co-variates. Although use of prior covariates in the second level can improve estimates, particularly when analysing a large number of first-level exposures, simulation studies have shown that a greater number of prior covariates leads to decreased precision of posterior estimates (Greenland, 1993; Witte & Greenland, 1996). The a-priori relevance of each prior covariate should therefore be considered carefully.

As more epidemiological studies incorporating susceptibility markers are conducted, it is likely that greater understanding of underlying toxico-logical mechanisms will allow more frequent integration of detailed toxicological data into prior distributions. The proposed E-G-D database could be useful in this regard by providing a site for compilation and links to toxicological data relevant to genotype-related effects. For example, in a study of multiple effects of specific dioxin congeners on the incidence of non-Hodgkin lymphoma (NHL), a hypothesis of the underlying toxicological mechanism might be that any true effect is occurring through the binding of dioxin to the intracellular aryl hydrocarbon (Ah) receptor and subsequent induction of various biological responses (NTP, 2001). In this example, the E-G-D database could provide data on the toxic equivalency quotient (TEQ) of each congener, where the TEQ is a measure of each congener's ability to bind to the Ah receptor, relative to the most toxic congener, 2,3,7,8-tetrachlorodibenzo-*para*-dioxin (TCDD) (IARC, 1997). Using these data in

regression modelling, the prior distribution for the effect of each specific dioxin congener could be defined using prior information on the TEQ of each congener. Thus, linked databases such as the proposed E-G-D databases could provide rich data sources with which to construct priors.

Table 3 shows statistical approaches to ana-lysing multiple gene variants in situations for which there are varying levels of prior infor-mation (the approaches outlined in the table could equally be applied to analyses of multiple expo-sures of any type, including toxicological agents, haplotypes or genotype–exposure interactions). Where there is little prior information on the gene variants about how they relate to disease, there is a high probability of generating some false-positive results using frequentist methods (approach 1). In this situation, the investigator can expect fewer false-positive results for an ensemble of estimates when using hierarchical regression compared with maximum likelihood estimation (Steenland *et al.*, 2000), because the magnitude of estimates can be adjusted towards a group mean and the precision of each estimate improved, lowering the total error (approach 2). Although shrinkage of all estimates towards a group mean may result in missing some true posi-tive results, this will usually only occur when esti-mates are based on very sparse data. Where prior information exists on the functional significance of gene variants or on how individual gene variants relate to the magnitude of effects for disease, this knowledge can be incorporated into an empirical Bayes or semi-Bayes analysis (approaches 4 and 5), resulting in adjusted esti-mates that may be more accurate than a hierar-chical regression approach using a less informed prior. Researchers may argue that the results of frequentist analytical approaches can be inter-preted using prior information (approach 3), thus resulting in the same conclusions as Bayesian approaches. The prior information applied to interpretation of results from frequentist analyses usually consists of a review of the relevant lite-rature, and can be useful in judging the impor-tance of results. The difference between the two approaches lies in the fact that by incorporating prior information into the analysis, as in hierar-

Table 3. Statistical approaches to analysis of multiple genotypes in relation to disease

	Prior information	Approach applied	What we learn	Benefit over other approaches	Downside
1	Little prior information: screening multiple genotypes (Gs) with little prior information on functional significance of variants	Frequentist approach: analysing one G at a time or groups of Gs simultaneously	Associations with certain Gs may give clues about potential aetiologic mechanisms or toxicological agents of interest	Relative ease of statistical computing compared to Empirical or semi-Bayes approaches	Where one G at a time is analysed, there is potential for confounding by related gene variants that aren't included in the model. High potential for false-positive results, particularly when sparse data results in imprecise estimates
2	Little prior information: screening multiple Gs with little prior information	Empirical- or semi-Bayes methods: defining one category of exchangeability for all screened Gs	Associations with certain Gs may give clues about potential aetiologic mechanisms or toxicological agents of interest	Greater overall accuracy and precision for ensemble of estimates compared to Approach 1, likely to avoid some false-positive results	Some false-positive results may be generated. True positive effects based on sparse data will be penalized toward the mean of all estimates; some may be missed
3	Some or detailed prior information, such as functional significance of Gs or prior epidemiological studies	Frequentist approach: analysing one genotype at a time or groups of Gs simultaneously	Associations with certain Gs may give clues about potential aetiologic mechanisms or toxicological agents of interest	Although false-positive results are likely to be generated, an advantage over Approach 1 is that prior information can assist in interpretation of results and in judging the importance of results	High potential for false-positive results, particularly when sparse data results in imprecise estimates

Table 3 (contd)

	Prior information	Approach applied	What we learn	Benefit over other approaches	Downside
4	Some prior information, such as groups of Gs that result in similar changes in gene function	Empirical- or semi-Bayes approach: defining prior distributions based on categories of exchangeability for Gs known to result in similar changes in function	Associations with certain Gs may give clues about potential aetiologic mechanisms or toxicological agents of interest	Greater overall accuracy and precision for ensemble of estimates compared to Approaches 1 or 3, particularly if categories of exchangeability are truly important in relation to disease Unlike Approach 3, prior information is incorporated into the analysis, thereby giving quantitative documentation of how prior information was thought to be relevant for the effects of Gs, and allowing judgment of the importance of results on strictly quantitative criteria	Some false-positive results may be generated True positive effects based on sparse data will be penalized toward the mean of the group; some true positives may be missed, although this is less likely than in Approach 2 if information used to define exchangeability is truly important in relation to disease
5	Detailed prior information, such as data on Gs that are thought to directly relate to the magnitude of G effects	Empirical or semi-Bayes approach: defining prior distributions based on data specific to each G as it relates to D (e.g. functional information)	Associations with certain Gs may give clues about potential aetiological mechanisms or toxicological agents of interest	If G-specific information on function is at least partially related to the magnitude of G effect on D, then estimates should be more accurate than in Approaches 1–4	Some false-positive results may be generated Possible to overspecify prior distribution using very specific prior information that in reality is not related to the magnitude of G effects on D, leading to spurious results

D, disease

chical regression, the investigator is providing formalized documentation of how the information was thought to be quantitatively relevant for the magnitude of the effects of interest. Also, because the prior information is used to adjust estimates and confidence limits, the importance of results can be judged by simple quantitative criteria rather than by interpreting results qualitatively in the context of existing literature.

The use of hierarchical models is attractive as a means to integrate prior information into analyses to improve estimates, although the methods do not provide a panacea for clarifying relationships that were previously obscured. At the very least, these methods will be useful in providing a means for more thoughtful interpretation of multiple effect estimates for which there is little prior information, by generating more reasonable estimates that help to prevent false-positive results and misinterpretation in the face of sparse data. At best, these methods can be useful in improving the accuracy of estimates for genotype and genotype–exposure combinations for which there are detailed underlying hypotheses about toxicological mechanisms, in order to estimate more realistically the magnitude of effects and potential public health importance.

Future considerations

Epidemiological studies incorporating susceptibility markers have the potential to elucidate relationships between toxicological exposures and disease by allowing for detection of different levels of risk among subgroups of exposed people in the population. The main effects of gene variants on disease can provide insight into pathways relevant to disease etiology, which may indicate certain groups of exposures as potentially important. Examination of the effect of exposure among people of differing genotypes can help to rule in or out any effect of the exposure convincingly, and can help to identify subgroups to target for public health intervention. Although epidemiology reaches its limits when attempting to interpret biological mechanisms underlying observed genotype–exposure interactions, replicated findings can provide a useful basis for toxicological research into mechanisms, using in-vitro or animal models.

Where in-vitro, animal and epidemiological studies have contributed to a well-developed hypothesis of a mechanism underlying a genotype–exposure effect, simple description of associations using standard epidemiological methods of analysis may be sufficient, although increasing understanding of biological relationships may warrant more complex modelling strategies. Standard epidemiological methods of data description are more likely to fail where studies are focused on screening large numbers of genotypes or genotype–exposure interactions for which there is little existing prior information on toxicological mechanisms. This is the area with the biggest potential for producing false leads due to false-positive results or misinterpretation. However, taking advantage of the available genetic technology to screen multiple variants in a non-mechanistic approach in relation to disease may hold some promise by providing leads in areas that are not restricted to the current state of scientific knowledge. In addition to using methods such as hierarchical regression to mitigate some of the problems inherent to studies incorporating susceptibility markers, the further development of several resources and methods could be an important approach to such studies in both the design and analysis phases.

Development of data resources

Coordination of exposure assessment and genotyping across various cohort and case–control studies will facilitate future pooling of studies. Data pooling will help to provide the sample size necessary for studies of modest main or joint effects, particularly for rare diseases and analyses by histological subtype. Several organized attempts are already underway, with consortia dedicated to pooling data from existing cohort studies. Communication between investigators and documentation of resources available within each study (e.g. exposure data, types of biological samples, histological information) will be important in assessing the feasibility of pooling data.

Linkage of existing databases or development of an E-G-D database, as described above, could aid researchers in choosing genotypes for study relevant to a certain disease or exposure, could assist researchers in consideration of toxicological agents or extraneous factors that may be important to consider as potential confounders or effect modifiers of a main effect of interest, and could lead the researcher to important sources of toxicological data that may be useful in analysis or interpretation. Development and linkage of such data resources will require considerable interpretation and synthesis of scientific information, and are thus unlikely to be available in the near future. However, with development and maintenance of other databases (e.g. OMIM) already occurring, coordination would be beneficial in streamlining and linking efforts to prevent duplication.

Because there are limited data regarding the effect of identified polymorphisms on gene function, further development and documentation on the functional significance of polymorphisms will aid in interpretation of epidemiological studies. In addition, epidemiological analyses of inherited susceptibility markers do not generally account for the fact that people with the same genotype will fall along a spectrum of expression. Factors affecting expression such as other genes, health, hormones, diet and other environmental exposures should be taken into account, usually by adjusting for such important factors in statistical analyses. Some data on variability of expression in the general population exist from phenotyping assays and toxicokinetic models; however, many more data are needed to understand the intrinsic variability in normal gene expression for the numerous polymorphisms that are now being studied. The recent development of DNA microarray technology for conducting genome-wide assessments of gene regulation has great potential for increasing the amount of useful data on environmental agents affecting expression (Afshari *et al.*, 1999). Compilation of increasing amounts of data on factors affecting variability in gene expression can provide important information on potential confounders and modifiers of effect when studying inherited susceptibility.

There is an additional need for the development of biologically based mechanistic models to guide interpretation of the available data (Portier, 2001). Mechanistic models would provide information about gene activity and genotype–exposure effects at different exposure dose levels. Such research could precede epidemiological research of the topic, in which case epidemiologists may glean clues from the toxicological literature about leads to pursue and strategies for analysing data. Conversely, results from epidemiological studies may inform toxicologists about potential genotype–exposure effects to investigate.

Methods of statistical analysis

With the increasing breadth of studies examining the effects of multiple exposures and multiple genotypes, and with potentially differing effects based on the numerous possible combinations of exposures and genotypes a person could have, it quickly becomes apparent that techniques capable of modelling complex relationships will be useful. The PBPK modelling approach described by Cortessis and Thomas (this volume) could be used to model complex relationships for which toxicological pathways between exposure and disease are well described, and where toxicokinetic data on factors affecting the fate of toxicological agents within the body are available. By modelling the creation of toxic metabolites within individuals on the basis of their multiple exposures and genotypes, the risk associated with the final metabolite on disease can be estimated. This approach is different from, but complementary to, the more empirical hierarchical regression modelling approach, which relies less heavily on specific mathematical models for the metabolic pathways. Both types of analyses would benefit from data in the proposed E-G-D database that could be used to inform the choice of prior covariates for the hierarchical modelling approach, and could provide toxicokinetic data on metabolic rates and other parameters for the PBPK modelling approach. Other types of statistical analyses, such as artificial neural networks, use pattern recognition techniques to look for patterns or clusters of variables that are associated with an outcome of interest (Duh *et al.*, 1998). Application in the realm of toxicological exposures and susceptibility markers could assist in studies in which a large number of exposures and genotypes are screened for associations with disease to help identify genotype–exposure combinations or combinations of polymorphisms (e.g. haplotypes) that confer susceptibility to disease (Curtis *et al.*, 2001). Although the applicability of these modelling techniques to epidemiology is as yet uncertain, the common theme is the recognition of a need for approaches to modelling multifactorial relationships in the realm of genetic susceptibility to toxicological agents and disease.

Acknowledgements

Martyn T. Smyth was supported by the National Institute of Environmental Health Sciences (grants P42ES04705, P30 ES01896 and R01ES06721) and the National Foundation for Cancer Research.

References

Afshari, C.A., Nuwaysir, E.F. & Barrett, J.C. (1999) Application of complementary DNA microarray technology to carcinogen identification, toxicology, and drug safety evaluation. *Cancer Res.*, **59**, 4759–4760

Aragaki, C.C., Greenland, S., Probst-Hensch, N. & Haile, R.W. (1997) Hierarchical modeling of gene-environment interactions: estimating NAT2* genotype-specific dietary effects on adenomatous polyps. *Cancer Epidemiol. Biomarkers Prev.*, **6**, 307–314

Bondy, M.L., Wang, L.E., El-Zein, R., de Andrade, M., Selvan, M.S., Bruner, J.M., Levin, V.A., Yung, W.K.A., Adatto, P. & Wei, Q. (2001) γ-Radiation sensitivity and risk of glioma. *J. natl Cancer Inst.*, **93**, 1553–1557

Botto, L.P. & Khoury, M.J. (2001) Facing the challenge of gene-environment interaction: the two-by-four table and beyond. *Am. J. Epidemiol.*, **153**, 1016–1020

Curtis, D., North, B.V. & Sham, P.C. (2001) Use of an artificial neural network to detect associations between a disease and multiple marker genotypes. *Ann. hum. Genet.*, **65**, 95–107

De Roos, A.J., Poole, C., Teschke, K. & Olshan, A.F. (2001) An application of hierarchical regression in the investigation of multiple paternal occupational exposures and neuroblastoma in offspring. *Am. J. ind. Med.*, **39**, 477–486

Dosemeci, M. & Stewart, P.A. (1996) Recommendations for reducing the effects of exposure misclassification on relative risk estimates. *Occup. Hyg.*, **3**, 169–176

Duh, M.S., Walker, A.M. & Ayanian, J.Z. (1998) Epidemiologic interpretation of artificial neural networks. *Am. J. Epidemiol.*, **147**, 1112–1122

Dunson, D.B. (2001) Commentary: practical advantages of Bayesian analysis of epidemiologic data. *Am. J. Epidemiol.*, **153**, 1222–1226

Fallin, D. & Schork, N.J. (2000) Accuracy of haplotype frequency estimation for biallelic loci, via the expectation-maximization algorithm for unphased diploid genotype data. *Am. J. hum. Genet.*, **67**, 947–959

Fallin, D., Cohen, A., Essioux, L., Chumakov, I., Blumenfeld, M., Cohen, D. & Schork, N.J. (2001) Genetic analysis of case/control data using estimated haplotype frequencies: application to APOE locus variation and Alzheimer's disease. *Genome Res.*, **11**, 143–151

Flegal, K.M., Brownie, C. & Haas, J.D. (1986) The effects of exposure misclassification on estimates of relative risk. *Am. J. Epidemiol.*, **123**, 736–751

Goodman, S.N. (1998) Multiple comparisons, explained. *Am. J. Epidemiol.*, **147**, 807–812

Greenland, S. (1992) A semi-Bayes approach to the analysis of correlated multiple associations, with an application to an occupational cancer-mortality study. *Statist. Med.*, **11**, 219–230

Greenland, S. (1993) Methods for epidemiologic analyses of multiple exposures: a review and comparative study of maximum-likelihood, preliminary-testing, and empirical-Bayes regression. *Statist. Med.*, **12**, 717–736

Greenland, S. (1994) Hierarchical regression for epidemiologic analyses of multiple exposures. *Environ. Health Perspect.*, **102** (Suppl 8), 33–39

Greenland, S. (1997) Introduction to regression models. In: Rothman, K. & Greenland, S., eds, *Modern Epidemiology*, Philadelphia, PA, Lippincott-Raven, pp. 359–399

Greenland, S. (2000a) Principles of multilevel modeling. *Int. J. Epidemiol.*, **29**, 158–167

Greenland, S. (2000b) When should epidemiologic regressions use random coefficients? *Biometrics*, **56**, 915–921

Greenland, S. & Poole, C. (1994) Empirical-Bayes and semi-Bayes approaches to occupational and environmental hazard surveillance. *Arch. environ. Health*, **49**, 9–16

IARC (1982) *IARC Monographs on the Evaluation of the Carcinogenic Risk of Chemicals to Humans*, Vol. 29, *Some Industrial Chemicals and Dyestuffs*, Lyon, IARC*Press*, pp. 93–148

IARC (1997) *IARC Monographs on the Evaluation of Carcinogenic Risks to Humans*, Vol. 69, *Polychlorinated Dibenzo-para-dioxins and Polychlorinated Dibenzofurans*, Lyon, IARC*Press*, pp. 33–630

Inskip, P.D., Linet, M.S. & Heineman, E.F. (1995) Etiology of brain tumors in adults. *Epidemiol. Rev.*, **17**, 382–414

Johnson, G.C.I., Esposito, L., Barratt, B.J., Smith, A.N., Heward, J., Di Genova, G., Ueda, H., Cordell, H.J., Eaves, I.A., Dudbridge, F., Twells, R.C.J., Payne, F., Hughes, W., Nutland, S., Stevens, H., Carr, P., Tuomilehto-Wolf, E., Tuomilehto, J., Gough, S.C.L., Clayton, D.G. & Todd, J.A. (2001) Haplotype tagging for the identification of common disease genes. *Nat. Genet.*, **29**, 233–237

Lang, N.P., Butler, M.A., Massengill, J., Lawson, M., Stotts, R.C., Hauer-Jensen, M. & Kadlubar, F.F. (1994) Rapid metabolic phenotypes for acetyltransferase and cytochrome P4501A2 and putative exposure to food-borne heterocyclic amines increase the risk for colorectal cancer or polyps. *Cancer Epidemiol. Biomarkers Prev.*, **3**, 675–682

Layton, D.W., Bogen, K.T., Knize, M.G., Hatch, F.T., Johnson, V.M. & Felton, J.S. (1995) Cancer risk of heterocyclic amines in cooked foods: an analysis and implications for research. *Carcinogenesis*, **16**, 39–52

Marchand, L.L., Wilkinson, G.R. & Wilkens, L.R. (1999) Genetic and dietary predictors of CYP2E1 activity: a phenotyping study in Hawaii Japanese using chlorzoxazone. *Cancer Epidemiol. Biomarkers Prev.*, **8**, 495–500

McCarver, D.G., Byun, R., Hines, R.N., Hichme, M. & Wegenek, W. (1998) A genetic polymorphism in the regulatory sequences of human CYP2E1: association with increased chlorzoxazone hydroxylation in the presence of obesity and ethanol intake. *Toxicol. appl. Pharmacol.*, **152**, 276–281

McMichael, A.J. (1988) Carcinogenicity of benzene, toluene and xylene: epidemiological and experimental evidence. In: Fishbein, L. & O'Neill, I.K., eds, *Environmental Carcinogens. Methods of Analysis and Exposure Assessment, Volume 10 – Benzene and Alkylated Benzenes* (IARC Scientific Publications No. 85), Lyon, IARC*Press*, pp. 3–18

NTP (National Toxicology Program) (2001) *Ninth Report on Carcinogens*, Research Triangle Park, NC, US Department of Health and Human Services, Public Health Service, National Institutes of Health

Portier, C.J. (2001) Linking toxicology and epidemiology: the role of mechanistic modelling. *Statist. Med.*, **20**, 1387–1393

Roberts-Thompson, I.C., Ryan, P., Khoo, K.K., Hart, W.J., McMichael, A.J. & Butler, R.N. (1996) Diet, acetylator phenotype, and risk of colorectal neoplasia. *Lancet*, **347**, 1372–1374

Rothman, N., Smith, M.T., Hayes, R.B., Traver, R.D., Hoener, B., Campleman, S., Li, G.L., Dosemeci, M., Linet, M., Zhang, L., Xi, L., Wacholder, S., Lu, W., Meyer, K.B., Titenko-Holland, N., Stewart, J.T., Yin, S. & Ross, D. (1997) Benzene poisoning, a risk factor for hematological malignancy, is associated with the NQO1 $^{609}C{\rightarrow}T$ mutation and rapid fractional excretion of chlorzoxazone. *Cancer Res.*, **57**, 2839–2842

Rothman, N., Garcia-Closas, M., Stewart, W.T. & Lubin, J. (1999) The impact of misclassification in case–control studies of gene-environment interactions. In: Vineis, P., Malats, N., Lang, M., d'Erico, A., Caporaso, N., Cuzick, J. & Boffetta, P., eds, *Metabolic Polymorphisms and Susceptibility to Cancer* (IARC Scientific Publications No. 148), Lyon, IARC*Press*, pp. 89–96

Sinha, R., Kulldorff, M., Chow, W.H., Denobile, J. & Rothman, N. (2001) Dietary intake of heterocyclic amines, meat-derived mutagenic activity, and risk of colorectal adenomas. *Cancer Epidemiol. Biomarkers Prev.*, **10**, 559–562

Steenland, K., Bray, I., Greenland, S. & Boffetta, P. (2000) Empirical Bayes adjustments for multiple results in hypothesis-generating or surveillance studies. *Cancer Epidemiol. Biomarkers Prev.*, **9**, 895–903

Strange, R.C. & Fryer, A.A. (1999) The glutathione S-transferases: influence of polymorphism on cancer susceptibility. In: Vineis, P., Malats, N., Lang, M., d'Errico, A., Caporaso, N., Cuzick, J. & Boffetta, P., eds, *Metabolic Polymorphisms and Susceptibility to Cancer* (IARC Scientific Publications No. 148), Lyon, IARC*Press*, pp. 231–249

Stubbins, M.J. & Wolf, C.R. (1999) Additional polymorphisms and cancer. In: Vineis, P., Malats, N., Lang, M., d'Errico, A., Caporaso, N., Cuzick, J. & Boffetta, P., eds, *Metabolic Polymorphisms and Susceptibility to Cancer* (IARC Scientific Publications No. 148), Lyon, IARC*Press*, pp. 271–302

Thomas, D., Langholz, B., Clayton, D., Pitkaniemi, J., Tuomilehto-Wolf, E. & Tuomilehto, J. (1992) Empirical-Bayes methods for testing associations with large numbers of candidate genes in the presence of environmental risk factors, with applications to HLA associations in IDDM. *Ann. Med.*, **24**, 387–392

Thomas, D.C., Morrison, J.L. & Clayton, D.G. (2001) Bayes estimates of haplotype effects. *Genet. Epidemiol.*, **21** (Suppl. 1), S712–S717

Thompson, W.D. (1991) Effect modification and the limits of biological inference from epidemiologic data. *J. clin. Epidemiol.*, **44**, 221–232

Toyota, M., Ushjima, T., Kakiuchi, H., Canzian, F., Watanabe, M., Imai, K., Sugimura, T. & Nagao, M. (1996) Genetic alterations in rat colon tumors induced by heterocyclic amines. *Cancer*, **77** (Suppl 8), 1593–1597

Vatsis, K.P., Weber, W.W., Bell, D.A., Dupret, J.M., Evans, D.A.P., Grant, D.M., Hein, D.W., Lin, H.J., Meyer, U.A., Relling, M.V., Sim, E., Suzuki, T. & Yamazoc, Y. (1995) Nomenclature for *N*-acetyltransferases. *Pharmacogenetics*, **5**, 1–17

Witte, J.S. & Greenland, S. (1996) Simulation study of hierarchical regression. *Statist. Med.*, **15**, 1161–1170

Witte, J.S., Greenland, S., Haile, R.W. & Bird, C.L. (1994) Hierarchical regression analysis applied to a study of multiple dietary exposures and breast cancer. *Epidemiology*, **5**, 612–621

Witte, J.S., Greenland, S., Kim, L.L. & Arab, L. (2000) Multilevel modeling in epidemiology with GLIMMIX. *Epidemiology*, **11**, 684–688

Corresponding author:

Nathaniel Rothman
Occupational Epidemiology Branch,
National Cancer Institute,
NIH/NCI/EPS 8116,
Bethesda, MD 20892, USA
rothmann@exchange.nih.gov

Mechanisms of Carcinogenesis: Contributions of Molecular Epidemiology
Patricia Buffler, Jerry Rice, Robert Baan, Michael Bird and Paolo Boffetta, eds
IARC Scientific Publications No. 157
International Agency for Research on Cancer, Lyon, 2004

Toxicokinetic Genetics: an Approach to Gene–Environment and Gene–Gene Interactions in Complex Metabolic Pathways

Victoria Cortessis and Duncan C. Thomas

Summary

We propose an approach to modelling the joint effects of multiple genes involved in metabolic activation and detoxification of environmental exposures. A physiologically based pharmacokinetic (PBPK) model is used, in which the various person-specific metabolic rates are related to measurements of the genotypes and/or phenotypes at the various stages of the relevant pathways. Markov chain Monte Carlo (MCMC) methods are used to fit the model. We illustrate the approach by application to case–control data on colorectal polyps in relation to consumption of well-done red meat and tobacco smoking via pathways involving heterocyclic amines (regulated by the genes *CYP1A2*, *NAT1* and *NAT2*) and polycyclic aromatic hydrocarbons (regulated by the genes *CYP1A1*, *EPHX1* (also called *mEH*) and *GSTM3*). In this chapter, we focus on the biochemical basis for our conceptual models, deferring detailed mathematical description of the models and simulation results to a separate paper.

Introduction

The field of molecular epidemiology is concerned with the effects of environmental exposures and the genes which modify their effects through metabolic activation and detoxification, DNA repair, cell cycle control and related mechanisms. It is now widely understood that the pathways leading from exposure to disease can involve numerous steps; there may be several competing pathways by which a single compound causes disease; and several different compounds may be metabolized by reactions occurring in a single biochemical pathway. Many of the genes regulating these pathways are known to be polymorphic, and some genotypes defined by known polymorphisms have been shown to be associated with disease risk, or to interact with environmental exposures or with variants of other genes. Although the relative risks (RRs) associated with such 'metabolic genes' tend to be relatively modest (1.5–3, for example) compared with the tens- or hundred-fold RRs for rare 'major susceptibility genes' such as *BRCA1*, the population attributable risk for metabolic genes could be much higher, because the variant alleles are often very common. Hence, there is great interest in better characterizing the effects of metabolic genes and their interactions with each other and with environmental agents.

Here we suggest an approach for examining joint effects of environmental compounds and metabolic genes that encode proteins involved in their biochemical conversion. For each compound of interest, a physiologically based pharmacokinetic (PBPK) model is used to estimate levels of one or more activated metabolites. An effects model relates these metabolite levels to occurrence of disease. An individual's genotypes and history of exposure are addressed in the PBPK model, in which they are treated as determinants of metabolite levels. The specific form of the PBPK model is based on prior information about how these factors participate in the relevant biochemical pathway. We illustrate the approach by exploring the joint effects of two procarcinogens and several genes involved in their metabolism on the occurrence of colorectal adenoma.

The etiology of colorectal cancer and its precursor lesion, colonic adenoma (polyps), probably involves activation of exogenous compounds by metabolic enzymes. Although findings are not entirely consistent, published epidemiological studies (reviewed by Potter, 1999) suggest that occurrence of these conditions is associated with meat consumption, perhaps particularly with habitual consumption of well-browned or well-done meat. Cooked meat contains both heterocyclic amines (HCAs), which form when protein-containing foods are cooked (Wakabayashi et al., 1992), and polycyclic aromatic hydrocarbons (PAHs), which originate from incomplete combustion (pyrolysis) of organic material by numerous processes, including preparation of food at high temperature. Smoking is an additional risk factor for polyps and a putative risk factor for colorectal cancer. Tobacco smoke also contains PAHs and HCAs. Both classes of compounds (PAHs and HCAs) include molecules that can be metabolized to reactive intermediates that have been shown to be mutagenic and to have other genotoxic effects. In this report, we describe a simplified metabolic pathway whereby a single compound of each class, the PAH benzo[a]pyrene and the HCA 2-amino-3,8-dimethylimidazo-[4,5-f]quinoxaline (MeIQx), is converted to its putatively most carcinogenic metabolite. Both pathways are illustrated in Figure 1, and the biochemical reactions are described below. These pathways immediately suggest that to understand the etiological effect of these environmental factors, PAHs and HCAs, we will wish to study them in conjunction with functionally polymorphic genes encoding their metabolic enzymes.

The conventional approach in molecular epidemiology has been to examine each of these factors – genetic and environmental – separately or in pairwise combinations, reasoning perhaps that the available sample size would not support finer stratification. For example, Table 1 summarizes RRs of colorectal polyps in relation to tobacco smoking, consumption of well-done red meat (WDRM) and the genes EPHX1 and GSTM3

estimated from a case–control study by Cortessis et al. (2001). Cases and controls were selected from patients at two Southern California Kaiser-Permanente facilities who had undergone sigmoidoscopy for routine screening (not indicated by symptoms). Cases ($n = 466$) were those found for the first time to have one or more polyps. Controls ($n = 509$) were selected at random from those found to be free of polyps (with no history of polyps), matched to cases on age, sex, date of sigmoidoscopy and facility. The study population and instruments used to assess environmental exposures have already been described in detail (Haile et al., 1997) and are briefly described in the Methods section below. In univariate analyses, WDRM was not significantly associated with risk of polyps, although smoking (current versus never) was. Similarly, neither EPHX1 (a composite measure of two polymorphisms in exons 3 and 4 which we interpret as a proxy for microsomal epoxide hydrolase activity (Cortessis et al., 2001)) nor GSTM3 alone (*A*A genotype versus *A*B and *B*B) was significantly associated with polyps univariately. However, amongst never smokers who eat meat, habitual WDRM consumption showed a significant interaction with EPHX1 ($p = 0.03$), and there was also a significant interaction between EPHX1 and GSTM3 ($p = 0.03$ marginally, 0.004 after adjusting for smoking).

Unfortunately, this approach to the analysis poses several problems. Why focus on just these two genes and two exposures when several other genes and exposures are also thought to be involved? Of the set of all possible interactions, how do we decide which ones to consider? Clearly the answer to both of these questions should be informed by prior knowledge of the biological mechanisms. Upon further stratification to incorporate other risk factors, one quickly encounters the inter-related problems of sparse data and multiple comparisons – as one examines more strata, there are greater opportunities for false-positive associations just by chance, while at the same time, the amount of data available becomes too small for stable effect estimates. Nevertheless, failure to account for other genes, exposures or real interaction effects could

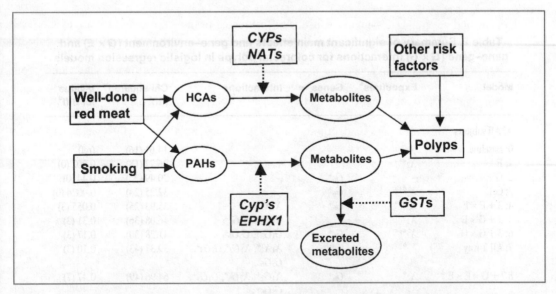

Figure 1. Conceptual model for heterocyclic amine (HCA) and polycyclic aromatic hydrocarbon (PAH) pathways leading from well-done red meat and tobacco smoking to colorectal polyps

Table 1. Descriptive associations of selected exposures and genes with colorectal polyps

Exposure	Level	Epoxide hydrolase activity predicted from *EPHX1* genotype[a]			All
Variable		Low	Medium	High	
All subjects		1.0	1.17 (0.87–1.57)	1.33 (0.93–1.91)	
Red meat	Not well done	1.0	0.81 (0.41–1.62)	0.57 (0.24–1.35)	1.0
cooking[b]	Well done	1.01 (0.53–1.93)	1.21 (0.58–2.53)	2.47 (0.99–6.19)	1.51 (0.96–2.38)
Smoking[c]	Never	1.0	0.92 (0.57–1.49)	1.13 (0.63–2.03)	1.0
	Current	1.58 (0.82–3.05)	2.56 (1.38–4.74)	4.27 (1.68–10.8)	2.22 (1.46–3.38)
GSTM3	*B*B	1.0	1.02 (0.82–1.26)	1.03 (0.67–1.58)	1.0
	*A*B	0.86 (0.62–1.21)	1.19 (0.87–1.62)	1.64 (1.06–2.52)	1.11 (0.80–1.55)
	*A*A	0.75 (0.38–1.47)	1.64 (1.06–2.52)	2.60 (1.28–2.58)	1.31 (0.75–2.28)

Adapted from Cortessis *et al.* (2001)

[a] Number of putatively more stable alleles at exons 3 (113Y) and 4 (139R): low = 0,1; medium = 2; high = 3,4.

[b] Among never-smoking subjects who eat red meat.

[c] Excluding ex-smokers.

lead to confounding of the effects of immediate interest. These concerns suggest the need for some kind of multivariate model, as opposed to simple descriptive analysis, but of course one must then be concerned about mis-specifying the form of the model.

A standard statistical alternative to simple description of finely stratified risk estimates is multivariate modelling. Table 2 provides a summary of a series of logistic regression models, in which main effects, gene–environment ($G \times E$) and gene–gene ($G \times G$) interactions, and higher-order

Table 2. Summary of significant main effects and gene–environment ($G \times E$) and gene–gene ($G \times G$) interactions for colorectal polyps in logistic regression models

Model	Exposures[a]	Genes[b] =	Interactions	Chi-squared (df)[c]	p-value for diff[d]
A. All subjects					
0: Baseline				14.61 (16)	(ref)
1: E	X_2***	–	–	26.72 (18)	0.002 (0)
2: G	–	G_6+	–	20.49 (22)	0.44 (0)
3: G,E	X_2***	G_6+	–	32.25 (24)	0.0024 (0)
4: 3 + E×E	X_2***	G_6+	X_1X_2+	35.93 (25)	0.055 (3)
5: 3 + G×E	X_2+		X_1G_2*, X_2G_6+	46.08 (36)	0.31 (3)
6: 3 + G×G	X_2***	G_6+	G_1G_3+, G_5G_6*	41.28 (30)	0.17 (3)
7: All 2-way	X_2*		X_1X_2*, X_1G_2*, G_1G_3*, G_5G_6*	59.37 (43)	0.10 (3)
8 7 + G×E×E	X_2*	G_6+	X_1G_2+, X_2G_6*, G_1G_3+, G_5G_6+	64.96 (49)	0.47 (7)
9: 7 + G×G×E	X_2+		X_1X_2*, X_1G_2**, X_2G_1+, G_1G_2+, G_1G_3*, $X_1G_1G_2$*, $X_2G_5G_6$**	79.56 (55)	0.063 (7)
10: 7 + G×G×G	X_2*	G_2+	X_1X_2*, X_1G_2*, G_1G_3*, $G_1G_2G_3$*	62.96 (45)	0.17 (7)
B. Non-smokers only					
0: Baseline				17.99 (15)	(ref)
1: E	X_1+	–	–	21.37 (16)	0.066 (0)
2: G	–		–	22.81 (21)	0.57 (0)
3: G,E	X_1+		–	26.31 (22)	0.31 (0)
5: 3 + G×E		G_2*, G_5+, G_6+	X_1G_2**, X_1G_6**	40.01 (28)	0.033 (3)
6: 3 + G×G	X_1+	G_1+	G_5G_6***	42.68 (28)	0.011 (3)
7: All 2-way		G_2*, G_4*, G_5*	X_1G_2**, X_1G_6*, G_5G_6***	56.80 (34)	0.002 (3)
9: 7 + G×G×E		G_1+, G_2*, G_6*	X_1G_2**, G_1G_2*, G_1G_3*, G_5G_6*, $X_1G_1G_2$**	71.97 (40)	0.019 (7)
10: 7 + G×G×G		G_2*, G_4+, G_5+	X_1G_2**, X_1G_6*, G_1G_3+	57.45 (36)	0.72 (7)

[a] X_1 = WDRM (well-done red meat); X_2 = smoking.

[b] G_1 = *CYP1A2* phenotype, G_2 = *NAT1* genotype, G_3 = *NAT2* genotype, G_4 = *CYP1A1* genotype, G_5 = *GSTM3* genotype, G_6 = *EPHX1* genotype; measured values are phenotypes for *CYP1A2* and genotypes for *NAT1, NAT2, CYP1A1, GSTM3*, and *EPHX1*.

[c] Likelihood ratio chi-squared for baseline model, containing age, sex, ethnicity, NSAIDs, exercise, dietary fibre, ex-smokers and missing value indicators for exposures and genotypes.

[d] p-value for the improvement in fit of the overall model, relative to the model shown in parentheses, including all terms of the indicated category (whether individually significant or not) +, $p < 0.10$; *, $p < 0.05$; **, $p < 0.01$; ***, $p < 0.001$

interactions suggested by the pathways were entered in succession. For this purpose, all variables were centred on zero, and missing values were replaced by zeros, so that the same subjects could be included in each analysis. Results of the univariate analysis of all subjects are shown in lines 1 and 2 of part A of Table 2. Smoking (X_2) was a highly significant predictor ($p < 0.001$), but WDRM (X_1) was not. *EPHX1* was the only gene that showed any effect univariately, and only at a very marginal level of significance ($p < 0.10$). As reported in lines 3–10 of part A of Table 2, a number of two- and three-way interactions were individually significant, but the number of comparisons should be borne in mind, as no overall test of each class of interactions was statistically significant. Because of the overwhelming strength of the smoking effect, we also analysed nonsmokers separately (part B of Table 2) and found no significant univariate effects, but a much stronger pattern of interactions among the remaining variables. The overall test of all two-way interactions was highly significant ($p = 0.002$), with the strongest individual contributions being $G \times E$ interactions of WDRM (X_1) with *NAT1* (G_2) and of WDRM with *EPHX1* (G_6), and a $G \times G$ interaction between *EPHX1* and *GSTM3* (G_5). The addition of the entire class of $G \times G \times E$ interactions also produced a significant improvement in fit ($p = 0.019$), mainly contributed by WDRM $\times$ *CYP1A2* (G_1) $\times$ *NAT1*. It is worth emphasizing that without having restricted this exploration of interaction effects to the subset of those suggested by the two pathways, the number of possible comparisons would have been considerably larger.

In this paper, we explore a new modelling approach which would allow us to examine all the relevant factors simultaneously, using elementary ideas from PBPK models. Mathematical details and a simulation study will be described elsewhere; the primary focus here is on the biochemical basis for our conceptual approach. The approach is illustrated by application of the model to the data on polyps. We suggest this approach as a potentially more informative alternative for exploring complex patterns of interactions where the underlying pathways are already understood to some extent.

Methods
Overview of the approach
In contrast to the purely empirical models described in the Introduction (descriptive RR estimates such as those shown in Table 1 or multivariate logistic regression models such as those shown in Table 2), we now explore more mechanistic approaches based on PBPK models. Specifically, we first describe the biochemical pathways for the metabolism of HCAs and PAHs and the various genes acting on these pathways. Next, we develop a statistical representation of these pathways in terms of a set of hypothesized random variables corresponding to the long-term averages of these metabolites and their relationships to the exposures, genes and the ultimate outcome of polyps. These relationships are expressed in terms of a hierarchical model, with a number of latent variables for each subject, which are in turn governed by a set of statistical models for the distribution of these variables across subjects. Such complex models are difficult to fit using standard maximum likelihood techniques, so instead we use Markov chain Monte Carlo (MCMC) methods within a Bayesian framework, thereby allowing all the different parts of the model to be fitted simultaneously.

Biochemical pathways
HCA pathway: Amino-3,8-dimethylimidazo-[4,5-*f*]quinoxaline (MeIQx) is one of the most abundant mutagenic HCAs present in cooked meat (Wakabayashi *et al.*, 1993). The MeIQx content of fried beef patties increases with cooking temperature and cooking time (Felton *et al.*, 1994), and can thus be assumed to be greater in well-done beef. MeIQx is a potent bacterial mutagen, a multisite rodent carcinogen and a precursor to electrophilic derivatives that can form DNA-binding adducts. Low doses of orally administered MeIQx have been shown to form DNA adducts in the human colon (Mauthe *et al.*, 1999). The most extensive studies of the metabolism of MeIQx have been conducted in animal models, and there are significant differences in the metabolism of

this compound by rodents versus humans (Turesky et al., 1994; Langouet et al., 2001); the major pathways of MeIQx metabolism in humans therefore remain to be elucidated fully (Langouet et al., 2001). Nonetheless, in-vitro heterologous expression and cytotoxicity studies (for example, Yanagawa et al., 1994; Potter, 1999) and in-vivo metabolic studies (for example, Boobis et al., 1994) have identified several human metabolic enzymes that appear to be important in the conversion of MeIQx to reactive metabolites that form DNA adducts.

On the basis of a limited review of recent literature, we propose a simplified pathway (part A of Figure 2) whereby ingested MeIQx forms MeIQx–DNA adducts in the colon. This 'HCA pathway' includes reactions that are catalysed by enzymes known to be polymorphic in humans. In the liver, an N-oxidation reaction catalysed primarily by CYP1A2 converts MeIQx to N-OH-MeIQx, which is transported to or reformed in the colon, where it can be O-acetylated by either of two N-acetyltransferases, NAT1 or NAT2. Both isozymes are functionally polymorphic in humans. The acetylation product, N-O-acetyl-MeIQx, is believed to degrade spontaneously into the highly reactive nitronium ion, which putatively binds DNA to form adducts. In heterologous expression studies in which recombinant human CYP1A2 was co-expressed with each of the human wild-type NATs (Minchin et al., 1992; Hein et al., 1994), this sequence of reactions was approximately 20 times more efficient in the presence of NAT2 versus NAT1, presumably due to higher specific activity of the former isoform.

PAH pathway: Exposure to high levels of benzo[a]pyrene occurs in some occupations, and the general population is exposed primarily through cooked food and tobacco smoke. Benzo[a]pyrene is considered to be one of the main contributors to the carcinogenic action of naturally occurring mixtures of PAHs, and it is often used as a surrogate for exposure to total PAHs. Benzo[a]-pyrene is a bacterial mutagen, and in eukaryotes it has been shown to induce numerous forms of genotoxic damage and mutations.

Reactions in the PAH pathway (part B of Figure 2) are illustrated by their action on the pro-carcinogen benzo[a]pyrene, which is metabolically activated by P450 enzymes such as CYP1A1 to benzo[a]pyrene 7,8-epoxide. This epoxide can be detoxified by glutathione conjugation catalysed by any of several glutathione S-transferases, or converted to benzo[a]pyrene 7,8-diol by microsomal epoxide hydrolase (encoded by *EPHX1*). The diol is subject to subsequent conversion to benzo[a]pyrene 7,8-dihydrodiol 9,10-epoxide, which has been shown experimentally to be a much more potent carcinogen than the 7,8-epoxide.

Both pathways are hypothesized to be involved in the etiology of colorectal polyps and colorectal cancer, through production of final activated metabolites that can form DNA adducts. Both HCA adducts and benzo[a]pyrene adducts have been detected in the human colon (Autrup et al., 1982).

Gene regulation: Although the long-term average metabolic rates of individuals are not directly observable, they are determined in part by their measurable genotypes and by factors that induce or inhibit their expression, some of which are also measurable (Figure 3). Several genes in these pathways are reportedly subject to regulation by environmental agents. Most notably, tobacco smoke has been shown to induce expression of both *CYP1A1* and *CYP1A2*; expression of *CYP1A2* has also been shown to be induced by HCAs (Sinha et al., 1994); and *NAT2* expression is inhibited by acetaminophen (Rothen et al., 1998). In addition to affecting the long-term expression of a gene, various covariates such as age or gender might also affect the validity or reproducibility of short-term measurements of the metabolic rates. We have not explicitly allowed for that in our primary analysis, although the methodology is sufficiently general to allow for this possibility by including covariates in either portion of the model (see Results for details of this sensitivity analysis).

Subjects and data

Haile et al. (1997) provided a detailed description of the study population, 466 cases with polyps and

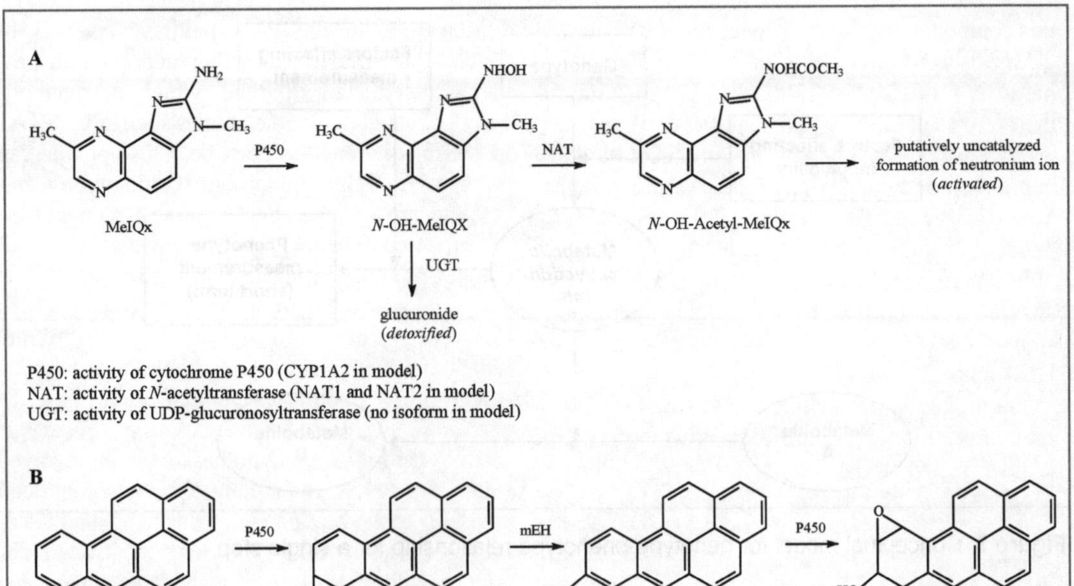

A

P450: activity of cytochrome P450 (CYP1A2 in model)
NAT: activity of *N*-acetyltransferase (NAT1 and NAT2 in model)
UGT: activity of UDP-glucuronosyltransferase (no isoform in model)

B

mEH: activity of microsomal epoxide hydrolase (EPHX1 in model)
P450: activity of cytochrome P450 (CYP1A in model)
GST: activity of glutathione *S*-transferase (GSTM3 in model)

Figure 2. Biochemical representation of the two pathways: A. HCA pathway (simplified schema illustrating conversion of 2-amino-3,8-dimethylimidazo[4,5-*f*]quinoxaline (MeIQx) to putatively activated and detoxified metabolites). B. PAH pathway (simplified schema illustrating conversion of benzo[a]pyrene to putatively activated and detoxified metabolites)

509 controls, and their questionnaire responses used as measures for exposure to PAHs, HCAs and compounds that induce or inhibit enzyme expression. In this analysis, we limit attention to cigarette smoking (pack–years and current status) and WDRM (a five-point ordinal classification based on usual consumption and cooking methods). For each gene in the model, measurements were made by genotyping, phenotyping or both. Genotypes were measured by assaying genomic DNA provided by study participants, to determine each individual's sequence for previously described

polymorphisms. *CYP1A1* genotypes for the non-coding 3′ T250C polymorphism and the exon 7 Ile462Val substitution were assayed essentially as described by Hayashi *et al.* (1991). *EPHX1* and *GSTM3* genotypes were measured as described by Cortessis *et al.* (2001). *NAT1* and *NAT2* genotypes were assayed and assigned to activity groups as described by Lin *et al.* (1994a) and Probst-Hensch *et al.* (1995), respectively. Phenotypic measurements were made by asking study participants to ingest a standard dose of a test substrate, wait for a specified time interval, then provide a urine

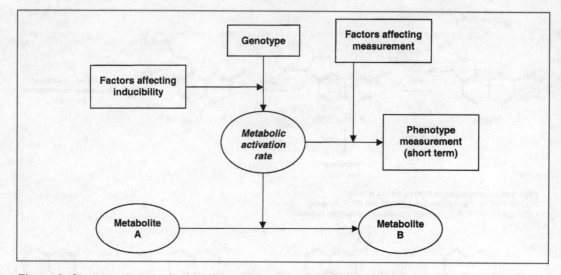

Figure 3. Conceptual model for genotype-phenotype relationship for a single step

sample from which ratios of the substrate's metabolites were measured. Using caffeine as a probe drug for activities of *NAT2* and *CYP1A2* and *para*-aminosalicylic acid as a probe drug for *NAT1* activity, phenotypes were concurrently measured as metabolic indices for these three enzymes as described by Grant *et al.* (1992).

Statistical methods
The basic statistical model and the MCMC method for fitting it are described in detail in the Appendix. Here we summarize the major features in a non-mathematical way. The central feature of our approach is a statistical idealization of the metabolic pathways summarized in Figures 1 and 2. In this representation, we treat the long-term average concentrations of each of the intermediate metabolites as a set of unobserved 'latent variables' for each subject. These seven intermediate metabolites are described in Table 3, together with the various genes that influence their respective activation and detoxification rates. In addition to these metabolite concentrations, the metabolic rates are also treated as latent variables for each subject. These rates are assumed to have statistical distributions related to the observable genotypes or phenotypes and to a further set of population parameters corresponding to their genotype-specific means and variances (Figure 3). Figure 4,

explained more fully in the Appendix, shows the relationship between the observable exposures (indicated by the boxes labelled X) genotypes (G), phenotypes (P), and outcome (polyps, Y), and the unobserved intermediate metabolites (indicated by the circles labelled Z). The quantitative relationships between the various metabolites is given by a set of first-order toxicokinetic equations, together with additional models for the relationship of initial and final metabolites to exposure and disease, respectively. Figure 5 provides the details of any one step in the metabolic process, namely the relationship between the metabolites, an activation or detoxification rate and the observable genotypes and phenotypes. The various unobservable long-term metabolic rates and the short-term measurements of these rates are related to the corresponding genotypes by lognormal distributions. To summarize, the model is comprised of the following six submodels (see Appendix):
- a linear model for the dependence of the first metabolite in each pathway on exposure (Equation 2)
- a logistic model for the risk of disease on the final metabolite in each pathway (Equation 3)
- a system of linear toxicokinetic equations for the dependence of each metabolite on its precursor and corresponding activation and detoxification rates (Equation 4)

Table 3. Intermediate metabolites and corresponding activation and detoxification genes shown in Figure 2

Pathway	Parent compound or metabolite	Gene[a]	
		Activation	Detoxification
HCA	Z_1 = MeIQx[b]	–	–
	Z_2 = N-OH-MeIQx[c]	P_1 = CYP1A2	–
	Z_3 = N-O-Acetyl-MeIQx[c]	G_2, P_2 = NAT1	–
		G_3, P_3 = NAT2	
PAH	Z_4 = Benzo[a]pyrene (BAP)[c]	–	–
	Z_5 = BAP 7,8-epoxide[c]	G_4 = CYP1A1	G_5 = GSTM3
	Z_6 = BAP 7,8-diol[c]	G_6 = EPHX1	
	Z_7 = BAP 7,8-dihydrodiol 9,10-epoxide[c]	G_4 = CYP1A1	G_5 = GSTM3

[a] P_n, phenotypic measurement; G_n, genotypic measurement
[b] Procarcinogen parent compound
[c] Metabolite

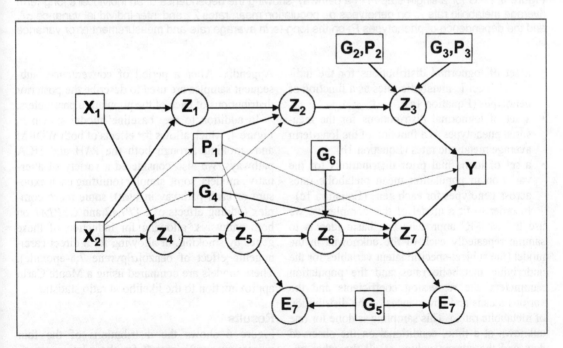

Figure 4. Directed acyclic graph (DAG) for the combined pathway model: Xs represent exposures, Y the disease phenotype, Z the procarcinogen parent compounds and their metabolites, G the genotypes determining metabolic rates, and P the phenotypes corresponding to these genes. The key to the parent compounds, metabolites and genes is given in Table 3. Dotted lines indicate additional relationships that were considered in alternative models, but not part of the main study results.

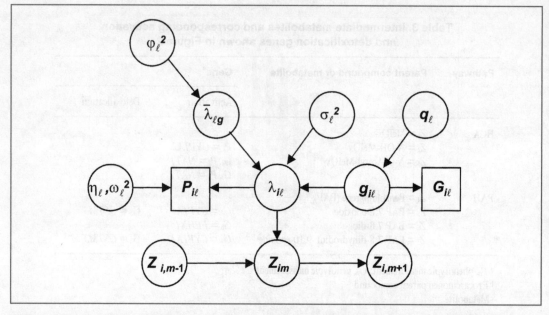

Figure 5. DAG for a single step m in a pathway, showing the dependence of an individual's long-term average metabolic rate λ_{il} on genotypes g_{il}, population mean rates $\bar{\lambda}_{lg}$ and inter-individual variance σ_l^2, and the dependence of phenotypes P_{il} on the long-term average rate and measurement error variance ω_l^2

- a set of lognormal distributions for the individual-specific metabolic rates as a function of genotypes (Equation 1a)
- a set of lognormal distributions for the measured phenotypes as a function of the long-term average metabolic rates (Equation 1b)
- a set of lognormal prior distributions for the variation in population mean metabolic rates across genotypes for each gene (Equation 1c)

In order to fit a model of this complexity, we use the MCMC approach. The basic idea is to sample repeatedly each of the unknowns in the model (the subject-specific latent variables for the underlying metabolic rates and the population parameters, the regression coefficients and the various means and covariances of the distribution of metabolic rates). This sampling is done for one unknown at a time, conditional on the observed data and the current values of all the other unknowns. (To improve performance, the metabolite concentrations are not sampled, but are handled deterministically.) The specific procedures for each of these samplings are described in the Appendix. After a period of convergence, subsequent samples are used to describe the posterior distributions of each of the population parameters.

In addition to the 'baseline' model shown in Figure 4, which allows for effects of both WDRM and smoking through both the PAH and HCA pathways, we also considered a variety of alternative models, some simpler (omitting each exposure or each pathway in turn), some more complex (adding effects of *CYP1A2* and *CYP1A1* on both pathways, allowing for induction of these genes by smoking, or allowing for a direct carcinogenic effect of benzo[a]pyrene 7,8-epoxide). These models are compared using a Monte Carlo approximation to the likelihood ratio statistic.

Results

Figure 6 shows the distributions of the four regression coefficients β for the relative contributions of WDRM and smoking to the HCA and PAH pathways, respectively. The shaded bars are the posterior densities, the open bars are the prior densities, and the solid bars are their ratios,

known as Bayes factors, which should be used to draw inference about the information from the data about each parameter. These can be thought of as the Bayesian analogue of likelihood ratios, except that they are constructed from the marginal distributions, rather than maximized over nuisance parameters, and do not have the same asymptotic distribution theory leading to chi-squared distributions. Kass and Raftery (1995) have suggested guidelines for interpretation of Bayes factors as follows: a Bayes factor of 1–3 can be considered as 'very mild evidence', 3–20 as 'positive', 20–150 'strong' and greater than 150 as 'very strong'. These criteria were suggested for comparison of alternative models rather than for parameter estimation purposes, but they suggest that inference on these parameters will be rather weak. Generally speaking, however, there appears to be somewhat stronger evidence for values of $\beta > 0$ for smoking than for WDRM on both pathways. However, the contributions of both exposures are somewhat diluted by being split into separate pathways, and the evidence for contributions of both exposures becomes stronger when the analysis is restricted to a single pathway at a time (results not shown).

Figure 7 provides similar plots of the distributions and Bayes factors for the parameters γ of the logistic model for polyps risk in terms of the final metabolites on both pathways. Not surprisingly, the intercept term γ_0 can be estimated with much greater precision than either of the relative risk parameters, although there is somewhat stronger evidence for the contribution γ_2 of the PAH pathway than for the HCA pathway γ_1.

Figure 8 summarizes the marginal means of the estimates of genotype-specific mean activity levels $\bar{\lambda}_{lg}$ for the six genes. The posterior means are shown on the left-hand side of the figure and the corresponding prior means on the right. For identifiability, we constrained these means to be monotonic across the genotype categories for each gene, and hence the trend even under the prior has a relatively broad range. This variability across genotypes was generally smaller in the posterior distribution, since a relatively uninformative prior was used, the strongest posterior gradients being seen for NAT2 and EPHX1.

By logistic regression of Y on $E(Z_3)$ and $E(Z_7)$, the average of the individuals' final metabolite assignments across MCMC samples, we could see that the PAH pathway appeared to be the more important contributor to risk of polyps. Similarly, linear regression of $E(Z_3)$ and $E(Z_7)$ on the various Xs and Gs indicated that smoking was the larger contributor to both pathways, and that NAT1 made a relatively minor contribution to the HCA pathway, whereas all three genes made very strong contributions to the PAH pathway (results not shown). Because the models are not nested and because the pathways analysis incorporates additional prior assumptions, a direct comparison of the fit of this model to the simpler logistic regression models described in the Introduction would not be appropriate.

Table 4 summarizes the fit of a number of alternative models that we considered. Model 1 is the 'baseline' model previously described in detail, against which each of the alternatives should be compared. The table provides the posterior means and posterior SDs of the four βs for the contributions of WDRM and pack-years of cigarette smoking to each of the two pathways, together with the corresponding contributions γ of the final metabolites in each pathway to risk of polyps. The final column provides the mean of the log likelihood ratios comparing $\Pr(Y \mid Z_3, Z_7)$ for the fitted model to that for the null model (constant risk of polyps); this statistic is intended only as a rough comparison of the relative predictive value of the alternative models and should not be construed as having a chi-squared distribution (Chib, 1995). In all the models considered, WDRM made a relatively small contribution to either pathway, even when only one or the other pathway was included in the model (e.g. models 2 and 3) or when the analysis was restricted to nonsmokers (model 5), whereas smoking had generally stronger effects, particularly when its contribution was limited to a single pathway. The fit of model 6, which restricted effects of WDRM to the HCA pathway and effects of smoking to the PAH pathway, was somewhat worse than the baseline model. Model 7 allows for induction of CYP1A2 and CYP1A1 by smoking status, age and sex; this model did not improve the overall fit and considerably inflated

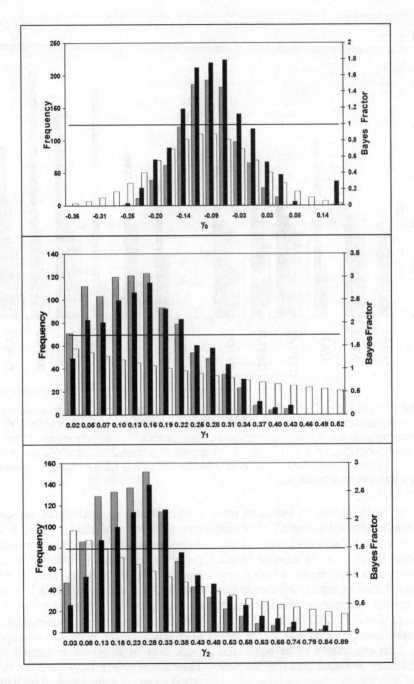

Figure 7. Posterior distributions (shaded bars), prior distributions (open bars) and Bayes factors (solid bars) for the regression coefficients γ giving the intercept (γ_0, upper panel) of the logistic model for risk of polyps and the log relative risk for the final metabolites in the HCA pathway (γ_1, middle panel) and the PAH pathway (γ_2, bottom panel), based on every 10th of 10 000 iterations following a burn-in period of 2000 iterations.

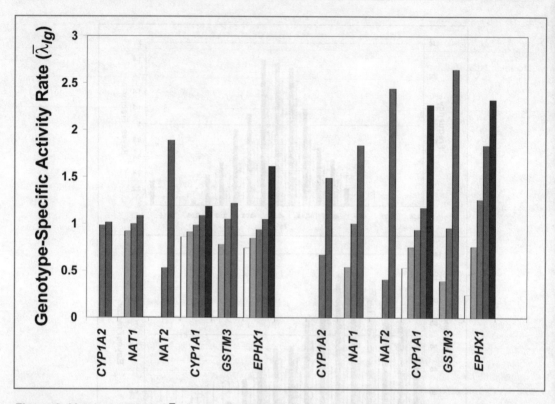

Figure 8. Marginal means of $\overline{\lambda}_{lg}$ for the six genes: left: posterior means; right prior means, based on lognormal distribution with order constraint. Order of genotypes from white to black: for *CYP1A2*, *NAT1* and *NAT2*: homozygous low-activity, heterozygous, homozygous high-activity imputed from phenotype among two level genotype; for *CYP1A1*: 0,1,2,3,4 copies of alleles 250C and 462Val in joint 3' non-coding/exon 7 genotype; for *GSTM3*: *B*B,*A*B,*A*A; for *EPHX1*: 0,1,2,3,4 copies of alleles 113Y and 139R in joint exon 3/exon 4 genotype.

the SEs of both the βs and the γs, indicating problems of identifiability. Allowing *CYP1A2* and *CYP1A1* to act on both pathways (model 8) also did not improve the fit over our baseline model, nor did allowing for a direct action of both Z_5 and Z_7 on Y (model 9). Finally, model 10 is the same as model 1 except that the relative contributions of *NAT1* versus *NAT2* to Z_3, *CYP1A1* to Z_5 and Z_7 and *GSTM3* to detoxification of Z_5 and Z_7 are estimated rather than constrained to be equal; this additional flexibility produced little improvement in fit.

Discussion

A great deal is known from experimental studies about the biochemical reactions by which

environmental procarcinogens are converted to carcinogenic metabolites (Vineis *et al.*, 1999). Although this information is frequently used to guide the selection of factors to be addressed in epidemiological analyses and to interpret the findings, it is seldom explicitly incorporated into the analysis. We have proposed a statistical approach to accomplish this aim. At this point, we offer this approach more as a conceptual framework than as a definitive method of analysis. There are of course many questions that could be raised about our formulation, from both statistical and biological perspectives.

From a biological perspective, the proposed model is necessarily simplified, due to incomplete understanding of human metabolic pathways and

Table 4. Summary of fits of alternative models

Model	HCA Pathway			PAH Pathway			Mean
	β_1 (WDRM)	β_2 (Smoking)	γ_1 Polyps	β_3 (WDRM)	β_4 (Smoking)	γ_2 Polyps	LLR (S.E.)
1	0.16 (0.18)	0.38 (0.30)	0.15 (0.10)	0.15 (0.21)	0.37 (0.33)	0.29 (0.22)	14.28 (0.15)
2	0.15 (0.17)	0.57 (0.38)	0.20 (0.10)	–	–	–	3.70 (0.03)
3	–	–	–	0.11 (0.15)	0.49 (0.39)	0.35 (0.19)	14.10 (0.14)
4	–	0.46 (0.36)	0.15 (0.09)	–	0.34 (0.30)	0.24 (0.16)	10.32 (0.10)
5[a]	0.18 (0.31)	–	0.09 (0.08)	0.19 (0.25)	–	0.19 (0.14)	1.00 (0.02)
6	0.18 (0.20)	–	0.10 (0.07)	–	0.48 (0.36)	0.31 (0.16)	11.41 (0.10)
7[b]	0.30 (0.32)	0.46 (0.37)	0.33 (0.27)	0.38 (0.35)	0.57 (0.75)	0.65 (0.65)	7.65 (0.05)
8[c]	0.17 (0.19)	0.47 (0.42)	0.14 (0.09)	0.13 (0.17)	0.37 (0.31)	0.25 (0.15)	10.88 (0.08)
9[d]	0.17 (0.19)	0.51 (0.36)	0.15 (0.09)	0.10 (0.13)	0.34 (0.29)	0.19 (0.11) 0.08 (0.06)	9.07 (0.07)
10[e]	0.16 (0.17)	0.35 (0.33)	0.14 (0.08)	0.12 (0.15)	0.47 (0.38)	0.27 (0.14)	10.51 (0.07)

[a] Never smokers only (Note: log LR is not comparable to the others because there are fewer subjects).
[b] Allows for induction of *CYP1A2* and *CYP1A1* by smoking status, age, and sex.
[c] Allows for action of *CYP1A2* and *CYP1A1* on both pathways.
[d] Allows for direct action of both Z_5 and Z_7 on Y (coefficient γ of Z_5 is shown below that of Z_7).
[e] Same as model 1 except relative contributions of *NAT1* versus *NAT2* to Z_3, *CYP1A1* to Z_5 and Z_7 and *GSTM3* to detoxification of Z_5 and Z_7 are estimated rather than constrained to be equal.
WDRM, well-done red meat; LLR, log likelihood ratio; SE, standard error

limitations in available data. We attempted to identify and model etiologically important steps in the process whereby exposure to xenobiotic compounds leads to formation of colorectal polyps. Elements of the pathways were suggested by published epidemiological, biochemical, genetic and gene-expression studies, and these will surely change as additional relevant findings emerge. However, even on the basis of what is now known, many additional variants of the proposed pathways might be considered to address limitations of these analyses, described below.

• First, to construct a model, one must identify the important environmental procarcinogens, and our list may not be complete. It may be argued, for example, that additional classes of compounds, such as aromatic amines (AAs) – which, together with PAHs and HCAs, are present in tobacco smoke – should be included.

• Second, we have not included all pathways for the metabolism and action of PAHs and HCAs, and one or more omitted pathways may be etio-

logically relevant. For example, some authors suggest that a proposed PAH pathway not considered in this report may be of particular interest for the induction of DNA damage in extrahepatic tissue such as the colon (De Kok & van Maanen, 2000). This proposed metabolic pathway involves 1-electron oxidation to 6-oxo benzo[*a*]pyrene radical leading to benzo[*a*]pyrene-3,6 dione, benzo[*a*]pyrene-1,6 dione, benzo[*a*]pyrene-6,12 dione, corresponding benzo[*a*]pyrene diols and reactive oxygen species.

• Third, there may be other important connections or steps we have not included in the pathways we described, and we have not included all the steps between exposure and occurrence of disease. In the PAH pathway, we have included only a single member of the cytochrome P450 class of activation genes and only a single member of the glutathione *S*-transferase detoxification genes, although others may be important. Although polymorphisms have been described in several distinct genes encoding human glutathione *S*-transferases, we measured *GSTM3*A/*B* because a previous report (Jourenkova-Mironova *et al.*, 2000) suggested that this polymorphism may be an important modifier of associations between *EPHX1* polymorphisms and smoking-related disease. However, the functional significance of this *GSTM3* polymorphism is not clear, and reported effects may arise from linkage disequilibrium with unmeasured variants in the *GSTM3* region, which contains five *GST* μ class genes. We did not include the human α class *GST*s in the HCA pathway, even though these enzymes inhibit the covalent binding of HCAs to DNA, with the greatest effect (90% inhibition) observed for the A1-1 isoenzyme (Lin *et al.*, 1994b). We do not address other possible activating enzymes, such as sulfotransferases in the HCA pathway, or additional transport and elimination steps such as that catalysed by UDP-glucuronosyltransferases. We do not address intermediate biomarkers including DNA adducts that could in theory be incorporated, or consider the action of cell cycle regulators or DNA repair mechanisms on PAH– or HCA–DNA adducts, before polyp formation. Hierarchical models, such as those discussed by De Roos *et al.* (this volume), might provide a suitable means for incorporating multiple genes which might potentially be acting at a particular stage of the model but which are *a priori* 'exchangeable'. Some genes whose products participate in these pathways have been studied, individually and in combinations, in epidemiological studies exploring the possibility that certain variants may predispose to colorectal carcinoma or polyps. Conflicting results are reported for associations of *NAT2* genotypes and phenotypes with these outcomes in numerous studies (e.g. Katoh *et al.*, 2000 and those reviewed by Hein *et al.*, 2000 and Brockton *et al.*, 2000). Some report no association; others report associations with rapid acetylator variants, with a tendency for strongest associations with rapid variants to be reported jointly with rapid CYP1A2 activity, in

studies addressing both loci. Bell *et al.* (1995) found an association between the *NAT1*10 allele and colorectal cancer, with risk highest among NAT2 rapid acetylators, and Chen *et al.* (1998) found the strongest effect of WDRM among rapid acetylators for both NAT1 and NAT2. However, in two studies of *NAT1* variants and polyps previously conducted using data included in the present analysis, no association was found (Probst-Hensch *et al.*, 1995; Lin *et al.*, 1998), and Katoh *et al.* (2000) did not find an association between *NAT1* variants and adenocarcinoma of the colon, in a joint analysis with *NAT2*. Finally, in contrast to our results suggesting that polyps are associated with more stable *EPHX1* variants in some subgroups, Ulrich *et al.* (2001) found no overall association between *EPHX1* exon 3 or 4 variants and polyps, but they did find an association between the exon 3 lower stability variant in some subgroups, with highest risks among those who reported eating fried, baked or broiled meat more than twice a week. We are not aware of other studies addressing genes whose products participate in both PAH and HCA pathways. The studies published to date illustrate the variety of approaches taken to address genes whose products participate in the HCA pathway, and exposures to parent compounds and inducers such as smoking. It is not possible at present to determine whether these conflicting results are attributable to model misspecification or other factors.

- Fourth, for those enzymes included in the model, we have not formally addressed all possible determinants of total activity. The measured polymorphisms may capture important differences in specific or total activity of individual protein variants, and we have included some indicators of induction and inhibition of gene expression. However, other determinants of total activity are not addressed. These include additional known or presumed inducers and inhibitors (environmental and endogenous) of gene expression, differential stability of variant transcripts and proteins, factors affecting assembly of holoenzyme and pre- and post-translational regulation of enzyme activity, availability of cofactors and possible competition between isoenzymes for coenzymes.

• Fifth, there are several notable limitations in the data on polyps. These include numerous limitations in the available data on genotype and phenotype. For example, among the 975 participants in the study, *CYP1A2*, *NAT1* and *NAT2* phenotypes were available for only 461, 462 and 530, respectively. Fortunately, data on genotype (*NAT1*, *NAT2*, *CYP1A1*, *GSTM3*, *EPHX1*) were available for the vast majority (929–958) of participants. Our measurements of the two exposure variables are extremely crude – pack–years of smoking and a five-point classification of WDRM combining frequency of meat consumption and usual cooking method. We use these definitions of smoking and meat consumption as proxy measures of exposure to PAHs and HCAs, respectively. However, the accuracy of these proxy measures is not known, as these exposures carry with them other classes of compounds (such as AAs), and they do not measure individual PAHs or HCAs. Thus we use benzo[*a*]pyrene and MeIQx to illustrate the action of enzymes in the pathways on classes of compounds (PAHs and HCAs), rather than on individual compounds. This seems reasonable because we presume that compounds within a class will be metabolized by the same set of enzymes. However, we are aware that, even within a class of compounds, an enzyme's affinities and kinetics may vary from one specific substrate to another. An example is provided by heterologous expression studies of recombinant human *NAT1* and *NAT2* (Minchin *et al.*, 1992; Hein *et al.*, 1994). These investigators measured specific activities for *O*-acetylation of three individual HCAs implicated in the etiology of colorectal adenoma and carcinoma: 2-amino-3-methylimidazo[4,5-*f*]quinolin (IQ), 2-amino-1-methyl-6-phenylimidazo[4,5-*b*]pyridine (PhIP) and MeIQx. Wild-type NAT1 was shown to have higher activity for N-OH-IQ than wild-type NAT2 but, conversely, NAT2 had higher activity for both N-OH-PhIP and N-OH-MeIQx. Sinha *et al.* (personal communication) and

Keating *et al.* (2000) have been developing more elaborate methods for quantifying HCAs, based on laboratory measurements of their individual concentrations in various foods following differing methods of preparation. Their measures have recently been included in several epidemiological studies (most notably Sinha *et al.*, 2001), and could be applied to future epidemiological studies. Once such data are available, pathways could in theory be refined to address exposure to individual compounds.

• Finally, even if these are the most important pathways and their biological components are appropriately specified, they may not be adequately described by our statistical idealization of them. As already discussed, our methods are restricted to linear kinetics models; with better measures of exposure, it would be worth exploring non-linear models such as the Hill equation (Denes *et al.*, 1996). The assumptions of linear exposure and logistic risk models could of course also be relaxed.

The primary statistical concerns are the identifiability of the parameters, and the influence of priors for parameters which cannot be estimated directly from the available data. Two examples were difficulties (1) in jointly estimating the regression coefficients (βs and γs), and (2) in jointly estimating the inter-individual and measurement error variances (σ^2 and ω^2, respectively). We also found that other parameters need to be constrained. Although our choice of priors for such parameters was arbitrary, it is in principle possible to develop meaningful priors for some of these parameters from additional measurements that could be made in a study that aimed to use this approach (e.g. replicate measurements of the metabolic phenotypes or measurements of the intermediate or excreted phenotypes), or from separate studies (e.g. studies of the population variance in metabolic rates or tissue culture studies of genotype-specific metabolic rates). De Roos *et al.* (this volume) propose the creation of an 'Exposure–Gene–Disease (E-G-D)' database which might assemble all the relevant information of the toxicology of various chemicals, their metabolic pathways and the genes they contain,

their polymorphisms and effects on their metabolic activity. Such data would be invaluable as a
basis for specifying informative priors for a PBPK
analysis like our approach. Alternatively, validation substudies (or even entirely separate
studies) aimed at measuring metabolic activities
or other components of the model could be analysed jointly with the main study data to narrow
the uncertainties about some of the constituent
parameters. Simulation would also be useful for
studying the potential information gain that could
be obtained by incorporating different types of
additional measurements. Recent simulation
studies (to be reported elsewhere) indicate that
both of the problems of identifiability described
above can be improved by having measurements
of some of the intermediate metabolites, for
example in the form of short-term measurements
of excreted metabolites.

We recognize that a sample of about 1000
subjects with a dichotomous outcome (in addition
to the other data limitations discussed above) may
be inadequate to fit a model of this complexity.
Unfortunately, there is no analytical way to determine sample size requirements for such models,
so investigators will have to rely on simulation for
this purpose. Our own simulation studies have
been based on model parameters estimated from
our already available data on polyps; by repeated
generation of new data using these parameters, we
can then estimate the sample sizes that would be
needed for a more definitive application of the
model to new data. For application in a new
setting, an investigator might use trial and error to
specify a range of parameter values that would
produce descriptive risk estimates for main effects
and interactions of the size anticipated, and then
use simulations to determine the sample size
requirements for mechanistic modelling.

Another complexity we have not attempted to
address is the time-dependent nature of the exposures. We have no data on changes in individuals'
diets – only the 'usual' consumption and cooking
methods of meats – but for cigarette smoking, we
have the ages at starting and quitting smoking and
the usual number of cigarettes per day. As is
conventional, we have used pack–years as the
measure of exposure, X_2, in our models, but an

ideal analysis would have made the calculations
separately for periods of smoking and not
smoking, using cigarettes per day as X_2, and then
integrated the resulting Z_M over the relevant time
periods. This would then entail consideration of
such effects as age and latency (Thomas, 1988)
that we considered beyond the scope of this
already complex analysis.

Despite many limitations in this early model
and the data to which we have applied it, we feel
that the approach has considerable potential to
provide insights into biological pathways that
cannot be obtained by standard statistical analysis. In fact, our enumeration of these limitations
highlights several potential strengths of the
approach.

• First, the statistical machinery is highly
  flexible and readily adapted to competing or
  emerging biochemical models. For example,
  although the linear PBPK formulation we have
  adopted might be suitable for modelling metabolic activation and detoxification of carcinogens, a very different form of mathematical
  model might be needed for other mechanisms,
  such as DNA damage and repair. We expect
  that this flexibility will be advantageous in
  both the planning and the conduct of studies.

• Second, in the process of specifying the model,
  important gaps in the supporting genetic and
  biochemical theory are explicitly revealed. The
  relative importance of various missing pieces
  can then be explored by simulation, as a basis
  for rational decisions about which avenues to
  pursue. Similarly, simulation can be used to
  evaluate the potential importance of new
  related findings – such as a novel genetic polymorphism or detection of enzyme expression in
  an additional cell compartment – in light of
  what is already established.

The hierarchical modelling approach described
by De Roos et al. (this volume) represents a very
different but complementary way of dealing with
complex problems involving multiple genes and
multiple exposures, possibly interacting in
complex ways. In their approach, a standard
logistic model for the observed data is specified
first, incorporating various main effects and interactions, and then a second-level model puts some

statistical structure on the regression coefficients from the first stage. This second-level model might, for example, group exposures or genes into classes that are considered *a priori* exchangeable, thereby assuming that their effect estimates have a common distribution, characterized by a mean and variance which is to be estimated or which has some prior distribution. As in our proposal above, the E-G-D database could be used to specify informative priors for this second-level model. The hierarchical modelling approach can be thought of as an empirical approach which is less reliant on specific mathematical models for the metabolic pathways, in contrast to our more mechanistic approach. It might thus be less powerful (if our mechanistic models were correctly specified) but more robust (if they were not). In our view, the two approaches are complementary and could be used in combination, the empirical models suggesting specific models that could then be fitted mechanistically.

The analyses described in this paper were based on a C++ programme written specifically for this purpose (available on request from the authors); considerable effort might be required to adapt the programme for different applications. However, it appears that standard MCMC software, such as the BUGS programme (Gilks *et al.*, 1994) might be adaptable for this purpose and a version specifically tailored for PBPK modelling is now available (http://www.med.ic.ac.uk/divisions/60/pkbugs_web/home.html). Unfortunately, it appears that the flexibility and generality of BUGS lead to some computational inefficiency, so that it runs much more slowly than our programme on large data sets, although it is very useful for designing analyses on data sets of modest size.

We hasten to point out that even a good fit of the model to data can never establish the truth of the model. Instead, we view the utility of a model in terms of the types of comparisons it can offer within a unified framework. For example, in the context of environmental epidemiology, 'empirical models' such as the logistic model have been widely used to estimate exposure–response relationships, but mechanistic models like the Armitage–Doll multistage model or the

Moolgavkar–Knudson two-event clonal expansion model offer an alternative approach that exploits our understanding of the carcinogenic process. Although the validity of such models cannot be determined by their fit to epidemiological data, they can be useful as a basis for inferring whether an exposure acts at an early or a late stage in a multistage process or as an initiator or promoter (Thomas, 1988). In the same manner, in the present context, one can test whether the effect of WDRM is stronger through the HCA or the PAH pathway by setting β_1 or β_3 to zero, or by eliminating various genes from the model one can test hypotheses about their effects and interactions. Similarly, we began to explore the hypotheses about the inducibility of *CYP1A2* and *CYP1A1* by adding links between X_2 and λ_{i1} and λ_{i4}.

Although there is an extensive literature on PBPK models, which have been widely used in carcinogenic risk assessment, very little attention has been paid to incorporation of genetic information into such models. We leave many questions unanswered in this preliminary report, but would like to encourage others to pursue this approach.

In principle, a similar approach could be taken to other applications. For example, we are currently exploring one involving aromatic amines and bladder cancer, a particularly appealing system because some intermediate metabolites may be assayed in urine. The basic process of developing such applications would entail first conceptualizing the relevant biological processes in the form of a statistical representation such as that shown in Figure 4, followed by developing the fitting algorithms. Although our programme is somewhat flexible in terms of the specific pathways, genes, exposures and outcomes, we anticipate that adapting it to other applications would require some sophistication and considerable effort, and that additional simulation studies might be needed to validate is performance on other model systems.

Acknowledgements

Supported by grants from the National Cancer Institute (CA-42949, CA-52862) and the National

Institute for Environmental Health Sciences (P30-ES-10421), U.S. Public Health Service.

Appendix: statistical methods
Models for metabolic pathways
Figure 4 provides a statistical idealization of a hypothetical metabolic pathway in the form of a directed acyclic graph (DAG). In this representation, squares represent observed quantities and circles represent unobserved quantities – latent variables and population parameters. Here, Y represents disease, and the Xs represent exposures (WDRM and pack–years of smoking), Gs genotypes and Ps phenotypes (the measured metabolic activity rates).

Figure 5 shows the details of the model for a single stage in the process as a DAG representation of the conceptual model shown in Figure 3. The circles containing Z_{im} represent the intermediate metabolites for the mth step ($m = 1, \ldots, 7$) for subject $i = 1, \ldots, n$. The circles containing λ_{il} denote the long-term average metabolic activation or detoxification rates for the various genetic loci $l = 1,\ldots,L$; in other words, λ_{il} denotes the rate at which Z_{m-1} is converted to Z_m (for an activating enzyme) or the rate at which Z_m is eliminated by pathways other than conversion to Z_{m+1} (for a detoxifying enzyme). These unobserved long-term rates λ_{il} are determined by the individual's genotypes G_{il} at the corresponding locus, and in turn are determinants of the short-term phenotypic measures P_{il} (i.e. assays of the enzyme activity levels). The circles containing g_{il} represent the subject's true genotypes, with population allele frequency $q_{l,}$ whereas the squares containing G_{il} represent the observed genotype (assumed to be the same as the true where available).

To allow for inter-individual variability, we assume that subjects' unobserved long-term average rates λ_{il} are distributed around the population average rate $\bar{\lambda}_{lg}$, corresponding to their genotypes G_{il} with some inter-individual variance σ_l^2. (In analyses incorporating induction effects, we adopted a log-linear model for the effects of current smoking status, age and gender on λ_{il}, with regression coefficients that were also estimated.) Detoxification rates for which we have no measurements of the relevant genes were

arbitrarily fixed at 1. We also assume that subjects' phenotypes P_{il} are distributed around λ_{il} with measurement-error variance τ_l^2. To the extent that measurable factors such as age, gender or smoking status modify an individual's metabolic rate, this could be accounted for by incorporating covariates into the models for λ_{il} and P_{il}. (In exploratory analyses, we included the current smoking status as a binary indicator variable in a linear model for $\ln(\lambda_{il})$ and pack–years of smoking as the exposure X_2. Age and gender were also considered as covariates in a linear model for $\ln(P_{il})$. However, these additional complexities appeared to produce some problems of identifiability and have been eliminated in the results.) Finally, the variance of the population mean rates $\bar{\lambda}_l$ across genotypes is determined by the population variance φ_l^2. Specifically, we assume that all the relevant variables have lognormal distributions, i.e.

$$\log \lambda_{il} \sim N(\log \bar{\lambda}_{lg_{il}}, \sigma_l^2), \tag{1a}$$

$$\log P_{il} \sim N[\log(\eta_l \lambda_{il}), \omega_l^2], \tag{1b}$$

$$\log \bar{\lambda}_{lg} \sim N(0, \varphi_l^2). \tag{1c}$$

Finally, since not all subjects have genotypes available at all loci, genotypes are assumed to have multinomial distributions with population frequencies q_l.

We begin by assuming that the first substrate on each pathway (Z_{i1} and Z_{i4} in our model) is related to exposure(s) via a simple linear model:

$$Z_{i1} = 1 + \beta_1 X_{i1} + \beta_2 X_{i2} \tag{2a}$$

$$Z_{i4} = 1 + \beta_3 X_{i1} + \beta_4 X_{i2} \tag{2b}$$

We also assume a logistic dependence of the disease phenotype on the final metabolites (Z_{i3} and Z_{i7}) of the form

$$logit \Pr(Y_i = 1 \mid Z_{iM}) =$$
$$\gamma_0 + \gamma_1[Z_{i3} - E(Z_{*3})] + \gamma_2[Z_{i7} - E(Z_{*7})] + \ldots, \tag{3}$$

where '...' indicates the possibility of including other pathways or covariates. Centring the final metabolites on their mean in this way improves the identifiability of the βs and γs. The simplest linear pharmacokinetic model is given by differential equations of the form

$$\frac{dZ_m}{dt} = \lambda_{m-1} Z_{m-1} - (\lambda_m + \mu_m) Z_m$$

where the rate of change of metabolite Z_m is the rate at which it is being created from its precursor by λ_{m-1} minus the rates at which it is transformed into its successor or detoxified by λ_m and μ_m, respectively. In this linear equation, the creation and elimination rates are treated as proportional to the concentration of the respective substrate, times the corresponding rate parameter. More complex Michaelis–Menton or receptor-binding models (Denes *et al.*, 1996; Moolgavkar *et al.*, 1999) could be used to allow for some nonlinear threshold or saturation effects, the shapes of which could depend in various ways upon genotype. The steady-state solution to this equation, obtained by setting $dZ_m/dt = 0$, is

$$Z_m = Z_{m-1} \left(\frac{\lambda_{m-1}}{\lambda_m + \mu_m} \right) \qquad (4)$$

By combining Equation (2) and successive applications of Equation (4) for each step in the two pathways, the concentrations of the final metabolites in our model can be written as

$$Z_3(\mathbf{X}_i, \boldsymbol{\beta}, \boldsymbol{\lambda}_i) =$$
$$(1 + \beta_1 X_1 + \beta_2 X_2)\left(\frac{\lambda_{i1}}{1 + \lambda_{i2} + \lambda_{i3}} \right)(\lambda_{i2} + \lambda_{i3}) \qquad (5a)$$

$$Z_7(\mathbf{X}_i, \boldsymbol{\beta}, \boldsymbol{\lambda}_i) =$$
$$(1 + \beta_3 X_1 + \beta_4 X_2)\left(\frac{\lambda_{i4}}{\lambda_{i5} + \lambda_{i6}} \right)\left(\frac{\lambda_{i6}}{1 + \lambda_{i4}} \right)\left(\frac{\lambda_{i4}}{1 + \lambda_{i5}} \right) \qquad (5b)$$

where the various λs depend upon the corresponding genotypes.

To complete the model specification, we place vague priors on the model parameters β, γ, φ^2, σ^2, η, ω^2 and q. For identifiability, we assume each of the βs and γs is positive, using exponential prior distributions. To minimize the influence of these prior specifications, we base our inferences on Bayes factors, as explained further below.

Model fitting methods

We use an MCMC approach to fit the model. Beginning with an initial assignment of all the unknowns, we visit each of the model parameters (β, γ, $\bar{\lambda}$, φ^2, σ^2, η, ω^2) and latent variables λ_i and any unobserved genotypes g_{il}, and propose small random perturbations. We then calculate the likelihood ratio under the new and old values to decide whether or not to accept the proposal using the Metropolis–Hastings algorithm. Thus the likelihood for a given set of rates is given by

$$L(\boldsymbol{\beta}, \boldsymbol{\gamma}, \boldsymbol{\lambda}) =$$
$$\prod_{i=1}^{n} \frac{\exp[\gamma_0 + \gamma_1 Z_3(\mathbf{X}_i, \boldsymbol{\beta}, \boldsymbol{\lambda}_i) + \gamma_2 Z_7(\mathbf{X}_i, \boldsymbol{\beta}, \boldsymbol{\lambda}_i)]^{Y_i}}{1 + \exp[\gamma_0 + \gamma_1 Z_3(\mathbf{X}_i, \boldsymbol{\beta}, \boldsymbol{\lambda}_i) + \gamma_2 Z_7(\mathbf{X}_i, \boldsymbol{\beta}, \boldsymbol{\lambda}_i)]}$$

where the Zs are given by Equations (5), subtracting their means. Specifically, the steps are as follows:

- For each i and each λ, update λ_{il} given the current assignments of $\bar{\lambda}_l$, σ_i^2, ω_i^2, G_{il}, P_{il}, X_i, Y_i, and all the other λs for the same subject.
- For each λ, update $\bar{\lambda}_l$, and σ_i^2 based on the λs for all subjects with the corresponding genotype at that locus and its prior variance φ_l^2. Then the prior variances φ_l^2 are updated given the current assignments of $\bar{\lambda}_l$.
- For each λ, update ω_l^2 and η_l given $\{\lambda_{il}, P_{il}\}$.
- For any subjects with missing genotypes (or for all subjects at the completely untyped *CYP1A2* locus), assign a random genotype G_{il}, given q_l, $\bar{\lambda}_l$, σ_i^2, ω_i^2, P_{il}, X_i, Y_i and all the other λs for the same subject.
- Update the global regression coefficients β and γ.

Details of these updating steps will be described in a subsequent statistical paper. This procedure is repeated many times until the resulting distributions have stabilized. The results are based on every 10th sample from 10 000 cycles, after discarding 2000 iterations to allow for convergence. Thereafter, samples can be captured at periodic intervals in order to summarize the marginal posterior distributions of the various parameters of interest. Here, we are interested in βs, which summarize the contributions of each environmental exposure to the two pathways, and the $\bar{\lambda}$s, which describe the effects of the genes on the various metabolic rates.

We have developed a unified C++ programme for both simulation and analysis purposes.

References

Autrup, H., Grafstrom, R.C., Brugh, M., Lechner, J.F., Haugen, A., Trump, B.F. & Harris, C.C. (1982) Comparison of benzo(a)pyrene metabolism in bronchus, esophagus, colon and duodenum from the same individual. *Cancer Res.*, **42**, 934–938

Bell, D.A., Badawi, A.F., Lang, N.P., Ilett, K.F., Kadlubar, F.F. & Hirvonen, A. (1995) Polymorphism in the N-acetyltransferase 1 (NAT1) polyadenylation signal: association of NAT1*10 allele with higher N-acetylation activity in bladder and colon tissue. *Cancer Res.*, **55**, 5226–5229

Boobis, A., Lynch, A., Murray, S., de la Torre, R., Solans, A., Farre, M., Segura, J., Gooderham, N.J. & Davies, D.S. (1994) CYP1A2-Catalyzed conversion of dietary heterocyclic amines to their proximate carcinogens is their major route of metabolism in humans. *Cancer Res.*, **54**, 89–94

Brockton, N., Little, J., Sharp, L. & Cotton, S.C. (2000) N-Acetyltransferase polymorphisms and colorectal cancer: a HuGE review. *Am. J. Epidemiol.*, **151**, 846–861

Chen, J., Stampfer, M.J., Hough, H.L., Garcia-Closas, M., Willett, W.C., Hennekens, C.H., Kelsey, K.T. & Hunter, D.J. (1998) A prospective study of N-acetyltransferase genotype, red meat intake, and risk of colorectal cancer. *Cancer Res.*, **58**, 3307–3311

Chib, S. (1995) Marginal likelihood from the Gibbs output. *J. Am. Statist. Assoc.*, **90**, 1311–1321

Cortessis, V., Siegmund, K., Chen, Q., Zhou, N., Diep, A., Frankl, H., Lee, E., Zhu, Q.S., Haile, R. & Levy, D. (2001) A case–control study of microsomal epoxide hydrolase, smoking, meat consumption, glutathione S-transferase M3, and risk of colorectal adenomas. *Cancer Res.*, **61**, 2381–2385

De Kok, T.M. & van Maanen, J.M. (2000) Evaluation of fecal mutagenicity and colorectal cancer risk. *Mutat. Res.*, **463**, 53–101

Denes, J., Blakey, D., Krewski, D. & Withey, J. (1996) Applications of receptor-binding models in toxicology. In: Fan, A. & Chang, L., eds, *Toxicology and Risk Assessment: Principles, Methods, and Applications*, New York, Marcel Dekker, pp. 447–472

Felton, J.S., Knize, M.G., Dolbeare, F.A. & Wu, R. (1994) Mutagenic activity of heterocyclic amines in cooked foods. *Environ. Health Perspect.*, **102** (Suppl. 6), 201–204

Gilks, W.K., Thomas, A. & Spiegelhalter, D.J. (1994) A language and program for complex Bayesian modelling. *Statistician*, **43**, 169–178

Grant, D.M., Vohra, P., Avis, Y. & Ima, A. (1992) Detection of a new polymorphism of human arylamine N-acetyltransferase NAT1 using p-aminosalicylic acid as an in vivo probe. *J. Basic clin. Physiol. Pharmacol.*, **3** (Suppl.), 244

Haile, R.W., Witte, J.S., Longnecker, M.P., Probst-Hensch, N., Chen, M.-J., Harper, J., Frankl, H.D. & Lee, E.R. (1997) A sigmoidoscopy-based case–control study of polyps: macronutrients, fiber, and meat consumption. *Int. J. Cancer*, **73**, 497–502

Hayashi, S., Watanabe, J., Nakachi, K. & Kawajiri, K. (1991) Genetic linkage of lung cancer-associated MspI polymorphisms with amino acid replacement in the heme binding region of the human cytochrome P450IA1 gene. *J. Biochem.*, **110**, 407–411

Hein, D.W., Rustan, T.D., Ferguson, R.J., Doll, M.A. & Gray, K. (1994) Metabolic activation of aromatic and heterocyclic N-hydroxyaralamines by wild-type and mutant recombinant human NAT1 and NAT2 acetyltransferases. *Arch. Toxicol.*, **68**, 129–133

Hein, D.W., Doll, M.A., Fretland, A.J., Leff, M.A., Webb, S.J., Xiao, G.H., Devanaboyina, U.S., Nangju, N.A. & Feng, Y. (2000) Molecular genetics and epidemiology of the NAT1 and NAT2 acetylation polymorphisms. *Cancer Epidemiol. Biomarkers Prev.*, **9**, 29–42

Jourenkova-Mironova, N., Mitrunen, K., Bouchardy, C., Dayer, P., Benhamou, S. & Hirvonen, A. (2000) High-activity microsomal epoxide hydrolase genotypes and the risk of oral, pharynx, and larynx cancers. *Cancer Res.*, **60**, 534–536

Kass, R. & Raftery, A. (1995) Bayes factors. *J. Am. Statist. Assoc.*, **90**, 773–795

Katoh, T., Boissy, R., Nagata, N., Kitagawa, K., Kuroda, Y., Itoh, H., Kawamoto, T. & Bell, D.A. (2000) Inherited polymorphism in the N-acetyltransferase 1 (NAT1) and 2 (NAT2) genes and susceptibility to gastric and colorectal adenocarcinoma. *Int. J. Cancer*, **85**, 46–49

Keating, G.A., Sinha, R., Layton, D., Salmon, C.P., Knize, M.G., Bogen, K.T., Lynch, C.F. & Alavanja, M. (2000) Comparison of heterocyclic amine levels in home-cooked meats with exposure indicators (United States). *Cancer Causes Control*, **11**, 731–739

Langouet, S., Welti, D.H., Kerriguy, N., Fay, L.B., Huynh-Ba, T., Markovic, J., Guengerich, F.P., Guiouzo, A. & Turesky, R.J. (2001) Metabolism of 2-amino-3,8-dimethylimidazo[4,5-*f*]-quinozaline in human hepatocytes: 2-amino-3-methylimidazo-[4,5-*f*]-quinozaline-8-carboxylic acid is a major detoxification pathway catalyzed by cytochrome P450 1A2. *Chem. Res. Toxicol.*, **14**, 211–221

Lin, H.J., Han, C.-Y., Bernstein, D.A., Hsaio, W., Lin, B.K. & Hardy, S. (1994a) Ethnic distribution of the glutathione transferase Mu 1–1 (GASTM1) null genotype in 1473 individuals and application to bladder cancer susceptibility. *Carcinogenesis*, **15**, 1077–1081

Lin, D., Meyer, D.J., Ketterer, B., Lang, N.P. & Kadlubar, F.F. (1994b) Effects of human and rat glutathione S-transferases on the covalent DNA binding of the *N*-acetoxy derivatives of heterocyclic amine carcinogens *in vitro*: a possible mechanism of organ specificity in their carcinogenesis. *Cancer Res.*, **54**, 4920–4926

Lin, H.J., Probst-Hensch, N.M., Hughes, N.C., Sakamoto, G.T., Louis, A.D., Kau, I.H., Lin, B.K., Lee, D.B., Lin, J., Frankl, H.D., Lee, E.R., Hardy, S., Grant, D.M. & Haile, R.W. (1998) Variants of *N*-acetyltransferase NAT1 and a case–control study of colorectal adenomas. *Pharmacogenetics*, **8**, 269–281

Mauthe, R.J., Dingley, K.H., Leveson, S.H., Freeman, S.P., Turesky, R.J., Garner, R.C. & Turteltaub, K.W. (1999) Comparison of DNA-adduct and tissue-available dose levels of MeIQx in human and rodent colon following administration of a very low dose. *Int. J. Cancer*, **80**, 539–545

Minchin, R.F., Reeves, P.T., Teitel, C.H., McManus, M.E., Mojarrabi, B., Ilett, K.F. & Kadlubar, F.F. (1992) *N*- and *O*-Acetylation of aromatic and heterocyclic amine carcinogens by human monomorphic and polymorphic acetyltransferases expressed in *COS-1* cells. *Biochem. biophys. Res. Commun.*, **185**, 839–844

Moolgavkar, S., Krewski, D., Zeise, L., Cardis, E. & Møller, H., eds (1999) *Quantitative Estimation and Prediction of Human Cancer Risks* (IARC Scientific Publications No. 131), Lyon, IARC*Press*

Potter, J.D. (1999) Colorectal cancer: molecules and populations. *J. natl Cancer Inst.*, **91**, 916–932

Probst-Hensch, N.M., Haile, R.W., Ingles, S.A., Longnecker, M.P., Han, C.-Y., Lin, B.K., Lee, D.B., Sakamoto, G.T., Frankl, H.D., Lee, E.R. & Lin, H.J. (1995) Acetylation polymorphism and prevalence of colorectal adenomas. *Cancer Res.*, **55**, 2017–2020

Rothen, J.-P., Haefeli, W.E., Meyer, U.A.., Todesco, L. & Wenk, M. (1998) Acetaminophen is an inhibitor of hepatic *N*-acetyltransferase 2 *in vitro* and *in vivo*. *Pharmacogenetics*, **8**, 553–559

Sinha, R., Rothman, N., Brown, E.D., Mark, S.D., Hoover, R.N., Caporaso, N.E., Levander, O.A., Knize, M.G., Lang, N.P. & Kadlubar, F.F. (1994) Pan-fried meat containing high levels of heterocyclic aromatic amines but low levels of polycyclic aromatic hydrocarbons induces cytochrome P4501A2 activity in humans. *Cancer Res.*, **54**, 6154–6159

Sinha, R., Kulldorff, M., Chow, W.H., Denobile, J. & Rothman, N. (2001) Dietary intake of heterocyclic amines, meat-derived mutagenic activity, and risk of colorectal adenomas. *Cancer Epidemiol. Biomarkers Prev.*, **10**, 559–562

Thomas, D.C. (1988) Models for exposure–time–response relationships with applications to cancer epidemiology. *Annu. Rev. public Health*, **9**, 451–482

Turesky, R.J., Gross, G.A., Stillwell, W.G., Skipper, P.L. & Tannenbaum, S.R. (1994) Species differences in metabolism of heterocyclic aromatic amines, human exposure, and biomonitoring. *Environ. Health Perspect.*, **102** (Suppl. 6), 47–51

Ulrich, C.M., Bigler, J., Whitton, J.A., Bostick, R., Fosdick, L. & Potter, J.D. (2001) Epoxide hydrolase Tyr113His polymorphism is associated with elevated risk of colorectal polyps in the presence of smoking and high meat intake. *Cancer Epidemiol. Biomarkers Prev.*, **10**, 875–882

Vineis, P., Malats, N., Lang, M., d'Errico, A., Caporaso, N., Cuzick, J. & Boffetta, P., eds (1999) *Metabolic Polymorphisms and Susceptibility to Cancer* (IARC Scientific Publications No. 148), Lyon, IARC*Press*

Wakabayashi, K., Nagao, M., Esumi, H. & Sugimura, T. (1992) Food-derived mutagens and carcinogens. *Cancer Res.*, **52** (Suppl. 7), 2092s–2098s

Wakabayashi, K., Ushiyama, H., Takahashi, M., Nukaya, H., Kim, S.B., Ochiai, M., Sugimura, T. & Nagao, M. (1993) Exposure to heterocyclic amines. *Environ. Health Perspect.*, **99**, 129–134

Yanagawa, Y., Sawada, M., Deguchi, T., Gonzalez, F.J. & Kamataki, T. (1994) Stable expression of human CYP1A2 and *N*-acetyltransferases in Chinese hamster CHL cells: mutagenic activation of 2-amino-3-methylimidazo[4,5-f]quinoline and 2-amino-3,8-dimethylimidazo[4,5-f]quinoxaline. *Cancer Res.*, **54**, 3422–3427

Corresponding author
Duncan C. Thomas
Biostatistics Division,
Verner Richter Chair in Cancer Research,
Department of Preventive medicine,
University of Southern California,
1540 Alcazar Street, CHP-220,
Los Angeles, CA 90089-9011, USA
dthomas@usc.edu

Genetic Issues

Mechanisms of Carcinogenesis: Contributions of Molecular Epidemiology
Patricia Buffler, Jerry Rice, Robert Baan, Michael Bird and Paolo Boffetta, eds
IARC Scientific Publications No. 157
International Agency for Research on Cancer, Lyon, 2004

Mechanistic Insights from Biomarker Studies: Somatic Mutations and Rodent/Human Comparisons Following Exposure to a Potential Carcinogen

Richard J. Albertini

Summary

The field of cancer molecular epidemiology is maturing rapidly. There is a vast armamentarium of biomarkers that is now used to assess human exposures to environmental carcinogens, the non-cancer effects of the exposures, and individual susceptibilities. There is also widespread realization that biomarkers must be validated before they are useful for human studies. One of the objectives of molecular epidemiology is the development of mechanistic insights into the carcinogenic process. Somatic mutations are biomarkers of effect that are proving useful in this regard. Mutations in reporter genes can serve as pre-disease mechanistic probes. A recent transitional epidemiological study of workers exposed to 1,3-butadiene evaluated a continuum of biomarkers of exposure, effect, and susceptibility. Results showed that relative concentrations of metabolites of this agent in humans are quite different from those in mice, which is the sensitive species for 1,3-butadiene carcinogenicity. Inter-species comparisons of the continuum of biological responses in mice, rats, and humans illustrate how these non-cancer endpoints might ultimately be used for making judgments as to cancer risk in humans.

Introduction

Molecular epidemiology

Epidemiology, as the study of disease distributions in human populations, investigates causes, outcomes, and pathogenic mechanisms. Studies based on disease endpoints easily detect disorders that are acute and relatively common, as well as chronic conditions, including cancers, that result from strong or unique causal agents. By contrast, other chronic diseases, including cancers, which are due to weak causal agents are much less amenable to study using this approach. For these diseases, alternative endpoints have been proposed, *e.g.* cellular or molecular endpoints. Studies of alternative endpoints in human populations may be called molecular epidemiological studies. Molecular epidemiology too is concerned with disease, but has its focus on biological responses rather than health outcomes. These biological responses, or biomarkers, reflect pre-disease processes. Biomarkers may be surrogates for pathogenic processes, identifying mechanisms by analogy, or may themselves be these processes. Studies of environmental carcinogenesis offer good examples of some applications of molecular epidemiology (Perera, 1996).

Tools

The molecular epidemiology of cancer is rapidly maturing. In part this is due to the number and availability of sophisticated assays of in-vivo biological responses, *i.e.* biomarkers (Albertini *et al.*, 1996; Toniolo *et al.*, 1997; Albertini, 1998a; Brooks, 1999; Albertini, 2001). Biomarkers are usually classified as measures of exposure, effect, or susceptibility in relation to environmental cancer-causing agents. This classification is, however, somewhat arbitrary, depending more on the question being asked than on intrinsic properties of the biomarker.

The presence of environmental chemicals or metabolites in tissues or body fluids is the most obvious biomarker of exposure. In-vivo concentrations of metabolites, in addition to assessing internal dose, are the first measures of response to environmental carcinogens. They describe pathways of activation or detoxification, define excretion patterns, and may indicate saturation kinetics. Finding urine or other body fluids containing genotoxic activity related to an exposure to a chemical demonstrates the in-vivo production of toxic materials. Covalent adducts of proteins or nucleic acids identify the in-vivo production of electrophilic substances capable of reacting with macromolecules. Both provide measures of steady state internal cumulative doses, with protein adducts being the better dosimeters because they are not repaired. DNA adducts, however, provide information about the penetration of chemicals to the actual targets of genotoxicity or carcinogenicity. The quantity, kind, and sites of DNA adducts begin a description of the mechanisms of genetic damage inflicted by these agents. For genotoxic carcinogens, biomarkers traditionally classified as measures of effect are irreversible changes in the structure of the genetic material. These genetic changes may be non-specific, being simple reporters of a genetic effect, or specific, reflecting precise changes that characterize particular malignancies. Non-specific reporter and specific cancer changes can be alterations at either the chromosome or gene level. Specific cancer changes may be measured in normal, non-cancer cells and tissues, or in actual tumours, with mutational patterns in the latter being used to infer causation.

Added to these conventional biomarkers are newly emerging measures of changes in gene expression, in protein production, or of inherited genetic polymorphisms (Caporaso & Goldstein, 1997; Nuwaysir et al., 1999; Steiner & Anderson, 2000). The latter provide information about predisposition and are widely employed as biomarkers of susceptibility. The paradigm of the progression from external exposure to the production of malignancy for environmental cancers

as proposed by the National Research Council (NRC) (Committee on Biological Markers of the National Research Council, 1987), with the superimposition of some of the currently available biomarkers, is shown in Figure 1.

Validation

Unfortunately, the simple availability of biomarkers does not indicate their usefulness for molecular epidemiological studies. No matter how sophisticated a measure may be, nor how easy it is to assess, a biomarker must be validated before it is informative. There are many kinds of validation, but that relevant to the current discussion is the demonstration that a biomarker truly reflects what it is intended to reflect. A biomarker of exposure must be a true measure of the exposure, allowing an assessment of internal dose. A biomarker of effect must first detect the effect and, if being used as a surrogate for disease outcome, must predict in some sense the subsequent occurrence of disease. Biomarkers of susceptibility must be shown to be effect modifiers in actual field studies.

Validation of the kind referred to here is achieved by another kind of epidemiological study, i.e. a transitional epidemiological study that bridges the gap between the laboratory and the field (Hulka, 1991; Hulka & Margolin, 1992; Schulte, 1993; Schulte & Perera, 1997). In a transitional study, the focus is on the biomarker, which is the dependent variable. The independent variable, i.e. the exposure, effect, or susceptibility state, is what the biomarker is supposed to reflect.

Objectives

Four objectives are usually identified for molecular epidemiological studies of cancer (Albertini, 2001):

• To increase the accuracy of exposure assessment to a potential environmental carcinogen, thereby reducing misclassifications in traditional epidemiological studies.

• To predict disease outcomes in populations, at least in a statistical sense. The goal is to identify individuals at increased risk for developing a disorder due to an environmental exposure by

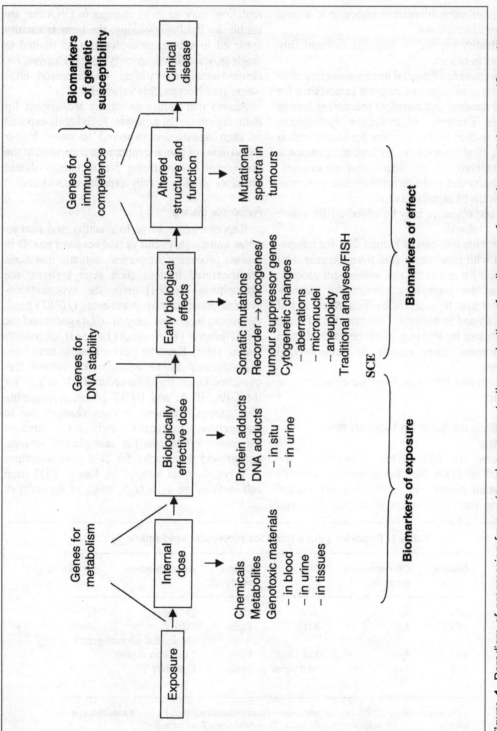

Figure 1. Paradigm of progression from external exposure to the production of malignancy for environmental cancer (Committee on Biological Markers of the National Research Council, 1987?) with superimposition of some of the currently available biomarkers. FISH, fluorescence in situ hybridization; SCE, sister chromatid exchange. From Albertini (2001)

means of some biomarker response at a time before disease onset.

- To identify genetic or acquired susceptibility factors in cancer.
- To discover fundamental mechanisms in pathogenesis – an objective of great importance for understanding and therefore preventing human cancer. Examples of molecular epidemiological studies in this area are the identification of critical metabolic pathways, genotoxic mechanisms, or the acquisition of genomic instability that underlie carcinogenic processes by means of biomarkers.

To this last objective may be added a fifth which is closely related:

- To provide non-cancer human data for comparison with non-cancer data from experimental animals for use in the risk assessment process. All of the steps in environmental carcinogenesis may be assessed by biomarkers in test animals and in humans. Comparisons of these events step by step may allow better prediction in humans from results in experimental animals.

The fourth and fifth objectives are considered in this chapter.

Somatic mutations as biomarkers
Overview

Mutations are irreversible changes in the sequence of DNA that fundamentally alter its information content. As such, they are central events in the development of cancer. Although mutations may be gross changes in DNA that are visible by light microscopy, the term is usually confined to sub-microscopic changes limited to single genes. Microscopically visible changes, *i.e.* chromosomal aberrations, are discussed elsewhere (see Norppa, this volume).

Agents that induce mutations are suspect for inducing cancer. In principle, individuals exposed to such agents are expected to show higher frequencies of somatic mutations compared to the non-exposed. Monitoring for mutations should therefore identify heavily exposed individuals.

Reporter genes

Reporter genes serve to quantify and characterize mutational events *in vivo* but have no role in disease processes. At present, somatic mutations are measured in four such gene systems: the glycophorin-A (*GPA*) gene, the hypoxanthine-guanine phosphoribosyltransferase (*HPRT*) gene, the human leukocyte antigen (*HLA*) genes and the T-cell receptor (*TCR*) genes (Table 1) (Albertini & Hayes, 1997). Reporter gene mutations have been characterized as to background mutant frequencies. These are of the order of 10^{-6} to 10^{-5} for the GPA, HLA, and HPRT genes, representing spontaneous mutations *in vivo*, changes due to endogenous mutagens and even random exogenous influences. For unexplained reasons, background frequencies for *TCR* gene mutations in T lymphocytes assayed by loss of CD3 from cell surface, are quite high, being of the order of 10^{-4}.

Table 1. Reporter genes used for molecular epidemiology

Gene(s)	Chromosome location	Size	Cells assayed	Assay method
GPA	4q	44 kb	RBC	Cytometry
HPRT	Xq	44 kb	T cells	Cell culture Cloning and autoradiography
HLA-A	6p	5 kb	T cells	Cell culture cloning
TCR	14q 7q	'Multi-gene'	T cells	Cytometry

GPA, glycophorin-A; *HPRT*, hypoxanthine-guanine phosphoribosyltransferase; HLA-A, human leukocyte antigen-A; TCR, T-cell receptor (assay is for loss of CD3 molecules from T-cell surface).

The current somatic mutation assays differ in the chromosomal locations of the reporter genes. *HPRT* is on the X chromosome; the others are autosomal (Table 1). Therefore, although the haploid *HPRT* gene (one actual copy in males; one functional copy in females) is a usable marker in all individuals because single mutational events produce selectable phenotypic changes, it cannot participate in events such as homologous recombination, *i.e.* transfer of genetic material between homologous chromosomes. As this is an important step in the loss of heterozygosity (LOH) often observed for tumour suppressor genes in tumours, it is a serious limitation. However, *HPRT* does participate in recombination events that underlie deletions and insertions within the X chromosome as well as translocations between the X chromosome and autosomal chromosomes, in addition, of course, to point mutations.

The recombination events seen in cancers, especially in leukaemia and lymphoma, probably have several underlying mechanisms. It is important that reporter genes should be capable of capturing these processes and others operative in carcinogenesis. Molecular analyses of *HPRT* deletion mutants have revealed changes at breakpoints that implicate several mechanisms of recombination. These include sequence homologies, topoisomerase II consensus cleavage sites, and V(D)J recombination signal sites (Fuscoe *et al.*, 1991; Rainville *et al.*, 1995; Finette *et al.*, 1996). Furthermore, deletions with the production of fusion genes between *HPRT* and other DNA regions – mimicking a phenomenon frequently seen in cancer – have also been observed (Lippert *et al.*, 1997). There is a common misconception that the *HPRT* gene cannot suffer a large deletion because of the loss of nearby essential genes due to its haploid location. However, the observation of deletions as large as 3.5 Mb by the use of pulsed field analysis has put this to rest (Lippert *et al.*, 1995). Actually, and initially paradoxically, population monitoring for large deletions in outbred populations such as humans is probably better done with a haploid rather than a diploid gene because mutations of essential genes are most likely eliminated in each generation in a haploid genetic region, *i.e.* from the X chromosome. By contrast, recessive lethals in essential autosomal genes can accumulate in the population. Heterozygosity and *cis–trans* relationships to the autosomal reporter gene being used must then be considered in monitoring. It is probable that different individuals in the population will have different mutational 'target sizes', resulting in different background mutant frequency values throughout the population.

Despite this, both the *GPA* and *HLA* genes reflect mutagenic mechanisms that *HPRT* cannot. These are mitotic recombination with the homologous chromosome, gene conversion, and chromosome reduplication. *GPA*, being a phenotypic assay, does not allow molecular characterization of the mutants. Mutational mechanisms are therefore inferred only. The assay can be performed only in individuals of the MN blood group, who constitute approximately 50% of the population. In the GPA assay, 'point mutations' occurring in haematopoietic stem cells are quantified from the frequencies of rare red blood cells that have lost expression of the M antigen in the peripheral blood of an MN heterozygous individual (Langlois *et al.*, 1990; Grant & Bigbee, 1993; Jensen & Bigbee, 1996). These NO red blood cells are called 'hemizygous variants'. Mitotic recombination, gene conversion, or chromosome loss with reduplication events are quantified from the frequencies of rare red blood cells in the heterozygous individual that have lost expression of the M antigen but doubled the expression of the N antigen. These NN red blood cells are called 'homozygous variants'. In contrast to GPA, HLA mutations arising in T lymphocytes can be characterized at the RNA/DNA level. In the limited molecular analyses conducted thus far, 2–8% of the background mutations have shown simple deletions and approximately 30% have shown changes compatible with mitotic homologous recombination (Turner *et al.*, 1988; Morley *et al.*, 1990; Grist *et al.*, 1992). Few have shown changes compatible with gene conversion. Sequencing of the HLA region has been difficult because of the complexity of the region. Although most mutants showed no molecular changes in these studies, the methods employed could not detect small alterations in the DNA. Most 'no change' mutants are assumed to have point mutations.

The reporter gene mutations assays except for GPA are laborious and expensive, especially when molecular analyses are required for identifying mechanisms. GPA, being a cytometric assay, is rapid, but lacks the potential for producing molecular information. There is a need for sensitive genotypic assays that can both quantify and characterize mutations by simple PCR-based methods. Two that detect translocation events are currently in use. One detects illegitimate V(D)J recombinase-mediated events (see below) by identifying hybrid TCR genes, *i.e.* VB–JG or VG–JB, formed *in vivo* by inversions of chromosome 7 (inv7[p13;q32]) in peripheral blood T-lymphocyte genomes (Lipkowitz *et al.*, 1992). The other method measures another aberrant V(D)J recombinase-mediated event of direct relevance to cancer (Liu *et al.*, 1994). It also employs a PCR-based method to quantify frequencies of B-lymphocyte genomes in peripheral blood that carry a translocation uniting chromosomes 14 and 18 (t[14:18][q32:q21]) – the *BCL-2* translocation. Data are now becoming available from both of these assays that will further mechanistic understanding of mutagenic events that arise *in vivo* in humans.

There remains a need for additional genotypic assays to identify translocational events with carcinogenic potential that are produced by environmental exposures. Perhaps methods using primers designed to amplify leukaemia-specific translocations in non-malignant cells will provide the reporters for the next generation of somatic mutation assays.

Mutations are now classified as biomarkers of effect. Of the four genes described above for human monitoring, only *GPA* and *HPRT* have been used to any extent. Reporter gene mutations were originally used to assess exposures. However, conventional biomarkers of exposure, being 'proximal' to the induction of genetic changes (Figure 1) are more sensitive for this application. Among the biomarkers now classified as measures of effect, chromosomal aberrations are more sensitive than somatic mutations for detecting certain genotoxic exposures, *i.e.* those

that produce chromosome breaks (clastogens). Chromosomes are large structures over which aberrations can occur; single genes are much smaller, with measurable changes being rare. Chromosomal aberrations remain the gold standard for assessing acute exposures to ionizing radiation. A study comparing several biomarkers for their sensitivity in reflecting an exposure to cyclophosphamide (a mutagenic and clastogenic alkylating chemical) found them to be in the following order:

haemoglobin adducts > sister chromatid exchanges (SCE > chromosomal aberrations > micronuclei > *HPRT* mutations,

even though each gave a positive response (Tates *et al.*, 1991).

If they are not sensitive endpoints for assessing exposures, then why measure somatic mutations at all in molecular epidemiology? An answer is gradually emerging (Albertini, 1994). Somatic mutations indicate unequivocally that in-vivo genotoxicity has occurred. An increase in the frequencies of mutations in a population with known exposure to a genotoxic agent is a warning that the exposure is having an effect in the setting that is being evaluated. Conversely, although with less certainty, the lack of an increase in somatic mutations in a heavily exposed population offers some evidence that the exposure is not having a deleterious effect. If the agent of concern is clastogenic as well as mutagenic, chromosomal changes must also be assessed to draw this conclusion. Induction of somatic mutations in humans exposed to an agent known to be a genotoxic carcinogen in experimental animals is evidence that the agent is also carcinogenic in humans, making this endpoint relevant in cancer risk assessments. Somatic mutations may also define 'safe' levels of exposure to genotoxic agents and assess the efficacy of measures taken to prevent genotoxicity in a population, *e.g.* in workers in hazardous occupations or cancer patients receiving radio- or chemotherapy. Finally, somatic mutations are probes for in-vivo cellular and mechanistic processes as discussed in detail below (Albertini, 1998b).

Somatic mutations are best used to describe effects. There may be instances however, when there are no other endpoints with which to identify exposures, especially if the potentially deleterious agents in an environment are unknown. One property of mutations useful for assessing exposures is almost unique to this endpoint, *i.e.* the variability of the underlying molecular changes. A given mutation results from one of a large number of possible alterations of the DNA.

Mutational spectra

The distribution and relative kinds of molecular alterations in a collection of independent mutations within a gene defines a mutational spectrum. Mutations arising from different exogenous causes frequently show different characteristic spectra (Van Houten & Albertini, 1994). For example, those due to low linear energy transfer (LET) ionizing radiation show relatively high frequencies of large deletions and translocations, G→T transversions (*i.e.* base substitution of a pyrimidine for a purine) and G→A transitions (*i.e.* base substitution of a purine for a purine). Both base substitution mutations may have other causes (see below), but a likely cause of G→A (C→T) transitions when ultraviolet (UV) radiation is not a consideration (see below) is radiation-induced oxidative damage to the DNA. The deletions and translocations result from DNA strand breaks, either direct or as a secondary effect of the repair of oxidative DNA damage. Mutations from high-LET radiation may also show multiple base changes clustered in DNA due to secondary ionizations arising in a small track.

UV radiation produces a characteristic mutational spectrum dominated by C→T and double C:C→T:T transitions, the latter being a signature mutation for UV (Miller, 1985; McGregor *et al.*, 1991). The important environmental chemicals that produce bulky DNA adducts, *i.e.* the polycyclic aromatic hydrocarbons (PAHs) and the mycotoxins, form adducts at the N^2 or N7 position of guanine, respectively, resulting in a G→T transversion due to mispairing or depurination, respectively (Van Houten & Albertini, 1994).

Other chemical agents produce other characteristic spectra. Exogenous intercalating agents result in base additions or subtractions and frameshift mutations (Ripley, 1991). Exogenous base analogues cause base substitution mutations because of altered base pairing. Exogenous chemicals may alter intracellular purine or pyrimidine pools and produce base substitution mutations characteristic of the altered pool. Direct-acting S_N1 alkylating agents produce spectra characterized by G→A transitions resulting from O^6 alkyl G adducts unless these are repaired. Fortunately, most cells have a robust repair mechanism for this kind of damage.

Repair is also an important determinant of final mutational change. In particular, exogenously produced bulky (and some other) DNA adducts cause blocks in transcription of the gene. Repair of DNA damage due to these DNA lesions is generally faster in actively transcribed genes than elsewhere in the genome (Bohr *et al.*, 1987; Xanthoudakis *et al.*, 1992; Evans *et al.*, 1993; Schaeffer *et al.*, 1993). Importantly, repair is more rapid on the transcribed or template strand than it is on the non-transcribed or coding strand of active genes (Mellon *et al.*, 1986; Hanawalt, 1989). An important result of preferential repair in transcribed DNA strands is strand bias for base substitution mutations. For practical applications, if strand bias is excluded for other reasons, *e.g.* differential occurrence of the normal base in one strand or functional constraints, bias for mutations in the non-transcribed strand of an actively transcribed gene is evidence of exogenous DNA damage, often due to a bulky adduct.

This is only a small fraction of the possible kinds of mutations. It is enough, however, to illustrate how mutational spectra provide insights in molecular epidemiological studies. Among the reporter genes, in-vivo spectra have been defined for *HPRT* mutations in T lymphocytes.

HPRT mutational spectra

Several laboratories have defined background in-vivo *HPRT* mutational spectra for different populations. There is now a large computerized database of these changes available to all workers in the field (Cariello & Skopek, 1993; Cariello, 1994). The background spectrum for adults includes less than 15% gross structural alterations of the gene, *i.e.* deletions, insertions, or other rearrangements, as determined by Southern blot analyses. More recent studies, using multiplex PCR of genomic DNA, put this frequency even lower, reflecting the ability of Southern blots to detect translocations missed by multiplex PCR (Clark *et al.*, 1997). The remainder of the background (over 85%) includes base substitutions and frameshifts, small deletions and insertions, complex alterations, and uncharacterized splice site changes. Transversions are at least as frequent as transitions, suggesting that random exogenous mutagens may be the cause of some of the background (Cole & Skopek, 1994; Albertini & Hayes, 1997; Curry *et al.*, 2000).

The background *HPRT* mutational spectrum in the fetus, as detected in placental blood T lymphocytes, and in young children, is remarkably different from that in adults (McGinniss *et al.*, 1989; Fuscoe *et al.*, 1991; Finette *et al.*, 1996). At these early stages of life, over 75% of the mutational changes are due to large structural alterations in the gene, most of which are deletions. One class of deletion constitutes the majority of these large alterations. Sequence analyses of their breakpoints have shown changes attributable to an illegitimate activity of the V(D)J recombinase mechanism – the mechanism that normally functions during this period of life to rearrange the T-cell receptor (TCR) genes for immunological maturity.

The frequencies of in-vivo *HPRT* mutations are increased by a variety of chemical and radiation exposures. In principle, such increases are used as indications of exposure. This is described in detail in several reviews, and is not reported here since specific studies are not within the scope of this discussion (Cole & Skopek, 1994; Albertini & Hayes, 1997). Spectra for in-vivo *HPRT* mutations induced by some exogenous agents have been described. Low-LET ionizing radiation produces a spectrum that becomes increasingly dominated by large structural alterations as radiation doses increase, with the frequency of deletions being a better reflection of dose than the actual *HPRT* MF (Nicklas *et al.*, 1990, 1991). High-LET ionizing radiation produces a different pattern, as judged both by analysis of mutations in former plutonium workers with current radioactivity body burdens and by in-vitro studies of

G_0 T-lymphocytes exposed to radon gas (Albertini *et al.*, 1997). Deletion frequencies associated with high-LET radiation are lower than those associated with low-LET radiation, perhaps reflecting a higher frequency of translocation events, and the deletions that are seen are smaller. Also, there are multiple tandem point mutations.

Chemical exposures also produce *HPRT* mutational spectra that differ from background. An early report indicated a high frequency of a specific base substitution that changed the sequence GTGT to ATGT in individuals exposed to ethylene oxide (Cariello *et al.*, 1992). Although G→A transitions are expected after exposure to this alkylating agent, the base affected (G_{197}) is also a mutational hotspot in the background spectrum. To date, this finding has not been confirmed. Passive exposures of pregnant women to cigarette smoke produces an increase in the V(D)J recombinase mediated *HPRT* deletions in the newborn – a finding that has been confirmed (Finette *et al.*, 1998; Bigbee *et al.*, 1999).

Specific experimental exposures of human T lymphocytes (or lymphoblastoid cells) *in vitro* can be used to generate characteristic mutational spectra for comparison with those found in humans exposed *in vivo* as indicated above for high-LET radiations. The insecticide malathion produces characteristic overlapping deletions of *HPRT in vitro* in human T lymphocytes (Pluth *et al.*, 1996). The monoepoxide metabolite of 1,3-butadiene induces *HPRT* mutations in cultured human lymphoblastoid cells that are characterized by an excess of changes at AT base pairs, whereas the diepoxide metabolite induces deletions in the gene (Cochrane & Skopek, 1994; Steen *et al.*, 1997a,b). These changes are being sought *in vivo* in humans with known exposures to these agents.

The several molecular changes that underlie oncogene or tumour suppressor gene mutations that are also reflected in *HPRT* have been described above. Studies of mutational spectra in reporter genes such as *HPRT* can detect skewed patterns of mutational changes compared to background, but they are unlikely to show a single change dominating the spectrum because all mutations arising among millions of normal cells are sampled. Except for clonal outgrowths of one or two mutants (see below), a specific mutational change caused by a specific environmental exposure must be read against a background of all *HPRT* mutations that have arisen in that individual. Mutational spectra in reporter genes such as *HPRT* differ from each other by statistical changes in distributions, not by single clonal mutations such as are those expressed in tumours.

Mechanistic insights from HPRT mutations

Several mechanistic insights have come from studies of *HPRT* mutations in human populations. The V(D)J recombinase-mediated deletions noted above are cases in point. These changes are significant because they capture a mutagenic mechanism that is frequent in human lymphoid malignancies (Finger *et al.*, 1986; Boehm & Rabbitts, 1989; Tycko & Sklar, 1990). Illegitimate V(D)J recombinase activity may produce chromosome translocations with one breakpoint near an immunoglobulin (Ig) or T-cell receptor (TCR gene) (in B or T cells respectively), and the other near an oncogene. This dysregulates the oncogene to constitutive expression, resulting in a lymphoid malignancy. More frequently in malignancies, a submicroscopic deletion event occurs (analogous to that in *HPRT*) with one breakpoint being near a constitutively expressed gene and the other near an oncogene, again resulting in dysregulation (Breit *et al.*, 1993). It is noteworthy that V(D)J recombinase-mediated deletions analogous to those seen in *HPRT* are observed in the *tal* gene (T-cell acute leukaemia gene) in this form of childhood malignancy (Van Dongen *et al.*, 1990). The *tal*[d] mutations are clonal in the leukaemia and are presumed to be of aetiological significance. The *HPRT* V(D)J recombinase-mediated deletions are, therefore, surrogate markers for this mutagenic event with carcinogenic potential. However, assuming that the *tal*[d] deletions arise at the frequency of the *HPRT* deletions (~10^{-7} in most normal newborns), something more than their occurrence must be required to produce this form of T-cell leukaemia.

The *HPRT* mutations in T lymphocytes permit even more fundamental mechanistic insights when analysed in the context of their in-vivo clonality, which can be determined from their specific *TCR* gene rearrangements. In addition, *TCR* gene rearrangements provide a reference point for temporally ordering events that occur in the clone. Such events, e.g. *HPRT* mutations, may occur before *TCR* gene rearrangement, generally in pre- or intra-thymic cells, or after *TCR* gene rearrangement, in post-thymic mature T cells. Mutational analysis in this way requires recovery a number of *HPRT* mutant T-cell isolates from an individual (*e.g.* 20–40) and a determination of both the *HPRT* mutational change and *TCR* gene rearrangement for each isolate. The combined *HPRT–TCR* patterns are then grouped. Four patterns may be observed for groups consisting of two or more mutant isolates. Each has its own interpretation(s).

1. Identity for both *HPRT* mutational change and *TCR* gene rearrangement defines 'sibling' *HPRT* mutants arising *in vivo* from a single mutational event in a post-thymic T cell, with subsequent clonal amplification. This frequently indicates an in-vivo stimulus for clonal T-cell proliferation.
2. Non-identity for *HPRT* mutational changes but identity for *TCR* gene rearrangements defines independent *HPRT* mutational events in the same post-thymic T-cell clone. This also indicates extensive in-vivo proliferation of the T-cell clone and, perhaps, depending on the distribution and order of *HPRT* mutational changes, the acquisition of a mutator phenotype.
3. Non-identity for both the *HPRT* mutational changes and the *TCR* gene rearrangements indicates independent in-vivo mutational events arising *in vivo* in different post-thymic T cells. This is the usual pattern that has indicated that the majority of mutations in most normal individuals arise independently.
4. Identity of *HPRT* mutational change but non-identity of *TCR* gene rearrangements usually indicates a single *HPRT* mutational event that arose *in vivo* in a pre- or intra-thymic cell before its *TCR* gene rearrangement. This pattern is frequently seen in children but rarely in adults, perhaps indicating the vulnerability of developing T cells to somatic mutation. An alternative interpretation of this

pattern is independent *in vivo HPRT* mutational events in a mutational hot spot in different post-thymic T cells. This interpretation requires that the same *HPRT* hot spot be observed in different individuals – something that has been observed rarely, if ever.

In-vivo proliferation of *HPRT* mutants, with or without the acquisition of multiple mutations within the clone (*i.e.* pattern 1 or 2 above) is not infrequent in individuals with ongoing immunological processes such as an autoimmune disease. This, coupled with the fact that it is rare to recover two non-mutant (wild type) T-cell isolates with the same *TCR* gene rearrangement from an individual has led to the concept that spontaneous T-cell mutations *in vivo* preferentially arise in dividing cells, *i.e.* that cell division is 'mutagenic'. Independent confirmation of this comes from the observation that background *HPRT* mutant frequencies are 3–5-fold higher in the CD45RO+ memory fraction than in the CD45RA+ naive fraction of T cells from the same individual (Baars *et al.*, 1995). These observations have led to a series of mutational studies in individuals with autoimmune diseases, including multiple sclerosis (Allegretta *et al.*, 1990, 1994; Sriram, 1994; Trotter *et al.*, 1997), systemic lupus erythematosus (Gmelig-Meyling *et al.*, 1992; Dawisha *et al.*, 1994), systemic sclerosis, mixed connective tissue disease (Holyst *et al.*, 1994), other demyelinating disorders (Van den Berg *et al.*, 1995), rheumatoid arthritis (Cannons *et al.*, 1998), and insulin-dependent diabetes mellitus (Falta *et al.*, 1999). Elevated mutant frequencies found in patients with malignant melanoma have suggested an ongoing immunological response to the tumour (Albertini *et al.*, 2001). Elevations of *HPRT* T-cell mutant frequency have predicted rejection episodes in heart transplant recipients (Ansari *et al.*, 1995). Selecting for *HPRT* mutants has been found to be a form of surrogate selection for candidate immunologically relevant T cells recognized by their specific *TCR* gene rearrangements in some of these disorders.

Mutant isolates from some individuals reveal that multiple *HPRT* mutational changes have arisen in the same in-vivo clone (pattern 2 above), but only a single *HPRT* change has occurred per mutant isolate. This pattern probably indicates extensive in-vivo clonal proliferation, the magnitude of which is a linear function of the number of different *HPRT* mutations that have occurred in the clone. For example, given a background mutation rate of 10^{-6}/cell generation, three independent mutations might arise in a clone that has undergone approximately 3×10^6 cell generations *in vivo*. However, the distribution of *HPRT* mutations in some individuals who show pattern 2 for *HPRT-PCR* changes is not so easily explained (Albertini *et al.*, 1998). Here, the different *HPRT* mutations arise sequentially, as evidenced by an ordering of their appearance in different mutant isolates from the same clone. The majority of isolates show a single 'founding' *HPRT* change. Fewer isolates show both this primary founding mutation plus a secondary change that coexists in the same allele (*i.e.* in the same molecule). Different secondary mutations might appear in different isolates, all with the same founding mutation. A tertiary mutation may also appear. The sequential *HPRT* mutations now define sublineages within the TCR defined clone. A background mutation rate of 10^{-6}/cell generation will require 10^{18} cell generations for three *HPRT* mutations to arise in this way, as the number of cell generations is now an exponential function of the number of mutations produced. As this is clearly unreasonable, an alternative explanation is required. One such explanation is an increase in the background mutation rate to 10^{-2} to 10^{-3}/cell generation. This defines clonally restricted genomic instability.

One clinical situation where clonally restricted genomic instability is not infrequent is in children after treatment for acute lymphocytic leukaemia (Finette *et al.*, 2000). These children receive multiple genotoxic chemotherapeutic agents, including prolonged 6-thioguanine treatment. 6-Thioguanine positively selects *in vivo* for cells that are deficient in *HPRT*, the precise mutational phenotype in *HPRT* mutant T cells. It is quite probable that the extensive chemotherapy these children receive results in extensive cell death, including death in the T-cell population. Restorative proliferation is then required to restore cell numbers. During this proliferation, *HPRT* mutations arise in the regenerating population.

Any *HPRT* mutant T cells will be positively selected because of the 6-thioguanine, with such mutants gaining a proliferative advantage. Importantly, if the underlying mutation rates in the *in vivo* T-cell population are different, the *HPRT* mutations are most likely to arise in those cells with the highest intrinsic rate of mutation. There are many possibilities for heterogeneity of mutation rates *in vivo* producing clones of cells with different mutation rates. One such possibility is an underlying constitutional heterozygosity for DNA repair gene mutations with the occurrence of rare 'null' cells arising from an earlier somatic mutation or recombinational event – perhaps during fetal development. Once an *HPRT* mutation occurs in a cell with pre-existing genomic instability, the process becomes progressive, resulting in secondary and tertiary non-selected *HPRT* mutations.

An important mechanistic insight deriving from this observation is the importance of in-vivo selection for determining the distributions of in-vivo cell populations. Perhaps molecular epidemiology should study in-vivo 'selectogens'. For genomic instability, selecting for any mutation (*e.g.* in these leukaemic children it was mutations in *HPRT*) in a heterogeneous population of cells (*e.g.* T cells) will also select for those cells most likely to mutate (*i.e.* rare cells with pre-existing genomic instability). There is ample evidence that this phenomenon occurs *in vitro* in both prokaryotic and eukaryotic systems (Miller, 1996; Mao *et al.*, 1997; Hunt *et al.*, 1998). Another insight from these in-vivo observations is that this process goes forward in apparently normal T cells and might be an inherent biological potential in all cells. Its apparent obligatory relationship to malignancy might be an artefact of previous studies that have involved malignant cells.

Biomarker responses in workers exposed to 1,3-butadiene

1,3-Butadiene

1,3-Butadiene (BD) is an air pollutant that affects large numbers of humans (European Centre for Ecotoxicity and Toxicology of Chemicals, 1997; Himmelstein *et al.*, 1997; IARC, 1999). The greatest exposures are in workplace settings but the general population is also exposed from mobile sources and other sources. BD is carcinogenic in rodent bioassays but with vastly different potencies in mice and rats. The former are by far the more susceptible, developing tumours at the lowest exposure concentrations tested (Huff *et al.*, 1985; Irons *et al.*, 1989; Melnick *et al.*, 1990). By contrast, rats developed tumours at 1000-fold higher exposure levels, although lower levels have not been tested (Owen *et al.*, 1987). Epidemiological investigations in humans have given mixed results, with indications of excess leukaemia in the largest and most complete study to date of styrene-butadiene rubber workers. Such excesses of leukaemia were not found in monomer production workers (Delzell *et al.*, 1996; Divine & Hartman, 1996; Macaluso *et al.*, 1996). These results have been considered insufficient by IARC to classify BD as a known human carcinogen (IARC Group 1). Its current classification is Group 2A, *i.e.* a probable human carcinogen (IARC, 1999).

BD is itself not biologically active, but it is metabolized *in vivo* to at least three electrophilic species: 1,2-epoxy-3-butene (EB) (the monoepoxide), 1,2,3,4-diepoxybutane (DEB) (the diepoxide), and 1,2-dihydroxy-3,4-epoxybutane (EBD) (the diol-epoxide) (reviewed in Himmelstein *et al.*, 1997). All three metabolites are genotoxic in all systems tested, with potencies in the order DEB > EB > EBD. BD metabolites are detoxified by conjugation or hydrolysis – the former mediated by glutathione-*S*-transferase (GST) and the latter by epoxide hydrolase (EH). The M_1 urinary excretion product (1,2-dihydroxy-4-*N*-(acetylcysteinyl)butane) is considered to be a biomarker of hydrolysis and the M_2 product (1-hydroxy-2-*N*-(acetylcysteinyl)-3-butene in racemic mixture with 1-(*N*-acetylcysteinyl)-2-hydroxy-3-butene) is considered to be a biomarker of conjugation. The ratio $M_1/(M_1 + M_2)$ in urine defines the relative importance of hydrolysis in detoxification (Henderson *et al.*, 1996).

Oxidation and hydrolysis of BD and its metabolites may also be assessed by haemoglobin adducts. The *N*-(2-hydroxy-3-butenyl)valine haemoglobin adduct (HBVal) is produced by EB

(Osterman-Golkar *et al.*, 1991; Osterman-Golkar *et al.*, 1993; Van Sittert & Van Vliet, 1994), whereas the *N*-(2,3,4-trihydroxy-butyl)valine adduct (THBVal) derives primarily from EBD (Perez *et al.*, 1997). The relative concentrations of these two adducts are measures of oxidation and hydrolysis, respectively.

Although there are common activation and detoxification steps for BD in all species, there are differences in the extent to which the pathways are utilized. Extensive research has been directed at interspecies comparisons to determine if differential metabolism can account for the different carcinogenic potencies of BD. Mice, which are the most susceptible to BD-induced cancer, are much more efficient than rats in oxidizing this agent to EB or DEB. Urinary M1/(M1 + M2) ratios for mice and rats exposed to BD by inhalation indicate that conjugation detoxification predominates in mice whereas hydrolysis is more important in rats (Henderson *et al.*, 1996).

Interspecies comparisons of haemoglobin and DNA adduct data are consistent with the results of the metabolic studies in mice and rats, indicating that the former is the more efficient species in oxidizing BD to its electrophilic intermediates. Interspecies comparisons of genotoxicity *in vivo* in the two species have shown both somatic chromosome and gene level mutations in mice but only gene level changes in rats (reviewed in Albertini *et al.*, 2001). Furthermore, even at the gene level, the mutagenic potency of BD is much greater in mice than in rats. Despite several studies of both somatic and germ cell effects *in vivo*, chromosomal aberrations have never been demonstrated in rats.

BD is clearly a genotoxic carcinogen in rodents. Animal studies reveal that metabolism produces the genotoxic intermediates, with carcinogen potency directly related to genotoxicity. The low-order carcinogenicity in rats relative to mice is due to the lower genotoxicity of the metabolites produced in that species. It is now possible to assess all of these parameters in humans, also perhaps allowing mechanistic insights and estimates of risk for BD in humans relative to rodents.

Molecular epidemiological studies in humans have assessed internal doses and genotoxicity in workers exposed to BD. One difficulty in relating these investigations to the cancer epidemiological studies is that modern exposure levels are probably much lower than those of the 1950s and 1960s when currently recognized malignancies may have been induced. Nonetheless, several recent investigations have measured exposure levels, urinary M1 metabolite concentrations, haemoglobin adducts and in-vivo genotoxicity. The last is of most relevance here. Three studies failed to find chromosome level changes in three different exposed worker populations, although re-analysis of one of these studies on the basis of GST genotypes showed the GST T1 null BD-exposed workers to have significantly higher aberration frequencies than the appropriate controls (Au *et al.*,1995; Sorsa *et al.*, 1994, 1996; Hayes *et al.*, 2000). A subsequent study of one of these populations also showed an increase in aberrations in exposed versus unexposed workers (Sram *et al.*, 1998). Mutagenicity studies have also yielded conflicting results. Two large studies failed to find increases in somatic *HPRT* gene mutations (Tates *et al.*, 1996; Hayes *et al.*, 2000), although an overlapping series of investigations from another laboratory in other populations using a different methodology did find increases (Ward *et al.*, 1994, 1996, 2001; Ma *et al.*, 2000; Albertini *et al.*, 2001; Ammenheuser *et al.*, 2001; Albertini *et al.*, 2003).

The overall results of genotoxicity studies in humans have therefore been mixed. Each investigation can be questioned, especially in terms of external exposure assessment, confounding exposures and time after exposure measurement that blood samples were obtained. As genotoxicity is an important endpoint for assessing the risks in humans of an agent that is a known genotoxic carcinogen in animals, this uncertainty is an important data gap in assessing the carcinogenic potential of modern worker exposures.

Mechanistic insights

A recent large-scale study of a continuum of biomarker responses – assessing exposure, effect, and susceptibility – was recently completed in

BD-exposed workers engaged in the production of monomer or styrene-butadiene rubber (Albertini *et al.*, 2001, 2003) (Figure 2). The primary objective of the study was to validate each of the biomarkers as a measure of exposure. External exposures, therefore, had to be determined with precision. Personal 8-h BD measurements were made on several occasions over a 60-day period for each potentially exposed worker in order to provide maximum accuracy for this independent variable and to accommodate the different expression intervals of the several biomarkers. Area BD levels and co-exposures to styrene, benzene, and toluene were also measured. A secondary objective of the study was to reconcile the inconsistencies in the human genotoxicity results noted above.

This molecular epidemiological study included 24 BD-monomer production workers, with a mean BD exposure of 0.291 ppm (0.642 mg/m^2), 34 styrene butadiene rubber workers, with a mean BD exposure of 0.796 ppm (1.794 mg/m^3) and 25 controls, with a mean BD exposure of 0.012 ppm (0.023 mg/m^3). In summary, urinary M1 and M2 metabolites and HBVal and THBVal haemoglobin adducts all correlated significantly with BD exposure levels, with the adducts being the most highly associated. All four biomarkers were therefore validated as measures of internal doses. Individual external BD exposure levels could be calculated from individual concentrations of haemoglobin adducts. There was no evidence for genotoxicity in this study at either the chromosome or the gene level. Molecular genotypes, including GST, did not influence these overall results. These results are summarized according to the NRC paradigm in Figure 3.

Several mechanistic insights were gleaned from this transitional study. The ratio of urinary metabolites $M_1/(M_1 + M_2)$ was approximately 0.99, indicating that humans rely almost entirely on the hydrolytic detoxification pathway for BD metabolites. This is in marked contrast to mice, the susceptible species for BD carcinogenicity. Furthermore, the THBVal haemoglobin adduct concentrations were 300- to 400-fold higher than the HBVal adduct concentrations, presumably reflecting this hydrolytic pathway with much

greater in-vivo accumulation of EBD than EB in humans. Even though the conjugation detoxification pathway is minor in humans, group mean urinary concentrations of M_2 were positively associated with group mean BD exposure levels, suggesting that even this minor pathway is stimulated with increasing BD (data not shown; Albertini *et al.*, 2001, 2003). However, in the groups of workers with the GST null genotypes, there were relative decreases in production of the M_2 metabolite, blunting this stimulatory effect. This clearly indicates the dependence of the conjugation pathway on GST.

Interspecies comparisons

Non-tumour data have now been obtained under comparable conditions for BD exposed mice, rats and humans, allowing for interspecies comparisons (Walker & Meng, 2000; Meng *et al.*, 2001; Swenberg *et al.*, 2001; Walker, personal communication). The relevant results from recent studies in mice and rats are shown in Figures 4A and 4B according to the NCR paradigm. These data may be compared to the human data described above to begin modelling BD's mode of action in inducing cancer and for assessing its cancer risks to humans (Figure 5).

Although the BD exposure levels to mice, rats, and humans have been vastly different over their entire ranges, they have been comparable at the lower levels. The relative detoxification metabolic pathways in the three species, as assessed by the ratio of metabolite concentrations in urine, $M_1/(M_1 + M_2)$, are 24% hydrolysis in mice, 51% hydrolysis in rats, and 99% hydrolysis in humans. The biologically effective doses achieved *in vivo* in the three species can be assessed by the haemoglobin adduct concentrations. Measures for both HBVal and THBVal show that mice and rats develop comparable levels of adduct concentrations at exposure levels up to 62.5 ppm, after which the mice show dramatically higher levels. It is noteworthy that mice have higher HBVal adduct concentrations (oxidative pathway) at all external exposure levels than do rats, whereas THBVal adduct concentrations are comparable except at the highest external exposure. Although the HBVal adduct concentrations are appreciable

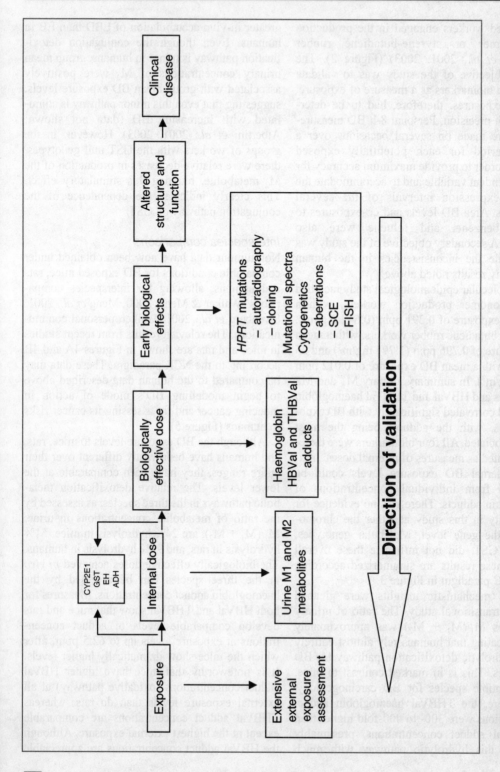

Figure 2. The continuum of biomarkers evaluated in a transitional epidemiological study of Czech workers exposed to 1,3-butadiene. ADH, alcohol dehydrogenase; CYP2E1, A P450 enzyme; EH, epoxide hydrolase; FISH, fluorescence *in situ* hybridization; GST, glutathione-*S*-transferase; HBVal, *N*-(2-hydroxy-3-butenyl)valine; M_1, 1,2-dihydroxy-4-(*N*-acetylcysteinyl)butane; M_2, 1-hydroxy-2-(*N*-acetylcysteinyl))-3-butene; THBVal, *N*-(2,3,4-trihydroxybutyl)valine.

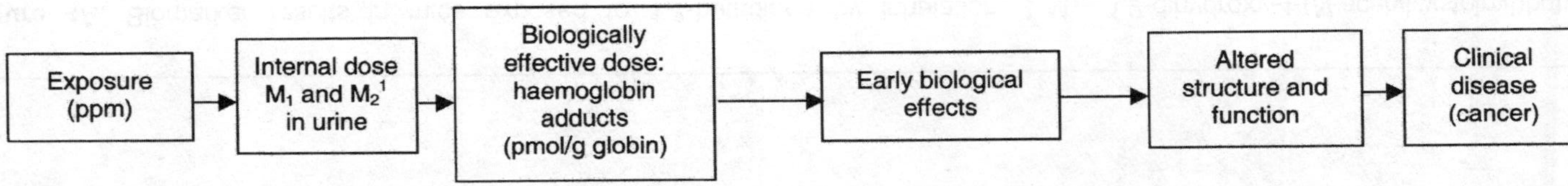

Figure 3. Partial results of transitional epidemiological study of Czech workers exposed to 1,3-butadiene. [1] M_1 = 1,2-dihydroxy-4-(N-acetylcysteinyl)butane; M_2 = 1-hydroxy-2-(N-acetylcysteinyl)-3-butene (mean concentration not shown); [2] influenced by GST genotype; [3] HBVal, N-(2-hydroxy-3-butenyl)valine; THBVal, N-(2,3,4-trihydroxybutyl)valine; [4] HPRT mutations assessed by both cloning and autoradiographic assay methods; no change in $HPRT$ mutational spectrum from background; [5] Chromosomal changes measured include sister chromatid exchanges (SCEs) and chromosomal aberrations measured by conventional methods and by FISH; [6] 0, no significant differences, compared to background controls; [7] 0, no significant differences, compared to background controls; [8] inconsistent epidemiological findings (see text).

Exposure (ppm)	$M_1/(M_1 + M_2)$ [2]	HBVal [3]	THBVal [3]	Hprt mutations [4] ($\times 10^{-6}$)		Chromosomal changes [5]
				Cloning	Autoradio-graphy	
0.012 (n = 25) (administrative controls)	0.996	0.22 ± 0.21	94.77 ± 38.71	13.0 ± 8.1 (n = 24)	10.8 ± 6.1 (n = 18)	
0.291 (n = 24) (monomer production workers)	0.989	0.47 ± 0.45	178.73 ± 101.31	0.8 × control (n = 18)	0.5 × control (n = 16)	0[7]
0.796 (n = 34) (polymerization workers)	0.985	2.23 ± 1.40	716 ± 425.72	1.3 × control[6] (n = 32)	0.6 × control (n = 15)	0

Flowchart: Exposure (ppm) → Internal dose M_1 and M_2[1] in urine → Biologically effective dose: haemoglobin adducts (pmol/g globin) → Early biological effects → Altered structure and function → Clinical disease (cancer)

?[8]

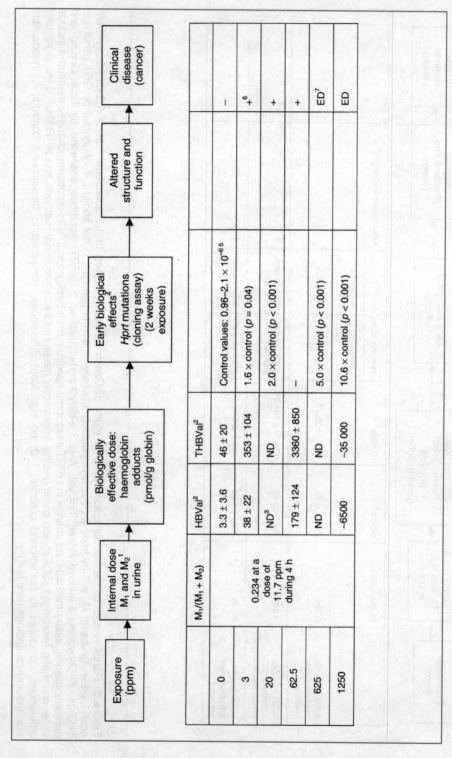

Figure 4A. Biomarker results in mice exposed to 1,3-butadiene by inhalation. [1] M_1, 1,2-dihydroxy-4-(N-acetylcysteinyl)butane; M_2, 1-hydroxy-2-(N-acetylcysteinyl)-3-butene (mean concentration not shown). [2] HBVal, N-(2-hydroxy-3-butenyl)valine; THBVal, N-(2,3,4-trihydroxybutyl)valine. [3] ND, not determined. [4] Chromosomal aberrations have frequently been demonstrated in mice exposed to BD by inhalation, but have never been demonstrated in rats exposed to BD by inhalation (but have been for EB or DEB). [5] Mean value range for different experiments. [6] +, positive tumour response in long-term bioassays (Huff et al., 1985; Melnick et al., 1990). [7] ED, early death in long term bioassays.

Exposure (ppm)	$M_1/(M_1 + M_2)$	HBVal[2]	THBVal[2]	Early biological effects[4] Hprt mutations (cloning assay) (2 weeks exposure)	Clinical disease (cancer)
0	0.234 at a dose of 11.7 ppm during 4 h	3.3 ± 3.6	46 ± 20	Control values: $0.96-2.1 \times 10^{-6}$ [5]	–
3		38 ± 22	353 ± 104	$1.6 \times$ control ($p = 0.04$)	+[6]
20		ND[3]	ND	$2.0 \times$ control ($p < 0.001$)	+
62.5		179 ± 124	3360 ± 850	–	+
625		ND	ND	$5.0 \times$ control ($p < 0.001$)	ED[7]
1250		~6500	~35 000	$10.6 \times$ control ($p < 0.001$)	ED

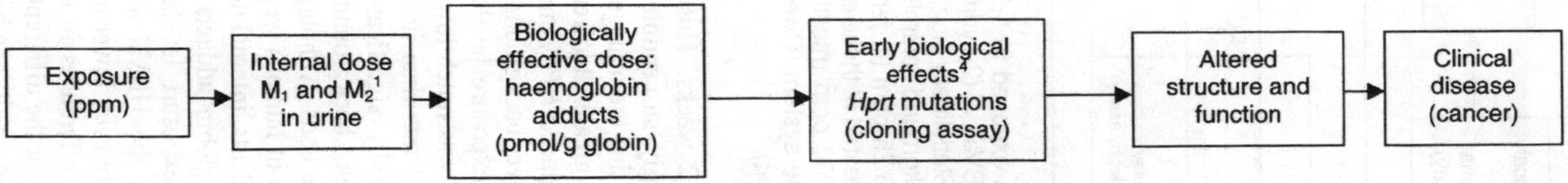

Exposure (ppm)	Internal dose M₁ and M₂ in urine	Biologically effective dose: haemoglobin adducts (pmol/g globin)		Early biological effects[4] Hprt mutations (cloning assay)	Altered structure and function	Clinical disease (cancer)
	$M_1/(M_1 + M_2)$	HBVal[2]	THBVal[2]			
0		5.3 ± 4.5	58.0 ± 8.0	Control value: $2.4{-}2.8 \times 10^{-6}$		–
3		14.0 ± 4.0	400 ± 37	–		NT[6]
20	0.510 at a dose of 11.7 ppm during 4 h	ND[3]	ND	0[5]		NT
62.5		85.0 ± 4.0	2990 ± 150	0		NT
625		ND	ND	1.7 × control (p = 0.028)		NT
1250		~1000	~6000	3.5 × control (p = 0.005)		benign only[7]

Figure 4B. Biomarker results in rats exposed to 1,3-butadiene by inhalation. [1] M_1, 1,2-dihydroxy-4-(N-acetylcysteinyl)butane. M_2, 1-hydroxy-2-(N-acetylcysteinyl)-3-butene (mean concentration not shown). [2] HBVal, N-(2-hydroxy-3-butenyl)valine; THBVal, N-(2,3,4-trihydroxybutyl)valine. [3] ND, not determined. [4] Chromosomal aberrations have **NEVER** been demonstrated in **RATS** exposed to BD by inhalation (but have been for EB or DEB). [5] 0, no significant differences, compared to background controls. [6] NT, not tested in long-term bioassays. [7] Finding at 1000 ppm for two years in long-term bioassay (Owen et al., 1987).

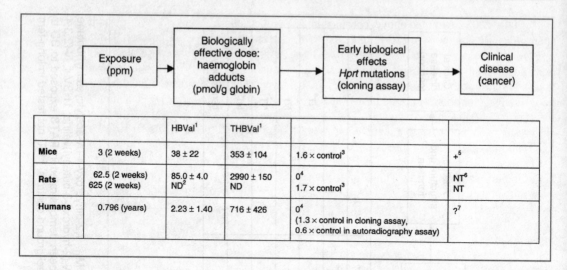

		HBVal[1]	THBVal[1]		
				Early biological effects *Hprt* mutations (cloning assay)	Clinical disease (cancer)
Mice	3 (2 weeks)	38 ± 22	353 ± 104	1.6 × control[3]	+[5]
Rats	62.5 (2 weeks) 625 (2 weeks)	85.0 ± 4.0 ND[2]	2990 ± 150 ND	0[4] 1.7 × control[3]	NT[6] NT
Humans	0.796 (years)	2.23 ± 1.40	716 ± 426	0[4] (1.3 × control in cloning assay, 0.6 × control in autoradiography assay)	?[7]

Figure 5. Comparison of biomarker results in mice, rats, and humans exposed to 1,3-butadiene by inhalation: minimal effective or maximal no-effect exposure doses. [1] HBVal, *N*-(2-hydroxy-3-butenyl)-valine; THBVal, *N*-(2,3,4-trihydroxybutyl)valine. [2] ND, not determined. [3] Statistically significant increase over background controls. [4] No statistically significant increase over background controls. [5] Positive for tumour induction at all exposure levels tested, including the lowest at 6.25 ppm (in females) in long-term bioassay in mice (Huff *et al.*, 1985; Melnick *et al.*, 1990). [6] NT = not tested at these exposure levels in long-term bioassay in rats. Increases in tumours were found at 1000 ppm (mostly benign) and 8000 ppm, with a pattern suggesting an indirect effect on the endocrine system (Owen *et al.*, 1987; Owen & Glaister, 1990). [7] Inconsistent epidemiological evidence (see text).

in both species, the THB concentrations are higher, indicating that hydrolysis, with production of EBD, occurs in both rodent species. Humans develop THBVal adduct concentrations at exposure levels below 1 ppm that are comparable to those in rodents at higher exposure levels – certainly up to 3 ppm and probably up to 20 ppm. However, HBVal adducts in humans are considerably lower than in rodents. As noted above, the concentrations of THBVal adducts are dramatically higher in humans than are the concentrations of HBVal adducts, illustrating the dominance of hydrolysis in BD metabolism in humans. The most important interspecies comparison seen in Figure 5 is that for genotoxic effects which, in these rodent studies, are represented only by *HPRT* mutations. Mice showed statistically significant increases in mutations over controls even at exposure levels as low as 3 ppm administered by inhalation for 2 weeks. Mutant frequencies became progressively higher to the highest level of BD exposure tested,

i.e. 1250 ppm for 2 weeks. This confirms that mice are exceedingly susceptible to the genotoxicity of BD and that the mutagenic potency of this agent in mice is greater at lower than at higher exposure levels. Induced *HPRT* mutations at frequencies elevated over background were not seen in rats below BD exposure levels of 625 ppm. Mutation induction was much lower, even at the higher BD levels in rats than in mice. Humans showed no statistically significant increases in *HPRT* mutations over background, as measured by two different methods. Although the external BD exposure levels in humans were much lower than those in the rodents, internal doses as judged by THBVal haemoglobin adducts were comparable at the lower exposure levels. However, at these lower levels, the HBVal adduct concentrations were actually even lower in humans than expected from the differences in external exposure concentrations for the different species.

These comparative results can be considered in the context of other studies (reviewed in Albertini *et al.*, 2001, 2003). As noted above, chromosomal aberrations are common *in vivo* in mice exposed to BD but have never been observed in rats. The transitional study in humans included several assays for chromosome level mutations, *i.e.* traditional analysis for aberrations, and FISH analyses for aberrations and measurements of SCEs. All chromosome endpoints were unequivocally negative (Albertini *et al.*, 2001, 2003).

Data gaps become apparent when viewing BD non-tumour data in this way. The animal studies were all conducted as is traditional, *i.e.* exposures at various levels followed by removal of the agent, allowing time for development of biomarkers, and then testing. It would be better if the animals were continuously exposed throughout the time of testing. This would allow biological responses to be determined in the animals under conditions that are exactly comparable to those in exposed humans. For humans, there is a lack of studies at BD exposure concentrations above 1 ppm. Heavily exposed human populations should be sought and studied with all relevant biomarkers. Efforts should be made to find evidence of genotoxicity in such heavily exposed individuals. Finding such evidence will allow the above paradigm to be used to extrapolate risk for cancer in humans quantitatively, using the combined human and animal data sets, including the animal cancer results. At present, a critical non-cancer early biological effect endpoint, genotoxicity, has not been found with certainty in humans to allow this extrapolation. In the human study presented here, there were 32 individuals in the high-exposure group who were compared with 24 control individuals in the low-exposure group for *HPRT* mutant frequencies determined by the cloning assay. Previous analyses of statistical considerations for the assay indicate the median ratio of mutant frequencies from two populations of these sizes that can be detected with a probability of 0.9 (range from about 1.46 to 1.94), depending on between-subject variance (Robinson *et al.*, 1994). For the autoradiographic assay, the exposed workers actually showed lower *HPRT* variant frequencies than did the administrative controls. None of several assays for chromosome-level genetic damage showed an effect in this study.

Nonetheless, weak but important genotoxic effects could have been missed. Finding a level of exposure to BD that does induce genotoxicity in humans is important. Such an exposure level will also identify critical concentrations for biomarkers of exposure, *e.g.* haemoglobin adducts, that indicate biologically effective doses for human monitoring aimed at disease prevention. From Figures 4 and 5, it might seem that the HBVal adduct concentrations are the critical markers of effective exposure. However, it is formally possible that genotoxicity will not be convincingly demonstrated in humans at any BD exposure level experienced or haemoglobin adduct concentration found. In that case, it must be questioned whether or not this agent is truly genotoxic in humans at realistic exposure levels. If it is not, its carcinogenicity for humans at these exposure levels must be questioned.

Conclusions

Many biomarkers have been developed for human molecular epidemiological studies. Once validated, these endpoints can be useful probes for developing a mechanistic understanding of the diseases in question. Somatic mutations, as the central events in carcinogenicity, are particularly valuable in this regard. Mutations in reporter genes can be used for the quantitative and qualitative measurement of exposures to environmental carcinogens, although this is not their best use. Mutations, even in reporter genes not on the pathway to cancer, capture the mechanisms that underlie them. Many of these mechanisms are the same for all genes, allowing effects in reporter genes to serve as surrogates for effects in cancer-related genes. Developing insights into the former provides understanding of the latter. Molecular epidemiological studies that employ a multiplicity of biomarkers spanning the continuum from exposure to effect allow additional insights into pathogenic mechanisms that range from metabolism to genotoxic consequences. This array of non-cancer endpoints can be compared among species. Such interspecies comparisons, using experimental animals for which actual carcinogenicity data are also available, should play an increasing role in the cancer risk assessment process.

References

Albertini, M.R., King, D.M., Newton, M.A. & Vacek, P.M. (2001) *In vivo* mutant frequency of thio-guanine-resistant T cells in the peripheral blood and lymph nodes of melanoma patients. *Mutat. Res.*, **476**, 83–97

Albertini, R.J. (1994) Why use somatic mutations for human biomonitoring? *Environ. Mol. Mutagen.*, **23** (Suppl 24), 18–22

Albertini, R.J. (1998a) The use and interpretation of biomarkers of environmental genotoxicity in humans. *Biotherapy*, **11**, 155–167

Albertini, R.J. (1998b) Somatic mutations as multi-purpose biomarkers. In: Mendelsohn, M.L., Mohr, L.C. & Peeters, J.P., eds, *Biomarkers, Medical and Workplace Applications*, Washington, DC, John Henry Press, pp. 167–185

Albertini, R.J. (2001) Developing sustainable studies on environmental health. *Mutat. Res.*, **480–481**, 317–331

Albertini, R.J. & Hayes, R.B. (1997) Somatic muta-tions in cancer epidemiology. In: Toniolo, P., Boffetta, P., Shuker, D.E.G, Rothman, N., Hulka, B. & Pearce, N., eds, *Application of Biomarkers in Cancer Epidemiology* (IARC Sci. Publ. No. 142), Lyon, IARC*Press*, pp. 159–184

Albertini, R.J., Nicklas, J.A. & O'Neill, J.P. (1996) Future research directions for evaluating human genetic and cancer risk from environmental exposures. *Environ.Health Perspect.*, **104** (Suppl. 3), 503–510

Albertini, R.J., Clark, L.S., Nicklas, J.A., O'Neill, J.P., Hui, T.E. & Jostes, R. (1997) Radiation quality affects the efficiency of induction and the mole-cular spectrum of *HPRT* mutations in human T cells. *Radiat. Res.*, **148** (Suppl. 5), S76–S86

Albertini, R.J., Nicklas, J.A., Skopek, T.R., Recio, L. & O'Neill, J.P. (1998) Genetic instability in human T lymphocytes. *Mutat. Res.*, **400**, 381–389

Albertini, R.J., Sram, R.J., Vacek, P.M., Lynch, J., Wright, M., Nicklas, J.A., Boogaard, P.J., Henderson, R.F., Swenberg, J.A., Tates, A.D. & Ward, J.B., Jr (2001) Biomarkers for assessing occupational exposures to 1,3-butadiene. *Chem.. Biol. Interact.*, **135–136**, 429–453

Albertini, R.J., Owen, P.E., Glaister, J.R., Gaunt, I.F. & Pullinger, D.H. (2003) Biomarker responses in butadiene exposed Czech workers: A transitional,

epidemiological study. Final Report. Cambridge MA, USA, Health Effects Institute

Allegretta, M., Nicklas, J.A., Sriram, S. & Albertini, R.J. (1990) T cells responsive to myelin basic protein in patients with multiple sclerosis. *Science*, **247**, 718–721

Allegretta, M., Albertini, R.J., Howell, M.D., Smith, L.R., Martin, R., McFarland, H.F., Sriram, S., Brostoff, S. & Steinman, L. (1994) Homologies between T-cell receptor junctional sequences unique to multiple sclerosis and T cells mediating experimental allergic encephalomyelitis. *J. Clin. Invest.*, **94**, 105–109

Ammenheuser, M.M., Bechtold, W.E., Abdel-Rahman, S.Z., Rosenblatt, J.I., Hastings-Smith, D.A. & Ward, J.B., Jr. (2001) Assessment of 1,3-butadiene exposure in polymer production workers using *HPRT* mutations in lymphocytes as a biomarker. *Environ. Health Perspect.*, **109**, 1249–1255

Ansari, A.A., Mayne, A., Sundstrom, J.B., Gravanis, M.B., Kanter K., Sell, K.W., Villinger, F., Siu, C.O. & Herskowitz, A. (1995) Frequency of hypo-xanthine guanine phophoribosyltransferase (HPRT⁻) T cells in the peripheral blood of cardiac transplant recipients: a non-invasive technique for the diagnosis of allograft rejection. *Circulation*, **92**, 862–874

Au, W.W., Bechtold, W.E., Whorton, E.B., Jr & Legator, M.S. (1995) Chromosome aberrations and response to gamma-ray challenge in lymphocytes of workers exposed to 1,3-butadiene by inhalation. *Mutat. Res.*, **309**, 315–320.

Baars, P.A., Maurice, M.M., Rep, M., Hooibrink, B. & van Lier, R.A.W. (1995) Heterogeneity of the circulating CD4⁺ T cell population: further evi-dence that the CD4⁺ CD45RA⁻ CD27⁻ T cell subset contains specialized primed T cells. *J. Immunol.*, **154**, 17–25

Bigbee, W.L., Day, R.D., Grant, S.G., Keohavong, P., Xi, L., Zhang, L. & Ness, R.B. (1999) Impact of maternal lifestyle factors on newborn *HPRT* mutant frequencies and molecular spectrum – initial results from the Pre-natal Exposures and Pre-eclampsia Prevention (PEPP) study. *Mutat. Res.*, **431**, 279–289

Boehm, T. & Rabbitts, T.H. (1989) The human T-cell receptor genes are targets for chromosomal abnormalities in T cell tumors. *FASEB J.*, **3**, 2344–2359

Bohr, V.A., Phillips, D.H. & Hanawalt, P.C. (1987) Heterogeneous DNA damage and repair in the mammalian genome. *Cancer Res.*, **47**, 6426–6436

Breit, T.M., Mol, E.J., Wolvers-Tettero, I.L.M., Ludwig, W.-D., van Wering, E.R. & Van Dongen, J.J.M. (1993) Site-specified deletions involving the *tal-1* and *sil* genes are restricted to cells of the T-cell receptor alpha/beta lineage: T-cell receptor delta gene deletion mechanism affects multiple genes. *J. Exp. Med.*, **177**, 965–977

Brooks, A.L. (1999) Biomarkers of exposure, sensitivity and disease. *Int. J. Radiat. Biol.*, **75**, 1481–1503

Cannons, J.L., Karsh, J., Birnboim, H.C. & Goldstein, R. (1998) *HPRT* ⁻ mutant T cells in the peripheral blood and synovial tissue of patients with rheumatoid arthritis. *Arthritis Rheum.*, **41**, 1772–1782

Caporaso, N. & Goldstein, A. (1997) Issues involving biomarkers in the study of the genetics of human cancer. In: Toniolo, P., Boffetta, P., Shuker, D.E.G., Rothman, N., Hulka, B. & Pearce, N., eds, *Application of Biomarkers in Cancer Epidemiology* (IARC Sci. Publ. No. 142), Lyon, IARC*Press*, pp. 237–250

Cariello, N.F. (1994) Software for the analysis of mutations at the human *HPRT* gene. *Mutat. Res.*, **312**, 173–185

Cariello, N.F. & Skopek, T.R. (1993) Analysis of mutations occurring at the human *HPRT* locus. *J. Mol. Biol.*, **231**, 41–57

Cariello, N.F., Craft, T.R., Vrieling, H., van Zeeland, A.A., Adams, T. & Skopek, T.R. (1992) Human *HPRT* mutant database: Software for data entry and retrieval. *Environ. Mol. Mutagen.*, **20**, 81–83

Clark, L.S., Albertini, R.J. & Nicklas, J.A. (1997) The aminothiol WR-1065 protects T lymphocytes from ionizing radiation-induced deletions of the *HPRT* gene. *Cancer Epidemiol. Biomarkers Prev.*, **6**, 1033–1037

Cochrane, J.E. & Skopek, T.R. (1994) Mutagenicity of butadiene and its epoxide metabolites: I. Mutagenic potential of 1,2-epoxybutene, 1,2,3,4-diepoxybutane and 3,4-epoxy-1,2-butanediol in cultured human lymphoblasts. *Carcinogenesis*, **15**, 713–717

Cole, J. & Skopek, T.R. (1994) International Commission for Protection against Environmental Muta-

gens and Carcinogens, Working Paper No. 3. Somatic mutant frequency, mutation rates and mutational spectra in the human population *in vivo*. *Mutat. Res.*, **304**, 33–105

Committee on Biological Markers of the National Research Council (1987) Biological markers in environmental health research. *Environ. Health Perspect.*, **74**, 3–9

Curry, J., Khaidakov, M. & Glickman, B.W. (2000) Russian mutational spectrum differs from that of their Western counterparts. *Hum. Mutat.*, **15**, 439–446

Dawisha, S.M., Gmelig-Meyling, F. & Steinberg, A.D. (1994) Assessment of clinical parameters associated with increased frequency of mutant T cells in patients with systemic lupus erythematosus. *Arthritis Rheum.*, **37**, 270–277

Delzell, E., Sathiakumar, N., Hovinga, M., Macaluso, M., Julian, J., Larson, R., Cole, P. & Muir, D.C.F. (1996) A follow-up study of synthetic rubber workers. *Toxicology*, **113**, 182–189

Divine, B.J. & Hartman, C.M. (1996) Mortality update of butadiene preduction workers. *Toxicology*, **113**, 169–181

European Centre for Ecotoxicity and Toxicology of Chemicals (1997) *1,3-Butadiene OEL Criteria Document, 2nd Ed.*, Brussels, European Centre for Ecotoxicity and Toxicology of Chemicals

Evans, M.K., Taffe, B.G., Harris, C.C. & Bohr, V.A. (1993) DNA strand bias in the repair of the p53 gene in normal human and xeroderma pigmentosum group C fibroblasts. *Cancer Res.*, **53**, 5377–5381

Falta, M.T., Magin, G.K., Allegretta, M., Steinman, L., Atkinson, M.A., Brostoff, S.W. & Albertini, R.J. (1999) Selection of *HPRT* mutant T cells as surrogates for dividing cells reveals a restricted T-cell receptor BV repertoire in insulin-dependent diabetes mellitus. *Clin. Immunol.*, **90**, 340–351

Finette, B.A., Poseno, T. & Albertini, R.J. (1996) V(D)J recombinase-mediated *HPRT* mutations in peripheral blood lymphocytes of normal children. *Cancer Res.*, **56**, 1405–1412

Finette, B.A., O'Neill, J.P., Vacek, P.M. & Albertini, R.J. (1998) Gene mutations with characteristic deletions in cord blood T lymphocytes associated with passive maternal exposure to tobacco smoke. *Nature Med.*, **4**, 1144–1151

Finette, B.A., Homans, A.C. & Albertini, R.J. (2000) Emergence of genetic instability in children treated for leukemia. *Science*, **288**, 514–517

Finger, L.R., Harvey, R.C., Moore, R.C.A., Showe, L.C. & Croce, C.M. (1986) Common mechanism of chromosomal translocation in T- and B-cell neoplasia. *Science*, **234**, 982–985

Fuscoe, J.C., Zimmerman, L.J., Lippert, M.L., Nicklas, J.A., O'Neill, J.P. & Albertini, R.J. (1991) V(D)J recombinase-like activity mediates *HPRT* gene deletion in human fetal T-lymphocytes. *Cancer Res.*, **51**, 6001–6005

Gmelig-Meyling, F., Dawisha, S. & Steinberg, A.D. (1992) Assessment of in-vivo frequency of mutated T cells in patients with systemic lupus erythematosis. *J. Exp. Med.*, **175**, 297–300

Grant, S.G. & Bigbee, W.L. (1993) In-vivo somatic mutation and segregation at the human glycophorin A (GPA) locus: phenotypic variation encompassing both gene-specific and chromosomal mechanisms. *Mutat. Res.*, **288**, 163–172

Grist, S.A., McCarron, M., Kutlaca, A., Turner, D.R. & Morley, A.A. (1992) In-vivo human somatic mutation: frequency and spectrum with age. *Mutat. Res.*, **266**, 189–196

Hayes, R.B., Zhang, L., Yin, S., Swenberg, J.A., Xi, L., Wiencke, J., Bechtold, W.E., Yao, M., Rothman, N., Haas, R., O'Neill, J.P., Wiemels, J., Dosemeci, M., Li, G. & Smith, M.T. (2000) Genotoxic markers among butadiene-polymer workers in China. *Carcinogenesis*, **21**, 55–62

Hanawalt, P.C. (1989) Concepts and models for DNA repair: from *Escherichia coli* to mammalian cells. *Environ. Mol. Mutagen.*, **14** (Suppl 16), 90–98

Henderson, R.F., Thornton-Manning, J.R., Bechtold, W.E. & Dahl, A.R. (1996) Metabolism of 1,3-butadiene: species differences. *Toxicology*, **113**, 17–22

Himmelstein, M.W., Acquavella, J.F., Recio, L., Medinsky, M.A. & Bond, J.A. (1997) Toxicology and epidemiology of 1,3-butadiene. *Crit. Rev. Toxicol.*, **27**, 1–108

Holyst, M.-M., Hill, D.L., Sharp, G.C. & Hoffman, R.W. (1994) Increased frequency of mutations in the *HPRT* gene of T cells isolated from patients with anti-U1–70 kD autoantibody-positive connective tissue disease. *Int. Arch. Allergy Immunol.*, **105**, 234–237

Huff, J.E., Melnick, R.L., Solleveld, H.A., Haseman, J.K., Powers, M. & Miller, R.A. (1985) Multiple organ carcinogenicity of 1,3-butadiene in B6C3F1 mice after 60 weeks of inhalation exposure. *Science*, **227**, 548–549

Hulka, B.S. (1991) Epidemiologic studies using biological markers: issues for epidemiologists. *Cancer Epidemiol. Biomarkers Prev.*, **1**, 13–19

Hulka, B.S. & Margolin, B.H. (1992) Methodological issues in epidemiologic studies using biologic markers. *Am. J. Epidemiol.*, **135**, 200–209

Hunt, C.R., Sim, J.E., Sullivan, S.J., Featherstone, T., Golder, W., Kapp-Herr, C.V., Hock, R.A., Gomez, R.A., Parsian, A.J. & Spitz, D.R. (1998) Genomic instability and catalase gene amplification induced by chronic exposure to oxidative stress. *Cancer Res.*, **58**, 3986–3992

IARC (1999) *IARC Monographs on the Evaluation of Carcinogenic Risks to Humans*, Vol. 71, *Re-evaluation of Some Organic Chemicals, Hydrazine and Hydrogen Peroxide, Part I*, Lyon, IARC*Press*, pp. 109–125

Irons, R.D., Cathro, H.P., Stillman, W.S., Steinhagen, W.H. & Shah, R.S. (1989) Susceptibility to 1,3-butadiene-induced leukemogenesis correlates with endogenous ecotropic retroviral background in the mouse. *Toxicol. Appl. Pharmacol.*, **101**, 170–176

Jensen, R.H. & Bigbee, W. (1996) Direct immunofluorescence labeling provides an improved method for the glycophorin A somatic cell mutation assay. *Cytometry*, **23**, 337–343

Langlois, R.G, Nisbet, B.A., Bigbee, W.L., Ridinger, D.N. & Jensen, R.H. (1990) An improved flow cytometric assay for somatic mutations at the glycophorin A locus in humans. *Cytometry*, **11**, 513–521

Lipkowitz, S., Garry, V.F. & Kirsch, I.R. (1992) Interlocus V-J recombination measures genomic instability in agriculture workers at risk for lymphoid malignancies. *Proc. Natl Acad. Sci. USA*, **89**, 5301–5305

Lippert, M.J., Nicklas, J.A., Hunter, T.C. & Albertini, R.J. (1995) Pulsed field analysis of *hprt* T-cell deletions: telomeric region breakpoint spectrum. *Mutat. Res.*, **326**, 51–64

Lippert, M.J., Rainville, I.R., Nicklas, J.A. & Albertini, R.J. (1997) Large deletions partially external to the human *HPRT* gene result in chimeric transcripts. *Mutagenesis*, **12**, 185–190

Liu, Y., Hernandez, A.M., Shibata, D. & Cortopassi, G.A. (1994) *BCL2* translocation frequency rises with age in humans. *Proc. Natl Acad. Sci. USA*, **91**, 8910–8914

Ma, H., Wood, T.G., Ammenheuser, M.M., Rosenblatt, J.I. & Ward, J.B., Jr. (2000) Molecular analysis of *HPRT* mutant lymphocytes from 1,3-butadiene exposed workers. *Environ. Mol. Mutagen.*, **36**, 59–71.

Macaluso, M., Larson, R., Delzell, E., Sathikumar, N., Hovinga, M., Julian, J., Muir, D. & Cole, P. (1996) Leukemia and cumulative exposure to butadiene, styrene and benzene among workers in the synthetic rubber industry. *Toxicology*, **113**, 190–202

Mao, E.F., Lane, L., Lee, J. & Miller, J.H. (1997) Proliferation of mutators in a cell population. *J. Bacteriol.*, **179**, 417–422

McGinniss, M.J., Nicklas, J.A. & Albertini, R.J. (1989) Molecular analyses of *in vivo HPRT* mutations in human T-lymphocytes. IV. Studies in newborns. *Environ. Mol. Mutagen.*, **14**, 229–237

McGregor, W.G., Chen, R.-H., Lukash, L., Maher, V.M. & McCormick, J.J. (1991) Cell cycle-dependent strand bias for UV-induced mutations in the transcribed strand of excision repair-proficient human fibroblasts but not in repair-deficient cells. *Mol. Cell Biol.*, **11**, 1927–1934

Mellon, I., Bohr, V., Smith, C.A. & Hanawalt, P. (1986) Preferential DNA repair of an active gene in human cells. *Proc. Natl Acad. Sci. USA*, **83**, 8878–8882

Melnick, R.L., Huff, J., Chou, B.J. & Miller, R.A. (1990) Carcinogenicity of 1,3-butadiene in C57BL/6 × C3H F$_1$ mice at low exposure concentrations. *Cancer Res.*, **50**, 6592–6599

Meng, Q., Henderson, R.F., Long, L., Blair, L., Walker, D.M., Upton, P.B., Swenberg, J.A. & Walker, V.E. (2001) Mutagenicity at the *HPRT* locus in T cells of female mice following inhalation exposures to low levels of 1,3-butadiene. *Chem.-Biol. Interact.*, **135–136**, 343–361

Miller, J.H. (1985) Mutagenic specificity of ultraviolet light. *J. Mol. Biol.*, **182**, 45–65

Miller, J.H. (1996) Spontaneous mutators in bacteria: insights into pathways of mutagenesis and repair. *Annu. Rev. Microbiol.*, **50**, 625–643

Morley, A.A., Grist, S.A., Turner, D.R., Kutlaca, A. & Bennett, G. (1990) Molecular nature of *in vivo* mutations in human cells at the autosomal HLA-A locus. *Cancer Res.*, **50**, 4584–4587

Nicklas, J.A., Falta, M.T., Hunter, T.C., O'Neill, J.P., Jacobson-Kram, D., Williams, J.R. & Albertini, R.J. (1990) Molecular analysis of *in vivo HPRT* mutations in human lymphocytes. V. Effects of total body irradiation secondary to radioimmunoglobulin therapy (RIT). *Mutagenesis*, **5**, 461–468

Nicklas, J.A., O'Neill, J.P., Hunter, T.C., Falta, M.T., Lippert, M.J., Jacobson-Kram, D., Williams, J.R. & Albertini, R.J. (1991) In-vivo ionizing irradiations produce deletions in the *HPRT* gene of human T lymphocytes. *Mutat. Res.*, **250**, 383–396

Nuwaysir, E.F., Bittner, M., Trent, J., Barrett, J.C. & Afshari, C.A. (1999) Microarrays and toxicology: the advent of toxicogenomics. *Mol. Carcinog.*, **24**, 153–159

Osterman-Golkar, S., Kautiainen, A., Bergmark, E., Hakansson, K. & Maaki-Paakkanen, J. (1991) Hemoglobin adducts and urinary mercapturic acids in rats as biological indicators of butadiene exposure. *Chem.-Biol. Interact.*, **80**, 291–302

Osterman-Golkar, S.M., Bond, J.A., Ward, J.B. & Legator, M.S. (1993) Use of haemoglobin adducts for biomonitoring exposure to 1,3-butadiene. In: Sorsa, M., Peltonen, K., Vainio, H. & Hemminki, K., eds, *Butadiene and Styrene – Assessment of Health Hazards* (IARC Sci. Publ. No. 127), Lyon, IARC*Press*, pp. 127–134

Owen, P.E., Glaister, J.R., Gaunt, I.F. & Pullinger, D.H. (1987) Inhalation toxicity studies with 1,3-butadiene. 3. Two-year toxicity/carcinogenicity study in rats. *Am. Ind. Hyg. Assoc. J.*, **48**, 407–413

Owen, P.E. & Glaister, J.R. (1990) Inhalation toxicity and carcinogenicity of 1,3-butadiene in Sprague-Dawley rats. *Environ. Health Perspect.*, **86**, 19–25.

Perera, F.P. (1996) Molecular epidemiology: insights into cancer susceptibility, risk assessment and prevention. *J. Natl Cancer Inst.*, **88**, 496–509

Perez, H.L., Lahdetie, J., Hindso-Landin, H., Kilpelainen, I., Koivisto, P., Peltonen, K. & Osterman-Golkar, S. (1997) Haemoglobin adducts of epoxybutanediol from exposure to 1,3-butadiene or butadiene epoxides. *Chem.-Biol. Interact.*, **105**, 181–198

Pluth, J.M., Nicklas, J.A., O'Neill, J.P. & Albertini, R.J. (1996) Increased frequency of specific genomic deletions resulting from in-vitro malathion exposure. *Cancer Res.*, **56**, 2393–2399

Rainville, I.R., Albertini, R.J., O'Neill, J.P. & Nicklas, J.A. (1995) Breakpoints and junctional regions of intragenic deletions in the *HPRT* gene in human T-cells. *Somat. Cell Mol. Genet.*, **21**, 309–326

Ripley, L.S. (1991) Mechanisms of gene mutations. In: Li, A.P. & Heflich, R.H., eds, *Genetic Toxicology*, Boca Raton, CRC Press, pp. ???

Robinson, D.R., Goodall, K., Albertini, R.J., O'Neill, J.P., Finette B., Sala-Trepat, M., Moustacchi, E., Tates, A.D., Beare, D.M., Green, M.H.L. & Cole, J. (1994) An analysis of in-vivo *hprt* mutant frequency in circulating T lymphocytes in the normal human population: a comparison of four datasets. *Mutat. Res.* **313**, 227–247

Schaeffer, L., Roy, R., Humbert, S., Moncollin, V., Vermeulen, W., Hoeijmakers, J.H., Chambon, P. & Egly, J.M. (1993) DNA repair helicase: A component of BTF2 (TFIIH) basic transcription factor. *Science*, **260**, 58–63

Schulte, P.A. (1993) Use of biological markers in occupational health research and practice. *J. Toxicol. Environ. Health*, **40**, 359–366

Schulte, P.A. & Perera, F.P. (1997) Transitional studies. In: Toniolo, P., Boffetta, P., Shuker, D.E.G., Rothman, N., Hulka, B. & Pearce, N., eds, *Application of Biomarkers in Cancer Epidemiology* (IARC Sci. Publ. No. 142), Lyon, IARC*Press*, pp. 19–29

Sorsa, M., Autio, K., Demopoulos, N.A., Jarventaus, H., Rössner, P., Šrám, R.J., Stephanou, G. & Vlachodimitropoulos, D. (1994) Human cytogenetic biomonitoring of occupational exposure to 1,3-butadiene. *Mutat. Res.*, **309**, 321–326

Sorsa, M., Osterman-Golkar, S., Peltonen, K., Saarikoski, S.T. & Šrám, R. (1996) Assessment of exposure to butadiene in the process industry. *Toxicology*, **113**, 77–83

Šrám, R.J., Rössner, P., Peltonen, K., Podrazilova, K., Mrackova, G., Demopoulos, N.A., Stephanou, G., Vlachodimitropoulos, D., Darroudi, F. & Tates, A.D. (1998) Chromosomal aberrations, sister-chromatid exchanges, cells with high frequency of SCE, micronuclei and comet assay parameters in 1,3-butadiene-exposed workers. *Mutat. Res.*, **419**, 145–154

Sriram, S. (1994) Longitudinal study of frequency of *HPRT* mutant T cells in patients with multiple sclerosis. *Neurology*, **44**, 311–315

Steen, A.M., Meyer, K.G. & Recio, O. (1997a) Analysis of *HPRT* mutations occurring in human TK6 lymphoblastoid cells following exposure to 1,2,3,4-diepoxybutane. *Mutagenesis*, **12**, 61–67

Steen, A.M., Meyer, K.G. & Recio, L. (1997b) Characterization of *HPRT* mutations following 1,2-epoxy-3-butene exposure of human TK6 cells. *Mutagenesis*, **12**, 359–364

Steiner, S. & Anderson, N.L. (2000) Expression profiling in toxicology–potentials and limitations. *Toxicol. Lett.*, **112-113**, 467–471

Swenberg, J.A., Koc, H., Upton, P.B., Georguieva, N., Ranasinghe, A., Walker, V.E. & Henderson, R. (2001) Using DNA and hemoglobin adducts to improve the risk assessment of butadiene. *Chem.-Biol. Interact.*, **135–136**, 387–403

Tates, A.D., Grummt, T., Tornqvist, M., Farmer, P.B., van Dam, F.J., van Mossel, H., Schoemaker, H.M., Osterman-Golkar, S., Uebel, C., Tang, Y.S., Zwinderman, A.H., Natarajan, A.T. & Ehrenberg, L. (1991) Biological and chemical monitoring of occupational exposure to ethylene oxide. *Mutat. Res.*, **250**, 483–497

Tates, A.D., van Dam, F.J., de Zwart, F.A., Darroudi, F., Natarajan, A.T., Rössner, P., Peterková, K., Peltonen, K., Demopoulos, N.A., Stephanou, G., Vlachodimitripoulos, D. & Šrám, R.J. (1996) Biological effect monitoring in industrial workers from the Czech Republic exposed to low levels of butadiene. *Toxicology*, **113**, 91–99

Toniolo, P., Boffetta, P., Shuker, D.E.G, Rothman, N., Hulka, B. & Pearce, N., eds (1997) *Application of Biomarkers in Cancer Epidemiology* (IARC Sci. Publ. No. 142), Lyon, IARC*Press*

Trotter, J.L., Damico, C.A., Cross, A.H., Pelfrey, C.M., Karr, R.W., Fu, X.T. & McFarland, H.F. (1997) *HPRT* mutant T-cell lines from multiple sclerosis patients recognize myelin proteolipid protein peptides. *J. Neuroimmunol.*, **75**, 95–103

Turner, D.R., Grist, S.A., Janatipour, M. & Morley, A.A. (1988) Mutations in human lymphocytes commonly involve gene duplication and resemble those seen in cancer cells. *Proc. Natl Acad. Sci. USA*, **85**, 3189–3192

Tycko, B. & Sklar, J. (1990) Chromosomal translocations in lymphoid neoplasia: a reappraisal of the recombinase model. *Cancer Cells*, **2**, 1–8

Van den Berg, L.H., Mollee, I., Wokke, J.H.J. & Logtenberg, T. (1995) Increased frequencies of *HPRT* mutant T lymphocytes in patients with Guillain–Barré syndrome and chronic inflammatory demyelinating polyneuropathy: further evidence for a role of T cells in the etiopathogenesis of peripheral demyelinating diseases. *J. Neuroimmunol.*, **58**, 37–42

Van Dongen, J.J.M., Comans-Bitter, W.M., Wolvers-Tettero, I.L.M. & Borst, J. (1990) Development of human T lymphocytes and their thymus-dependency. *Thymus*, **16**, 207–234

Van Houten, B. & Albertini, R.J. (1994) DNA damage and repair. In: Craighead, J.E., ed., *Pathology of Environmental and Occupational Disease*, St. Louis, Mosby-Year Book, Inc., pp. 311–327

Van Sittert, N.J. & Van Vliet, E.W.N. (1994) Monitoring occupational exposure to some industrial chemicals by determining hemoglobin adducts. *Clin. Chem.*, **40**, 1472–1475

Walker, V.E. & Meng, Q. (2000) 1,3-Butadiene: cancer, mutations and adducts. Part III: In-vivo mutation of the endogenous *HPRT* genes of mice and rats by 1,3-butadiene and its metabolites. *Res. Rep. Health Eff. Inst.*, **92**, 89–139

Ward, J.B., Jr, Ammenheuser, M.M., Bechtold, W.E., Whorton, E.B., Jr & Legator, M.S. (1994) *HPRT* mutant lymphocyte frequencies in workers at a 1,3-butadiene production plant. *Environ. Health Perspect.*, **102**, 79–85

Ward, J.B., Jr, Ammenheuser, M.M., Whorton, E.B.Jr, Bechtold, W.E., Kelsey, K.T. & Legator, M.S. (1996) Biological monitoring for mutagenic effects of occupational exposure to butadiene. *Toxicology*, **113**, 84–90

Ward, J.B. Jr, Abdel-Rahman, S.Z., Henderson, R.F., Stack, T.H., Morandi, M., Rosenblatt, J.I. & Ammenheuser, M.M. (2001) Assessment of butadiene exposure in synthetic rubber manufacturing workers in Teas using frequencies of *HPRT* mutant lymphocytes as a biomarker. *Chem. Biol. Interact.*, **135–136**, 465–483

Xanthoudakis, S., Miao, G., Wang, F., Pan Y.C. & Curran, T. (1992) Redox activation of Fos-Jun DNA binding activity is mediated by a DNA repair enzyme. *EMBO J.*, **11**, 3323–3335

Corresponding author:

Richard J. Albertini
Genetic Toxicology Laboratory,
University of Vermont,
32 North Prospect Street,
Burlington, VT 05401, USA
ralberti@zoo.uvm.edu

Mechanisms of Carcinogenesis: Contributions of Molecular Epidemiology
Patricia Buffler, Jerry Rice, Robert Baan, Michael Bird and Paolo Boffetta, eds
IARC Scientific Publications No. 157
International Agency for Research on Cancer, Lyon, 2004

Cytogenetic Biomarkers

Hannu Norppa

Summary

Cytogenetic biomarkers in peripheral blood lymphocytes such as chromosomal aberrations, sister chromatid exchanges and micronuclei have long been applied in surveillance of human genotoxic exposure and early effects of genotoxic carcinogens. The use of these biomarker assays is based on the fact that most established human carcinogens are genotoxic in short-term tests and capable of inducing chromosomal damage. The relevance of chromosomal aberrations as a biomarker has been further emphasized by epidemiological studies suggesting that a high frequency of chromosomal aberrations is predictive of an increased risk of cancer. Structural and numerical chromosomal aberrations are typical of cancer cells, probably as a manifestation of genetic instability of such cells, but may also represent mechanisms leading to such instability. The frequency of all three biomarkers increases with age, and this effect is particularly clear for micronuclei in women. Tobacco smoking is known to increase the level of sister chromatid exchanges and chromosomal aberrations, but its effect on micronuclei is unclear. Several studies have recently examined the influence of genetic polymorphisms of xenobiotic metabolizing enzymes on cytogenetic biomarkers. The lack of glutathione S-transferase M1 (*GSTM1* null genotype) appears to be associated with increased sensitivity to genotoxicity of tobacco smoking. *N*-Acetyltransferase (*NAT2*) slow acetylation genotypes seem to elevate baseline level of chromosomal aberrations, whereas deletion of glutathione S-transferase T1 gene (*GSTT1* null genotype) has been found to yield an increase in baseline sister chromatid exchange frequency. These findings may be explained by reduced detoxification capacity rendered by the altered gene and may be linked with exposure to, for example, heterocyclic amines in the case of *NAT2* and endogenously formed ethylene oxide in
the case of *GSTT1*. Recently discovered polymorphisms affecting DNA repair may be expected to be of special importance in modulating genotoxic effects, but, as yet, there is very little information about the significance of these polymorphisms or about their impact on cytogenetic biomarkers.

Introduction

Cytogenetic alterations in peripheral blood lymphocytes, such as chromosomal aberrations, sister chromatid exchanges and micronuclei have been used as biomarkers of human genotoxic exposure and early effects of genotoxic carcinogens for many years (Albertini *et al.*, 2000). The main rationale of using these assays is the fact that most established human carcinogens are genotoxic in short-term tests and capable of inducing chromosome damage (Waters *et al.*, 1999). Accordingly, an increased frequency of cytogenetic alterations in a well-designed and controlled study of occupationally exposed workers, for example, is usually considered a strong indication of exposure to genotoxic carcinogens that may suggest the need for hygienic improvements and the institution of other protective measures. Such considerations are further supported by epidemiological studies suggesting that a high frequency of chromosomal aberrations is predictive of an increased risk of cancer (see Hagmar *et al.*, this volume).

The present chapter provides a review of the rationales of using cytogenetic biomarkers in studies of human genotoxic exposure and effects, and discusses the various factors that may influence the level of cytogenetic damage, especially genetic polymorphisms.

Cytogenetic biomarkers

Various aspects relevant for the use of the three cytogenetic biomarkers in monitoring of genotoxic effects of carcinogens have been described in detail by Albertini *et al.* (2000). In humans, chromosomal aberrations are usually scored from metaphases of phytohaemagglutinin (PHA)-stimulated lymphocytes after cell culture. The chromosomal aberration assay is primarily used for the analysis of structural aberrations which are classified into two main categories, chromosome-type and chromatid-type aberrations. In both categories, breaks and various types of rearrangements are distinguished.

- **Chromosome-type aberrations** (induced in G_0 lymphocytes by ionizing radiation and radiomimetic chemicals) involve the same locus on both sister chromatids on one or multiple chromosomes; they are generated in G_0 lymphocytes *in vivo* and attain their typical appearance after DNA replication *in vitro*.
- **Chromatid-type aberrations** (induced by most chemical clastogens) affect one or several sister chromatids of a chromosome or several chromosomes; in cultured lymphocytes, they are formed *in vitro* when damaged DNA template is replicated.

Chromosome-type interchanges such as translocations can be identified by chromosome banding, which is very tedious and seldom used (see Tawn & Whitehouse, 2001) or by fluorescence in-situ hybridization (FISH, chromosome painting) techniques (see Ramsey *et al.*, 1995). Chromosome-type breaks in chromosomes 1 and 9 can be detected by tandem DNA probe labelling methods (Rupa *et al.*, 1995; Marcon *et al.*, 1999).

Numerical chromosomal aberrations, representing deviation by one or a few chromosomes (aneuploidy) or by multiplication (polyploidy) from the normal human diploid chromosome number ($2N = 46$), can be scored from metaphases, or from interphases by FISH using chromosome-specific centromeric DNA probes (Eastmond *et al.*, 1995; Zijno *et al.*, 1996; Surrallés *et al.*, 1997; Marcon *et al.*, 1999; Zhang *et al.*, 1999).

Sister chromatid exchanges are scored in humans from second-division metaphases of PHA-stimulated lymphocytes after cell culture in the presence of bromodeoxyuridine which facilitates differential staining of sister chromatids. Sister chromatid exchanges are formed during DNA replication *in vitro* by interchange of DNA replication products between sister chromatids at

apparently homologous loci. It has been suggested that the exchange process represents repair of DNA double-strand breaks by homologous recombination (Sonoda *et al.*, 1999; Johnson & Jasin, 2000).

Micronuclei are small additional nuclei that are formed from chromosomal fragments or whole chromosomes that have lagged behind in the anaphase/telophase stage of the cell cycle and have been excluded from either of the daughter nuclei. Micronuclei contain either chromosome or chromatid fragments or whole chromosomes consisting of one or both sister chromatids. In humans, micronuclei are usually detected in cultured peripheral lymphocytes by the cytokinesis-block method, which allows identification of cells after their first in-vitro mitosis (Fenech & Morley, 1985). Micronuclei formed *in vivo* can be analysed from exfoliated epithelial cells, such as those from the buccal mucosa. The presence of fragments or whole chromosomes in micronuclei can be identified by pancentromeric FISH (Norppa *et al.*, 1993).

Cytogenetic biomarkers in lymphocytes are surrogate end-points in surrogate cells

Two basic assumptions are made when cytogenetic alterations in peripheral lymphocytes are used as biomarkers of carcinogen exposure and effects.

- First, peripheral lymphocytes (differentiated cells that are not themselves targets for carcinogenesis) are examined as a surrogate for tissues where cancer can develop, assuming that similar genotoxic damage occurs in cancer-prone tissue. The justification for this assumption depends on the similarities of the surrogate and target tissue, as regards carcinogen distribution, uptake, metabolism and cellular response. Lymphocytes circulate throughout the body and can, therefore, be considered to represent systemic exposure in general. Their relevance as a model for actual target tissue largely depends on the agent to which they are exposed. Lymphocytes may not properly reflect exposure to substances that exert their effects at the site of entry into the body, such as some reactive compounds that may preferentially act on the upper airways (e.g. formaldehyde). In general, blood lymphocytes probably resemble more closely lymphatic tissue than, say, liver cells, which have a much higher metabolic capacity. There may also be differences between lymphocytes and target cells of carcinogenesis (most cancers are epithelial in origin) in cellular responses to genotoxic damage, such as DNA repair, cell proliferation, apoptosis and necrosis.

- Second, cytogenetic biomarkers depict unspecific cytogenetic damage in the whole genome, presuming that it reflects the more specific alterations expected to lead to cancer development. Thus, the rather common sporadic chromosomal aberrations observed in the assay are surrogates for the more specific and rare alterations relevant for carcinogenesis that may occur sequentially during carcinogenesis. Yet, the mechanism of formation for the unspecific and specific chromosomal alterations may be the same.

Cytogenetic biomarkers reveal effects of genotoxic carcinogens

Although it has long been known that some carcinogens are not genotoxic and that some in-vitro genotoxins are not carcinogens (Zeiger, 2001), the majority of chemicals classified by the International Agency for Research on Cancer (IARC) as human carcinogens are genotoxic (Waters et al., 1999). This is not surprising, since many genotoxic carcinogens are relatively potent and induce tumours at multiple sites. Most IARC human carcinogens also induce cytogenetic alterations. In 1999, data on at least two independent cytogenetic assays were available for 55 Group 1 (human carcinogen) and 2A (probable human carcinogen) chemicals; of these, 48 were able to induce chromosomal aberrations or micronuclei, three were negative and four inconclusive (Waters et al., 1999). This fact provides a strong justification for the use of cytogenetic end-points as biomarkers of the early effects of genotoxic carcinogens.

The potency of genotoxins to induce chromosomal damage varies, and many in-vitro genotoxins are not effective in vivo (Zeiger, 2001). On the other hand, benzene is an example of a carcinogen that shows mostly negative results in genotoxicity tests in vitro, and it is still argued whether benzene is really a genotoxic carcinogen (Golding & Watson, 1999). The toxicology and metabolism of benzene are highly complex (and probably impossible to reproduce in vitro), and the exact mechanism of benzene-associated leukaemia is unclear. In vivo, benzene is certainly genotoxic, since it is clearly clastogenic (i.e. it induces chromosomal aberrations) in experimental animals and exposed humans. In such a situation, negative data in vitro are of limited value (Eastmond, 2000).

The spectrum of genotoxic damage induced depends on the agent of exposure: some are primarily clastogenic (e.g. benzene, ethylene oxide, DNA cross-linking agents) whereas others preferentially induce gene mutations (e.g. N-ethyl-N-nitrosourea). The carcinogenic potency of clastogens may reflect the initial DNA alterations they produce. For instance, DNA cross-linking agents (e.g. melphalan) appear to be strong clastogens and carcinogens, whereas chemicals primarily inducing N-alkylations in DNA (e.g. methyl methanesulfonate) are moderate clastogens and weak carcinogens (Nivard & Vogel, 2001).

Chromosomal aberrations predict cancer risk

During the last few years, evidence has accumulated from Nordic, Italian, Taiwanese and Czech studies suggesting that a high frequency of chromosomal aberrations in peripheral lymphocytes is predictive of increased risk of cancer (Hagmar et al., 1994; Bonassi et al., 1995a; Hagmar et al., 1998; Liou et al., 1999; Bonassi et al., 2000; Hagmar et al., 2000; Smerhovsky et al., 2001; 2002; Hagmar et al., this volume). The Nordic and Italian studies indicated that the predictivity of chromosomal aberrations for cancer risk is not restricted to tobacco smokers or subjects with occupational exposure to carcinogens, but also concerns nonsmokers and subjects with no known occupational carcinogen exposure (Bonassi et al., 2000; Hagmar et al., 2000; Hagmar et al., this volume). In a small Taiwanese study on subjects apparently exposed to arsenic, cancer risk was associated with chromosome-type aberrations but not chromatid-type aberrations (Liou et al., 1999).

However, a Czech study (Smerhovsky *et al.*, 2001, 2002) suggested differential predictivity of cancer risk in a subgroup of radon-exposed miners. The cancer predictivity concerned the frequency of chromatid-type breaks (and total frequency of aberrant cells) which also correlated with exposure to radon. However, as chromatid-type aberrations are not expected to result from exposure of G_0 lymphocytes to radon, the result appears difficult to explain.

The Nordic–Italian findings of chromosomal aberrations predicting cancer risk also in the 'unexposed' population (Bonassi *et al.*, 2000) suggest a general significance for chromosomal aberrations as a biomarker for cancer risk: whatever the initial reason, high chromosomal aberration frequency seems to indicate increased cancer risk. As predictivity of cancer risk did not depend on the time that had elapsed between the chromosome analysis and cancer diagnosis, indirect effects of undetected cancer did not seem to explain the findings. Several factors could explain the chromosomal aberration–cancer risk association in the 'unexposed', such as unidentified common exposure to genotoxic carcinogens (e.g. in diet), deficiency of micronutrients (e.g. folate) and individual susceptibility factors. The latter aspect is dealt with more detail later in this chapter.

Data on chromosomal aberration frequency are usually not accurate enough to provide a risk estimate for an individual. In general, cytogenetic data are exclusively interpreted at the group level, by comparison with a reference group; individual results are considered only in exceptional cases, for example in biological radiation dosimetry and when particularly high frequencies are encountered. Nevertheless, the observed association between level of chromosomal aberration and cancer risk adds more weight for positive findings in cytogenetic biomarker studies, even though the nature of this association is not yet fully understood.

On the other hand, it has not been possible to show an association between cancer risk and sister chromatid exchanges and micronuclei (Hagmar *et al.* 1994, 1998, 2000, this volume). This does not necessarily mean that the association does not exist. Purely methodologically, the chromosomal aberration assay is more robust than the sister chromatid exchange and micronuclei assays, at least with regard to historical data used in existing epidemiological studies.

Unlike data on chromosomal aberrations, results for sister chromatid exchanges are very difficult to classify in tertiles (high, medium and low categories) or quartiles, as is done in studies of cancer predictivity. The difference between control level and a positive exposure effect, say in smokers, is usually only about 10% in the sister chromatid exchange assay, whereas it may be twofold or higher in the chromosomal aberration assay. Furthermore, there seems to be more variation among culture batches and scorers in the sister chromatid exchange assay than in the chromosomal aberration assay. As a consequence, standardization of data on sister chromatid exchanges between laboratories and among different studies within a laboratory is difficult. Nevertheless, in single studies where variation in level of sister chromatid exchanges can be controlled, sister chromatid exchanges may be a good biomarker for genotoxic exposures (such as ethylene oxide) that are efficient inducers of sister chromatid exchanges (Laurent *et al.*, 1984; Yong *et al.*, 2001).

The problem with data on micronuclei in existing studies of cancer predictivity has primarily been the variable methods used for evaluation of micronuclei, which – together with the small sample size and young cohort age – has precluded firm conclusions. A new evaluation, based on a single technique (the cytokinesis-block method) that is supposed to avoid the problem of scoring cells that have not divided in culture, is under way (Bonassi *et al.*, 2001) as part of an effort funded by the European Commission.

Chromosomal alterations are typical of cancer cells

The relevance of cytogenetic alterations to cancer is supported by the fact that cancer cells typically have structural and numerical chromosomal aberrations and micronuclei. These alterations may reflect the genomic instability and clonal evolution of cancer cells rather than immediate effects of genotoxic exposure (Duesberg *et al.*, 1998; Rasnick & Duesberg, 1999; Jackson & Loeb, 2001), although it can be envisaged that induced genotoxic insult may influence carcinogenesis at various stages.

It is actually unclear what phenomenon is the cause and what is the consequence. Structural chromosomal aberrations and chromosome loss may have a role in inducing genetic instability or a mutator phenotype if they affect key genes regulating genomic integrity or cellular control, or, if the resulting massive changes in the balance of cellular proteins lead to general failure of homeostasis, facilitating generation of further sequential genetic alterations, thus paving the way to a neoplastic phenotype (Duesberg *et al.*, 1998; Rasnick & Duesberg, 1999; Jackson & Loeb, 2001; Loeb, 2001). Genome reorganization may also result from telomere dysfunction (Gisselsson *et al.*, 2001), breakage–fusion–bridge cycle and disorganized division of polyploid and binucleated cells. The breakage–fusion–bridge cycle may create gene amplification. Structural chromosomal aberrations and chromosome loss occur much more often than specific gene mutations and are potential sources of loss of heterozygosity (LOH); micronucleation and non-disjunction are probable mechanisms for the elimination (or gain) of chromosomes and their fragments.

Many types of cancer carry specific balanced chromosomal alterations that are used in the diagnosis of the disease and are considered to have a role in its etiology. These balanced rearrangements appear to act via deregulation of a gene by relocation to an immunoglobulin or T-cell receptor gene, or the creation of a hybrid gene by the fusion of parts of two genes (Mitelman, 2000).

There is little evidence suggesting involvement of sister chromatid exchanges in carcinogenesis, besides the fact that sister chromatid exchanges depict exposure to genotoxic carcinogens. As sister chromatid exchanges have been proposed to represent a manifestation of double-strand DNA break repair by homologous recombination (Sonoda *et al.*, 1999; Johnson & Jasin, 2000), they would depict repaired damage rather than events that could themselves be in the pathway to cancer. Sister chromatid exchanges may, therefore, be expected to reflect genotoxic exposure, but, at an equivalent exposure level, a high frequency of sister chromatid exchanges might indicate better management of DNA lesions than a low frequency.

Predisposition to cancer is often observed in various human syndromes showing spontaneous or inducible chromosomal instability (Taylor, 2001). Six of these disorders appear to be due to mutations in different helicase genes: *XPB* and *XPD* mutations can result in xeroderma pigmentosum, Cockayne syndrome or trichothiodystrophy, and mutations in the RecQ-like genes *BLM*, *WRN* and *RECQL4* give rise to Bloom syndrome, Werner syndrome and Rothmund–Thomson syndrome, respectively (van Brabant *et al.*, 2000). Ataxia telangiectasia is due to mutations in *ATM* which encodes a protein kinase, a central regulator of responses to DNA double-strand breaks (Khanna *et al.*, 2001). Mutations in at least eight genes (*FANCA, B, C, D1, D2, E, F* and *G*) have been described in Fanconi anaemia; the exact role of these genes has not yet been defined, but also they appear to function primarily in response to DNA damage (Grompe & D'Andrea, 2001). Similarly, Nijmegen breakage syndrome protein (NBS) is part of a DNA repair complex and has been suggested to be an accessory protein for telomere extension (Ranganathan *et al.*, 2001). An ataxia telangiectasia-like disorder involves mutation in double-strand break repair gene *hMRE11* (Stewart *et al.*, 1999).

Factors affecting the level of cytogenetic biomarkers

Exposure to genotoxic agents is expected to increase the frequency of chromosomal aberrations, sister chromatid exchanges and micronuclei, but the efficiency of different agents in affecting the three biomarkers differs. Ionizing radiation induces chromosomal aberrations and micronuclei but not sister chromatid exchanges in G_0 lymphocytes (Wolff, 1991; Müller *et al.*, 1996; Gutierrez *et al.*, 1999; Jones *et al.*, 2001).

Age is known to affect the frequency of structural and numerical chromosomal aberrations, sister chromatid exchanges and micronuclei (Bonassi *et al.*, 1995b; Ramsey *et al.*, 1995;

Thierens *et al.*, 1996; Bolognesi *et al.*, 1997; Pressl *et al.*, 1999; Tawn & Whitehouse, 2001). Its effect is particularly clear on micronuclei, apparently mostly because of the age-dependent micronucleation of sex chromosomes (see Catalán *et al.*, 1998). Women have a higher frequency of micronuclei than men; this difference appears to be primarily due to the X chromosome. Some studies have also indicated a marginally higher sister chromatid exchange frequency in women than in men.

Smoking is known to increase both chromosomal aberrations and sister chromatid exchanges, but does not appear to have a clear effect on frequency of micronuclei (Lambert *et al.*, 1978; Obe *et al.*, 1982; Milillo *et al.*, 1996; Thierens *et al.*, 1996; Barale *et al.*, 1998; Tawn & Whitehouse, 2001). This is puzzling, considering that chromosomal fragments form a large proportion of micronuclei.

Much of the individual variation in cytogenetic biomarkers is due to unknown factors. However, micronutrients can be expected to have a marked effect. High plasma homocysteine, vitamin B_{12} deficiency and low folic acid intake have recently been associated with increased frequencies of micronuclei (Odagiri & Uchida, 1998; see Fenech, 2001); these findings may reflect increased misincorporation of uracil into DNA.

Genetic polymorphisms and cytogenetic parameters

During the last few years, increasing attention has been focused on genetic polymorphisms that could modulate human response to genotoxic insult (see Norppa, 1997; Au *et al.*, 1999; Autrup, 2000; Norppa, 2000; Norppa & Hirvonen, 2000; Pavanello & Clonfero, 2000; Au *et al.*, 2001; Norppa, 2001). In principle, any polymorphisms that affect xenobiotic metabolism or cellular response to DNA damage could alter individual sensitivity to genotoxins. Many studies have addressed the question of whether a particular genotype of a xenobiotic-metabolizing enzyme is over-represented among cancer patients (see Hirvonen, 1999a; Strange & Fryer, 1999; Wormhoudt *et al.*, 1999; Au *et al.*, 2001). Such investigations require a large number of cases and

controls, and relationship to past exposure is often difficult to establish because of insufficient information and the long time elapsed between the exposure and the disease. It is easier to study the role of genetic polymorphisms using biomarkers such as cytogenetic alterations, because biomarker levels, instead of numbers of individuals, in different genotype groups are compared, and information on exposure is usually available.

Several studies have implied that genetic polymorphisms can influence the level of chromosomal damage associated with some genotoxic exposures, but may also affect the apparent background level of cytogenetic alterations (see references in the following sections and in Tables 1–5). Thus, genetic polymorphisms might partly explain the association between levels of chromosomal aberrations and cancer risk.

The genetic polymorphisms potentially important for a biomarker largely depend on the agent of exposure, the biological material examined and ethnicity of the population under study. Individual exposure level may vary considerably, and a reliable estimate of the exposure is essential for correct interpretation of genotype–exposure interaction. Cytogenetic biomarkers may reflect genotoxic exposures that occurred months or even years before cell sampling, and spot measurements of urinary metabolites or ambient concentrations may not be representative of the relevant exposure period. In some cases, the exposed subjects can be divided into groups with distinct exposure levels, but usually comparison with an unexposed control group is needed. Differences in genotype in the exposed group that are not seen in the control group may suggest exposure–genotype interactions; those that are seen in both the exposed and the controls (or only in the controls) may represent genotype effects on the baseline level of the cytogenetic biomarker.

Another important factor determining whether the effect of a genetic polymorphism is seen in a cytogenetic biomarker is the expression of differences in genotype in the cells examined. For example, glutathione *S*-transferase M1 (GSTM1) and T1 (GSTT1) are expressed in leukocytes and erythrocytes, respectively, in proficient individuals (*GSTM1*- and *GSTT1*-positive subjects)

(Wiencke *et al.*, 1990; Brockmöller *et al.*, 1992; Pemble *et al.*, 1994; Norppa *et al.*, 1995). Theoretically, the cytogenetic effects of the genotoxic substrates of GSTM1 or GSTT1 could be expected to be elevated in blood cells in *GSTM1*- and *GSTT1*-null subjects who totally lack the respective enzyme activities.

Effect of genetic polymorphisms on cytogenetic alterations in tobacco smokers

Tobacco smoke contains a multitude of genotoxic carcinogens that undergo metabolic activation or detoxification in the body. Polymorphisms of enzymes involved in these reactions could be expected to influence the genotoxic effects and carcinogenicity of tobacco smoking. GSTM1 takes part in the metabolic detoxification of various reactive chemicals, along with other members of the glutathione *S*-transferase (GST) superfamily (see Strange *et al.*, 2000). GSTM1 activity is present in individuals who have at least one copy of either the *GSTM1*A* or *GSTM1*B* allele, but is lacking in *GSTM1*-null individuals who are homozygous for *GSTM1* gene deletion (Brockmöller *et al.*, 1992; Strange *et al.*, 2000). The *GSTM1* null genotype is found in roughly 50% of the white population (see Hirvonen, 1999a).

The role of the *GSTM1*-null genotype as a risk factor in various types of human cancer has been studied extensively. Although the results have been somewhat conflicting, the homozygous *GSTM1* deletion has been observed to cause a slight increase in the risk of lung and bladder cancer in tobacco smokers (see Brockmöller *et al.*, 1994; McWilliams *et al.*, 1995; Hirvonen, 1999a; Strange & Fryer, 1999), and has also been suggested to play a role in lung cancer among nonsmokers exposed to environmental tobacco smoke (Bennett *et al.*, 1999).

Studies on cytogenetic biomarkers have supported the idea that *GSTM1*-null individuals have a reduced capacity to detoxify genotoxins in tobacco smoke. Table 1 shows that *GSTM1*-null (or GSTM1-deficient) subjects had an increased frequency of chromosomal aberrations (Scarpato *et al.*, 1997; Norppa *et al.*, 2001) and sister chromatid exchanges (van Poppel *et al.*, 1992) in their peripheral lymphocytes. Studies on DNA

adducts have suggested that these findings may reflect differences in genotype in DNA binding of reactive metabolites of polycyclic aromatic hydrocarbons (PAHs) present in tobacco smoke. In comparison with *GSTM1*-positive (or GSTM1-proficient) smokers, *GSTM1*-null (or GSTM1-deficient) smokers showed an elevated level of aromatic DNA adducts in their leukocytes and lung tissue (Shields *et al.*, 1993; Ryberg *et al.*, 1994, 1997; Butkiewicz *et al.*, 1998; Rojas *et al.*, 1998; Soni *et al.*, 1998; Butkiewicz *et al.*, 1999; Viezzer *et al.*, 1999; Butkiewicz *et al.*, 2000; Rojas *et al.*, 2000; Godschalk *et al.*, 2001; Hou *et al.*, 2001). Lymphocytes from *GSTM1*-null donors were also more sensitive to induction of chromosomal aberration (tandem probe assay) and sister chromatid exchange by 4-(methylnitrosamino)-1-(3-pyridyl)-1-butanone (NNK), a tobacco-specific nitrosamine (Salama *et al.*, 1999).

The fact that several studies have not observed a connection between *GSTM1* genotype and sister chromatid exchanges in smokers may reflect the fact that the effect of smoking itself on the mean number of sister chromatid exchanges per cell, although reproducible and proven, is usually small (only about a 10% increase). In such a situation, the demonstration of an interaction between smoking and *GSTM1* phenotype or genotype would require that either the smoking effect is seen exclusively in the deficient subjects, or there are enough subjects in the study to allow a small difference to be detected. Van Poppel *et al.* (1992), who originally described the association between *GSTM1* phenotype and sister chromatid exchange frequency in smokers, saw a 5.4% increase in mean sister chromatid exchanges/cell among 78 heavy smokers, when studying a total of 154 smokers. An almost identical increase in sister chromatid exchange was also observed by Scarpato *et al.* (1996), Cheng *et al.* (1999) and Wu *et al.* (2000), but they studied fewer individuals (with no separate analysis of heavy smokers), and statistical significance was not reached. Results of one study have suggested that *GSTM1* polymorphism could also influence sister chromatid exchange levels in nonsmokers (Cheng *et al.*, 1995a,b; Duell *et al.*, 2000).

Table 1. Genetic polymorphisms and chromosomal aberrations, sister chromatid exchanges and micronuclei in human peripheral lymphocytes in response to tobacco smoking

Study groups	No. of subjects (% smokers)	Genotypes studied	Risk genotype or phenotype associated with smoking	Reference
Chromosomal aberrations				
Floriculturists	23 (26)	GSTM1	— [a]	Scarpato et al. (1996)
Controls	22 (41)	GSTT1		
		NAT2		
Floriculturists	30 (27)	GSTM1	GSTM1-null [b]	Scarpato et al. (1997)
Controls	32 (31)	GSTT1		
Nuclear power plant workers and controls	56 (43)	GSTM1 GSTT1 NAT2	GSTM1-null	Norppa et al. (2001)
Lung cancer patients	22 (100)	GSTM1	GSTT1-null or GSTM1-	Conforti-Froes et al.
Controls	22 (100)	GSTT1	null or both (in patients)	(1997); El-Zein et al. (1997)
Lung cancer patients [a]	17 (100)	GSTM1	GSTT1-null or GSTM1-	Abdel-Rahman et al.
Controls [a]	24 (71)	GSTT1	null or both (in patients)	(1998)
Controls (chromosome painting)	65 (43)	GSTM1 GSTT1 GSTP1 CYP1A1 CYP2D6 NAT1 NAT2	NAT2 rapid [c]	Pluth et al. (2000a)
Sister chromatid exchanges				
Volunteers	220 (70)	GSTM1 phenotype	GSTM1-deficient	van Poppel et al. (1992)
Volunteers	194 (80)	GSTM1 phenotype	GSTM1-deficient	van Poppel et al. (1993)
Floriculturists	23 (26)	GSTM1	— [d]	Scarpato et al. (1996)
Controls	22 (41)	GSTT1		
		NAT2		
Cr electroplaters	35 (25)	GSTM1	— [d]	Wu et al. (2000)
Controls	35 (25)	GSTT1		
Resin synthesis workers	85 (49)	GSTM1 GSTT1	— [d]	Cheng et al. (1999)
Lung cancer cases	136 (42)	GSTM1	—	Tang et al. (1998)
Controls	115 (25)			

Table 1 (contd)

Study groups	No. of subjects (% smokers)	Genotypes studied	Risk genotype or phenotype associated with smoking	Reference
Controls	78 (23)	CYP1A1 CYP2D6	–	Cheng et al. (1995b)
Habitual drinkers	58 (64)	ALDH2	ALDH2 1-2 (smoking	Morimoto & Takeshita
Others	52 (42)		habitual drinkers), 1-1 (other smokers)	(1996)
Controls	76 (26)	XRCC1 ERCC2	XRCC1 Gln/Gln (in 3 current smokers)	Duell et al. (2000)
Micronuclei				
Volunteers (buccal cells)	194 (80)	GSTM1 phenotype	–	van Poppel et al. (1993)
Lung cancer cases	55 (31)	GSTM1	–	Cheng et al. (1996)
Controls	41 (33)			
Floriculturists	30 (29)	GSTM1	NAT2 rapid	Falck et al. (1999)
Controls	33 (30)	GSTT1 NAT2		

[a] A non-significant increase in chromosomal aberrations in GSTM1-null smokers.
[b] Additionally, GSTM1-null/GSTT1-null subjects ($n = 5$) showed a higher chromosomal aberration frequency than GSTM1-positive/GSTT1-null subjects ($n = 4$).
[c] Only in 6 smokers > 60 years of age, 4 of them GSTM1-null.
[d] Difference in sister chromatid exchange frequency between GSTM1-null and GSTM1-positive smokers same as for the respective phenotypes in van Poppel et al. (1992), but not significant.

NAT2 is an important polymorphic phase II enzyme that metabolizes xenobiotics with primary aromatic amine and hydrazine structures. Various variant alleles lead to amino acid changes in the NAT2 enzyme, and the different genotypes are usually classified as either rapid or slow in terms of their acetylation capacity (see Hirvonen, 1999b). Rapid acetylators have inherited at least one *NAT2*4* allele; slow acetylators have two slow acetylation-associated alleles. Slow acetylators have been observed to have an increased risk of bladder cancer, whereas rapid acetylators are over-represented among colon cancer patients (see Hirvonen, 1999b). The prevalence of the NAT2 slow acetylator genotype is 50–63% among white people, but Japanese and Chinese are mostly (92% and 80%, respectively) rapid acetylators.

A recent study (Pluth et al., 2000a) using chromosome painting for the analysis of stable chromosomal aberrations (translocations and insertions) suggested that, among heavy smokers 60 years of age or older, NAT2 rapid acetylator genotypes have a higher frequency of chromosomal aberrations than slow acetylator genotypes. This finding was based on only six slow acetylators, of whom four were GSTM1-null. NAT2 rapid acetylator genotypes were also associated with an increased frequency of micronuclei among smokers in a study of pesticide-exposed workers and controls (Falck et al., 1999). On the other hand, results on DNA adducts in smokers have suggested increased levels among subjects with the NAT2 slow acetylation genotypes (Dallinga et al., 1998; Godschalk et al., 2001;

Hou *et al.*, 2001). A recent study on DNA adducts and *HPRT* (hypoxanthine-guanine phosphoribosyl transferase) mutations suggested that the effect of *NAT2* genotype in lung cancer patients may depend on the amount smoked, so that high mutation frequency is associated with higher pack–years and the *NAT2* slow genotype with lower pack–years (Hou *et al.*, 2001).

Genetic polymorphisms and cytogenetic biomarkers in various environmental exposures

Tables 2–4 summarize studies published on the effects of genetic polymorphisms on cytogenetic biomarkers in individuals with various environmental exposures.

Knudsen *et al.* (1999) observed that *GSTM1*-null bus drivers (all nonsmokers), who are exposed to city air containing vehicle exhaust and other pollutants, have a higher frequency of chromosomal aberrations than *GSTM1*-positive drivers (see Table 2). There is some indication that such findings could reflect differences in genotype in genotoxic response to PAHs. Studies of DNA adducts (Nielsen *et al.*, 1996; Brescia *et al.*, 1999; Pavanello *et al.*, 1999; Šrám *et al.*, 1999) have indicated that the *GSTM1*-null genotype predisposes its carriers to the genotoxic effects of air pollutants containing PAHs. Ichiba *et al.* (1994) observed that the frequency of micronuclei in lymphocytes of chimney sweeps correlated with the level of DNA adducts only in *GSTM1*-null subjects.

A single study indicated that microsomal epoxide hydrolase (*EPHX*) exon 3 genotype could affect micronuclei frequency in aluminium extraction workers exposed to PAHs (Carstensen *et al.*, 1999). Among the exposed subjects, a correlation between airborne PAH concentration and the frequency of micronucleated CD8$^+$ lymphocytes was found only in workers with the *EPHX* exon 3 *Tyr/Tyr* genotype. This finding would agree with the role of EPHX in the metabolic activation of PAHs, as it has been suggested that the *Tyr* (wild-type) allele is associated with a higher EPHX activity than the exon 3 variant allele *His* (Hassett *et al.*, 1994). However, carriers of another variant allele (*Arg* in

exon 4), supposed to confer increased EPHX activity (Hassett *et al.*, 1994), did not show a similar correlation (Carstensen *et al.*, 1999). Thus, the role of the *EPHX* genotype in determining cytogenetic response to exposure to PAH requires further studies.

A homozygous deletion of the *GSTT1* gene (null genotype) is found in 10–20% of white people, making them unable to perform GSTT1-mediated detoxification reactions. The best known example of genotype-dependent response to an in-vitro chemical treatment is probably the sensitivity of glutathione *S*-transferase (*GSTT1*)-null donors to 1,2:3,4-diepoxybutane (DEB; a metabolite of 1,3-butadiene) (Wiencke *et al.*, 1991; Norppa *et al*, 1995; Wiencke *et al.*, 1995; Landi *et al.*, 1996; Pelin *et al.*, 1996; Vlachodimitropoulos *et al.*, 1997; Landi *et al.*, 1998; Kligerman *et al.*, 1999; Hayes *et al.*, 2000; Schlade-Bartusiak *et al.*, 2000). In-vitro sister chromatid exchange induction by 1,2-epoxy-3-butane, another metabolite of 1,3-butadiene, was found to be elevated in both *GSTT1*-null and *GSTM1*-null subjects (Uusküla *et al.*, 1995; Bernardini *et al.*, 1998; Sasiadek *et al.*, 1999). These genotypes also appear to play a role in 1,3-butadiene metabolism in humans *in vivo*, although glutathione conjugation is a minor metabolic detoxification route for 1,3-butadiene in humans (Albertini *et al.*, 2001). Workers exposed to 1,3-butadiene had a lower ratio of urinary metabolites M_2 (measure of glutathione conjugation pathway) and sum of M_1 (measure of hydrolytic detoxification pathway) and M_2, if they were *GSTT1*- and *GSTM1*-null than if they were *GSTT1*- and *GSTM1*-positive (Albertini *et al.*, 2001). Results on the possible effect of *GSTT1* and *GSTM1* genotypes on cytogenetic biomarkers in 1,3-butadiene-exposed workers have, however, been conflicting (Kelsey *et al.*, 1995; Sorsa *et al.*, 1996; Šrám *et al.*, 1998; Hayes *et al.*, 2000). For instance, an elevated frequency of chromosomal aberrations was observed in *GSTT1*-null workers in one study (Sorsa *et al.*, 1996) but in *GSTM1*-positive workers in another study (Šrám *et al.*, 1998).

The cytochrome P450 (CYP) superfamily of monooxygenases is involved in the metabolic activation of various precarcinogens. Studies on the toxicological influence of polymorphisms

Table 2. Genetic polymorphism and chromosomal aberrations in human peripheral lymphocytes in association with various exposures

Study groups	No. of subjects	Genotypes studied	Risk genotype or phenotype associated with the exposure studied	Reference
PAH				
Coke oven workers	64	GSTM1	–	Kalina *et al.* (1998)
Controls	34	NAT2		
Polluted air				
From polluted region	19	GSTM1	–	Binková *et al.* (1996)
From control region	30			
From polluted area	67	CYP1A1	–	Motykiewicz *et al.*
From less polluted area	72	GSTM1		(1998)
Bus drivers	106	GSTM1	GSTM1-null	Knudsen *et al.* (1999)
Postal workers	101	NAT2		
Pesticides				
Floriculturists	23	GSTM1	–	Scarpato *et al.* (1996)
Controls	22	GSTT1		
		NAT2		
Farmers	20	CYP1A1	–[a]	Au *et al.* (1999)
Controls	20	GSTM1		
		GSTT1		
		PON		
Butadiene				
Butadiene producers	53	GSTM1	GSTT1-null	Sorsa *et al.* (1996)
Controls	46	GSTT1		
Butadiene producers	20	GSTM1	GSTM1-positive	Šrám *et al.* (1998)
Controls	19	GSTT1		
Butadiene rubber producers[b]	39	GSTM1	–	Hayes *et al.* (2000)
		GSTT1		
Mixed exposures				
Ethylene producers	10	CYP1A1	–	Kure *et al.* (1999)
Cable manufacturers	31	CYP2E1		
Controls	39	EPHX		
		GSTM1		
		GSTP1		
		GSTT1		

Table 2 (contd)

Study groups	No. of subjects	Genotypes studied	Risk genotype or phenotype associated with the exposure studied	Reference
Styrene				
Reinforced plastics workers	39	*CYP1A1*	– [c]	Vodicka *et al.* (2001)
Controls	12	*CYP2E1*		
		EPHX		
		GSTM1		
		GSTT1		
		GSTP1		

[a] *PON* AA (paraoxonase AA gene) subjects had increased frequencies of dicentric chromosomes after in-vitro radiation treatment.
[b] Aneuploidy studied instead of structural chromosomal aberrations.
[c] Concerns only comparison of *EPHX* 'low' and 'medium activity' subjects; influence of the other genotypes could not be distinguished from exposure effect.

affecting various CYP species are complicated by, for example, unclear associations between CYP genotype and phenotype (see Hirvonen 1999a; Norppa, 2000). Although low levels of several types of CYPs are found in lymphocytes (Raucy et al., 1999), CYP2E1 is probably among the most important ones (Hukkanen et al., 1997). A base substitution in the 5′ flanking region ($C_{1017}T$) of *CYP2E1* gene, expected to result in CYP2E1 over-expression, has been associated with a (non-significantly) increased sister chromatid exchange frequency in workers exposed to vinyl chloride (Wong et al., 1998). This study also reported that aldehyde dehydrogenase (*ALDH2*) genotype may influence lymphocyte sister chromatid exchange frequency in the exposed workers.

Genetic polymorphism affecting the 'baseline' level of cytogenetic biomarkers
Several studies have addressed the question of whether genetic polymorphisms affect the 'baseline' (or 'spontaneous') level of cytogenetic biomarkers, irrespective of specific genotoxic exposures (Table 5). Such an effect can be assumed if genotype is shown to modulate the frequency of a biomarker in an 'unexposed' control population, or in controls and exposed alike (Norppa &

Hirvonen, 2000). Polymorphism that affects fundamental cellular processes responsible for maintaining the genomic integrity, such as DNA repair or folate metabolism, could be expected to have this kind of effect.

Various proteins involved in DNA repair are polymorphic (Shen et al., 1998). However, the actual influence of many of the recently discovered repair protein polymorphisms on DNA repair capacity is still unclear and very little is known about their effects on cytogenetic biomarkers in humans. The $Arg_{399}Gln$ substitution at exon 10 of *XRCC1* (X-ray repair cross-complementing group 1) gene has been suggested to be associated with reduced DNA repair efficiency (Lunn et al., 1999; Duell et al., 2000). XRCC1 is considered to be involved in the repair of DNA single-strand breaks after base excision repair of damage produced by ionizing radiation, alkylating agents and reactive oxygen species. Homozygous carriers of the variant allele who smoked showed increased frequencies of sister chromatid exchanges, although the findings were based on only three *Gln/Gln* subjects (Duell et al., 2000).

Polymorphisms of xenobiotic-metabolizing enzymes may also influence the 'baseline' level of chromosomal damage, if they participate in

Table 3. Genetic polymorphism and sister chromatid exchanges in human peripheral lymphocytes, in association with various exposures

Study groups	No. of subjects	Genotypes studied	Risk genotype associated with the exposure studied	Reference
PAH				
Coke oven workers	64	GSTM1	–	Kalina *et al.* (1998)
Controls	34	NAT2		
Coke oven workers	35	GSTM1	–	van Delft *et al.* (2001)
Controls	37	GSTT1		
Polluted air				
From polluted region	19	GSTM1	–	Binková *et al.* (1996)
From control region	30			
From polluted area	67	CYP1A1	–	Motykiewicz *et al.* (1998)
From less polluted area	72	GSTM1		
Pesticides				
Floriculturists	23	GSTM1	– a	Scarpato *et al.* (1996)
Controls	22	GSTT1		
		NAT2		
Butadiene				
Butadiene producers	40	GSTT1	– b	Kelsey *et al.* (1995)
Butadiene producers	53	GSTM1	–	Sorsa *et al.* (1996)
Controls	46	GSTT1		
Butadiene producers	20	GSTM1	–	Šrám *et al.* (1998)
Controls	19	GSTT1		
Polybutadiene rubber		GSTM1	–	Hayes *et al.* (2000)
producers	41	GSTT1		
Controls	38			
Ethylene oxide				
Sterilization workers	51	GSTM1	GSTT1-positive (all	Yong *et al.* (2001)
Controls	5	GSTT1	GSTT1-nulls were exposed)	
Vinyl chloride				
Polyvinyl chloride	44	ALDH2	ALDH2 1-2 or 2-2 c	Wong *et al.* (1998)
workers		CYP2E1	CYP2E1 c1c2 or c2c2 a	
		GSTM1		
		GSTT1		

Table 3 (contd)

Study groups	No. of subjects	Genotypes studied	Risk genotype associated with the exposure studied	Reference
Benzene				
Painters	23	*GSTT1*	–	Xu *et al.* (1998)
Factory controls	22			
Organic solvents				
Shoe workers	52	*GSTM1*	–	Pitarque *et al.* (2002)
Controls	36	*GSTT1*		
Epichlorohydrin, dimethylformamide				
Resin producers	85	*GSTT1*	–	Cheng *et al.* (1999)
Chromium				
Electroplaters	35	*GSTM1*	–	Wu *et al.* (2000)
Controls	35	*GSTT1*		

[a] Effect of *CYP2E1* was not statistically significant.

[b] Six *GSTT1*-null (DEB-sensitive) workers had a higher mean frequency of sister chromatid exchanges than 34 *GSTT1*-positive (DEB-resistant) workers, but this was considered a baseline effect, since no associations were observed between sister chromatid exchanges, on the one hand, and urinary M_1, breathing-zone concentrations of 1,3-butadiene or exposure history, on the other hand. Unexposed controls were not included.

[c] Statistically significant in all subjects and in smokers; an effect of smoking was obvious only in *ALDH2* 1–2/2–2 subjects.

inborn metabolism important for chromosome integrity, or if their substrate is a genotoxin to which most people are exposed.

Subjects with the *NAT2* slow acetylator genotype had an increased baseline frequency of lymphocyte chromosomal aberrations, not associated with known exposures (Knudsen *et al.*, 1999). This effect seemed to be reproducible, as it was also seen in two other studies (Norppa *et al.*, 2000, 2001). It might be explained by common exposure to genotoxins, such as heterocyclic amines in heated food. *N*-Acetylation might function as a detoxification route in peripheral blood cells (Norppa, 2001) where the activities of CYPs (e.g. CYP1A2) capable of metabolically activating heterocyclic amines are low (Hukkanen *et al.*, 1997; Raucy *et al.*, 1999). Earlier studies have suggested that the *NAT2* slow genotype is associated with an increased level of aromatic DNA adducts in white blood cells, regardless of smoking (Peluso *et al.*, 1998, 2000). Alterna-tively, NAT2 may detoxify important (as yet unknown) endogenously formed genotoxins(s). Acetyltransferases are involved in the inter-conversion of polyamines (Seiler *et al.*, 1985) and acetylation of histones (Grunstein, 1997), but there is no evidence for the involvement of NAT2 in such reactions. Another polymorphic acetyl-transferase, NAT1, appears to have a role in the catabolism of folate (Minchin, 1995), but NAT2 is not known to be involved.

The *GSTT1*-null genotype has been associated with an increased 'baseline' level of sister chro-matid exchanges in lymphocytes, not associated with smoking or other known exposures (Schröder *et al.*, 1995; Wiencke *et al.*, 1995; Norppa *et al.*, 2000). The finding might reflect an interaction between the genotype and some common endo-genous or exogenous exposure; ethylene oxide generated from endogenous ethylene was pro-posed as a possible explanation (Schröder *et al.*, 1995). This interpretation is supported by data

Table 4. Genetic polymorphism and micronuclei in human peripheral lymphocytes, in association with various exposures

Study groups	No. of subjects	Polymorphism studied	Risk genotype associated with the exposure studied	Reference
PAH				
Chimney sweeps	71	CYP1A1 GSTM1	–	Carstensen *et al.* (1993)
Chimney sweeps Controls	48–67 29–35	GSTM1	GSTM1-null [a]	Ichiba *et al.* (1994)
Coke-oven workers Controls	76 18	CYP1A1 GSTM1	–	Brescia *et al.* (1999)
Potroom workers Controls		CYP1A1 EPHX GSTM1 GSTP1 GSTT1	EPHX exon 3 Tyr/Tyr [b]	Carstensen *et al.* (1999)
Coke oven workers Controls	21 11	GSTM1 GSTT1	–[c]	van Delft *et al.* (2001)
Pesticides				
Floriculturists Controls	23 22	GSTM1 GSTT1 NAT2	–	Scarpato *et al.* (1996)
Floriculturists Controls	30 33	GSTM1 GSTT1 NAT2	–	Falck *et al.* (1999)
Greenhouse workers Controls	64 50	GSTM1 GSTT1	–[d]	Lucero *et al.* (2000)
Butadiene				
Butadiene producers Controls	53 46	GSTM1 GSTT1	GSTT1-positive	Sorsa *et al.* (1996)
Butadiene producers Controls	20 19	GSTM1 GSTT1	–	Šrám *et al.* (1998)
Organic solvents				
Shoe workers Controls	52 36	GSTM1	GSTM1-null [e]	Pitarque *et al.* (2002)

[a] Correlation between micronuclei in T lymphocytes and DNA adduct level in white blood cells was significant only for GSTM1-null subjects (all subjects included).
[b] After adjustment for age, correlation observed between micronuclei in CD8+ lymphocytes and airborne particulate PAH, airborne gas phase PAH and length of employment in the potroom only in exon 3 Tyr/Tyr subjects (wild-type homozygotes).
[c] Micronuclei were studied in urothelial cells.
[d] Genotype effects were also not seen for micronuclei in buccal cells.
[e] In smokers, occupational exposure was associated with increased frequency of micronuclei in GSTM1-null subjects, but not in GSTM1-positive subjects.

Table 5. Genetic polymorphism and baseline level of chromosomal aberrations, sister chromatid exchanges and micronuclei in human peripheral lymphocytes

Studied groups	No. of subjects (% smokers)	Genotypes studied	Risk genotype (affected group)	Reference
Chromosomal aberrations				
Controls	46 (ND)	*GSTM1* *GSTT1*	*GSTM1*-positive	Sorsa *et al.* (1996)
Culture controls	109 (27)	*GSTM1* *GSTP1* *GSTT1*	*GSTT1*-null [a]	Landi *et al.* (1998)
Controls	19(47)	*GSTM1* *GSTT1*	*GSTT1*-null [b]	Šrám *et al.* (1998)
Floriculturists Controls	23 (26) 22 (41)	*GSTM1* *GSTT1* *NAT2*	– [c]	Scarpato *et al.* (1996)
Bus drivers Postal workers	106 (0) 101 (0)	*GSTM1* *NAT2*	*NAT2* slow (all)	Knudsen *et al.* (1999)
Polyurethane workers Controls	73 (36) 70 (41)	*GSTM1* *GSTT1* *NAT1* *NAT2*	*NAT2* slow (all)	Norppa *et al.* (2000)
Nuclear power plant workers and controls	56 (43)	*GSTM1* *GSTT1* *NAT2*	*NAT2* slow (all)	Norppa *et al.* (2001)
Newborns (chromosome painting)	26 (0)	*GSTM1* *GSTT1* *GSTP1* *CYP1A1* *CYP2D6* *NAT1* *NAT2*	*CYP1A1* MspI heterozygotes	Pluth *et al.* (2000b)
Culture controls	34 (100) 36 (100)	*CYP2D6* *CYP2E1*	*CYP2E1* WT/*5B	Abdel-Rahman *et al.* (2000)
Controls	12 (ND)	*CYP1A1* *CYP2E1* *EPHX* *GSTM1* *GSTT1* *GSTP1*	*EPHX* 'low activity' [d]	Vodicka *et al.* (2001)

Table 5 (contd)

Studied groups	No. of subjects (% smokers)	Genotypes studied	Risk genotype (affected group)	Reference
Sister chromatid exchanges				
Culture controls	45 (8)	GSTM1 phenotype	–	Wiencke et al. (1990)
Lung cancer cases	74 (23)	GSTM1	GSTM1-null (never-smokers)	Cheng et al. (1995a,b)
Controls	77 (22)			
Culture controls	20 (5)	GSTM1 GSTT1	GSTT1-null	Norppa et al.(1995)
Volunteers	30 (43)	GSTT1	GSTT1-null	Schröder et al. (1995)
Culture controls	78 (10)	GSTT1	GSTT1 null	Wiencke et al. (1995)
Polyurethane workers	73 (36)	GSTM1	GSTT1-null (all)	Norppa et al. (2000)
Controls	70 (41)	GSTT1 NAT1 NAT2		
Floriculturists	23 (26)	GSTM1	GSTT1-positive (all) [b]	Scarpato et al. (1996)
Controls	22 (41)	GSTT1 NAT2		
Culture controls	18 (0)	GSTT1	–	Bernardini et al. (1998)
Culture controls	109 (27)	GSTM1 GSTP1 GSTT1	–	Landi et al. (1998)
Culture controls	20 (0)	GSTM1 GSTT1	–	Bernardini et al. (2001)
Micronuclei				
Floriculturists	30 (29)	GSTM1	GSTM1-positive (all)	Falck et al. (1999)
Controls	33 (30)	GSTT1 NAT2		

[a] Not quite statistically significant ($p = 0.06$).

[b] Based on only 4 GSTT1-null subjects.

[c] NAT2 slow subjects showed 1.4-fold higher chromosomal aberration frequencies than NAT2 rapid subjects in two samplings, but the difference was not statistically significant.

[d] Based on 2 'high', 2 'medium' and 8 'low activity' subjects; influence of the other genotypes was not shown separately for the controls.

showing that ethylene oxide–haemoglobin adducts are increased in GSTT1-null subjects among nonsmokers, smokers and occupationally exposed workers (Müller et al., 1998; Thier et al., 1999; Fennell et al., 2000; Thier et al., 2001; Yong et al., 2001). However, in one study (Yong et al., 2001), sister chromatid exchange frequencies in workers exposed to ethylene oxide showed a negative correlation with ethylene oxide–haemoglobin adducts.

The effect of *GSTT1* genotype on baseline sister chromatid exchange level was roughly the size of the effect of smoking (i.e. quite small), which may explain why it has not been detected in all studies (see Norppa, 2000). In general, the low frequency of the *GSTT1*-null genotype in Caucasians has complicated the evaluation of the influence of *GSTT1* in many studies. Two papers have suggested that the *GSTT1*-null genotype is also associated with an increase in 'spontaneous' chromosomal aberrations in lymphocytes (Landi *et al.*, 1998; Šrám *et al.* 1998).

Single studies (see Table 5) have indicated an increase in baseline chromosomal aberrations among *GSTM1*-positive subjects, *CYP1A1 msp*I heterozygotes (translocations in newborns), *CYP2E1* wt/*5B heterozygotes and *EPHX* 'low activity' genotype, in baseline sister chromatid exchanges among *GSTT1* positive genotype and in micronuclei in *GSTM1*-positive subjects. These findings are based on a few individuals and need to be examined further in future studies.

Conclusions

Cytogenetic biomarkers reflect the cellular effects of exposure to genotoxic carcinogens and represent mechanisms that are believed to have an important role in carcinogenesis. A high level of chromosomal aberrations (but not sister chromatid exchanges or micronuclei) in peripheral lymphocytes has been observed to be predictive of increased cancer risk, irrespective of tobacco smoking or occupational exposure to carcinogens. These findings might be explained by individual susceptibility factors, such as genetic polymorphisms affecting DNA repair, genomic stability and carcinogen metabolism. Although studies on the polymorphisms of the first two factors are scant, polymorphisms of some xenobiotic-metabolizing enzymes have been observed to affect both cancer risk and cytogenetic biomarkers. If genetic polymorphisms are important modifiers of genotoxic effects, their control in cytogenetic biomarker studies is expected to help in managing individual variability, detection of exposure effects and identification of sensitive subgroups. The importance of various genetic polymorphisms is expected to depend on the exposure agent, cell type examined and ethnicity of the population studied.

Acknowledgements

This paper was partly supported by Commission of the European Communities Contract No. QLK4-CT-2000-00628, 'Cytogenetic Biomarkers and Human Cancer Risk' (CancerRiskBiomarkers).

References

Abdel-Rahman, S.Z., El-Zein, R.A, Zwischenberger, J.B. & Au, W.W. (1998) Association of the NAT1*10 genotype with increased chromosome aberrations and higher lung cancer risk in cigarette smokers. *Mutat. Res.*, **398**, 43–54

Abdel-Rahman, S.Z., Salama, S.A., Au, W.W. & Hamada, F.A. (2000) Role of polymorphic *CYP2E1* and *CYP2D6* in NNK-induced chromosome aberrations in cultured human lymphocytes. *Pharmacogenetics*, **10**, 239–249

Albertini, R.J., Anderson, D., Douglas, G.R., Hagmar, L., Hemminki, K., Merlo, F., Natarajan, A.T., Norppa, H., Shuker, D.E., Tice, R., Waters, M.D. & Aitio, A. (2000) IPCS guidelines for the monitoring of genotoxic effects of carcinogens in humans. *Mutat. Res.*, **463**, 111–172

Albertini, R.J., Šrám, R.J., Vacek, P.M., Lynch, J., Wright, M., Nicklas, J.A., Boogaard, P.J., Henderson, R.F., Swenberg, J.A., Tates, A.D. & Ward, J.B., Jr (2001) Biomarkers for assessing occupational exposures to 1,3-butadiene. *Chem.-biol. Interact.*, **135–136**, 429–453

Au, W.W., Sierra-Torres, C.H., Cajas-Salazar, N., Shipp, B.K. & Legator, M.S. (1999) Cytogenetic effects from exposure to mixed pesticides and the influence from genetic susceptibility. *Environ. Health Perspect.*, **107**, 501–505

Au, W.W., Oh, H.Y., Grady, J., Salama, S.A. & Heo, M.Y. (2001) Usefulness of genetic susceptibility and biomarkers for evaluation of environmental health risk. *Environ. mol. Mutag.*, **37**, 215–225

Autrup, H. (2000) Genetic polymorphisms in human xenobiotica metabolizing enzymes as susceptibility factors in toxic response. *Mutat. Res.*, **464**, 65–76

Barale, R., Chelotti, L., Davini, T., Del Ry, S., Andreassi, M.G, Ballardin, M., Bulleri, M., He, J., Baldacci, S., Di Pede, F., Gemignani, F. & Landi, S.

(1998) Sister chromatid exchange and micronucleus frequency in human lymphocytes of 1,650 subjects in an Italian population: II. Contribution of sex, age, and lifestyle. *Environ. mol. Mutag.*, **31**, 228–242

Bennett, W.P., Alavanja, M.C., Blomeke, B., Vähakangas, K.H., Castren, K., Welsh, J.A., Bowman, E..D., Khan, M.A., Flieder, D.B. & Harris, C.C. (1999) Environmental tobacco smoke, genetic susceptibility, and risk of lung cancer in never-smoking women. *J. natl Cancer Inst.*, **91**, 2009–2014

Bernardini, S., Hirvonen, A., Pelin, K. & Norppa, H. (1998) Induction of sister chromatid exchange by 1,2-epoxy-3-butene in cultured human lymphocytes: influence of *GSTT1* genotype. *Carcinogenesis*, **19**, 377–380

Bernardini, S., Hirvonen, A., Järventaus, H. & Norppa, H. (2001) *trans*-Stilbene oxide-induced sister chromatid exchange in cultured human lymphocytes: influence of *GSTM1* and *GSTT1* genotypes. *Mutagenesis*, **16**, 277–281

Binková, B., Lewtas, J., Mišková, I., Rössner, P., Cerná, M., Mrácková, G., Peterková, K., Mumford, J., Meyer, S. & Šrám, R. (1996) Biomarker studies in Northern Bohemia. *Environ. Health Perspect.*, **104** (Suppl. 3), 591–597

Bolognesi, C., Abbondandolo, A., Barale, R., Casalone, R., Dalpra, L., De Ferrari, M., Degrassi, F., Forni, A., Lamberti, L., Lando, C., Migliore, L., Padovani, P., Pasquini, R., Puntoni, R., Sbrana, I., Stella, M. & Bonassi, S. (1997) Age-related increase of baseline frequencies of sister chromatid exchanges, chromosome aberrations, and micronuclei in human lymphocytes. *Cancer Epidemiol. Biomarkers Prev.*, **6**, 249–256

Bonassi, S., Abbondandolo, A., Camurri, L., Dal Prá, L., De Ferrari, M., Degrassi, F., Forni, A., Lamberti, L., Lando, C., Padovani, P., Sbrana, I., Vecchio, D. & Puntoni, R. (1995a) Are chromosome aberrations in circulating lymphocytes predictive of a future cancer onset in humans? Preliminary results of an Italian cohort study. *Cancer Genet. Cytogenet.*, **79**, 133–135

Bonassi, S., Bolognesi, C., Abbondandolo, A., Barale, R., Bigatti, P., Camurri, L., Dal Prá, L., De Ferrari, M., Forni, A., Lando, C., Padovani, P., Pasquini, R., Stella, M. & Puntoni, R. (1995b) Influence of sex

on cytogenetic end points: evidence from a large human sample and review of the literature. *Cancer Epidemiol. Biomarkers Prev.*, **4**, 671–679

Bonassi, S., Hagmar, L., Strömberg, U., Montagud, A.H., Tinnerberg, H., Forni, A., Heikkilä, P., Wanders, S., Wilhardt, P., Hansteen, I.L., Knudsen, L.E. & Norppa, H. (2000) Chromosomal aberrations in lymphocytes predict human cancer independently of exposure to carcinogens. *Cancer Res.*, **60**, 1619–1625

Bonassi, S., Fenech, M., Lando, C., Lin, Y.P., Ceppi, M., Chang, W.P., Holland, N., Kirsch-Volders, M., Zeiger, E., Ban, S., Barale, R., Bigatti, M.P., Bolognesi, C., Jia, C., Di Giorgio, M., Ferguson, L.R., Fucic, A., Lima, O.G., Hrelia, P., Krishnaja, A.P., Lee, T.K., Migliore, L., Mikhalevich, L., Mirkova, E., Mosesso, P., Muller, W.U., Odagiri, Y., Scarffi, M.R., Szabova, E., Vorobtsova, I., Vral, A. & Zijno, A. (2001) Human Micronucleus project: international database comparison for results with the cytokinesis-block micronucleus assay in human lymphocytes: I. Effect of laboratory protocol, scoring criteria, and host factors on the frequency of micronuclei. *Environ. mol. Mutag.*, **37**, 31–45

van Brabant, A.J., Stan, R. & Ellis, N.A. (2000) DNA helicases, genomic instability, and human genetic disease. *Ann. Rev. Genomics hum. Genet.*, **1**, 409–459

Brescia, G., Celotti, L., Clonfero, E., Neumann, G.H., Forni, A., Foà, V., Pisoni, M., Ferri, G.M. & Assennato, G. (1999) The influence of cytochrome P450 1A1 and glutathione S-transferase M1 genotypes on biomarker levels in coke-oven workers. *Arch. Toxicol.*, **73**, 431–439

Brockmöller, J., Gross, D., Kerb, R., Drakoulis, N. & Roots, I. (1992) Correlation between *trans*-stilbene oxide-glutathione conjugation activity and the deletion mutation in the glutathione S-transferase class mu gene detected by polymerase chain reaction. *Biochem. Pharmacol.*, **43**, 647–650

Brockmöller, J., Kerb, R., Drakoulis, N., Staffeldt, B. & Roots, I. (1994) Glutathione S-transferase M1 and its variants A and B as host factors of bladder cancer susceptibility: a case-control study. *Cancer Res.*, **54**, 4103–4111

Butkiewicz, D., Grzybowska, E., Hemminki, K., Øvrebrø, S., Haugen, A., Motykiewicz, G. & Chorazy, M. (1998) Modulation of DNA adduct levels in human mononuclear white blood cells and granulocytes by *CYP1A1*, *CYP2D6* and *GSTM1* genetic polymorphisms. *Mutat. Res.*, **415**, 97–108

Butkiewicz, D., Cole, K.J., Phillips, D.H., Harris, C.C. & Chorazy, M. (1999) GSTM1, GSTP1, CYP1A1 and CYP2D6 polymorphisms in lung cancer patients from an environmentally polluted region of Poland: correlation with lung DNA adduct levels. *Eur. J. Cancer*, **8**, 315–323

Butkiewicz, D., Grzybowska, E., Phillips, D.H., Hemminki, K. & Chorazy, M. (2000) Polymorphisms of the *GSTP1* and *GSTM1* genes and PAH-DNA adducts in human mononuclear white blood cells. *Environ. mol. Mutag.*, **35**, 99–105

Carstensen, U., Alexandrie, A.K., Högstedt, B., Rannug, A., Bratt, I. & Hagmar, L. (1993) B- and T-Lymphocyte micronuclei in chimney sweeps with respect to genetic polymorphism for CYP1A1 and GST1 (class mu). *Mutat. Res.*, **289**, 187–195

Carstensen, U., Hou, S.M., Alexandrie, A.K., Högstedt, B., Tagesson, C., Warholm, M., Rannug, A., Lambert, B., Axmon, A. & Hagmar, L. (1999) Influence of genetic polymorphisms of biotransformation enzymes on gene mutations, strand breaks of deoxyribonucleic acid, and micronuclei in mononuclear blood cells and urinary 8-hydroxyguanosine in potroom workers exposed to polyaromatic hydrocarbons. *Scand. J. Work Environ. Health*, **25**, 351–360

Catalán, J., Autio, K., Kuosma, E. & Norppa, H. (1998) Age-dependent inclusion of sex chromosomes in lymphocyte micronuclei of man. *Am. J. hum. Genet.*, **63**, 1464–1472

Cheng, T.-J., Christiani, D.C., Wiencke, J.K., Wain, J.C., Xu, X., & Kelsey, K.T. (1995a) Comparison of sister chromatid exchange frequency in peripheral lymphocytes in lung cancer cases and controls. *Mutat. Res.*, **348**, 75–82

Cheng, T.-J., Christiani, D.C., Xu, X., Wain, J.C., Wiencke, J.K. & Kelsey, K.T. (1995b) Glutathione *S*-transferase μ genotype, diet, and smoking as determinants of sister chromatid exchange frequency in lymphocytes, *Cancer Epidemiol. Biomarker Prev.*, **4**, 535–542

Cheng, T.-J., Christiani, D.C., Xu, X., Wain, J.C., Wiencke, J.K. & Kelsey, K.T. (1996) Increased micronucleus frequency in lymphocytes from smokers with lung cancer. *Mutat. Res.*, **349**, 43–50

Cheng, T.-J., Hwang, S.-J., Kuo, H.-W., Luo, J.-C. & Chang, M.J.W. (1999) Exposure to epichlorohydrin and dimethylformamide, glutathione *S*-transferases and sister chromatid exchange frequencies in peripheral lymphocytes. *Arch. Toxicol.*, **73**, 282–287

Conforti-Froes, N., El-Zein, R., Abdel-Rahman, S.Z., Zwischenberger, J.B. & Au, W.W. (1997) Predisposing genes and increased chromosome aberrations in lung cancer cigarette smokers. *Mutat. Res.*, **379**, 53–59

Dallinga, J.W., Pachen, D.M.F.A., Wijnhoven, S.W.P., Breedijk, A., van 't Veer, L., Wigbout, G., van Zandwijk, N., Maas, L.M., van Agen, E., Kleinjans, J.C.S. & van Schooten, F.-J. (1998) The use of 4-aminobiphenyl hemoglobin adducts and aromatic DNA adducts in lymphocytes of smokers as biomarkers of exposure. *Cancer Epidemiol. Biomarkers Prev.*, **7**, 571–577

van Delft, J.H.M., Steenwinkel, M.-J.S.T., van Asten, J.G., de Vogel, N., Bruijntjes-Rozier, T.C., Schouten, T., Cramers, P., Maas, L., van Herwijnen, M.H., van Schooten, F.-J. & Hopmans, P.M.J. (2001) Biological monitoring the exposure to polycyclic aromatic hydrocarbons of coke oven workers in relation to smoking and genetic polymorphisms for *GSTM1* and *GSTT1*. *Ann. Occup. Hyg.*, **45**, 395–408

Duell, E.J., Wiencke, J.K., Cheng, T.-J., Varkonyi, A., Zuo, Z.F., Ashok, T.D.S., Mark, E.J., Wain, J.C., Christiani, D.C. & Kelsey, K.T. (2000) Polymorphisms in the DNA repair genes *XRCC1* and *ERCC2* and biomarkers of DNA damage in human blood mononuclear cells. *Carcinogenesis*, **21**, 965–971

Duesberg, P., Rausch, C., Rasnick, D. & Hehlmann, R. (1998) Genetic instability of cancer cells is proportional to their degree of aneuploidy. *Proc. natl Acad. Sci. USA*, **95**, 13692–13697

Eastmond, D.A. (2000) Benzene-induced genotoxicity: a different perspective. *J. Toxicol. environ. Health*, Part A, **61**, 353–356

Eastmond, D.A., Schuler, M. & Rupa, D.S. (1995) Advantages and limitations of using fluorescence in situ hybridisation for the detection of aneuploidy in interphase human cells. *Mutat. Res.*, **348**, 153–162

El-Zein, R., Conforti-Froes, N. & Au, W.W. (1997) Interactions between genetic predisposition and environmental toxicants for development of lung cancer. *Environ. mol. Mutag.*, **30**, 196–204

Falck, G.C.-M., Hirvonen, A., Scarpato, R., Saarikoski, S.T., Migliore, L. & Norppa, H. (1999) Micronuclei in blood lymphocytes and genetic polymorphism for GSTM1, GSTT1 and NAT2 in pesticide-exposed greenhouse workers. *Mutat. Res.*, **441**, 225–237

Fenech, M. (2001) The role of folic acid and vitamin B12 in genomic stability of human cells. *Mutat. Res.*, **475**, 57–67

Fenech, M. & Morley, A. (1985) Measurement of micronuclei in lymphocytes. *Mutat. Res.*, **147**, 29–36

Fennell, T.R., MacNeela, J.P., Morris, R.W., Watson, M., Thompson, C.L. & Bell, D.A. (2000) Hemoglobin adducts from acrylonitrile and ethylene oxide in cigarette smokers: effects of glutathione *S*-transferase T1-null and M1-null genotypes. *Cancer Epidemiol. Biomarkers Prev.*, **9**, 705–712

Gisselsson, D., Jonson, T., Petersén, Å., Strömbeck, B., Dal Cin, P., Höglund, M., Mitelman, F., Mertens, F. & Mandahl, N. (2001) Telomere dysfunction triggers extensive DNA fragmentation and evolution of complex chromosome abnormalities in human malignant tumors. *Proc. natl Acad. Sci. USA*, **98**, 12683–12688

Godschalk, R.W.L., Dallinga, J.W., Wikman, H., Risch, A., Kleinjans, J.C., Bartsch, H. & Van Schooten, F.-J. (2001) Modulation of DNA and protein adducts in smokers by genetic polymorphisms in GSTM1, GSTT1, NAT1 and NAT2. *Pharmacogenetics*, **11**, 389–398

Golding, B.T. & Watson, W.P. (1999) Possible mechanisms of carcinogenesis after exposure to benzene. In: Singer, B. & Bartsch, H., eds, *Exocyclic DNA Adducts in Mutagenesis and Carcinogenesis* (IARC Scientific Publications No. 150), Lyon, IARC*Press*, pp. 75–88

Grompe, M. & D'Andrea, A. (2001) Fanconi anemia and DNA repair. *Hum. mol. Genet.*, **10**, 2253–2259

Grunstein, M. (1997) Histone acetylation in chromatin structure and transcription. *Nature*, **389**, 349–352

Gutierrez, S., Carbonell, E., Galofre, P., Creus, A. & Marcos, R. (1999) Low sensitivity of the sister chromatid exchange assay to detect the genotoxic effects of radioiodine therapy. *Mutagenesis*, **14**, 221–226

Hagmar, L., Brøgger, A., Hansteen, I.-L., Heim, S., Högstedt, B., Knudsen, L., Lambert, B., Linnainmaa, K., Mitelman, F., Nordenson, I., Reuterwall, C., Salomaa, S., Skerfving, S. & Sorsa, M. (1994) Cancer risk in humans predicted by increased levels of chromosome aberrations in lymphocytes: Nordic Study Group on the Health Risk of Chromosome Damage. *Cancer Res.*, **54**, 2919–2922

Hagmar, L., Bonassi, S., Strömberg, U., Brøgger, A., Knudsen, L.E., Norppa, H., Reuterwall, C., Forni, A., Hansteen, I.-L., Högstedt, B., Huici Montagud, A., Lambert, B., Mitelman, F., Nordenson, I., Salomaa, S. & Skerfving, S. (1998) Chromosomal aberrations in lymphocytes predict human cancer – a report from the European Study Group on Cytogenetic Biomarkers and Health (ESCH). *Cancer Res.*, **58**, 4117–4121

Hagmar, L., Tinnerberg, H., Mikoczy, Z., Strömberg, U., Bonassi, S., Huici Montagud, A., Hansteen, I.-L., Knudsen, L. & Norppa, H. (2000) Do cytogenetic biomarkers, used for occupational health surveillance, predict cancer? In: Anderson, D., Karakaya, A.E. & Šrám, R.J., eds, *Human Monitoring after Environmental and Occupational Exposure to Chemical and Physical Agents* (NATO Science Series, Series A: Life Sciences No. 313), Amsterdam, IOS Press, pp. 1–6

Hasset, C., Aicher, L., Sidhu, J.S. & Omiecinski, C.J. (1994) Human microsomal epoxide hydrolase: genetic polymorphism and functional expression *in vitro* of amino acid variants. *Hum. mol. Genet.*, **3**, 421–428

Hayes, R.B., Zhang, L., Yin, S., Swenberg, J.A., Xi, L., Wiencke, J., Bechtold W.E., Yao, M, Rothman, N., Haas, R., O'Neill, J.P.O., Zhang, D., Wiemels, J., Dosemeci, M., Li, G. & Smith M.T. (2000) Genotoxic markers among butadiene polymer workers in China. *Carcinogenesis*, **21**, 55–62

Hirvonen, A. (1999a) Polymorphisms of xenobiotic-metabolizing enzymes and susceptibility to cancer. *Environ. Health Perspect.*, **107** (Suppl. 1), 37–47

Hirvonen, A. (1999b) Polymorphic NATs and cancer predisposition. In: Vineis, P., Malats, N., Lang, M., d'Errico, A., Caporaso, N., Cuzick, J. & Boffetta, P., eds, *Metabolic Polymorphisms and Susceptibility to Cancer* (IARC Scientific Publications No. 148), Lyon, IARC*Press*, pp. 251–270

Hou, S.-M., Fält, S., Yang, K., Nyberg, F., Pershagen, G., Hemminki, K. & Lambert, B. (2001) Differential interactions between GSTM1 and NAT2 genotypes on aromatic DNA adduct level and HPRT mutant frequency in lung cancer patients and population controls. *Cancer Epidemiol. Biomarkers Prev.*, **10**, 133–140

Hukkanen, J., Hakkola, J., Anttila, S., Piipari, R., Karjalainen, A., Pelkonen, O. & Raunio, H. (1997) Detection of mRNA encoding xenobiotic-metabolizing cytochrome P450s in human bronchoalveolar macrophages and peripheral blood lymphocytes. *Mol. Carcinog.*, **20**, 224–230

Ichiba, M., Hagmar, L., Rannug, A., Högstedt, B., Alexandrie, A.-K., Carstensen, U. & Hemminki, K. (1994) Aromatic DNA adducts, micronuclei and genetic polymorphism for CYP1A1 and GST in chimney sweeps. *Carcinogenesis*, **15**, 1347–1352

Jackson, A.L. & Loeb, L.A. (2001) The contribution of endogenous sources of DNA damage to the multiple mutations in cancer. *Mutat. Res.*, **477**, 7–21

Johnson, R.D. & Jasin, M. (2000) Sister chromatid gene conversion is a prominent double-strand break repair pathway in mammalian cells. *EMBO J.*, **19**, 3398–3407

Jones, I.M., Tucker, J.D., Langlois, R.G., Mendelsohn, M.L., Pleshanov, P. & Nelson, D.O. (2001) Evaluation of three somatic genetic biomarkers as indicators of low dose radiation effects in clean-up workers of the Chernobyl nuclear reactor accident. *Radiat. Prot. Dosimetry*, **97**, 61–67

Kalina, I., Brezáni, P., Gajdošová, D., Binková, B., Šalagovic, J., Habalová, V., Mrackova, G., Dobiáš, L. & Šrám, R.I. (1998) Cytogenetic monitoring in coke oven workers. *Mutat. Res.*, **417**, 9–17

Kelsey, K.T., Wiencke, J.K., Ward, J., Bechtold, W. & Fajen, J. (1995) Sister-chromatid exchanges, glutathione S-transferase θ deletion and cytogenetic sensitivity to diepoxybutane in lymphocytes from butadiene monomer production workers. *Mutat. Res.*, **335**, 267–273

Khanna, K.K., Lavin, M.F., Jackson, S.P. & Mulhern, T.D. (2001) ATM, a central controller of cellular responses to DNA damage. *Cell Death Differ.*, **8**, 1052–1065

Kligerman, A.D., DeMarini, D.M., Doerr, C.L., Hanley, N.M., Milholland, V.S. & Tennant, A.H. (1999) Comparison of cytogenetic effects of 3,4-epoxy-1-butene and 1,2:3,4-diepoxybutane in mouse, rat and human lymphocytes following in-vitro G_0 exposures. *Mutat. Res.*, **439**, 13–23

Knudsen, L.E., Norppa, H., Gamborg, M.O., Nielsen, P.S., Okkels, H., Soll-Johanning, H., Raffn, E., Järventaus, H. & Autrup, H. (1999) Chromosomal aberrations in humans induced by urban air pollution: influence of DNA repair and polymorphisms of glutathione S-transferase M1 and N-acetyltransferase 2. *Cancer Epidemiol. Biomarkers Prev.*, **8**, 303–310

Kure, E., Thorsen, M. & Hansteen, I.-L. (1999) Gene–exposure interaction in occupational and environmental epidemiology: results from an ongoing study. *Norsk Epidemiol.*, **9**, 39–46

Lambert, B., Lindblad, A., Nordenskjöld, M. & Werelius, B. (1978) Increased frequency of sister chromatid exchanges in cigarette smokers. *Hereditas*, **88**, 147–149

Landi, S., Ponzanelli, I., Hirvonen, A., Norppa, H. & Barale, R. (1996) Repeated analysis of sister chromatid exchange induction by diepoxybutane in cultured human lymphocytes: effect of glutathione S-transferase T1 and M1 genotypes. *Mutat. Res.*, **351**, 79–85

Landi, S., Norppa, H., Frenzilli, G., Cipollini, G., Ponzanelli, I., Barale, R. & Hirvonen, A. (1998) Individual sensitivity to cytogenetics effects of 1,2:3,4-diepoxybutane in cultured human lymphocytes: influence of glutathione S-transferases M1, P1 and T1 genotypes. *Pharmacogenetics*, **8**, 461–471

Laurent, C., Frederic, J. & Leonard, A.Y. (1984) Sister chromatid exchange frequency in workers exposed to high levels of ethylene oxide, in a hospital sterilization service. *Int. Arch. occup. environ. Health*, **54**, 33–43

Liou, S.H., Lung, J.C., Chen, Y.H., Yang, T., Hsieh, L.L., Chen, C.J. & Wu, T.N. (1999) Increased chromosome-type chromosome aberration frequencies as biomarkers of cancer risk in a blackfoot endemic area. *Cancer Res.*, **59**, 1481–1484

Loeb, L.A. (2001) A mutator phenotype in cancer. *Cancer Res.*, **61**, 3230–3239

Lucero, L., Pastor, S., Suárez, S., Durbán, R., Gómez, C., Parrón, T., Creus, A. & Marcos, R. (2000) Cytogenetic biomonitoring of Spanish greenhouse workers exposed to pesticides: micronuclei analysis in peripheral blood lymphocytes and buccal epithelial cells. *Mutat. Res.*, **464**, 255–262

Lunn, R.M., Langlois, R.G., Hsieh, L.L., Thompson, C.L. & Bell, D.A. (1999) *XRCC1* polymorphisms: effect on aflatoxin B_1-DNA adducts and glycophorin A variant frequency. *Cancer Res.*, **59**, 2557–2561

Marcon, F., Zijno, A., Crebelli, R., Carere, A., Veidebaum, T., Peltonen, K., Parks, R., Schuler, M. & Eastmond, D. (1999) Chromosome damage and aneuploidy detected by interphase multicolour FISH in benzene-exposed shale oil workers. *Mutat. Res.*, **445**, 155–166

McWilliams, J.E., Sanderson, B.J., Harris, E.L., Richert-Boe, K.E. & Henner, W.D. (1995) Glutathione *S*-transferase M1 (GSTM1) deficiency and lung cancer risk. *Cancer Epidemiol. Biomarkers Prev.*, **4**, 589–594

Milillo, C.P., Gemignani, F., Sbrana, I., Carrozzi, L., Viegi, G. & Barale, R. (1996) Chromosome aberrations in humans in relation to site of residence. *Mutat. Res.*, **360**, 173–179

Minchin, R.F. (1995) Acetylation of *p*-aminobenzoylglutamate, a folic acid catabolite, by recombinant human arylamine *N*-acetyltransferase and U937 cells. *Biochem. J.*, **307**, 1–3

Mitelman, F. (2000) Recurrent chromosome aberrations in cancer. *Mutat. Res.*, **462**, 247–253

Morimoto, K. & Takeshita, T. (1996) Low K_m aldehyde dehydrogenase (ALDH2) polymorphism, alcohol-drinking behaviour, and chromosome alterations in peripheral lymphocytes. *Environ. Health Perspect.*, **104** (Suppl. 3), 563–567

Motykiewicz, G., Michalska, J., Pendzich, J., Malusecka, E., Strózyk, M., Kalinowska, E., Butkiewicz, D., Mielzynska, D., Midro, A., Santella, R.M. & Chorazy, M. (1998) A molecular epidemiology study in women from Upper Silesia, Poland. *Toxicol. Lett.*, **96–97**, 195–202

Müller, W.U., Nusse, M., Miller, B.M., Slavotinek, A., Viaggi, S. & Streffer, C. (1996) Micronuclei: a biological indicator of radiation damage. *Mutat. Res.*, **366**, 163–169

Müller, M., Krämer, A., Angerer, J. & Hallier, E. (1998) Ethylene oxide–protein adduct formation in humans: influence of glutathione *S*-transferase polymorphisms. *Int. Arch. occup. environ. Health*, **71**, 499–502

Nielsen, P.S., de Pater, N., Okkels, H. & Autrup, H. (1996) Environmental air pollution and DNA adducts in Copenhagen bus drivers – effect of GSTM1 and NAT2 genotypes on adduct levels. *Carcinogenesis*, **17**, 1021–1027

Nivard, M.J.M. & Vogel, E.W. (2001) The relationship between DNA adduct formation , repair, hereditary genetic damage and cancer formation of genotoxic agents. *Mutat. Res.*, **483** (Suppl. 1), S46

Norppa, H. (1997) Cytogenetic markers of susceptibility: influence of polymorphic carcinogen-metabolizing enzymes. *Environ. Health Perspect.*, **105** (Suppl. 4), 829–835

Norppa, H. (2000) Influence of genetic enzyme polymorphisms on cytogenetic biomarkers. In: Anderson, D., Karakaya, A.E. & Šrám, R.J., eds, *Human Monitoring after Environmental and Occupational Exposure to Chemical and Physical Agents* (NATO Science Series, Series A: Life Sciences No. 313), Amsterdam, IOS Press, pp. 300–311

Norppa, H. (2001) Genetic polymorphisms and chromosome damage. *Int. J. Hyg. environ. Health*, **204**, 31–38

Norppa, H. & Hirvonen, A. (2000) Metabolic polymorphisms of importance in biomonitoring. In: Anderson, D., Karakaya, A.E. & Šrám, R.J., eds, *Human Monitoring after Environmental and Occupational Exposure to Chemical and Physical Agents* (NATO Science Series, Series A: Life Sciences No. 313), Amsterdam, IOS Press, pp. 289–299

Norppa, H., Renzi, L. & Lindholm, C. (1993) Detection of whole chromosomes in micronuclei of cytokinesis-blocked human lymphocytes by antikinetochore staining and in situ hybridization. *Mutagenesis*, **8**, 519–525

Norppa, H., Hirvonen, A., Järventaus, H., Uusküla, M., Tasa, G., Ojajärvi, A. & Sorsa, M. (1995) Role of GSTT1 and GSTM1 genotypes in determining individual sensitivity to sister chromatid exchange induction by diepoxybutane in cultured human lymphocytes. *Carcinogenesis*, **16**, 1261–1264

Norppa, H., Bernardini, S., Wikman, H., Järventaus, H., Rosenberg, C., Bolognesi, C. & Hirvonen, A. (2000) Cytogenetic biomarkers in occupational exposure to diisocyanates: influence of genetic polymorphisms of metabolic enzymes. *Environ. mol. Mutag.*, **35** (Suppl. 31), 45

Norppa, H., Lindholm, C., Ojajärvi, A., Salomaa, S. & Hirvonen, A. (2001) Metabolic polymorphisms and frequency of chromosomal aberrations. *Environ. mol. Mutag.*, **37** (Suppl. 32), 58

Obe, G., Vogt, H.-J., Madle, S., Fahning, A. & Heller, W.D. (1982) Double-blind study on the effect of cigarette smoking on the chromosomes of human peripheral blood lymphocytes *in vivo*. *Mutat. Res.*, **92**, 309–319

Odagiri, Y. & Uchida, H. (1998) Influence of serum micronutrients on the incidence of kinetochore-positive or -negative micronuclei in human peripheral blood lymphocytes. *Mutat. Res.*, **415**, 35–45

Pavanello, S. & Clonfero, E. (2000) Biological indicators of genotoxic risk and metabolic polymorphisms. *Mutat. Res.*, **463**, 285–308

Pavanello, S., Gabbani, G., Mastrangelo, G., Brugnone, F., Maccacaro, G. & Clonfero, E. (1999) Influence of GSTM1 genotypes on anti-BPDE–DNA adduct levels in mononuclear white blood cells of humans exposed to PAH. *Int. Arch. environ. Health*, **72**, 238–246

Pelin, K., Hirvonen, A. & Norppa, H. (1996) Influence of erythrocyte glutathione S-transferase T1 on sister chromatid exchanges induced by diepoxybutane in cultured human lymphocytes. *Mutagenesis*, **11**, 213–215

Peluso, M., Airoldi, L., Armelle, M., Martone, T., Coda, R., Malaveille, C., Giacomelli, G., Terrone, C., Casetta, G. & Vineis, P. (1998) White blood cell DNA adducts, smoking, and NAT2 and GSTM1 genotypes in bladder cancer: a case control study. *Cancer Epidemiol. Biomarkers Prev.*, **7**, 341–346

Peluso, M., Airoldi, L., Magagnotti, C., Fiorini, L., Munnia, A., Hautefeuille, A., Malaveille, C. & Vineis, P. (2000) White blood cell DNA adducts and fruit and vegetable consumption in bladder cancer. *Carcinogenesis*, **21**, 183–187

Pemble, S., Schroeder, K.R., Spencer, S.R., Meyer, D.J., Hallier, E., Bolt, H.M., Ketterer, B. & Taylor, J.B. (1994) Human glutathione S-transferase theta (GSTT1): cDNA cloning and the characterization of a genetic polymorphism. *Biochem. J.*, **300**, 271–276

Pitarque, M., Vaglenov, A., Nosko, M., Pavlova, S., Petkova, V., Hirvonen, A., Creus, A., Norppa, H. & Marcos, R. (2002) Sister chromatid exchanges and micronuclei in peripheral lymphocytes shoe factory workers exposed to solvents. *Environ. Health Perspect.*, **110**, 399–404

Pluth, J.M., Nelson, D.O., Ramsey, M.J. & Tucker J.D. (2000a) The relationship between genotype and chromosome aberrations frequencies in a normal adult population. *Pharmacogenetics*, **10**, 311–319

Pluth, J.M., Ramsey, M.J. & Tucker, J.D. (2000b) Role of maternal exposures and newborn genotypes on newborn chromosome aberration frequencies. *Mutat. Res.*, **465**, 101–111

van Poppel, G., de Vogel, N., van Bladeren, P.J. & Kok, F.J. (1992) Increased cytogenetic damage in smokers deficient in glutathione S-transferase isozyme μ. *Carcinogenesis*, **13**, 303–305

van Poppel, G., Verhagen, H., van 't Veer, P. & van Bladeren, P.J. (1993) Markers for cytogenetic damage in smokers: associations with plasma antioxidants and glutathione S-transferase μ. *Cancer Epidemiol. Biomarkers Prev.*, **2**, 441–447

Pressl, S., Edwards, A. & Stephan, G. (1999) The influence of age, sex and smoking habits on the background level of FISH-detected translocations. *Mutat. Res.*, **442**, 89–95

Ramsey, M.J., Moore, D.H., II, Briner, J.F., Lee, D.A., Olsen, L., Senft, J.R. & Tucker, J.D. (1995) The effects of age and lifestyle factors on the accumulation of cytogenetic damage as measured by chromosome painting. *Mutat. Res.*, **338**, 95–106

Ranganathan, V., Heine, W.F., Ciccone, D.N., Rudolph, K.L., Wu, X., Chang, S., Hai, H., Ahearn, I.M., Livingston, D.M., Resnick, I., Rosen, F., Seemanova, E., Jarolim, P., DePinho, R.A. & Weaver, D.T. (2001) Rescue of a telomere length defect of Nijmegen breakage syndrome cells requires NBS and telomerase catalytic subunit. *Curr. Biol.*, **11**, 962–966

Rasnick, D. & Duesberg, P.H. (1999) How aneuploidy affects metabolic control and causes cancer. *Biochem. J.*, **340**, 621–630

Raucy, J.L., Ingelman-Sundberg, M., Carpenter, S., Rannug, A., Rane, A., Franklin, M. & Romkes, M. (1999) Drug metabolizing enzymes in lymphocytes. *J. Biochem. mol. Toxicol.*, **13**, 223–226

Rojas, M., Alexandrov, K., Cascorbi, I., Brockmöller, J., Likhachev, A., Pozharisski, K., Bouvier, G., Auburtin, G., Mayer, L., Kopp-Schneider, A., Roots, I. & Bartsch, H. (1998) High benzo(a)pyrene diol-epoxide DNA adduct levels in lung and blood cells from individuals with combined *CYP1A1 Msp*I/*Msp*I-*GSTM1*0/*0* genotypes. *Pharmacogenetics*, **8**, 109–118

Rojas, M., Cascorbi, I., Alexandrov, K., Kriek, E., Auburtin, G., Mayer, L., Kopp-Schneider, A., Roots, I. & Bartsch, H. (2000) Modulation of benzo(a)pyrene diolepoxide-DNA adduct levels in human blood cells by *CYP1A1*, *GSTM1* and *GSTT1* polymorphism. *Carcinogenesis*, **21**, 35–41

Rupa, D.S., Hasegawa, L. & Eastmond, D.A. (1995) Detection of chromosomal breakage in the 1cen-1q12 region of interphase human lymphocytes using multicolor fluorescence in situ hybridisation with tandem DNA probes. *Cancer Res.*, **55**, 640–645

Ryberg, D., Hewer, A., Phillips, D.H. & Haugen, A. (1994) Different susceptibility to smoking-induced DNA damage among male and female lung cancer patients. *Cancer Res.*, **54**, 5801–5803

Ryberg, D., Skaug, V., Hewer, A., Phillips, D.H., Harries, L.W., Wolf, C.R., Øgreid, D., Ulvik, A., Vu, P. & Haugen, A. (1997) Genotypes of glutathione transferase M1 and P1 and their significance for lung DNA adduct levels and cancer risk. *Carcinogenesis*, **18**, 1285–1289

Salama, S.A., Abdel-Rahman, S.Z., Sierra-Torres, C.H., Hamada, F.A. & Au, W.W. (1999) Role of polymorphic *GSTM1* and *GSTT1* genotypes on NNK-induced genotoxicity. *Pharmacogenetics*, **9**, 735–743

Sasiadek, M., Hirvonen, A., Noga, L., Paprocka-Borowicz, M. & Norppa, H. (1999) Glutathione S-transferase M1 genotype influences sister chromatid exchange induction but not adaptive response in human lymphocytes treated with 1,2-epoxy-3-butene. *Mutat. Res.*, **439**, 207–212

Scarpato, R., Migliore, L., Hirvonen, A., Falck, G. & Norppa, H. (1996) Cytogenetic monitoring of occupational exposure to pesticides: characterization of *GSTM1*, *GSTT1* and *NAT2* genotypes. *Environ. mol. Mutag.*, **27**, 263–269

Scarpato, R., Hirvonen, A., Migliore, L., Falck, G. & Norppa, H. (1997) Influence of *GSTM1* and *GSTT1* polymorphisms on the frequency of chromosome aberrations in lymphocytes of smokers and pesticide-exposed greenhouse workers. *Mutat. Res.*, **389**, 227–235

Schlade-Bartusiak, K., Sasiadek, M. & Kozlowska, J. (2000) The influence of *GSTM1* and *GSTT1* genotypes on the induction of sister chromatid exchanges and chromosome aberrations by 1,2:3,4-diepoxybutane. *Mutat. Res.*, **465**, 69–75

Schröder, K.R., Wiebel, F.A., Reich, S., Dannappel, D., Bolt, H.M. & Hallier, E. (1995) Glutathione-S-transferase (GST) theta polymorphism influences background SCE rate. *Arch. Toxicol.*, **69**, 505–507

Seiler, N., Knodgen, B. & Bartholeyns, J. (1985) Polyamine metabolism and polyamine excretion in normal and tumour bearing rodents. *Anticancer Res.*, **5**, 371–377

Shen, M.R., Jones, I.M. & Mohrenweiser, H. (1998) Nonconservative amino acid substitution variants exist at polymorphic frequency in DNA repair genes in healthy humans. *Cancer Res.*, **58**, 604–608

Shields, P.G., Bowman, E.D., Harrington, A.M., Doan, V.T. & Weston, A. (1993) Polycyclic aromatic hydrocarbon–DNA adducts in lung and cancer susceptibility genes. *Cancer Res.*, **53**, 3486–3492

Smerhovsky, Z., Landa, K., Rössner, P., Brabec, M., Zudova, Z., Hola, N., Pokorna, Z., Mareckova, J. & Hurychova, D. (2001) Risk of cancer in an occupationally exposed cohort with increased level of chromosomal aberrations. *Environ. Health Perspect.*, **109**, 41–45

Smerhovsky, Z., Landa, K., Rössner, P., Juzova, D., Brabec, M., Zudova, Z., Hola, N., Zarska, H. & Nevsimalova, E. (2002) Increased risk of cancer in radon-exposed miners with elevated frequency of chromosomal aberrations. *Mutat. Res.*, **514**, 165–176

Soni, M., Madurantakan, M. & Krishnaswamy, K. (1998) Glutathione S-transferase Mu (GST Mu) deficiency and DNA adducts in lymphocytes of smokers. *Toxicology*, **126**, 155–162

Sonoda, E., Sasaki, M., Morrison, C., Yamaguchi-Iwai, Y., Takata, M. & Takeda, S. (1999) Sister chromatid exchanges are mediated by homologous recombination in vertebrate cells. *Mol. cell. Biol.*, **19**, 5166–5169

Sorsa, M., Osterman-Golkar, S., Peltonen, K., Saarikoski, S.T. & Šrám, R. (1996) Assessment of exposure to butadiene in the process industry. *Toxicology*, **113**, 77–83

Šrám, R.J., Rössner, P., Peltonen, K., Podrazilová, K., Mracková, G., Demopoulos, N.A., Stephanou, G., Vlachodimitropoulos, D., Darroudi, F. & Tates, A.D. (1998) Chromosomal aberrations, sister-chromatid exchanges, cells with high frequency of SCE, micronuclei and comet assay parameters in 1,3-butadiene-exposed workers. *Mutat. Res.*, **419**, 145–154

Šrám, R., Binková, B., Rössner, P., Rubeš, J., Topinka, J. & Dejmek, J. (1999) Adverse reproductive outcomes from exposure to environmental mutagens. *Mutat. Res.*, **428**, 203–215

Stewart, G.S., Maser, R.S., Stankovic, T., Bressan, D.A., Kaplan, M.I., Jaspers, N.G., Raams, A., Byrd, P.J., Petrini, J.H. & Taylor, A.M. (1999) The DNA double-strand break repair gene hMRE11 is mutated in individuals with an ataxia-telangiectasia-like disorder. *Cell*, **99**, 577–587

Strange, R.C. & Fryer, A.A. (1999) The glutathione *S*-transferases: influence of polymorphism on cancer susceptibility. In: Vineis, P., Malats, N., Lang, M., d'Errico, A., Caporaso, N., Cuzick, J. & Boffetta, P., eds, *Metabolic Polymorphisms and Susceptibility to Cancer* (IARC Scientific Publications No. 148), Lyon, IARC*Press*, pp. 231–249

Strange, R.C., Jones, P.W. & Fryer, A.A. (2000) Glutathione *S*-transferase: genetics and role in toxicology. *Toxicol. Lett.*, **112–113**, 357–363

Surrallés, J., Autio, K., Nylund, L., Järventaus, H., Norppa, H., Veidebaum, T., Sorsa, M. & Peltonen, K. (1997) Molecular cytogenetic analysis of buccal cells and lymphocytes from benzene-exposed workers. *Carcinogenesis*, **18**, 817–823

Tang, D.L., Rundle, A., Warburton, D., Santella, R.M., Tsai, W.-Y., Chiamprasert, S., Hsu, Y.Z. & Perera, F.P. (1998) Associations between both genetic and environmental biomarkers and lung cancer: evidence of a greater risk of lung cancer in women smokers. *Carcinogenesis*, **19**, 1949–1953

Tawn, E.J. & Whitehouse, C.A. (2001) Frequencies of chromosome aberrations in a control population determined by G banding. *Mutat. Res.*, **490**, 171–177

Taylor, A.M. (2001) Chromosome instability syndromes. *Best Pract. Res. clin. Haematol.*, **14**, 631–644

Thier, R., Lewalter, J., Kempkes, M., Selinski, S., Brüning, T. & Bolt, H.M. (1999) Haemoglobin adducts of acrylonitrile and ethylene oxide in acrylonitrile workers, dependent on polymorphisms of the glutathione transferases GSTT1 and GSTM1. *Arch. Toxicol.*, **73**, 197–202

Thier, R., Balkenhol, H., Lewalter, J., Selinski, S., Dommermuth, A. & Bolt, H.M. (2001) Influence of polymorphisms of the human glutathione transferases and cytochrome P450 2E1 enzyme on the metabolism and toxicity of ethylene oxide and acrylonitrile. *Mutat. Res.*, **482**, 41–46

Thierens, H., Vral, A. & De Ridder, L. (1996) A cytogenetic study of radiological workers: effect of age, smoking and radiation burden on the micronucleus frequency. *Mutat. Res.*, **360**, 75–82

Uusküla, M., Järventaus, H., Hirvonen, A., Sorsa, M. & Norppa, H. (1995) Influence of GSTM1 genotype on sister chromatid exchanges induced by styrene-7,8-oxide and 1,2-epoxy-3-butene in cultured human lymphocytes. *Carcinogenesis*, **16**, 947–950

Viezzer, C., Norppa, H., Clonfero, E., Gabbani, G., Mastrangelo, G., Hirvonen, A. & Celotti, L. (1999) Influence of *GSTM1*, *GSTT1*, *GSTP1* and *EPHX* gene polymorphisms on DNA adduct level and *HPRT* mutant frequency in coke-oven workers. *Mutat. Res.*, **431**, 259–269

Vlachodimitropoulos, D., Norppa, H., Autio, K., Catalán, J., Hirvonen, A., Tasa, G., Uusküla, M., Demopoulos, N.A. & Sorsa, M. (1997) GSTT1-dependent induction of centromere-negative and -positive micronuclei by diepoxybutane in cultured human lymphocytes. *Mutagenesis*, **12**, 397–403

Vodicka, P., Soucek, P., Tates, A.D., Dusinska, M., Sarmanova, J., Zamecnikova, M., Vodickova, L., Koskinen, M., de Zwart, F.A., Natarajan, A.T. & Hemminki, K. (2001) Association between genetic polymorphisms and biomarkers in styrene-exposed workers. *Mutat. Res.*, **482**, 89–103

Waters, M.D., Stack, H.F. & Jackson, M.A. (1999) Genetic toxicology data in the evaluation of potential human environmental carcinogens. *Mutat. Res.*, **437**, 21–49

Wiencke, J.K., Kelsey, K.T., Lamela, R.A. & Toscano, W.A., Jr (1990) Human glutathione *S*-transferase as a marker of susceptibility to epoxide-induced cytogenetic damage. *Cancer Res.*, **50**, 1585–1590

Wiencke, J.K., Christiani, D.C. & Kelsey, K.T. (1991) Bimodal distribution of sensitivity to SCE induction by diepoxybutane in human lymphocytes.

I. Correlation with chromosomal aberrations. *Mutat. Res.*, **248**, 17–26

Wiencke, J.K., Pemble, S., Ketterer, B. & Kelsey, K.T. (1995) Gene deletion of glutathione *S*-transferase θ: correlation with induced genetic damage and potential role in endogenous mutagenesis. *Cancer Epidemiol. Biomarker Prev.*, **4**, 253–259

Wolff, S. (1991) Biological dosimetry with cytogenetic endpoints. *Prog. clin. biol. Res.*, **372**, 351–362

Wong, R.-H., Wang, J.-D., Hsieh, L.-L., Du, C.-L. & Cheng, T.-J. (1998) Effects on sister chromatid exchange frequency of acetaldehyde dehydrogenase 2 genotype and smoking in vinyl chloride workers. *Mutat. Res.*, **420**, 99–107

Wormhoudt, L.W., Commandeur, J.N. & Vermeulen, N.P. (1999) Genetic polymorphisms of human *N*-acetyltransferase, cytochrome P450, glutathione *S*-transferase, and epoxide hydrolase enzymes: relevance to xenobiotic metabolism and toxicity. *Crit. Rev. Toxicol.*, **29**, 59–124

Wu, F.-Y., Tsai, F.-J., Kuo, H.-W., Tsai, C.-H., Wu, W.-Y., Wang, R.-Y. & Lai, J.-S. (2000) Cytogenetic study of workers exposed to chromium compounds. *Mutat. Res.*, **464**, 289–296

Xu, X., Wiencke, J.K., Niu, T., Wang, M., Watanabe, H., Kelsey, K.T. & Christiani, D.C. (1998) Benzene exposure, glutathione *S*-transferase theta homozygous deletion, and sister chromatid exchanges. *Am. J. ind. Med.*, **33**, 157–163

Yong, L.C., Schulte, P.A., Wiencke, J.K., Boeniger, M.F., Connally, L.B., Walker, J.T., Whelan, E.A. &

Ward, E.M. (2001) Hemoglobin adducts and sister chromatid exchanges in hospital workers exposed to ethylene oxide: effects of glutathione *S*-transferase T1 and M1 genotypes. *Cancer Epidemiol. Biomarkers Prev.*, **10**, 539–550

Zeiger, E. (2001) Mutagens that are not carcinogens: faulty theory or faulty tests? *Mutat. Res.*, **492**, 29–38

Zhang, L., Rothman, N., Wang, Y., Hayes, R.B., Yin, S., Titenko-Holland, N., Dosemeci, M., Wang, Y.Z., Kolachana, P., Lu, W., Xi, L., Li, G.L. & Smith, M.T. (1999) Benzene increases aneuploidy in the lymphocytes of exposed workers: a comparison of data obtained by fluorescence in situ hybridization in interphase and metaphase cells. *Environ. mol. Mutag.*, **34**, 260–268

Zijno, A., Leopardi, P., Marcon, F. & Crebelli, R. (1996) Analysis of chromosome segregation by means of fluorescence in situ hybridization: application to cytokinesis-blocked human lymphocytes. *Mutat. Res.*, **372**, 211–219

Corresponding author
Hannu Norppa
Department of Industrial Hygiene and Toxicology, Finnish Institute of Occupational Health, Topeliuksenkatu 41 aA, 00250 Helsinki, Finland
hannu.norppa@ttl.fi

Mechanisms of Carcinogenesis: Contributions of Molecular Epidemiology
Patricia Buffler, Jerry Rice, Robert Baan, Michael Bird and Paolo Boffetta, eds
IARC Scientific Publications No. 157
International Agency for Research on Cancer, Lyon, 2004

Epidemiological Evaluation of Cytogenetic Biomarkers as Potential Surrogate End-points for Cancer

Lars Hagmar, Ulf Strömberg, Håkan Tinnerberg and Zoli Mikoczy

Summary

Various occupational exposures have been monitored by chromosomal aberrations, sister chromatid exchanges and micronuclei in peripheral
blood lymphocytes. During the last decade, epidemiological studies have evaluated whether any of
these markers foreshadows cancer risk. Results
from Nordic, Italian and Czech cohorts support an
approximately twofold cancer risk among
subjects with high frequencies of chromosomal
aberrations, but no such association was seen for
any of the other biomarkers. The estimated attributable proportion of high frequencies of chromosomal aberrations for overall cancer risk is 0.25,
which gives a quantitative estimate of the chromosomal aberration assay as a surrogate end-
point of cancer. The results from the different
cohort studies are contradictory in terms of
whether or not the predictive value of the chromosomal aberration assay for cancer is differential
with respect to occupational exposure to clastogens. Genetic susceptibility factors are known to
affect the frequency of chromosomal aberrations
in peripheral blood lymphocytes. It is quite
possible that such factors might also affect the frequency of chromosomal aberrations directly or
might modify the impact of exposures to clasto-
gen. There is no other biomarker for general
cancer risk that is applicable to healthy subjects
from the general population with such a high attributable proportion. However, at present only a
simplified and tentative model can be proposed
for the role of the chromosomal aberration marker
in the pathogenesis of cancer.

Introduction

Since the 1960s, various occupational exposures
have been monitored by cytogenetic studies.
Thousands of papers have been published on the
effect of DNA-damaging agents in inducing chromosomal damage assessed by the frequency of
structural chromosomal aberrations in peripheral
blood lymphocytes. As well as chromosomal
aberrations, sister chromatid exchanges and
micronuclei in peripheral blood lymphocytes
have also been used as biomarkers of exposure to
clastogens.

It has been assumed that the macroscopic
damage to chromosomes reflected in the cytogenetic tests indicates an increased probability of
mutational events, which carry an increased risk
for cancer. Some circumstantial evidence has
supported this hypothesis, but no direct proof has
been provided until recent years. During the last
decade, epidemiological studies have evaluated
the predictive value for cancer of all three cytogenetic tests. In this overview, we will outline the
design and results of these studies and also discuss
briefly discuss the implications of the findings
with respect to future research within this field.

Nordic study

In the late 1980s, a cohort of 3182 adult subjects
who had been examined cytogenetically in 10
different laboratories in Sweden, Finland,
Norway or Denmark in 1970–88 was established
by a group of researchers in cytogenetics and epidemiology (Nordic Study Group, 1990a,b). The
inclusion criteria for the cohort are displayed in
Table 1. Of the 3182 subjects included, 1984 had
been studied for chromosomal aberrations, 2019

Table 1. Inclusion criteria employed for the Nordic cohort and the joint Nordic–Italian study base of subjects examined for chromosomal aberrations, sister chromatid exchanges or micronuclei in peripheral blood lymphocytes

Full personal identity

Known date for cytogenetic testing

At least 15 years of age at testing

The test had been performed because of potentially harmful exposures or because the subjects had served as unexposed controls

No cancer diagnosis before cytogenetic testing

for sister chromatid exchanges and 760 for micronuclei.

At least 100 metaphases had been scored with respect to chromosomal aberrations (gaps not included) for each individual. The culture time was 48 or 72 h at the different laboratories. The scoring of mean sister chromatid exchanges, after replication of a DNA template containing bromodeoxyuridine, was based on the analysis of 20–50 cells/individual. The estimate of micronuclei was based on at least 1000 interphase cells. In order to standardize for interlaboratory variation, the results for the different cytogenetic end-points were, for each laboratory and each culture, divided into tertiles: 'low' (1–33rd percentile), 'medium' (34–66th percentile) or 'high' (67–100th percentile) (Nordic Study Group, 1990b).

Linkages to national cancer registries in each country revealed 66 incident cancer cases in the cohort (Hagmar et al., 1994). Standardized incidence ratios (SIRs) were calculated using expected numbers based on age-, gender- and calendar year-specific incidence rates for each country.

Italian study

An Italian cohort was established made up of 1455 subjects examined for chromosomal aberrations in 1965–88 at 10 different laboratories (Bonassi et al., 1995). The inclusion criteria were similar to those employed in the Nordic study, and the subjects were classified in chromosomal aberration tertiles in the same manner as in that

study. Owing to the lack of a nationwide cancer incidence register, cancer mortality was studied instead. The cause of death for deceased subjects was obtained from the municipality of residence. Standardized mortality ratios (SMRs) were calculated by applying age-, sex-, cause- and calendar year-specific death rates of the Italian population.

Results of the two initial cohort studies

In the Nordic study, the SIR for those with 'high' chromosomal aberration frequency was 2.1 (95% CI, 1.5–2.8) as compared with 0.8 (0.5–1.1) for those with 'low' or 'medium' frequencies (Hagmar et al., 1994). In contrast, there was no indication of such an association for sister chromatid exchanges. The observations for micronuclei were too sparse to allow any firm conclusions. In the Italian study, subjects with 'medium' or 'high' chromosomal aberration frequencies had an SMR for overall cancer mortality of 1.8 (1.1–2.8) compared with 0.8 among those with 'low' chromosomal aberration frequencies (Bonassi et al., 1995). Thus, the results from both studies supported the hypothesis that the chromosomal aberration frequency indicated a risk for cancer.

European collaborative study

The results from the independent Nordic and Italian cohort studies supported the notion that chromosomal aberration frequency in peripheral blood lymphocytes may predict cancer. This conclusion was, however, based on relatively few cancer cases. Moreover, the mechanistic rationale for such an association remained obscure. One possibility is that the chromosomal aberration frequency in both peripheral blood lymphocytes and target cells reflects carcinogenic exposure and that these unstable aberrations give rise to chromosomal rearrangements directly involved in the pathogenesis of malignant neoplasms. Another possibility is that the chromosomal aberration frequency merely reflects carcinogenic exposures and that the aberrations observed are not in themselves involved in the mechanistic chain leading to cancer. A third possibility is that the chromosomal aberration frequency reflects individual susceptibility traits for cancer, independently of carcinogenic exposures.

In order to increase the statistical power of the epidemiological analyses and to gain further insights into the mechanistic aspects, a collaborative study was initiated and a joint Nordic and Italian database of cytogenetically examined subjects was created. The same inclusion criteria as those employed in the Nordic study were used (Table 1). The Nordic cohort was the same as that reported previously, but the Italian cohort differed slightly from the earlier one. Altogether, 5271 subjects examined in 1965–88 for at least one cytogenetic biomarker (3540 for chromosomal aberrations, 2702 for sister chromatid exchanges and 1496 for micronuclei) constituted the joint study database (Hagmar et al., 1998a). Each cytogenetic end-point was divided into tertiles as described previously. A more detailed description of the cohorts examined for chromosomal aberrations is given in Table 2. Register linkages for case identification and calculations of expected numbers were made in the same manner as before.

In the Nordic cohort, an elevated SIR of 1.5 (1.1–2.1) for subjects with 'high' chromosomal aberration frequency was observed compared with SIRs of 0.8 for subjects with both 'medium' and 'low' chromosomal aberration frequency levels (Figure 1; Hagmar et al., 1998b). In the Italian cohort, an SMR of 2.0 (1.4–2.9) was obtained for subjects with a 'high' chromosomal aberration frequency level, whereas the SMRs for the 'medium' and 'low' groups were 1.2 and 0.8, respectively (Figure 2). The Italian data on sister

chromatid exchange and cancer mortality were too sparse to allow any conclusion, but, for the 73 subjects from the Nordic cohort who had been monitored for sister chromatid exchanges before their cancer diagnosis, no association was seen between the sister chromatid exchange frequency and subsequent cancer incidence. Neither cancer incidence nor cancer mortality was associated with the outcome of the micronuclei test, however, based on altogether only 27 cancer cases.

Whether factors such as gender, age at test, time since test and country confounded or modified the associations between chromosomal aberrations and cancer incidence and cancer mortality was tested by means of Cox regression modelling. In the Nordic cohort, the adjusted incidence ratio between the 'high' and 'low' chromosomal aberration groups was estimated to be 2.1 (1.3–3.4) (Figure 1). The corresponding Italian mortality ratio was 2.6 (1.4–4.9) (Figure 2). These figures are quite similar to the relative risk estimates obtained for the crude cohort comparisons. None of the potential effect modifiers significantly affected the risk estimates.

Because of the lack of valid data from the original cytogenetic studies, the impact of occupational exposures and smoking habits on the association between chromosomal aberration frequency and cancer risk could not be assessed in the cohort study. In order to solve this problem, a cohort-based case–referent study was carried out. This included all the incident cancer cases and, for each of them, four controls from the cohort,

Table 2. Basic characteristics of the cohort studies evaluating the cancer predictive value of chromosomal aberrations in peripheral blood lymphocytes

Country	N	% females	Median age at test	Inclusion period	Follow-up period	Person–years at risk	Subjects with cancer diagnosis
Sweden	749	27	35	1970–88	1970–93	8687	33
Norway	471	22	38	1970–88	1970–94	6563	30
Finland	557	31	34	1974–88	1974–95	7740	26
Denmark	191	0	39	1987	1987–93	1285	2
Italy	1573	25	39	1965–87	1965–96	55 192	64
Czech Republic	3973	47	36	1975–98	1975–99	37 775	144

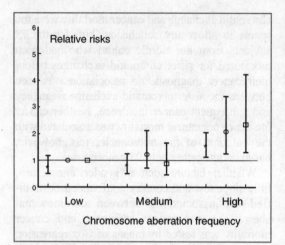

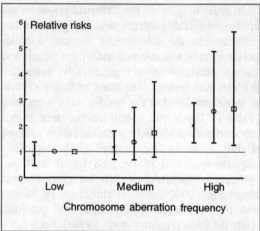

Figure 1. Relative risks for cancer incidence with respect to chromosomal aberration frequency categories in the Nordic cohort. *, standardized incidence ratios (SIRs) for the cohort analysis; O, incidence ratios adjusted for age, gender, country and time since test in a Cox regression analysis; □, odds ratios adjusted for occupational exposure and smoking habits, derived from a cohort-based case–control study. The point estimates for the relative risk measures are given with 95% confidence intervals.

Figure 2. Relative risks for cancer mortality with respect to chromosomal aberration frequency categories in the Italian cohort. *, standardized mortality ratios (SMRs) for the cohort analysis; O, incidence ratios adjusted for age, gender and time since test in a Cox regression analysis; □, odds ratios adjusted for occupational exposure and smoking habits, derived from a cohort-based case–control study. The point estimates for the relative risk measures are given with 95% confidence intervals.

matched with respect to country, gender, calendar year at birth and calendar time at chromosomal aberration testing (Bonassi *et al.*, 2000). Occupational hygienists collected information for the exposure assessment from telephone interviews with cases and controls or, if deceased, with their next of kin with respect to work history and smoking habits. Available exposure measurements, company records, medical records or interviews with former co-workers were also used for the exposure assessment. An exposure matrix was constructed with respect to 22 potentially hazardous occupational agents. Data were analysed with conditional logistic regression models. The chromosomal aberration frequency was clearly associated with smoking habits, but the associations with different measures of occupational exposure were weak and ambiguous. Significant odds ratios above 2 were estimated for the association between 'high' chromosomal aberration frequency and cancer. These odds ratios did not change noticeably when occupational exposure

and smoking habits were included in the models (Nordic cohort — odds ratio, 2.4; 95% CI, 1.3–4.2; Italian cohort — odds ratio, 2.7; 95% CI, 1.3–5.6) (Figures 1 and 2).

Czech Republic study

Another attempt to assess the predictive value of the chromosomal aberration assay for cancer has recently been made in the Czech Republic (Smerhovsky *et al.*, 2001). A cohort or 3973 subjects, examined at least once with the chromosomal aberration assay during the period 1975–98, was followed up until 1999 (Table 2). The inclusion criteria were the same as those in the European collaborative study. The categorization of the individual chromosomal aberration scores followed the previous model in creating tertiles of 'low', 'medium' and 'high', but categorization into quartiles was also used as well as treating the chromosomal aberration score distribution as a continuous variable. Unlike the earlier studies, this categorization was made without standardizing for the four participating laboratories. An important difference with the earlier studies was that in the Czech study, the mean chromosomal aberration score for each subject, calculated from the results of different examinations, and not the result of the first chromosomal aberration score was used for the calculations. In total, 8962 tests were performed on the 3973 subjects.

Adjusting for gender, age at test and occupational exposure (eight broad categories defined on the exposure at the time of cytogenetic testing) using a Cox regression model showed a hazard ratio of 1.6 (1.0–2.4) for those with 'high' chromosomal aberration scores compared with those with 'low' scores. So far, the results were completely in agreement with what had earlier been observed in the Nordic and Italian cohorts. However, when the analysis of the Czech cohort was stratified for exposure, the increased cancer risk for subjects with a 'high' chromosomal aberration score was confined to radon-exposed workers. This is in contrast to the earlier studies, where no significant effect modification of occupational exposure was observed. The potential effect of modification of smoking habits could not be assessed in the Czech study, owing to lack of data on smoking habits.

Taiwan study
Results from a small case–control study nested within a prospective Taiwanese cohort study of inhabitants in an area with arsenic-contaminated well-water supported the hypothesis of differential cancer predictivity between chromosomal and chromatid aberrations in peripheral blood lymphocytes (Liou et al., 1999). The chromosomal aberration frequency at the start of the cohort study was compared for 22 inhabitants who had developed cancer and 21 controls matched for sex, age, smoking habits and residential village. Those who had developed cancer during the 4-year follow-up period had had significantly higher chromosomal aberrations, but not chromatid aberrations, than the controls.

Discussion and conclusions
Results from all available studies clearly indicate that an elevated chromosomal aberration frequency in peripheral blood lymphocytes of healthy subjects predicts increased overall cancer risk. In contrast, available data for sister chromatid exchange and micronuclei assays do not support such predictivity. In the European collaborative study, the classifications of subjects into tertiles for each cytogenetic end-point agreed only poorly (Hagmar et al., 1998c). For those 1553 subjects examined for both chromosomal aberrations and sister chromatid exchanges, the correlation coefficient (κ) was as low as 0.03, and, for those 773 examined for both chromosomal aberrations and micronuclei, it was similarly low ($\kappa = 0.07$). It was therefore expected that the cancer predictivity of the chromosomal aberration assay differed from that of the two other cytogenetic techniques. The cancer predictivity of the micronuclei marker should not, however, be repudiated without careful consideration. The evaluation has been made only for subjects undergoing previous, conventional micronuclei analysis, which has been suggested to be sensitive to variation in lymphocyte proliferation rate (Albertini et al., 2000). No conclusions can therefore be drawn with respect to the cytokinesis-block technique, which is thought to overcome this problem.

A most interesting incoherence in results between the studies performed is that no effect due to occupational exposure is seen in the Nordic or Italian cohorts (Bonassi et al., 2000), whereas, in the Czech cohort, the association between chromosomal aberration frequency and cancer was confined to workers exposed to radon (Smerhovsky et al., 2001). Thus, the results from the Nordic and Italian cohorts support the impact of interindividual differences in susceptibility on chromosomal aberration formation and subsequent cancer risk, whereas the Czech data rather emphasize the role of the chromosomal aberration marker as an intermediate step between exposure to clastogens and cancer risk. There are some methodological differences that have to be considered between the Nordic and Italian cohort studies on the one hand, and the Czech cohort on the other. It can be assumed that the radon-exposed miners in the Czech study might have been more heavily exposed to clastogens than any of the exposure groups in the Nordic and Italian cohorts, but unfortunately this assumption cannot be validated as no exposure data are provided for the Czech study. Moreover, in the Czech cohort no attempt is made to take into account the importance of lifelong occupational exposures (i.e. exposures also before and after the time of cytogenetic testing) or smoking habits. This might result in a differential misclassification of exposure that can be illustrated by some data from the case–control study within the joint Nordic and Italian study base. At time of chromosomal aberration testing 328 subjects were classified as exposed to any of 22 potentially hazardous occupational agents. The remaining 239 subjects were unexposed at time of the test, but 117 of them had been exposed earlier to at least one of the 22 agents. Finally, the use of the mean chromosomal aberration score in the Czech cohort is slightly strange, as the chromosomal aberration frequency measure used for the follow-up study is affected by measurements made not only before but also during the risk period. It is, however, not obvious that any of these methodological discrepancies might explain the different findings in the cohort studies.

It is noteworthy that, in the small study from Taiwan, chromosomal aberrations but not chromatid aberrations had a predictive value for cancer (Liou *et al.*, 1999). Ionizing radiation causes chromosome-type aberrations (Albertini *et al.*, 2000). An interesting question is therefore whether the association between chromosomal aberration frequency and cancer in the Czech cohort study, confined to workers exposed to radon (Smerhovsky *et al.*, 2001), was mediated through chromosomal, but not chromatid, aberrations. In an ongoing follow-up of the Nordic and Italian cohorts, this hypothesis will be tested.

At present only a simplified and tentative model can be proposed for the role of the chromosomal aberration marker in cancer pathogenesis (Figure 3). The relative importance of different factors in this model is not very clear. Chromosomal aberration in peripheral blood lymphocytes is a proxy measure of chromosomal damage in target cells, but we do not know whether this proxy measure is similarly correlated with chromosomal damage in different organs in

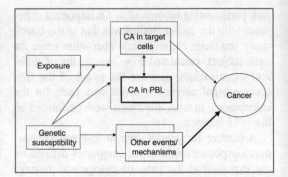

Figure 3. Tentative model of the interplay between clastogenic exposures, genetic susceptibility, chromosomal aberrations (CA) in peripheral blood lymphocytes (PBL) and cancer.

the body. Thus, the cancer predictivity of chromosomal aberrations in peripheral blood lymphocytes may well differ with respect to organ and type of neoplasm. The previous cohort analyses have included too few incident cancer cases to allow a tumour-specific risk assessment. With prolonged follow-up times, such analyses will be available. It will, however, still take a considerable number of years before such analyses can be made in a meaningful way.

Previous studies have suggested that various common polymorphisms of carcinogen-metabolizing enzymes influence both the level of chromosomal damage (cf. Norppa, 1997) and cancer risk (cf. Hirvonen 1999a, 1999b). Furthermore, evidence has started to appear on the association with cancer of the newly discovered polymorphisms of enzymes affecting DNA repair and genome stability (e.g. folate metabolism) (Chen *et al.*, 1996; Ma *et al.*, 1997; Price *et al.*, 1997; Shen *et al.*, 1998; Shinmura *et al.*, 1998; Chen *et al.*, 1999; Ishida *et al.*, 1999; Lunn *et al.*, 1999; Sturgis *et al.*, 1999; Skibola *et al.*, 1999). Genetic susceptibility factors might therefore directly affect the chromosomal aberration frequency in peripheral blood lymphocytes but also modify the impact of exposures on chromosomal aberration formation. Exposure to dietary carcinogens is another tentative factor that might affect both chromosomal aberration formation and cancer risk. In a planned continuation of the European collaborative project, measured relevant genetic polymorphisms in stored cell samples from cancer cases and matched controls from the cohorts will be used to test these hypotheses.

The theme of this paper is whether cytogenetic biomarkers are potential surrogate end-points for cancer. Available data limit this discussion to the role of the chromosomal aberration assay in peripheral blood lymphocytes. If the validity of a surrogate end-point marker for cancer is primarily determined by the extent to which it is a necessary event on the causal pathway to cancer (Schatzkin et al., 1997), the chromosomal aberration marker is not a precise enough surrogate end-point from a cancer screening perspective. The main problem is not the proxy nature of the assay. A biomarker may not be directly on the causal pathway to cancer but may be closely linked to a component of that causal pathway such that it still makes a reasonable surrogate end-point. The problem is rather that both the specificity and the sensitivity of a positive test (defined as being among one third of the subjects with the highest chromosomal aberration frequencies) are too low to enable meaningful cancer screening programmes. On the other hand, from a population perspective, the attributable proportion (AP) of a positive test was as high as 0.25 (based on the assumption of an overall relative risk for cancer of 2 among those with a positive test). In other words, tentatively, around 25% of incident cancer cases could be prevented if 'high' chromosomal aberration frequencies, by some unknown means, could be avoided. It should be emphasized that there is no other biomarker for general cancer risk, applicable to healthy subjects from the general population, with such a high AP. From a mechanistic point of view, an AP substantially lower than 1.0 for the chromosomal aberration test, as in this case, suggests that one or more alternative causal pathways for cancer is indeed operative (Schatzkin et al., 1997).

Acknowledgments

The studies performed within the ESCH collaboration have been supported by grants from European Union Biomed 2 Program (Contract No PL950874), Quality of Life and Management of Living Resources Program (Contract No QLK42-0000-0628), the Swedish Medical Research Council, the Swedish Cancer Society, the Swedish Council for Work Life Research, the Academy of Finland, Associazione Italiana per la Ricerca sul Cancro (AIRC), the Italian Ministry of Health, and the Italian Ministry of the University and Scientific and Technological Research. We are indebted to the other members of the ESCH group: Stefano Bonassi, Department of Environmental Epidemiology, Istituto Nazionale per la Ricerca sul Cancro, Genova, Italy; Alicia Huici Montagud, Centro Nacional de Condiciones de Trabajo, Instituto Nacional de Seguridad e Higiene en el Trabajo, Barcelona, Spain; Allesandra Forni, Dipartimento di Medicina del Lavoro, Clinica del Lavoro 'Luigi Devoto', Milan University, Milan, Italy; Pirjo Heikkilä and Hannu Norppa, Finnish Institute of Occupational Health, Helsinki, Finland; Inger-Lise Hansteen and Saskia Wanders, Department of Occupational and Evironmental Medicine, Telemark Central Hospital, Skien, Norway; Lisbeth E. Knudsen and Peter Wilhardt, Danish National Institute of Occupational Health, Copenhagen, Denmark; Felix Mitelman, Department of Clinical Genetics, and Staffan Skerfving, Department of Occupational and Environmental Medicine, Lund University, Lund, Sweden; Anton Brøgger, Norwegian Radium Hospital, Oslo, Norway; Benkt Högstedt, Department of Occupational Medicine, Central Hospital, Halmstad, Sweden; Christina Reuterwall, National Institute of Work Life, Solna, Sweden; Bo Lambert, Department of Biosciences, CNT/Novum, Karolinska Institute, Stockholm, Sweden; Ingrid Nordenson, National Institute of Work Life, Umeå, Sweden; and Sisko Salomaa, Finnish Centre for Radiation and Nuclear Safety, Helsinki, Finland.

References

Albertini, R.J., Anderson, D., Douglas, G.R., Hagmar, L., Hemminiki, K., Merlo, F., Natarajan, A.T., Norppa, H., Shuker, D.E.G., Tice, R., Waters, M.D. & Aitio, A. (2000) IPCS guidelines for the monitoring of genotoxic effects of carcinogens in humans. Mutat. Res., 463, 111–172

Bonassi, S., Abbondandolo, A., Camurri, L., Dal Prá, L., De Ferrari, M., Degrassi, F., Forni, A.,

Lamberti, L., Lando, C., Padovani, P., Sbrana, I., Vecchio, D. & Puntoni, R. (1995) Are chromosome aberrations in circulating lymphocytes predictive of a future cancer onset in humans? Preliminary results of an Italian cohort study. *Cancer Genet. Cytogenet.*, **79**, 133–135

Bonassi, S., Hagmar, L., Strömberg, U., Huici Montagud, A.H., Tinnerberg, H., Forni, A., Heikkilä, P., Wanders, S., Wilhardt, P., Hansteen, I.-L., Knudsen, L.E. & Norppa, H. (2000) Chromosomal aberrations in lymphocytes predict human cancer independently from exposure to carcinogens. European Study Group on Cytogenetic Biomarkers and Health. *Cancer Res.*, **60**, 1619–1625

Chen, J., Giovannucci, E., Kelsey, K., Rimm, E.B., Stampfer, M.J., Colditz, G.A., Spiegelman, D., Willett, W.C. & Hunter, D.J. (1996) A methylenetetrahydrofolate reductase polymorphism and the risk of colorectal cancer. *Cancer Res.*, **56**, 4862–4864

Chen, J., Giovannucci, E.L. & Hunter, D.J. (1999) MTHFR polymorphism, methyl-replete diets and the risk of colorectal carcinoma and adenoma among US men and women: an example of gene-environment interactions in colorectal tumorigenesis. *J. Nutr.*, **129**, 560s–564s

Hagmar, L., Brøgger, A., Hansteen, I.-L., Heim, S., Högstedt, B., Knudsen, L., Lambert, B., Linnainmaa, K., Mitelman, F., Nordenson, I., Reuterwall, C., Salomaa, S., Skerfving, S. & Sorsa, M. (1994) Cancer risk in humans predicted by increased levels of chromosome aberrations in lymphocytes: Nordic Study Group on the Health Risk of Chromosome Damage. *Cancer Res.*, **54**, 2919–2922

Hagmar, L., Bonassi, S., Strömberg, U., Micoczy, Z., Lando, C., Hansteen, I.L., Huici-Montagud, A., Knudsen, L., Norppa, H., Reuterwall, C., Tinnerburg, H., Brugger, A., Forni, A., Hogstedt, B., Lambert, B., Mittelman, F., Nordenson, I., Salomaa, S. & Skerfving, S. (1998a) Cancer predictive value of cytogenetic markers used in occupational health surveillance programs: a report from an ongoing study by the European Study Group on Cytogenetic Biomarkers and Health (ESCH). *Mutat. Res.*, **405**, 171–178

Hagmar, L., Bonassi, S., Strömberg, U., Brøgger, A., Knudsen, L., Norppa, H. & Reuterwall, C. (1998b) Chromosomal aberrations in lymphocytes predict human cancer – a report from the European Study Group on Cytogenetic Biomarkers and Health (ESCH). *Cancer Res.*, **58**, 4117–4121

Hagmar, L., Bonassi, S., Strömberg, U., Micoczy, Z., Lando, C., Hansteen, I.L., Huici-Montagud, A., Knudsen, L., Norppa, H., Reuterwall, C., Tinnerberg, H., Brøgger, A., Forni, A., Högstedt, B., Lambert, B., Mitelman, F., Nordenson, I., Salomaa, S. & Skerfving, S. (1998c) Cancer predictive value of cytogenetic markers used in occupational health surveillance programs. *Recent Results Cancer Res.*, **154**, 177–184

Hirvonen, A. (1999a) Polymorphic NATs and cancer predisposition. In: Vineis, P., Malats, N., Lang, M., d'Errico, A., Caporaso, N., Cuzick, J. & Boffetta, P., eds, *Metabolic Polymorphisms and Susceptibility to Cancer* (IARC Scientific Publications No. 148), Lyon, IARC*Press*, pp. 251–270

Hirvonen, A. (1999b) Polymorphisms of xenobiotic-metabolizing enzymes and susceptibility to cancer. *Environ. Health Perspect.*, **107** (Suppl 1), 37–47

Ishida, T., Takashima, R., Fukayama, M., Hamada, C., Hippo, Y., Fujii, T., Moriyama, S., Matsuba, C., Nakahori, Y., Morita, H., Yazaki, Y., Kodama, T., Nishimura, S. & Aburatani, H. (1999) New DNA polymorphisms of human MMH/OGG1 gene: prevalence of one polymorphism among lung-adenocarcinoma patients in Japan. *Int. J. Cancer*, **80**, 18–21

Liou, S.H., Lung, J.C., Chen, Y.H., Yang, T., Hsieh, L.L., Chen, C.J. & Wu, T.N. (1999) Increased chromosome-type chromosome aberration frequencies as biomarkers of cancer risk in a blackfoot endemic area. *Cancer Res.*, **59**, 1481–1484

Lunn, R.M., Langlois, R.G., Hsieh, L.L., Thompson, C.L. & Bell, D.A. (1999) XRCC1 polymorphisms: effect on aflatoxin B_1-DNA adducts and glycophorin A variant frequency. *Cancer Res.*, **59**, 2557–2561

Ma, J., Stampfer, M.J., Giovannucci, E., Artigas, C., Hunter, D.J., Fuchs, C., Willett, W.C., Selhub, J., Hennekens, C.H. & Rozen, R. (1997) Methylenetetrahydrofolate reductase polymorphism, dietary interactions, and risk of colorectal cancer. *Cancer Res.*, **57**, 1098–1102

Nordic Study Group on the Health Risk of Chromosome Damage (1990a) An inter-Nordic prospective study on cytogenetic endpoints and cancer risk. *Cancer Genet. Cytogenet.*, **45**, 85–92

Nordic Study Group on the Health Risk of Chromosome Damage (1990b) A Nordic data base on somatic chromosome damage in humans. *Mutat. Res.*, **241**, 325–337

Norppa, H. (1997) Cytogenetic markers of susceptibility: influence of polymorphic carcinogen-metabolizing enzymes. *Environ. Health Perspect.*, **105** (Suppl. 4), 829–835

Price, E.A., Bourne, S.L., Radbourne, R., Lawton, P.A., Lamerdin, J., Thompson, L.H. & Arrand, J.E. (1997) Rare microsatellite polymorphisms in the DNA repair genes XRCC1, XRCC3 and XRCC5 associated with cancer in patients of varying radiosensitivity. *Somat. cell. mol. Genet.*, **23**, 237–247

Schatzkin, A., Freedman, L.S., Dorgan, J., McShane, L., Schiffman, M.H. & Dawsey, S.M (1997) Using and interpreting surrogate end-points in cancer research. In: Toniolo, P., Boffetta, P., Shuker, D.E.G, Rothman, N., Hulka, B. & Pearce N., eds, *Application of Biomarkers in Cancer Epidemiology* (IARC Scientific Publications No. 142), Lyon, IARC*Press*, pp. 265–271

Shen, M.R., Jones, I.M. & Mohrenweiser, H. (1998) Nonconservative amino acid substitution variants exist at polymorphic frequency in DNA repair genes in healthy humans. *Cancer Res.*, **58**, 604–608

Shinmura, K., Kohno, T., Kasai, H., Koda, K., Sugimura, H. & Yokota, J. (1998) Infrequent mutations of the hOGG1 gene, that is involved in the excision of 8-hydroxyguanine in damaged DNA, in human gastric cancer. *Jpn J. Cancer Res.*, **89**, 825–828

Skibola, C.F., Smith, M.T., Kane, E., Roman, E., Rollinson, S., Cartwright, R.A. & Morgan, G. (1999) Polymorphisms in the methylenetetrahydrofolate reductase gene are associated with susceptibility to acute leukemia in adults. *Proc. natl Acad. Sci. USA*, **96**, 12810–12815

Smerhovsky, Z., Landa, K., Rossner, P., Brabec, M., Zudova, Z., Hola, N., Pokorna, Z., Mareckova, J. & Hurychova, D. (2001) Risk of cancer in an occupationally exposed cohort with increased level of chromosomal aberrations. *Environ. Health Perspect.*, **109**, 41–45

Sturgis, E.M., Castillo, E.J., Li, L., Zheng, R., Eicher, S.A., Clayman, G.L., Strom, S.S., Spitz, M.R. & Wei, Q. (1999) Polymorphisms of DNA repair gene XRCC1 in squamous cell carcinoma of the head and neck. *Carcinogenesis*, **20**, 2125–2129

Corresponding author:

L. Hagmar
Department of Occupational and Environmental Medicine, University Hospital,
22185 Lund, Sweden
lars.hagmar@ymed.lu.se

Mechanisms of Carcinogenesis: Contributions of Molecular Epidemiology
Patricia Buffler, Jerry Rice, Robert Baan, Michael Bird and Paolo Boffetta, eds
IARC Scientific Publications No. 157
International Agency for Research on Cancer, Lyon, 2004

Implications of Results of Molecular Epidemiology on DNA Adducts, their Repair and Mutations for Mechanisms of Human Cancer

Kari Hemminki and William G. Thilly

Summary

This review covers human data on DNA adducts, their repair and induced mutations. The new data on human studies *in vivo* challenge some widely held notions relating to cancer and ageing. These data collected from humans of different ages show no age-dependent change in levels of diverse DNA adducts in peripheral lymphocytes, no deterioration of global DNA excision repair in skin *in situ* and no change in mutation rate, because the *HPRT* mutant fraction increases linearly by age. These molecular epidemiological results argue against earlier animal and in-vitro data, but are in line with multistage models for cancer. A further application of DNA adducts as an intermediary tool for genotyping studies, for both metabolic enzyme and DNA repair system genotypes, is recommended. As the common polymorphisms are likely to cause at most moderate increases in the risk of cancer, the intermediary adduct end-point is a necessary proof of causal relationships. The mechanistic data on the mutational spectra induced by important human DNA adducts may be helpful in the characterization, not only of carcinogenic exposures, but also of protective factors, such as dietary ingredients. Examples are shown of the application of mutational spectra on the von Hippel Lindau (*VHL*) gene in kidney cancer in relation to dietary intake. Some fruit and vegetables provide protection against mutations and the effect is stronger among smokers who have both endogenous and exogenous mutagenic exposures.

Introduction

The field of molecular epidemiology has developed during the last decade as tools have become available for the assay of relevant biomarkers in humans. The study of DNA adducts has moved from the chemical characterization of new types of adducts to the understanding of their biology and levels in human tissues. It was in the 1990s that quantitative methods first became available for the study of chemically defined DNA adducts in humans. Complex mechanisms for DNA repair have been characterized, and a number of cancer syndromes have been linked to deficiencies in DNA repair. In replicating cells, DNA adducts may cause mutations, and great hopes have been expressed for interpreting tumour-specific mutations to the agents causing them. In this chapter, we review some mechanistic aspects of DNA adducts and their repair, and challenge some concepts relating to cancer and ageing that do not seem to withstand the evidence from human studies *in vivo*. We will also describe how certain types of DNA damage may be expressed as mutations and how mutational spectra of the *VHL* gene can be used in the molecular epidemiology of kidney cancer.

Multistage carcinogenesis and ageing

Understanding of the carcinogenic mechanisms has increased enormously in the past 10–15 years. The old epidemiological findings about the multistage nature of human cancer, based on the analysis of age–incidence relationships, have gained substance, and tens of cancer-related genes have been identified (Armitage & Doll, 1957; Hanahan & Weinberg, 2000). There is overwhelming evidence that mutations in oncogenes and tumour suppressor genes play a role in the carcinogenic process. Mutations constitute an axiomatic proof for a gene to be cancer-related: segregation with or altered expression in affected individuals need to be demonstrated in a family pedigree. The detection of germline mutations in tumour-related genes in families affected by hereditary cancer-prone syndromes and reproduction of cancer phenotypes in studies with tumour suppressor gene knockout animals provide evidence for the essential role of these genes in cancer development (Fearon, 1997).

According to the multistage theory of cancer, the clonal tumour emerges as a result of two or more mutations in a single cell (Armitage & Doll, 1954, 1957; Moolgavkar & Knudson, 1981; Moolgavkar & Luebeck, 1992; Herrero-Jimenez et al., 1998; Herrero-Jimenez et al., 2000; Hemminki & Mutanen, 2001; Loeb, 2001). The first mutation(s) occur in normal cells creating a slowly growing preneoplastic colony. Additional changes in a cell of the preneoplastic colony are believed to be necessary to create a neoplastic cell capable of growing as a tumour without further rate-limiting genetic changes. The number of required mutations may vary and probably depends on the genes and tissues affected. An initial mutant clone may arise and thus increase the target size for subsequent promotional mutations. It is important for the present discussion that the adoption of known mutation rates, number of stem cells and normal human life-span can accommodate a carcinogenic process with three or more mutations, for instance two in the initiation stage and one or more in the promotional stage (Herrero-Jimenez et al., 1998, 2000). Even though research into ageing, often through in-vitro and experimental animal studies, has suggested a number of metabolic processes that deteriorate with advancing age, including increasing oxidative damage, decreasing DNA repair and detoxification, these need not be invoked for understanding of the carcinogenic process. Ageing is commensurate with accumulation of mutations, and the known mutation rates appear to be sufficient to explain fully cancer formation in humans.

A large body of human in-vivo mutation data exists on the hypoxanthine-guanine phosphoribosyltransferase gene (HPRT), which shows a linear increase in mutant fraction (mutants/all cells) by age (Cole & Skopek, 1994; Podlutsky et al., 1999; Herrero-Jimenez et al., 2000). Data on 740 individuals, collected from several studies, are shown in Figure 1 (Herrero-Jimenez et al., 2000). This increase is compatible with a constant mutation rate (mutants/time, calculated in Figure 1 to be 2.1×10^{-7} HPRT mutants per cell year) on lymphopoietic stem cells over the human lifespan. In contrast, any cumulative process that increased with age would give an exponential, supralinear increase in mutant fraction. These data provide strong evidence against age-induced metabolic deterioration, and some direct evidence against such deterioration will be given below. A further question is the cause of the HPRT mutations. This remains unsettled, but the available data show little if any difference in the pattern of mutations among the young and the old, suggesting that the mutagenic process is largely independent of age (Podlutsky et al., 1999), and arguing further against age-induced 'catabolism'.

DNA adducts in humans

Over the years, a great deal of discussion has been devoted to the relationships of DNA adducts and risk of cancer (Hemminki, 1993; Hemminki et al., 2000a; Vineis & Perera, 2000; Hemminki et al., 2001a). Although there are no solid human data to resolve the question, the putative role of DNA adducts in causing mutations is the basis for their mechanistic links to cancer. However, cancer is a multistage disease affecting many genes, as discussed above, and the likelihood of targeting adducts to many critical genes and transforming them to mutations in sensitive tissues is always very small. The often heard argument that 'DNA adducts are not important for cancer because they are found at equal levels in target and non-target organs' is comparable to claiming that retinoblastoma gene mutations are not important in cancer because in members of retinoblastoma

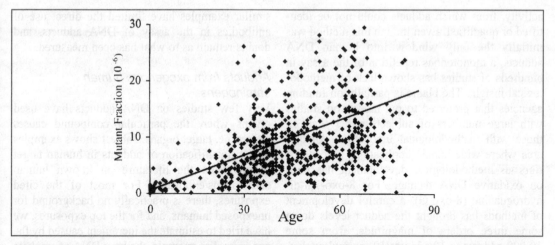

Figure 1. Human lymphocyte HPRT mutations in relation to age of the 740 subjects included; the slope shows the derived average constant mutation rate of 2.1×10^{-7} mutations per cell year (Herrero-Jimenez *et al.*, 2000).

families they occur in all cells but cause only eye cancers.

Successes and failures in adduct identification

Quantification of low levels of DNA adducts in humans requires sophisticated methods with high sensitivity and specificity. Consequently, the detection of DNA adducts in humans has so far been limited to fewer than 30 specific adducts (Hemminki *et al.*, 2000a). The useful methods include ^{32}P-postlabelling, fluorescence detection methods, gas chromatography/mass spectrometry (GC/MS) and immunoassay. Each method has advantages and disadvantages, depending on the type of adduct studied. DNA adducts have been determined in humans exposed to environmental, occupational, medicinal, lifestyle and endogenous sources of mutagens. The tissues obtained for adduct analysis are the total white blood cells or peripheral blood lymphocytes, which are readily accessible from humans. Other tissues that have been used include skin, placenta, kidney, liver, lung, breast and pancreas.

At present, the ^{32}P-postlabelling technique is the most versatile method, but it does not provide structural identification. This deficiency is mended by using structurally characterized standards of adducts as internal or external markers. Examples

of quantification with the help of adduct standards include 7-methyl-guanine (G), 7-hydroxyethyl-G (Zhao *et al.*, 1999), 1,3-butadiene (Zhao *et al.*, 2000), acrolein and crotonaldehyde DNA adducts (Nath *et al.*, 1996), the heterocyclic aromatic amine PhIP (Friesen *et al.*, 1994) and UV-photo-products (Bykov *et al.*, 1998). Mass spectrometry (MS) is more useful as a tool for the structural characterization of adducts, but relatively large quantities of DNA are required for analysis. MS has been applied to human biomonitoring in the analysis of DNA adducts of PhIP (Friesen *et al.*, 1994), 4-aminobiphenyl (Lin *et al.*, 1994) and malondialdehyde (Chaudhary *et al.*, 1994). Very few calibration studies have been carried out using different methods. Among the few, the coded comparisons between GC/MS and ^{32}P-post-labelling methods on 7-alkylguanine adducts of ethylene oxide in rat tissues showed excellent qualitative agreement between the methods and the laboratories, with a correlation coefficient of about 0.95 (Eide *et al.*, 1999).

However, there have also been less successful aspects of the assay of human DNA adducts. The postlabelling method was initially developed by Randerath and co-workers to analyse bulky aromatic types of DNA adducts using thin-layer chromatography. When applied to human samples, the results were diffuse smears of radioactivity, from which adducts could not be identified or quantified. Even though this method was initially the only window into human DNA adducts, a monotonous repetition of the assay in hundreds of studies has shown lack of methodological insight. The blame is partially on funding agencies that preferred to put money on studies with large numbers of subjects rather than on those with methodological innovation. Another area where wide human applications preceded a rigorous methodological development has been on oxidative DNA damage. For 8-oxo-7,8-dihydroguanine (8-oxo-G), a careful development of methods has brought the adduct levels down some three orders of magnitude, from some 10 000 adducts to 10 adducts/10^8 normal nucleotides, and the final call on the true human tissue levels is yet to come (Helbock *et al.*, 1998; Frelon *et al.*, 2000; Pouget *et al.*, 2000). Even though the problems in the analysis of 8-oxo-G were known for a long time, tens of papers were published and statements were made about the significance of this adduct in human disease and ageing (Helbock *et al.*, 1998; Beckman *et al.*, 2000). Even the earlier data on age-dependent decline in repair of 8-oxo-G in experimental animals have not held against the recent evidence (de Souza-Pinto *et al.*, 2001a,b). A third area where a careful comparison of methods identified a major problem was in the use of antibodies to DNA adducts (Fichtinger-Schepman *et al.*, 1989). Neither this nor other

similar examples have limited the direct use of antibodies in the assay of DNA adducts, and doubts remain as to what has been measured.

Adducts from exogenous human carcinogens

Very few studies on DNA adducts have used organs where the particular compound causes cancer, i.e. target organs. Table 1 shows examples of the quantification of adducts in human target tissues from the literature on known human carcinogens/exposures. For most of the cited exposures, there is practically no background for unexposed humans, and for the top exposures, we have tried to estimate the increment caused by the exposure. For example, the lung DNA of smokers contains methylation and hydroxyethylation products and benzo[*a*]pyrene-type adducts at levels 100 and 10 adducts/10^8 normal nucleotides, respectively. Benzidine, a potent bladder carcinogen, and PhIP, a food-derived heterocyclic aromatic amine associated with colorectal cancer, have been found at a level of 3 adducts/10^8 normal nucleotides, and the tamoxifen adduct is present in endometrial tissue at 0.3/10^8 normal nucleotides. An erythemal dose of UV induces dipyrimidine dimers in skin at 1000/10^8 normal nucleotides. The high level of UV damage in human DNA is a likely reason for UV carcinogenesis and for the extreme sensitivity of Xeroderma pigmentosum patients to solar UV-induced skin cancer.

Table 1. Levels of human DNA adducts in target organs by exogenous human carcinogens

Adduct	Tissue	Level (per 10^8 bases)	Exposure
7-Methyl-G	Lung	100	Smokers
7-Hydroxyethyl-G	Lung	10	Smoker
Benzo[*a*]pyrene-G	Lung	10	Smoker
Benzidine-G	Urothelium	3	Dye workers
1,3-Butadiene-A	Lymphocyte	0.5	Production
PhIP-G	Colon	3	Roasted meat
Tamoxifen-DNA	Endometrium	0.3	ca. 40 mg/d
Cyclobutane T = T	Skin	1000	400 J/m² UV

Modified from Hemminki *et al.* (2000a). A, adenine; G, guanine; T, thymine; T = T, cyclobutane dimer.

The background levels of 7-methyl-guanine (G) and 7-hydroxyethyl-G in human DNA are approximately similar to those cited in Table 1, i.e. smoking can almost double the levels of the adducts (Zhao et al., 1999). 7-Hydroxyethyl-G is likely to be the result of lipid peroxidation, releasing ethene as an end-product, which in turn undergoes oxidation to ethylene oxide. Other endogenous adducts are 8-oxo-G and etheno adducts. As discussed above, the true levels of 8-oxo-G adducts in humans have not been established but in cultured cells they are present from a non-detectable level to some 10 adducts/10^8 normal nucleotides (Beckman et al., 2000; Frelon et al., 2000; Pouget et al., 2000). A number of different types of etheno adducts exist and they are present at levels of $1/10^8$ normal nucleotides, but with a wide range (Nair et al., 1997; Kadlubar et al., 1998). Although some authors have considered only endogenous DNA damage to be a major factor in human cancer, the conclusion could be misleading because these authors used their own results, with 8-oxo-G levels probably 1000 times too high, as the point of reference (Ames et al., 1995; Helbock et al., 1998; Beckman et al., 2000).

Adducts and ageing

Considering the generally held view that ageing is associated with metabolic deterioration (Helbock et al., 1998), it is surprising that few human DNA adduct studies have tested the association of adduct levels and age. In a series of studies on lung cancer cases and controls, presenting with a large age-range, lymphocyte DNA adducts and HPRT mutations were determined (Figure 2). The adducts constituted aromatic products which were detected by the postlabelling method. Among the 343 subjects, HPRT mutant fractions increased linearly with age whereas for DNA adducts a weak but significant opposite trend was observed (Hou et al., 1999). The negative correlation was due to never or former smokers and controls; smoking controls showed no trend and smoking cases showed a significant positive age effect. In a later study, the latter association was found to be due to certain metabolic genotypes (Hou et al., 2001). The conclusion from these studies was

that, among healthy subjects, independent of their smoking status, lymphocyte aromatic DNA adducts were not positively correlated with age.

We have recently carried out an ad-hoc study to test the effect of age on the assumed endogenous adducts of 7-methyl-G and 7-hydroxymethyl-G in lymphocytes of healthy individuals. As was discussed for Table 1, these DNA adducts are among the most abundant background adducts detected in humans and animals. The data for 34 individuals are shown in Figure 3 (Zhao & Hemminki, 2002). There was a large inter-individual variation between adduct levels: 20-fold for 7-methyl-G and 15-fold for 7-hydroxyethyl-G. The results show that no age dependence can be observed in these chemically defined endogenous adducts. The data shown in Figures 2 and 3 provide strong evidence that the levels of these types of DNA adducts in peripheral lymphocytes are either independent of or decrease with age. The qualification is that lymphocytes are dormant cells, probably with slow DNA repair activity.

Adduct, phenotype and genotype

In addition to being indicators for exposure, DNA adducts appear to be excellent tools in carcinogen metabolism and DNA repair work (as shown later). However, this area has been underdeveloped because the methods for adduct determination have not been available for specific adducts in humans. Large amounts of work have been devoted to studying relationships between metabolic phenotypes or genotypes and cancer, with an implied assumption that DNA-damaging metabolites are involved (Vineis et al., 1999a). The results have been a bewildering collection of contradictory data. Recently, however, when specific DNA methods have been applied, coherent results on the effects of certain metabolic genotypes have emerged (Bartsch et al., 1998; Lunn et al., 1999; Thompson et al., 1999).

DNA repair

The sequencing work on the human genome is approaching completion and the compiled map has been published (International Human Genome Sequencing Consortium, 2001; Venter et al., 2001). Just over 1% of the human genome

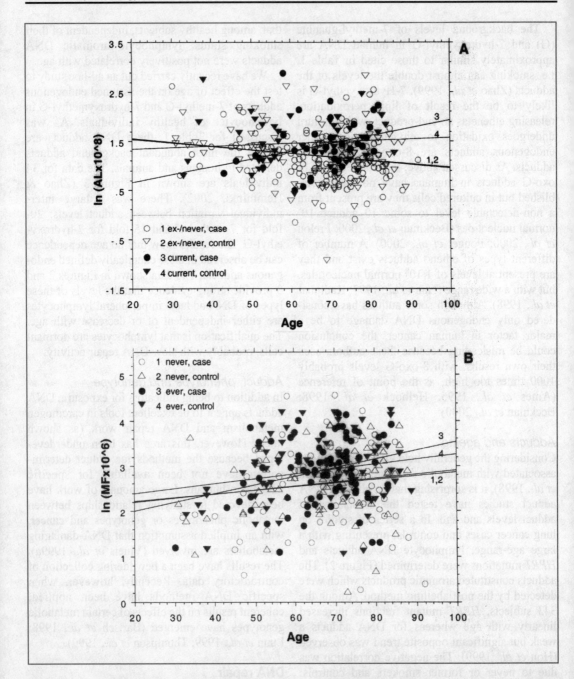

Figure 2. Age dependence of aromatic type of DNA adducts (A) and HPRT mutant frequency (B) in lymphocytes from 4 groups of subjects (numbered 1–4) separated by smoking and lung cancer status (*n*, 35–136). Each point represents one individual; the numbered regression lines refer to the specific group (Hou *et al.*, 1999). In A, the decrease in adduct levels by age was significant for the total population (*p* = 0.03), and for groups 1 and 2 (*p* = 0.04 and 0.01, respectively).

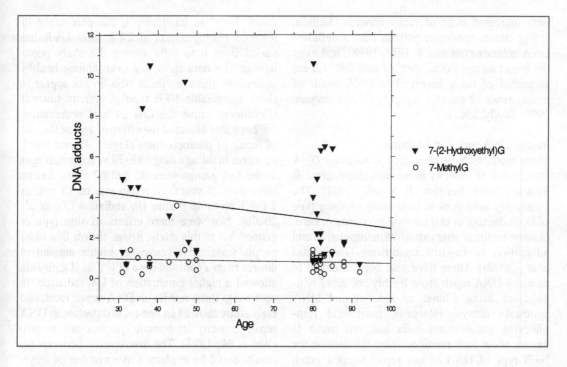

Figure 3. The level of in-vivo 7-methyl-G and 7-(2-hydroxyethyl)-G DNA adducts assayed in human lymphocytes and correlated with the age of the subject (Zhao & Hemminki, 2002). The slopes were not significant.

codes for proteins, and these sequences are the primary targets for mutations. Many DNA repair processes exist, and at least 130 genes are known to take part in human DNA repair (Wood *et al.*, 2001). UV-induced DNA damage and many bulky DNA lesions are repaired by means of the nucleotide excision repair (NER) enzyme system, which is a complex process involving about 30 different gene products (Balajee & Bohr, 2000). NER contains two sub-pathways, global genomic repair and transcription-coupled repair. The latter process surveys the small proportion of transcribed genes in any particular cell; as only 1% of the genome codes for proteins, and only a small proportion is active, transcription-coupled repair surveys perhaps of the order of 0.1% of the genome, depending on the cell type and physiological and developmental state. Transcription-coupled repair works on the transcribed strand of DNA, which is the cause for mutations often being targeted on the non-transcribed strand of

DNA (Greenblatt *et al.*, 1994; Podlutsky *et al.*, 1999; Balajee & Bohr, 2000; Hainault & Hollstein, 2000; Spatz *et al.*, 2001).

Many DNA repair deficiency syndromes involve vast increases in risk of cancer (Balajee & Bohr, 2000). Xeroderma pigmentosum patients experience some 1000-fold increase in the incidence of non-melanoma skin cancer and melanoma (Spatz *et al.*, 2001). Hereditary non-polyposis colorectal cancer (HNPCC), due to germline DNA mismatch repair gene mutations, predisposes affected individuals to a 70-fold excess risk of colorectal and endometrial cancer (Aarnio *et al.*, 1999). This syndrome is characterized by genetic instability at simple DNA repeat sequences because of DNA mismatch repair deficiency (Lynch & de la Chapelle, 1999). The tumour suppressor gene *TP53* has a role in arresting the cell cycle after DNA damage and thus allowing time for DNA repair; a germline mutation in the Li–Fraumeni families is consonant with increased risks of many cancers (Malkin, 1998). Bloom syndrome patients have a deficient DNA helicase (German & Ellis, 1998), and even the breast cancer genes, *BRCA1* and *BRCA2*, are suspected of being involved in DNA repair or maintenance of genome integrity (Venkitaraman, 1999; Scully, 2001).

In-situ DNA repair in humans

Many methods have been used to measure DNA repair rates or capacity in humans (Benhamou & Sarasin, 2000; Berwick & Vineis, 2000). The commonly used ones include assay of some type of DNA damage or cell survival in culture *in vitro*, in some methods after extensive manipulation and adaptation to in-vitro conditions (Hemminki *et al.*, 2000b). There have also been attempts to measure DNA repair from freshly collected lymphocytes using Comet or unscheduled DNA synthesis assays. However, peripheral lymphocytes are dormant cells and not much is known about their repair activity; the data on the NER type of DNA adduct repair suggest much slower rates than in skin (cf. Hou *et al.*, 1999). As a 'gold standard' of DNA repair has been lacking, it has not been possible to validate any of the methods used. An in-situ DNA repair method has been developed based on the above ^{32}P-post-labelling technique: volunteers are exposed to one or a few erythemal dose(s) of UV radiation and skin biopsies are taken after various periods of time to show the rate of removal of photoproducts. Based on this method, 50% of the damage was removed in some 20 h for cyclobutane dimers and in 5 h for 6–4 photoproducts (Bykov *et al.*, 1999). However the repair process is composed of many components and in recent experiments unrepaired T = T dimers have been detected even 3 weeks after exposure (Hemminki *et al.*, 2002a; Zhao *et al.*, 2002). As the method measures total DNA repair, it reflects global genomic repair.

We have used this method to study some parameters and skin diseases in relation to the rate of repair in humans *in situ*. The heterogeneity of global genomic repair of photoproducts has displayed substantial interindividual rate differences in these studies (Xu *et al.*, 2000a,b,c). Taking a

dimer T = C as an example, the percentage of repaired photoproducts at 24 h after UVR has varied from 0 to 90% among the study populations. The data show that even among healthy individuals there are those who do not appear to show appreciable NER type of activity towards UV dimers within the first 24 h of observation. We have also assessed the effect of age on the rate of repair of photoproducts (Figure 4), and found no effect in the age range 32–78 years (mean ages in the two groups were 42 and 63 years, i.e. no more than 21 years) on repair rate of TT = C or TT = T up to 48 h after UV radiation (Xu *et al.*, 2000b). Nor were there effects of skin type or gender. Yet in this study, it was shown that older people sustained a somewhat higher amount of dimers from a constant dose of UV, as if their skin allowed a higher penetration of UV radiation. In contrast to these results on DNA repair rates, one early study showed an age-related decline in DNA repair capacity in human lymphocytes *in vitro* (Wei *et al.*, 1993). The discrepancy between the results could be explained in a number of ways: different methods (in-situ rate or in-vitro capacity) or different cell types (epidermal cells or in-vitro stimulated lymphocytes). However, there is hardly any doubt as to which types of experiments are most relevant for repair of UV-induced DNA damage in human skin.

We have measured the rate of global genomic repair in sporadic melanoma and basal-cell carcinoma patients but we observed no difference between the patients and matched controls up to 48 h, and recently among melanoma patients up to 3 weeks (Xu *et al.*, 2000a,c). The results suggest that these patient groups are not deficient in the NER type of global genomic repair, and they disagree with previous studies using indirect in-vitro methods (reviewed by Berwick & Vineis, 2000). Obviously the data are not informative about transcription-coupled repair because that would account for such a small proportion of the total repair and would go unnoticed in the present experiments.

DNA repair genotypes

Polymorphisms have been found in many genes coding for DNA repair proteins, including those

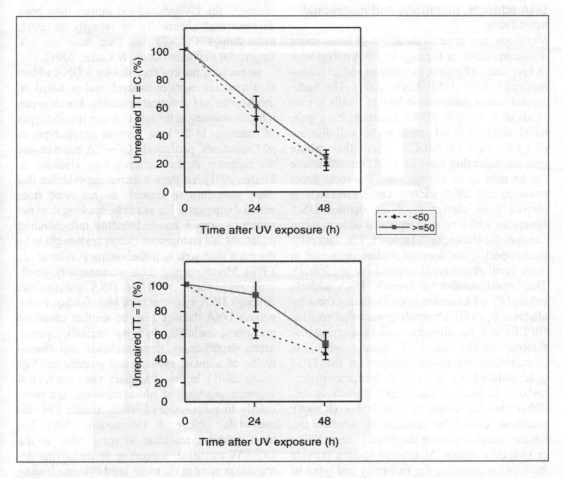

Figure 4. Repair of 2 cyclobutane dimers (TT=C, top and TT=T bottom) in human skin *in situ* among 16 subjects < 50 years of age (mean age, 42 years) and 13 older subjects (mean age, 63 years). The results are means and standard errors for the percentage of dimer remaining unrepaired after 24 and 48 h (Xu *et al.*, 2000b). The only significant difference (*p* < 0.05) was for TT=T at 24 h.

involved in the NER process, and the data are accumulating rapidly (Shen *et al.*, 1998). As a result, many genotypes will be ascertained without data on their functional significance, the same dilemma that was discussed in the context of metabolic genotypes. Again there is a temptation to test the effects of the genotypes against cancers, because genotyping a group of patients and controls is easier than finding out whether a genotype changes DNA repair function. As in the metabolic area, the result will be numerous false-positive associations.

Testing of the DNA repair genotypes with the DNA repair assay is a functional test and it is highly relevant to global genomic repair because the assay is carried out on humans. We have applied this so far to *XPD* and *XPG* polymorphisms. Exon 23, codon 751 A to C polymorphism in the *XPD* gene showed a decreased repair in the repair assay, and the results on lung and head and neck cancers appear to show that this may be a susceptibility genotype (Sturgis *et al.*, 2000; Hemminki *et al.*, 2001b; Spitz *et al.*, 2001).

DNA adducts, mutations and mutational specificity

Mutations may arise when adducted bases cause misincorporation or slippage by DNA polymerase in a replicative by-pass, or when an adduct is mis-repaired (Thilly, 1983; Loeb, 2001). The background rate of mutations in human T cells *in vivo* is about 7×10^{-11} *HPRT* mutations/base pair, which amounts to 0.4 mutations per cell division $(7 \times 10^{-11} \cdot 6 \times 10^9 = 0.42)$ over the whole genome, assuming that the *HPRT* mutation rate can be used as an average rate. The most direct evidence that DNA adducts cause mutations is derived from studies involving defined DNA sequences with single incorporated adducts using site-specific techniques (Table 2). The data refer to site-specific mutagenesis studies, discussed in more detail elsewhere (Hemminki *et al.*, 2000a). The largest number of specific DNA adducts induce GC→TA transversions, including those by aflatoxin B_1 (AFB$_1$), benzo[*a*]pyrene diol epoxide (BPDE) and the aromatic amines acetylamino-fluorene (AAF) and PhIP. Recent work has characterized mutational hotspots in the *TP53* gene induced by polycyclic aromatic hydro-carbons in lung carcinogenesis (Smith *et al.*, 2000). Another common type is the GC→AT transition, caused for example by nitrosoureas, tobacco-specific nitroso compounds (e.g. NNK) or oxidative agents. Mutational spectra provide information regarding the frequency and types of mutations that arise from a particular DNA damaging agent. However, linking a specific adduct to a mutation may be difficult because a particular DNA-reactive agent usually reacts at several sites in DNA to generate a variety of adducts. For example, mutational spectra related to oxidative DNA damage have most commonly revealed GC→AT transitions and GC→TA trans-versions (Wang *et al.*, 1998). The assessment of these lesions from the mutational spectra is espe-cially difficult, if not impossible, because of the multiplicity of lesions formed by an oxidative agent. However, by using single lesion substrates, it has been possible to relate 8-oxo-G adducts to GC→TA mutations, and 5-hydroxy-deoxycyti-dine, 5-hydroxy-deoxyuridine, and uridine glycol to GC→AT mutations (Wang *et al.*, 1998). Inte-restingly, the UV-induced CC dimers have been demonstrated chemically as recently as 2001, even though CC→TT has long been the UV fingerprint mutation (Douki & Cadet, 2001).

In humans, the evidence linking a DNA adduct to a mutation is more indirect, and is based on mechanistic and statistical reasoning. For example, tobacco smoking is thought to cause specific types of mutations in the lung, because certain types of *p53* mutations, particularly GC→TA transversion, are common in the smoker's lung (Hainaut & Pfeifer, 2001). Yet there is increasing evidence that many mutations in humans do not arise from external exposures. For example, smoking does not appear to increase human bronchial mitochondrial mutations and endogenous factors are thought to be the main mutagens in mitochondria (Coller *et al.*, 1998). Mutations may arise spontaneously, invol-ving replication errors by DNA polymerase, although DNA synthesis is of high fidelity. Endo-genous DNA damage may be another cause for mutations, including hydroxy radicals, sponta-neous depurination, depyrimidation and deami-nation of adenine, cytosine and guanine residues (Loeb, 2001). In the *TP53* gene, there are several sequence positions at which mutations are parti-cularly frequent, most of which include CpG di-nucleotides (Pfeifer & Denissenko, 1998). The most frequent mutation at these sites is the GC→AT transition, suggesting an underlying de-amination event at the methylated cytosine leading to thymine; cytosines at the CpG sequences are often methylated in human and animal cells (Pfeifer & Denissenko, 1998). In addition to the methylation pathway, the GC→AT mutations can be related to nitric oxide-induced deamination of cytosine and guanine in DNA (Caulfield *et al.*, 1998). Mutations in the *p53* gene at the CpG sites do not display strand bias, unlike other types of mutations (Hainaut & Hollstein, 2000).

Mutational specificity of the *ras* genes has also been studied in animals and humans (Marion & Boivin-Angele, 1999). A recent study from the occupational environment reported association of codon 12 *KRAS* mutations in pancreatic cancer with exposure to a number of solvents (Alguacil *et al.*, 2002). The results from these studies on *ras* genes have been difficult to interpret because the

Table 2. Frequent mutations induced by some exogenous and endogenous DNA damaging agents, mainly obtained by site-specific techniques (from Hemminki et al., 2000a)

Site of pre-mutagenic lesion	Mutagen	Mutations	Reference
N7-G	AFB₁	GC→TA	Bailey et al. (1996)
N²-G	BPDE	GC→TA	Jelinsky et al. (1995)
N²-G	Tamoxifen	GC→TA	Terashima et al. (1999)
O⁶-G	N-Methyl-N-nitrosourea	GC→AT [a]	Jansen et al. (1994)
O⁶-G	NNK	GC→AT [b]	Hecht (1998)
C8-G	1-Nitrosopyrene	GC→AT, GC→TA [a]	McGregor et al. (1994)
C8-G	4-Aminobiphenyl	GC→TA	Verghis et al. (1997)
C8-G	2-AAF	GC→TA	Shibutani et al. (1998)
C8-G	PhIP	GC→TA	Schut & Snyderwine (1999)
8-oxo-G	Oxidative agents	GC→TA	Wang et al. (1998)
1,N²-G	Malondialdehyde	GC→TA, GC→AT	Moriya et al. (1994)
N⁶-A	Styrene oxide	AT→CG [a]	Bastlová & Podlutsky (1996)
N⁶-A	Benzo[c]phenanthrene diol epoxide	AT→TA, AT→GC	Pontén et al. (1999)
N⁶-A	BPDE	AT→GC	Lavrukhin & Lloyd, (1998)
O²-T	N-Ethyl-N-nitrosourea	AT→TA [a]	Jansen et al. (1994)
3,N⁴-C	Vinyl chloride	GC→AT	Cheng et al. (1991)
5-OH-C, 5-OH-U, uridine glycol	Oxidative agents	GC→AT	Wang et al. (1998)
N³-U	Propylene oxide	GC→AT	Zhang et al. (1995)
Pyrimidine dimers	UV	CC→TT tandem mutation, GC→AT [c]	Ziegler et al. (1993)
Apurinic sites	Depurinating agents	GC→TA, AT→TA	Loeb & Preston (1986)

[a] hprt mutations from cell cultures
[b] K-ras mutations from mouse lung tumours
[c] TP53 mutations from basal-cell carcinomas

tissues apparently harbour clones of pre-existing *ras* mutations that exposure to carcinogens may propagate but in the absence of such stimulation no clonal expansion may take place (Cha *et al.*, 1996).

Mutations in the VHL *gene*

Human cancers are of clonal origin, implying that a particular mutation has been selected. Because of the distinctive features of the mutational spectra specific to different tumours, it has been suggested that it is possible to trace the causative agent for the tumours, especially in the *TP53* gene (Vogelstein & Kinzler, 1992; Greenblatt *et al.*, 1994; Pfeifer & Denissenko, 1998; Bennett *et al.*, 1999; Vineis *et al.*, 1999b), as reviewed by Olivier *et al.* (this volume). We have worked on the *VHL* gene mutation patterns in relation to various human exposures. Mutations in the *VHL* gene are thought to be initiating events for clear-cell renal carcinoma and they are often missense mutations, which are interesting for mutational spectra (Gnarra *et al.*, 1994). Occupational exposure to trichloroethylene has been associated with an increased risk of renal-cell carcinoma. Brauch *et al.* (1999) studied patients with renal-cell carcinoma who had known, high industrial exposure to trichloroethylene and found *VHL* mutations in 75% of cases. The mutations associated with exposure were often multiple and had a unique pattern compared with cases without the exposure. Information on some 750 diverse types of *VHL* mutations is available electronically (Universal *VHL*-Mutation Database, http://www. umd.necker.fr).

We have studied *VHL* mutations in kidney cancer from 102 Swedish patients identified in a case–control study (Ma *et al.*, 2001). Mutations were found in 46% of the patients, and included many recurrent mutations or polymorphism. The most common type of mutation was the GC→AT transition, which was found in 54% of all mutational events. The study was continued by examining associations between patient characteristics, including dietary habits, and mutations (Hemminki *et al.*, 2002b). The results are given as odds ratios in Table 3. In univariate analysis, consumption of vegetables and citrus fruit decreased the frequency of *VHL* mutations among smokers and consumption of citrus fruit decreased these mutations among all patients. In multivariate analysis, the most common single mutation that citrus fruit intake protected against was the GC→AT transition (odds ratio, 0.22) (data not shown). The results provided evidence that intake of vegetables and particularly of citrus fruit protected the renal *VHL* gene from mutational insults that could be endogenous, or at least common in the population. In the cases of smokers, the protection appears to be stronger, probably because smoking adds to the

mutagenic load, stimulates cell division or lowers endogenous resistance towards mutations.

The *VHL* study has several special features that should increase its validity: it was nested into the Swedish part of a well-conducted international case–control study; *VHL* is a gatekeeper gene for renal-cell carcinoma and the mutations may signal early events in tumorigenesis; and the results from mutation analysis were reported before the epidemiological analysis, excluding any unintentional bias in the interpretation of the mutation data (Yang *et al.*, 1999; Ma *et al.*, 2001).

The type of mutations may give some etiological clues. The most common mutation, GC→AT transition, was found in 25 patients (53% of patients with mutations and also 53% of all 84 mutations found). This is the most common mutation type in the *VHL* Mutation Database also, but it represents only 24% of all the listed events (http:// www.umd.necker.fr). Most of these mutations in our material (56% of patients and 49% of mutations) took place at CpG dinucleotides, in line with the VHL Mutation Database, where 51% of GC→AT mutations target CpG dinucleotides. In the *TP53* gene, CpG sites are involved in only between 5% and 40% of all GC→AT transitions, depending on the organ (Hainaut & Hollstein, 2000). In the *TP53* Database (R4, April 2000, www.IARC.fr) only 79 kidney cancers were recorded. However among these, 15/29 (52%) were GC→AT transitions at CpG sites, suggesting that kidney cancer deviates from other cancers in *TP53* mutations with regard to the unusually high share of CpG sites. Oxidative stress, particularly nitric oxide, enhances the rate of deamination, and these types of mutations are associated with endogenous mutagenic processes (Greenblatt *et al.*, 1994; Hainaut & Hollstein, 2000; Hemminki *et al.*, 2000a; Hussain *et al.*, 2000a,b). Any CpG sequence located adjacent to A, i.e. CGA, would then create a stop codon, TCA, which may be a general cause of inactivation mutations (Tomita-Mitchell *et al.*, 2000).

Conclusions

In-vivo data collected from humans of different ages show no age-dependent change in levels of diverse DNA adducts, no deterioration of global

Table 3. Association of *VHL* mutations with dietary intake in renal cancer patients based on univariate analysis

Variables	Intake g/month	VHL mutation in smokers						VHL mutation in all					
		No	Yes	OR	95% CI		P	No	Yes	OR	95% CI		P
Vegetables	< 1039	6	12	1.00			**0.04**	10	15	1.00			0.11
	= 1039	32	20	**0.31**	**0.10**	**0.97**		45	32	0.47	0.19	1.19	
Cruciferous vegetables	< 166	12	11	1.00			0.81	15	15	1.00			0.61
	= 166	26	21	0.88	0.32	2.40		40	32	0.80	0.34	1.88	
Fruits	< 1616	10	10	1.00			0.65	13	13	1.00			0.64
	= 1616	28	22	0.79	0.28	2.22		42	34	0.81	0.33	1.98	
Citrus	< 421	5	12	1.00			**0.02**	8	17	1.00			**0.01**
	= 421	33	20	**0.25**	**0.08**	**0.82**		47	30	**0.30**	**0.12**	**0.78**	

VHL, von Hippel Lindau; OR, odds ratio; 95% CI, 95% confidence interval
There were 102 renal tumour patients.
Figures in **bold** indicate that the 95% CIs do not overlap with 1.00.

DNA excision repair and no change in mutation rate because the *HPRT* mutant fraction is increasing linearly. These molecular epidemiological results, still partially limited to lymphocytes, argue against some animal and in-vitro data but are in line with multistage models for cancer. However, data are needed on human target cells. A further application of DNA adducts as an intermediary tool for genotyping studies, both for metabolic enzyme and DNA repair system genotypes, is recommended. As the common polymorphisms are likely to cause at most moderate increases in the risk of cancer, the intermediary adduct end-point is a necessary proof of causal relationships. The mechanistic data on the mutational spectra induced by important human DNA adducts may be helpful in the characterization, not only of carcinogenic exposures, but also of protective factors, such as dietary ingredients.

References

Aarnio, M., Sankila, R., Pukkala, E., Salovaara, R., Aaltonen, L.A., de la Chapelle, A., Peltomäki, P., Mecklin, J.-P. & Järvinen, H.J. (1999) Cancer risk in mutation carriers of DNA-mismatch-repair genes. *Int. J. Cancer*, **81**, 214–218

Alguacil, J., Porta, M., Malats, N., Kauppinen, T., Kokevinas, M., Benavides, F.G., Partanen, T. & Carrato, A. (2002) Occupational exposure to organic solvents and K-*ras* mutations in exocrine pancreatic cancer. *Carcinogenesis*, **23**, 101–106

Ames, B.N., Gold, L.S. & Willett, W.C. (1995) The causes and prevention of cancer. *Proc. natl Acad. Sci. USA*, **92**, 5258–5265

Armitage, P. & Doll, R. (1954) The age distribution of cancer and a multi-stage theory of carcinogenesis. *Br. J. Cancer*, **8**, 1–12

Armitage, P. & Doll, R. (1957) A two-stage theory of carcinogenesis in relation to the age distribution of human cancer. *Br. J. Cancer*, **11**, 161–169

Bailey, E.A., Iyer, R.S., Stone, M.P., Harris, T.M. & Essigmann, J.M. (1996) Mutational properties of the primary aflatoxin B_1–DNA adduct. *Proc. natl Acad. Sci. USA*, **93**, 1535–1539

Balajee, A.S. & Bohr, V.A. (2000) Genomic heterogeneity of nucleotide excision repair. *Gene*, **250**, 15–30

Bartsch, H., Rojas, M., Alexandrov, K. & Risch, A. (1998) Impact of adduct determination on the assessment of cancer susceptibility. *Recent Results Cancer Res.*, **154**, 86–96

Bastlová, T. & Podlutsky, A. (1996) Molecular analysis of styrene oxide-induced *hprt* mutations in human T lymphocytes. *Mutagenesis*, **11**, 581–591

Beckman, K.B., Saljoughi, S., Mashiyama, S.T. & Ames, B.N. (2000) A simpler, more robust method for the analysis of 8-oxoguanine in DNA. *Free Radic. Biol. Med.*, **29**, 357–367

Benhamou, S. & Sarasin, A. (2000) Variability in nucleotide excision repair and cancer risk: a review. *Mutat. Res.*, **462**, 149–158

Bennett, W.P., Hussain, S.P., Vahakangas, K.H., Khan, M.A., Shields, P.G. & Harris, C.C. (1999) Molecular epidemiology of human cancer risk: gene–environment interactions and p53 mutation spectrum in human lung cancer. *J. Pathol.*, **187**, 8–18

Berwick, M. & Vineis, P. (2000) Markers of DNA repair and susceptibility to cancer in humans: an epidemiological review. *J. natl Cancer Inst.*, **92**, 874–897

Brauch, H., Weirich, G., Hornauer, M.A., Störkel, S., Wöhl, T. & Bruning, T. (1999) Trichloroethylene exposure and specific somatic mutations in patients with renal cell carcinoma. *J. natl Cancer Inst.*, **91**, 854–861

Bykov, V.J, Jansen, C.T. & Hemminki, K. (1998) High levels of dipyrimidine dimers are induced in human skin by solar-simulating UV radiation. *Cancer Epidemiol. Biomarkers Prev.*, **7**, 199–202

Bykov, V.J., Sheehan, J.M., Hemminki, K. & Young, A.R. (1999) *In situ* repair of cyclobutane pyrimidine dimers and 6–4 photoproducts in human skin exposed to solar simulating radiation. *J. invest. Dermatol.*, **112**, 326–331

Caulfield, J.L., Wishnok, J.S. & Tannenbaum, S.R. (1998) Nitric oxide-induced deamination of cytosine and guanine in deoxynucleosides and oligonucleotides. *J. biol. Chem.*, **273**, 12689–12695

Cha, R.S., Guerra, L., Thilly, W.G. & Zarbl, H. (1996) Ha-ras-1 oncogene mutations in mammary epithelial cells do not contribute to initiation of spontaneous mammary tumorigenesis in rats. *Carcinogenesis*, **17**, 2519–2524

Chaudhary, A.K., Nokubo, M., Reddy, G.R., Yeola, S.N., Morrow, J.D., Blair, I.A. & Marnett, L.J. (1994) Detection of endogenous malondialdehyde-deoxyguanosine adducts in human liver. *Science*, **265**, 1580–1582

Cheng, K.C., Preston, B.D., Cahill, D.S., Dosanjh, M.K., Singer, B. & Loeb, L.A. (1991) The vinyl chloride DNA derivative N^2,3-ethenoguanine produces G→A transitions in *Escherichia coli*. *Proc. natl Acad. Sci. USA*, **88**, 9974–9978

Cole, J. & Skopek, T.R. (1994) Somatic mutant frequency, mutation rates and mutational spectra in

the human population *in vivo*. *Mutat. Res.*, **304**, 33–105

Coller, H.A., Khrapko, K., Torres, A., Frampton, M.W., Utell, M.J. & Thilly, W.G. (1998) Mutational spectra of a 100-base pair mitochondrial DNA target sequence in bronchial epithelial cells: a comparison of smoking and nonsmoking twins. *Cancer Res.*, **58**, 1268–1277

Douki, T. & Cadet, J. (2001) Individual determination of the yield of the main UV-induced dimeric pyrimidine photoproducts in DNA suggests a high mutagenicity of CC photolesions. *Biochemistry*, **40**, 2495–2501

Eide, I., Zhao, C., Kumar, R., Hemminki, K., Wu, K. & Swenberg, J. (1999) Comparison of ^{32}P-postlabelling and high resolution GC/MS in quantifying N7-(2-hydroxyethyl)guanine adducts. *Chem. Res. Toxicol.*, **12**, 979–984

Fearon, E.R. (1997) Human cancer syndromes: clues to the origin and nature of cancer. *Science*, **278**, 1043–1050

Fichtinger-Schepman, A.M., Baan, R.A & Berends, F. (1989) Influence of the degree of DNA modification on the immunochemical determination of cisplatin–DNA adduct levels. *Carcinogenesis*, **10**, 2367–2369

Frelon, S., Douki, T., Ravanat, J.L., Pouget, J.P., Tornabene, C. & Cadet, J. (2000) High-performance liquid chromatography–tandem mass spectrometry measurement of radiation-induced base damage to isolated and cellular DNA. *Chem. Res. Toxicol.*, **13**, 1002–1010

Friesen, M.D., Kaderlik, K., Lin, D., Garren, L., Bartsch, H., Lang, N.P. & Kadlubar, F.F. (1994) Analysis of DNA adducts of 2-amino-1-methyl-6-phenylimidazo[4,5-*b*]pyridine in rat and human tissues by alkaline hydrolysis and gas chromatography/electron capture mass spectrometry: validation by comparison with ^{32}P-postlabeling. *Chem. Res. Toxicol.*, **7**, 733–739

German, J. & Ellis, N. (1998) Bloom syndrome. In: Vogelstein, B. & Kinzler, K., eds, *The Genetic Basis of Human Cancer*, New York, McGraw-Hill, pp. 301–315

Gnarra, J.R., Tory, K., Weng, Y., Schmidt, L., Wei, M.H., Li, H., Latif, F., Liu, S., Chen, F., Duh, F.-M., Lubensky, I., Duan, D.R., Florence, C., Pozzatti, R., Walther, M.M., Bander, N.H., Grossman, H.B.,

Brauch, H., Pomer, S., Brooks, J.D., Isaacs, W.B., Lerman, M.I., Zbar, B. & Linehan, V.M. (1994) Mutations of the *VHL* tumour suppressor gene in renal carcinoma. *Nature Genet.*, **7**, 85–90

Greenblatt, M.S., Bennett, W.P., Hollstein, M. & Harris, C.C. (1994) Mutations in the *p53* tumor suppressor gene: clues to cancer etiology and molecular pathogenesis. *Cancer Res.*, **54**, 4855–4878

Hainaut, P. & Hollstein, M. (2000) p53 and human cancer: the first ten thousand mutations. *Adv. Cancer Res.*, **77**, 81–137

Hainaut, P. & Pfeifer, G. (2001) Patterns of p53 G to T transversions in lung cancers reflect the primary mutagenic signature of DNA-damage by tobacco smoke. *Carcinogenesis*, **22**, 367–374

Hanahan, D. & Weinberg, R.A. (2000) The hallmarks of cancer. *Cell*, **100**, 57–70

Hecht, S.S. (1998) Biochemistry, biology, and carcinogenicity of tobacco-specific *N*-nitrosoamines. *Chem. Res. Toxicol.*, **11**, 559–603

Helbock, H.J., Beckman, K.B., Shigenaga, M.K., Walter, P.B., Woodall, A.A., Yeo, H.C. & Ames, B.N. (1998) DNA oxidation matters: the HPLC-electrochemical detection assay of 8-oxo-deoxy-guanosine and 8-oxo-guanine. *Proc. natl Acad. Sci. USA*, **95**, 288–293

Hemminki, K. (1993) DNA adducts, mutations and cancer. *Carcinogenesis*, **14**, 2007–2012

Hemminki, K. & Mutanen, P. (2001) Genetic epidemiology of multistage carcinogenesis. *Mutat. Res.*, **473**, 11–21

Hemminki, K., Koskinen, M., Rajaniemi, H. & Zhao, C. (2000a) DNA adducts, mutations, and cancer 2000. *Regul. Toxicol. Pharmacol.*, **32**, 264–75

Hemminki, K., Xu, G. & Le Curieux, F. (2000b) Re: Markers of DNA repair and susceptibility to cancer in humans: an epidemiologic review. *J. natl Cancer Inst.*, **92**, 1536–1537

Hemminki, K., Koskinen, M. & Zhao, C. (2001a) DNA adducts as a marker for cancer risk? *Int. J. Cancer*, **92**, 923–926

Hemminki, K., Xu, G., Angelini, S., Snellman, E., Jansen, C.T., Lambert, B. & Hou, S.M. (2001b) XPD exon 10 and 23 polymorphisms and DNA repair in human skin in situ. *Carcinogenesis*, **22**, 1185–1188

Hemminki, K., Xu, G., Kause, L., Koulu, L.M., Zhao, C. & Jansen, C.T. (2002a) Demonstration of UV-dimers in human skin DNA in situ 3 weeks after exposure. *Carcinogenesis*, **23**, 605–609

Hemminki, K., Jiang, Y., Ma, X., Yang, K., Egevad, L. & Lindblad, P. (2002b) Molecular epidemiology of *VHL* gene mutations in renal cell carcinoma patients: relation to dietary and other factors. *Carcinogenesis*, **23**, 809–815

Herrero-Jimenez, P., Thilly, G., Southam, P.J., Tomita-Mitchell, A., Morgenthaler, S., Furth, E.E. & Thilly, W.G. (1998) Mutation, cell kinetics, and subpopulations at risk for colon cancer in the United States. *Mutat. Res.*, **400**, 553–578

Herrero-Jimenez, P., Tomita-Mitchell, A., Furth, E.E., Morgenthaler, S. & Thilly, W.G. (2000) Population risk and physiological rate paramenters for colon cancer. The union of an explicit model for carcinogenesis with the public health records of the United States. *Mutat. Res.*, **447**, 73–116

Hou, S.M., Yang, K., Nyberg, F., Hemminki, K., Pershagen, G. & Lambert, B. (1999) Hprt mutant frequency and aromatic DNA adduct level in non-smoking and smoking lung cancer patients and population controls. *Carcinogenesis*, **20**, 437–444

Hou, S.M., Falt, S., Yang, K., Nyberg, F., Pershagen, G., Hemminki, K. & Lambert, B. (2001) Differential interactions between GSTM1 and NAT2 genotypes on aromatic DNA adduct level and HPRT mutant frequency in lung cancer patients and population controls. *Cancer Epidemiol. Biomarkers Prev.*, **10**, 133–140

Hussain, S.P., Amstad, P., Raja, K., Ambs, S., Nagashima, M., Bennett, W.P., Shields, P.G., Ham, A.J., Swenberg, J.A., Marrogi, A.J. & Harris, C.C. (2000a) Increased p53 mutation load in noncancerous colon tissue from ulcerative colitis: a cancer-prone chronic inflammatory disease. *Cancer Res.*, **60**, 3333–3337

Hussain, S.P., Raja, K., Amstad, P.A., Sawyer, M., Trudel, L.J., Wogan, G.N., Hofseth, L.J., Shields, P.G., Billiar, T.R., Trautwein, C., Hohler, T., Galle, P.R., Phillips, D.H., Markin, R., Marrogi, A.J. & Harris, C.C. (2000b) Increased p53 mutation load in nontumorous human liver of Wilson disease and hemochromatosis: oxyradical overload diseases. *Proc. natl Acad. Sci. USA*, **97**, 12770–12775

International Human Genome Sequencing Consortium (2001) Initial sequencing and analysis of the human genome. *Nature*, **409**, 860–921

Jansen, J.G., Mohn, G.R., Vrieling, H., van Teijlingen, C.M.M., Lohman, P.H.M. & van Zeeland, A.A. (1994) Molecular analysis of *hprt* gene mutations in skin fibroblast of rats exposed *in vivo* to *N*-methyl-*N*-nitrosourea or *N*-ethyl-*N*-nitrosourea. *Cancer Res.*, **54**, 2478–2485

Jelinsky, S.A., Liu, T., Geacintov, N.E. & Loecler, E.L. (1995) The major N^2-Gua adduct of the (+)-*anti*-benzo[*a*]pyrene diol epoxide is capable of inducing G→A and G→C, in addition to G→T, mutations. *Biochemistry*, **34**, 13545–13553

Kadlubar, F.F., Anderson, K.E., Haussermann, S., Lang, N.P., Barone, G.W., Thompson, P.A., MacLeod, S.L., Chou, M.W., Mikhailova, M., Plastaras, J., Marnett, L.J., Nair, J., Velic, I. & Bartsch, H. (1998) Comparison of DNA adduct levels associated with oxidative stress in human pancreas. *Mutat. Res.*, **405**, 125–133

Lavrukhin, O.V. & Lloyd, R.S. (1998) Mutagenic replication in a human cell extract of DNAs containing site-specific and stereospecific benzo[*a*]pyrene-7,8-diol-9,10-epoxide DNA adducts placed on the leading and lagging strands. *Cancer Res.*, **58**, 887–891

Lin, D., Lay, J.O., Jr, Bryant, M.S., Malaveille, C., Friesen, M., Bartsch, H., Lang, N.P. & Kadlubar, F.F. (1994) Analysis of 4-aminobiphenyl–DNA adducts in human urinary bladder and lung by alkaline hydrolysis and negative ion gas chromatography-mass spectrometry. *Environ. Health Perspect.*, **102** (Suppl. 6), 11–16

Loeb, L.A. (2001) A mutator phenotype in cancer. *Cancer Res.*, **61**, 3230–3239

Loeb, L.A. & Preston, B.D. (1986) Mutagenesis by apurinic/apyrimidinic sites. *Annu. Rev. Genet.*, **20**, 201–230

Lunn, R.M., Langlois, R.G., Hsieh, L.L., Thompson, C.L. & Bell, D.A. (1999) XRCC1 polymorphisms: effects on aflatoxin B1-DNA adducts and glycophorin A variant frequency. *Cancer Res.*, **59**, 2557–2561

Lynch, H. & de la Chapelle, A. (1999) Genetic susceptibility to non-polyposis colorectal cancer. *J. med. Genet.*, **36**, 801–818

Ma, X., Yang, K., Lindblad, P., Egevad, L. & Hemmiki, K. (2001) VHL gene alterations in renal cell carcinoma patients: novel hotspot or founder mutations and linkage disequilibrium. *Oncogene*, **20**, 5393–5400

Malkin, D. (1998) The Li–Fraumeni syndrome. In: Vogelstein B. & Kinzler, K., eds, *The Genetic Basis of Human Cancer*, New York, McGraw-Hill, pp. 393–407

Marion, M.J. & Boivin-Angele, S. (1999) Vinyl choride-specific mutations in humans and animals. In: Singer, B. & Bartsch, H., eds, *Exocyclic DNA Adducts in Mutagenesis and Carcinogenesis* (IARC Scientific Publications No. 150), Lyon, IARC*Press*, pp. 315–324

McGregor, W.G., Maher, V.M. & McCormick, J.J. (1994) Kinds and locations of mutations induced in the hypoxanthine-guanine phosphoribosyltransferase gene of human T-lymphocytes by 1-nitrosopyrene, including those caused by V(D)J recombinase. *Cancer Res.*, **54**, 4207–4213

Moolgavkar, S.H. & Knudson, A.G., Jr (1981) Mutation and cancer: a model for human carcinogenesis. *J. natl Cancer Inst.*, **66**, 1037–52

Moolgavkar, S.H. & Luebeck, E.G. (1992) Multistage carcinogenesis: population-based model for colon cancer. *J. natl Cancer Inst.*, **84**, 610–618

Moriya, M., Zhang, W., Johnson, F. & Grollman, A.P. (1994) Mutagenic potency of exocyclic DNA adducts: marked differences between *Escherichia coli* and simian kidney cells. *Proc. natl Acad. Sci. USA*, **91**, 11899–11903

Nair, J., Vaca, C.E., Velic, I., Mutanen, M., Valsta, L.M. & Bartsch, H. (1997) High dietary omega-6 polyunsaturated fatty acids drastically increase the formation of etheno-DNA base adducts in white blood cells of female subjects. *Cancer Epidemiol. Biomarkers Prev.*, **6**, 597–601

Nath, R.G., Ocando, J.E. & Chung, F.L. (1996) Detection of 1,N^2-propanodeoxyguanosine adducts as potential endogenous DNA lesions in rodent and human tissues. *Cancer Res.*, **56**, 452–456

Pfeifer, G.P. & Denissenko, M.F. (1998) Formation and repair of DNA lesions in the *p53* gene: relation to cancer mutation. *Environ. mol. Mutag.*, **31**, 197–205

Podlutsky, A., Hou, S.-M., Nyberg, F., Pershagen, G. & Lambert, B. (1999) Influence of smoking and donor age on the spectrum of in vivo mutation at the HPRT-locus in T lymphocytes of healthy adults. *Mutat. Res.*, **431**, 325–339

Pontén, I., Sayer, J.M., Pilcher, A.S., Yagi, H., Kumar, S., Jerina, D.M. & Dipple, A. (1999) Sequence context effects on mutational properties of *cis*-opened benzo[a]phenanthrene diol epoxide-deoxyadenosine adducts in site-specific mutation studies. *Biochemistry*, **38**, 1144–1152

Pouget, J.P., Douki, T., Richard, M.J. & Cadet, J. (2000) DNA damage induced in cells by gamma and UVA radiation as measured by HPLC/GC-MS and HPLC-EC and Comet assay. *Chem. Res. Toxicol.*, **13**, 541–549

Schut, H.A.J. & Snyderwine, E.G. (1999) DNA adducts of heterocyclic amine food mutagens: implications for mutagenesis and carcinogenesis. *Carcinogenesis*, **20**, 353–368

Scully, R. (2001) Interactions between BRCA proteins and DNA structure. *Exp. Cell Res.*, **264**, 67–73

Shen, M.R., Jones, I.M. & Mohrenweiser, H. (1998) Nonconservative amino acid substitution variants exist at polymorphic frequency in DNA repair in healthy humans. *Cancer Res.*, **58**, 604–608

Shibutani, S., Suzuki, N. & Grollman, A.P. (1998) Mutagenic specificity of (acetylamino)fluorene-derived DNA adducts in mammalian cells. *Biochemistry*, **37**, 12034–12041

Smith, L.E., Denissenko, M.F., Bennett, W.P., Li, H., Amin, S., Tang, M. & Pfeifer, G.P. (2000) Targeting of lung mutational hotspots by polycyclic aromatic hydrocarbons. *J. natl Cancer Inst.*, **92**, 803–811

de Souza-Pinto, N.C., Eide, L., Hogue, B.A., Thybo, T., Stevnsner, T., Seeberg, E., Klungland, A. & Bohr, V.A. (2001a) Repair of 8-oxodeoxyguanosine lesions in mitochondrial DNA depends on the oxoguanine DNA glycosylase (*OGG1*) gene and 8-oxoguanine accumulates in the mitochondrial DNA of *OGG1*-defective mice. *Cancer Res.*, **61**, 5378–5381

de Souza-Pinto, N.C., Hogue, B.A. & Bohr, V.A. (2001b) DNA repair and aging in mouse liver: 8-oxodG glycosylase activity increase in mitochondrial but not in nuclear extracts. *Free Radic. Biol. Med.*, **30**, 916–923

Spatz, A., Giglia-Mari, G., Benhamou, S. & Sarasin, A. (2001) Association between DNA repair-deficiency and high level of p53 mutations in melanoma of xeroderma pigmentosum. *Cancer Res.*, **61**, 2480–2486

Spitz, M.R., Wu, X., Wang, Y., Wang, L.E., Shete, S., Amos, C.I., Guo, Z., Lei, L., Mohrenweiser, H. & Wei, Q. (2001) Modulation of nucleotide excision repair capacity by XPD polymorphisms in lung cancer patients. *Cancer Res.*, **61**, 1354–1357

Sturgis, E.M, Zheng, R., Li, L., Castillo, E.J., Eicher, S.A., Chen, M., Strom, S.S., Spitz, M.R. & Wei, Q. (2000) XPD/ERCC2 polymorphisms and risk of head and neck cancer: a case–control analysis. *Carcinogenesis*, **21**, 2219–2223

Terashima, I., Suzuki, N. & Shibutani, S. (1999) Mutagenic potential of α-(N^2-deoxyguanosinyl)-tamoxifen lesions, the major DNA adducts detected in endometrial tissues of patients treated with tamoxifen. *Cancer Res.*, **59**, 2091–2095

Thilly, W.G. (1983) Analysis of chemically induced mutation in single cell populations. *Basic Life Sci.*, **23**, 337–378

Thompson, P.A., Seyedi, F., Lang, N.P., MacLeod, S.L., Wogan, G.N., Anderson, K.E., Tang, Y.M., Coles, B. & Kadlubar, F.F. (1999) Comparison of DNA adduct levels associated with exogenous and endogenous exposures in human pancreas in relation to metabolic genotype. *Mutat. Res.*, **424**, 263–274

Tomita-Mitchell, A., Kat, A.G., Marcelino, L.A., Li-Sucholeiki, X.C., Goodluck-Griffith, J. & Thilly, W.G. (2000) Mismatch repair deficient human cells: spontaneous and MNNG-induced mutational spectra in the HPRT gene. *Mutat. Res.*, **450**, 125–138

Venkitaraman, A.R. (1999) Cancer: breast cancer genes and DNA repair. *Science*, **286**, 1100–1102

Venter, J.C., Adams, M.D., Myers, E.W., Li, P.W., Mural, R.J., Sutton, G.G., Smith, H.O., Yandell, M., Evans, C.A., Holt, R.A., Gocayne, J.D., Amanatides, P., Ballew, R.M., Huson, D.H., Wortman, J.R., Zhang, Q., Kodira, C.D., Zheng, X.H., Chen, L., Skupski, M., Subramanian, G., Thomas, P.D., Zhang, J., Gabor Miklos, G.L., Nelson, C., Broder, S., Clark, A.G., Nadeau, J., McKusick, V.A., Zinder, N., Levine, A.J., Roberts, R.J., Simon, M., Slayman, C., Hunkapiller, M., Bolanos, R., Delcher, A., Dew, I., Fasulo, D., Flanigan, M., Florea, L., Halpern, A., Hannenhalli, S., Kravitz, S., Levy, S., Mobarry, C., Reinert, K., Remington, K., Abu-Threideh, J., Beasley, E., Biddick, K., Bonazzi, V., Brandon, R., Cargill, M., Chandramouliswaran, I., Charlab, R., Chaturvedi, K., Deng, Z., Di Francesco, V., Dunn, P., Eilbeck,

K., Evangelista, C., Gabrielian, A.E., Gan, W., Ge, W., Gong, F., Gu, Z., Guan, P., Heiman, T.J., Higgins, M.E., Ji, R.R., Ke, Z., Ketchum, K.A., Lai, Z., Lei, Y., Li, Z., Li, J., Liang, Y., Lin, X., Lu, F., Merkulov, G.V., Milshina, N., Moore, H.M., Naik, A.K., Narayan, V.A., Neelam, B., Nusskern, D., Rusch, D.B., Salzberg, S., Shao, W., Shue, B., Sun, J., Wang, Z., Wang, A., Wang, X., Wang, J., Wei, M., Wides, R., Xiao, C., Yan, C., Yao, A., Ye, J., Zhan, M., Zhang, W., Zhang, H., Zhao, Q., Zheng, L., Zhong, F., Zhong, W., Zhu, S., Zhao, S., Gilbert, D., Baumhueter, S., Spier, G., Carter, C., Cravchik, A., Woodage, T., Ali, F., An, H., Awe, A., Baldwin, D., Baden, H., Barnstead, M., Barrow, I., Beeson, K., Busam, D., Carver, A., Center, A., Cheng, M.L., Curry, L., Danaher, S., Davenport, L., Desilets, R., Dietz, S., Dodson, K., Doup, L., Ferriera, S., Garg, N., Gluecksmann, A., Hart, B., Haynes, J., Haynes, C., Heiner, C., Hladun, S., Hostin, D., Houck, J., Howland, T., Ibegwam, C., Johnson, J., Kalush, F., Kline, L., Koduru, S., Love, A., Mann, F., May, D., McCawley, S., McIntosh, T., McMullen, I., Moy, M., Moy, L., Murphy, B., Nelson, K., Pfannkoch, C., Pratts, E., Puri, V., Qureshi, H., Reardon, M., Rodriguez, R., Rogers, Y.H., Romblad, D., Ruhfel, B., Scott, R., Sitter, C., Smallwood, M., Stewart, E., Strong, R., Suh, E., Thomas, R., Tint, N.N., Tse, S., Vech, C., Wang, G., Wetter, J., Williams, S., Williams, M., Windsor, S., Winn-Deen, E., Wolfe, K., Zaveri, J., Zaveri, K., Abril, J.F., Guigo, R., Campbell, M.J., Sjolander, K.V., Karlak, B., Kejariwal, A., Mi, H., Lazareva, B., Hatton, T., Narechania, A., Diemer, K., Muruganujan, A., Guo, N., Sato, S., Bafna, V., Istrail, S., Lippert, R., Schwartz, R., Walenz, B., Yooseph, S., Allen, D., Basu, A., Baxendale, J., Blick, L., Caminha, M., Carnes-Stine, J., Caulk, P., Chiang, Y.H., Coyne, M., Dahlke, C., Mays, A., Dombroski, M., Donnelly, M., Ely, D., Esparham, S., Fosler, C., Gire, H., Glanowski, S., Glasser, K., Glodek, A., Gorokhov, M., Graham, K., Gropman, B., Harris, M., Heil, J., Henderson, S., Hoover, J., Jennings, D., Jordan, C., Jordan, J., Kasha, J., Kagan, L., Kraft, C., Levitsky, A., Lewis, M., Liu, X., Lopez, J., Ma, D., Majoros, W., McDaniel, J., Murphy, S., Newman, M., Nguyen, T., Nguyen, N., Nodell, M., Pan, S., Peck, J., Peterson, M., Rowe, W., Sanders, R., Scott, J., Simpson, M., Smith, T.,

Sprague, A., Stockwell, T., Turner, R., Venter, E., Wang, M., Wen, M., Wu, D., Wu, M., Xia, A., Zandieh, A. & Zhu, X. (2001) The sequence of the human genome. *Science*, **291**, 1304–1351

Verghis, S.B.M., Essigmann, J.M., Kadlubar, F.F., Morningstar, M.L. & Lasko, D.D. (1997) Specificity of mutagenesis by 4-aminobiphenyl: mutations at G residues in bacteriophage M13 DNA and G→C transversions at a unique dG (8-ABP) lesion in single-stranded DNA. *Carcinogenesis*, **18**, 2403–2414

Vineis, P. & Perera, F. (2000) DNA adducts as markers of exposure to carcinogens and risk of cancer. *Int. J. Cancer*, **88**, 325–328

Vineis, P., Malats, N., Lang, M., d'Errico, A., Caporaso, N., Cuzick, J. & Boffetta, P., eds (1999a) *Metabolic Polymorphisms and Susceptibility to Cancer* (IARC Scientific Publications No. 148), Lyon, IARC*Press*

Vineis, P., Malats, N., Porta, M. & Real, F.X. (1999b) Human cancer, carcinogenic exposures and mutation spectra. *Mutat. Res.*, **436**, 185–194

Vogelstein, B. & Kinzler, K.W. (1992) Carcinogens leave fingerprints. *Nature*, **355**, 209–210

Wang, D., Kreutzer, D.A. & Essigman, J.M. (1998) Mutagenicity and repair of oxidative DNA damage: insights from studies using defined lesions. *Mutat. Res.*, **400**, 99–115

Wei, Q., Matanoski, G.M., Farmer, E.R., Hedayati, M.A. & Grossman, L. (1993) DNA repair and aging in basal cell carcinoma: a molecular epidemiology study. *Proc. natl Acad. Sci. USA*, **90**, 1614–1618

Wood, R., Mitchell, M., Sgouros, J. & Lindahl, T. (2001) Human DNA repair genes. *Science*, **291**, 1284–1289

Xu, G., Snellman, E., Bykov, V.J., Jansen, C.T. & Hemminki, K. (2000a) Cutaneous melanoma patients have normal repair kinetics of ultraviolet-induced DNA repair in skin *in situ*. *J. invest. Dermatol.*, **114**, 628–631

Xu, G., Snellman, E., Bykov, V.J., Jansen, C.T. & Hemminki, K. (2000b) Effect of age on the formation and repair of UV photoproducts in human skin in situ. *Mutat. Res.*, **459**, 195–202

Xu, G., Snellman, E., Jansen, C.T. & Hemminki, K. (2000c) Levels and repair of cyclobutane pyrimidine dimers and 6–4 photoproducts in skin of sporadic basal cell carcinoma patients. *J. invest. Dermatol.*, **115**, 95–99

Yang, K., Lindblad, P., Egevad, L. & Hemminki, K. (1999) Novel somatic mutations in the *VHL* gene in Swedish archived sporadic renal cell carcinomas. *Cancer Lett.*, **141**, 1–8

Zhang, W., Johnson, F., Grollman, A.P. & Shibutani, S. (1995) Miscoding by exocyclic and related DNA adducts 3,N⁴-etheno-2′-deoxycytidine, 3,N⁴-ethano-2′-deoxycytidine, and 3-(2-hydroxyethyl)-2′-deoxyuridine. *Chem. Res. Toxicol.*, **8**, 157–163

Zhao, C. & Hemminki, K. (2002) The in vivo levels of DNA alkylation products in human lymphocytes are not age-dependent: an assay of 7-methyl- and 7-(2-hydroxyethyl)-guanine DNA adducts. *Carcinogenesis*, **23**, 307–310

Zhao, C., Tyndyk, M., Eide, I. & Hemminki, K. (1999) Endogenous and background DNA adducts by methylating and 2-hydroxyethylating agents. *Mutat. Res.*, **424**, 117–125

Zhao, C., Vodicka, P., Šrám, R.J. & Hemminki, K. (2000) Human DNA adducts of 1,3-butadiene, an important environmental carcinogen. *Carcinogenesis*, **21**, 107–111

Zhao, C., Snellman, E., Jansen, C.T. & Hemminki, K. (2002) In situ repair of cyclobutane pyrimidine dimers in skin and melanocytic nevi of cutaneous melanoma patients. *Int. J. Cancer*, **98**, 331–334

Ziegler, A., Leffell, D.J., Kunala, S., Sharma, H.W., Gailani, M., Simon, J.A., Halperin, A.J., Baden, H.P., Shapiro, P.E., Bale, A.E. & Brash, D.E. (1993) Mutational hotspots due to sunlight in the *p53* gene of nonmelanoma skin cancers. *Proc. natl Acad. Sci. USA*, **90**, 4216–4220

Corresponding author:

Kari Hemminki
Department of Biosciences at Novum,
Karolinska Institute, Hälsovagen 7,
141 57 Huddinge, Sweden
kari.hemminki@cnt.ki.se

Mechanisms of Carcinogenesis: Contributions of Molecular Epidemiology
Patricia Buffler, Jerry Rice, Robert Baan, Michael Bird and Paolo Boffetta, eds
IARC Scientific Publications No. 157
International Agency for Research on Cancer, Lyon, 2004

Toxicological Considerations in the Application and Interpretation of DNA Adducts in Epidemiological Studies

James A. Swenberg

Summary

This chapter will review a variety of issues related to the use of biomarkers in molecular epidemiological studies. It will draw upon experience gained from related mechanistic research in toxicological studies. This includes important methodological issues that impact on the type of assays that can be used and how these issues affect the selection of the method and the biological sample. It will also address issues affecting the use of biomarkers as measures of exposure and effect, and discuss inferences for causality and the selection of target organ versus surrogate tissues. Combining information from toxicological studies can also aid in the interpretation of epidemiological studies, such as tissues with and without strong biological plausibility and relationships between observed DNA adducts and those that arise from endogenous processes. Finally, it will discuss issues related to important pathways of metabolism and implications of genetic polymorphisms. These critical issues affect both the design and interpretation of molecular epidemiological studies.

Introduction

DNA adducts have been a primary subject in cancer research for more than 30 years (Singer & Grunberger, 1983; La & Swenberg, 1997; Vainio, 1998). Most of this research has focused on the characterization, formation, repair and biology of individual adducts in experimental systems (Groopman & Kensler, 1999). More recently, DNA adducts have been investigated in DNA from tissues of humans exposed to a variety of

carcinogenic substances (van Delft *et al.*, 1998). In some cases, these investigations have been well-conducted molecular epidemiological studies that included environmental measurements in the workplace, or known exposures to drugs, radiation or pollutants. The techniques for measuring DNA adducts vary greatly in both sensitivity and specificity. Modern ^{32}P-postlabelling techniques can detect 1 adduct per 10^9 to 10^{10} nucleotides. When coupled with high-performance liquid chromatographic methods, these exquisitely sensitive methods can also provide relatively good specificity. Mass spectrometric methods have limits of detection down to 1 adduct per 10^8 nucleotides and provide good structural information on the chemistry of the adduct. Accelerator mass spectrometry is the most sensitive method available today, but relies on clean-up methods for its specificity. Still, there are many techniques being used that have lower sensitivity and specificity, or that are subject to high levels of artefact. This chapter focuses on some of the issues that impact on the interpretation and use of DNA adducts in molecular epidemiological studies.

Methods for measurement of DNA adducts

There are many reviews that evaluate the different methods available for analysing DNA adducts. No attempt is made here to re-analyse this large literature. Rather, this chapter will focus on pointing out various aspects of such measurements that affect the application and interpretation of data on DNA adducts in molecular epidemiological studies. The earliest studies on DNA adducts relied on chemical characterization of in-vitro reactions, and the administration of radio-isotopes to animals and cell cultures followed by radiochromatography. Such radioisotope methods used liquid chromatography and had limits of detection around 1 adduct per 10^6 nucleotides. The studies were very expensive, with radioiso-tope costs around $100 per animal, and each sample took 1–2 days to analyse. Studies using radiolabelled material were almost always confined to single dose administration, so infor-mation on steady-state concentrations of adducts was not obtained.

These methods were followed by a variety of immunological assays such as ELISA that did not require expensive radioisotopes and could exa-mine both single- and multiple-dose studies. Some of the immunoassays, however, were plagued by issues of cross-reactivity between related DNA adducts, making real quantitation impossible when the assays were applied to samples from animals or humans exposed to chemical mixtures. Since both highly mutagenic and poorly mutagenic DNA adducts reacted with the antibodies, accurate quantitation was not possible. This same lack of specificity exists today for ^{32}P-postlabelling studies on polycyclic aromatic hydrocarbons (PAH), where measure-ments of 'diagonal zones' are used for quanti-tation of PAH adducts. In this case, the 'diagonal zone' represents a smear of related PAH adducts.

Studies on experimental animals allow the investigation of almost any tissue, but that is not usually possible in human studies. Not only are many tissues inaccessible, the amount of DNA available for analysis is also frequently limited to the 25–50 µg of DNA that can be obtained from a blood sample. In contrast, samples ranging up to a milligram or more of DNA are often available in experimental studies. It is important to remember that the ability to measure DNA adducts depends both on the sensitivity of the method and on the amount of DNA available for analysis. The ^{32}P-postlabelling method is one of the most sensitive DNA adduct assays, but it is usually limited to applications of 1–10 µg of DNA. The ^{32}P-post-labelling method can measure 1 adduct in 10^9 nucleotides, but, if another method can

measure 1 adduct in 10^8 nucleotides and use a sample of 100 µg of DNA, it may be more sen-sitive. An exception to the limitation of the amount of DNA for the ^{32}P-postlabelling method is when various clean-up strategies can be incor-porated into the assay prior to the ^{32}P-post-labelling. This includes general chemical sepa-rations such as butanol/water extraction of the nucleotide digest, eliminating normal nucleotides with nuclease P1, and applying immunoaffinity chromatography to the samples before ^{32}P-post-labelling. Slot blot assays have similar restrictions on the amount of DNA that can be applied to a membrane, which again limits the ability of these assays to quantitate DNA damage. Unfortunately, selective clean-up strategies cannot be applied to slot blot assays since the DNA itself is applied to the membrane. Clean-up strategies remain a critical issue in most studies of DNA adducts, as one is truly looking for the proverbial needle in a haystack. In the case of mass spectrometry, there are important issues related to signal suppression when large amounts of normal nucleosides or bases are present in the sample. Strategies such as selective depurination of labile N7 guanine or N3 adenine adducts by neutral thermal hydrolysis, immunoaffinity chromatography and column switching for the elimination of normal nucleo-tides or nucleobases can greatly decrease both background and signal suppression.

DNA adducts as biomarkers of exposure and effect

DNA adducts are frequently used as biomarkers of exposure to chemicals that are either electrophilic or are metabolized to electrophiles. This is readily possible in experimental systems with known exposures and duration, but it is a much more complex issue in molecular epidemiological studies. For the information to be useful in a quan-titative manner, the exposure history and the half-life of the specific type of DNA adduct need to be known. Experimental studies have shown that with constant dosing, a steady-state concentration of DNA adducts will occur, where the number of new adducts formed each day equals the number of adducts that are lost due to repair or instability. Thus, if exposure is relatively constant in a molecular epidemiological study, it can be reasonably assumed that the adducts are at a steady-state concentration. In contrast, if exposures are intermittent and of unknown and variable amount, little inference can be made other than that exposure occurred. This points out an important difference between DNA adducts and haemoglobin adducts as surrogate biomarkers of exposure. Since haemoglobin adducts are not subject to repair, they accumulate for the lifetime of the protein. In the human, that is about 120 days. Thus, a measurement of haemoglobin adducts provides the cumulative exposure over this period of time. Neither haemoglobin adducts nor DNA adducts provide accurate estimates of exposure beyond the lifespan of the protein or several half-lives of the DNA adduct. Therefore, neither is likely to improve estimates of exposure in previous years.

Do DNA adducts convey causality?

Many different DNA adducts are now being measured, but a major issue in interpretation relates to their meaning. The presence of a chemical-specific DNA adduct in human DNA is a good indication that exposure to that chemical occurred. Exactly what that means for the prediction of outcome is an important question. Individuals participating in a molecular epidemiological study frequently want to know the results and what they mean. Similarly, when a study is completed, the implications of such measurements represent a key feature of the discussion section of reports and manuscripts.

DNA adducts have vastly different potentials for causing mutations. Some adducts are highly promutagenic, causing a mutation 8 out of 10 times that a DNA polymerase encounters an adduct in the template strand. Other DNA adducts are not promutagenic and do not lead to heritable effects. In the latter case, the presence of such adducts is simply a measure of exposure. The chemical causing the non-mutagenic adducts can, however, also cause other DNA adducts that are promutagenic.

DNA adducts are selected as biomarkers of exposure for several reasons:

- The adduct may be formed in the greatest amount, yielding the greatest likelihood of being measurable, even if it is not promutagenic.
- An adduct may be selected because it is promutagenic and a lesion of interest and concern.
- An adduct may be selected because it is known to be repaired poorly and is expected to accumulate.

These factors are not mutually exclusive, and impact on the interpretation of what the measurements mean.

New research is providing additional understanding of the biology of $N7$ alkylguanine DNA adducts. These adducts are not promutagenic, but are chemically unstable, depurinate and form apurinic sites in DNA as an intermediate step in the base excision repair pathway. Although the $N7$ alkylguanine adduct is not promutagenic, abasic (AP) sites have been shown to cause mutations in vitro when DNA polymerase passes the lesion. The critical issue is whether DNA repair of such lesions is balanced or unbalanced, i.e. do AP sites accumulate or are they repaired immediately after formation? AP sites are the most common form of endogenous DNA damage, with 50 000–100 000 abasic sites being present in every cell as a steady-state level of damage (Nakamura & Swenberg, 1999). Most of these appear to be a specific type of AP site resulting from oxidative attack (Nakamura et al., 2000). We have examined DNA from tissues of animals exposed to propylene oxide or ethylene oxide to investigate the kinetics of depurination and the formation and repair of AP sites. In the case of propylene oxide, measurements of 7-hydroxypropylguanine (7-OHPG) at the end of 4 weeks of inhalation exposure of rats to 500 ppm propylene oxide and 3 days later gave quantitative data on the number of adducts that were lost due to depurination or repair (Ríos-Blanco et al., 2000). The number of 7-OHPG adducts in the nasal respiratory mucosa was extremely high (606 7-OHPG per 10^6 guanines). The number of depurinations that occurred in these animals was increased 10-fold over the normal rate of spontaneous depurination in DNA. Even with this large increase in depurination that resulted in the formation of AP sites, there was no increase in AP sites in the nasal tissue, indicating that the repair of AP sites is highly efficient and has a large capacity. Similar data were obtained with ethylene oxide, where AP sites were examined in tissues of rats exposed to 100 ppm for up to 4 weeks (Asakura *et al.*, 2002). Thus, the presence of 7-alkylguanine adducts themselves does not connote a mutagenic risk. Recently, similar studies were carried out in animals on a folate-deficient diet. This leads to increased uracil incorporation into DNA which is removed by uracil glycosylase, forming AP sites. Again, no increase in AP sites was detectable. The AP sites formed by spontaneous depurination, chemical depurination and the action of glycosylase are chemically identical. The repair of these AP sites appears to be extremely efficient and rapid, suggesting that they are not likely to be an important source of mutagenesis *in vivo*. In contrast, the oxidized AP sites that are formed from oxidative attack appear to be less well repaired and may represent an important source of mutagenesis.

As methods for the measurement of DNA adducts become more sensitive, another issue that deserves attention relates to the implications for causality. It is well known that many DNA adducts are formed endogenously, with steady-state concentrations in the range of 1 adduct per 10^6 nucleotides. What then does a finding of a chemical-specific adduct in a human at 1 adduct per 10^9 nucleotides mean? An example is tamoxifen, an anti-estrogen used in the treatment of human breast cancer. Several ^{32}P-postlabelling studies have detected tamoxifen adducts at 1 per 10^9 to 10^8 nucleotides in human tissues (Carthew *et al.*, 1995; Hemminki *et al.*, 1996; Shibutani *et al.*, 2000). Rats that develop liver cancer have 3 adducts per 10^5 nucleotides (Carthew *et al.*, 1995). However, mice exposed to similar high doses of tamoxifen had 30–40% fewer DNA adducts than rats and 1000 times more than the human samples, but did not get cancer (White *et al.*, 1992). How then can any statements related to causality be made? Extensive scientific evidence is necessary for any suggestion of causality, such as identical hot spots for adduct formation and point mutations in cancers, where the point mutations are of the same type as has been associated with the adduct (Denissenko *et al.*, 1996).

Target organ versus surrogate tissue

As mentioned earlier, it is the exception rather than the rule that the tissue of major concern is available for molecular epidemiological studies. Instead, DNA from peripheral blood lymphocytes or haemoglobin samples is analysed for molecular evidence of exposure. In contrast, most experimental studies analyse adducts in the target organ, but not in peripheral blood lymphocytes. The likelihood that a surrogate such as lymphocyte DNA will provide a reasonable estimate of other tissues is dependent on the chemistry and metabolism of the chemical and its electrophile(s). If the ultimate carcinogen is highly unstable and formed only in target tissues with specific metabolic capacity, lymphocytes are not likely to provide data that are predictive for the target organ. An example of this is vinyl chloride, where the ultimate carcinogen, chloroethylene oxide, is formed in tissues rich in CYP2E1, but does not circulate to other tissues (Morinello *et al.*, 2002a,b). On the other hand, if the chemical is directly reactive and circulates in the blood, lymphocyte data should be quite good. An example of this is ethylene oxide (Wu *et al.*, 1999). Similarly, if the reactive metabolite(s) of a procarcinogen circulate(s) in the blood, lymphocyte data should be predictive. 1,3-Butadiene is a good example of this. Most of the metabolism is thought to occur in the liver, yet all tissues examined have similar levels of DNA adducts (Koc *et al.*, 1999).

Experimental studies can be very useful for determining the likely success of a molecular epidemiological study using a surrogate tissue. Examples of such studies are those comparing DNA adducts in liver and lymphocytes of rats exposed to *N*-nitrosodimethylamine (NDMA) (Souliotis *et al.*, 1995). Although the ultimate carcinogen of NDMA is highly reactive and not very stable, it was surprising to see that lymphocyte DNA adducts were quite predictive of the molecular dose measured in the liver. The lymphocytes exhibited approximately 60% of the adduct concentration found in livers at all doses and times in rats exposed to 0.2–2.64 ppm NDMA in the drinking-water for up to 4 weeks.

Another important consideration when selecting a surrogate tissue for molecular epidemiological studies is related to the lifespan of the surrogate and target tissues. There are huge differences in the lifespan of peripheral blood lymphocytes and neutrophils. Lymphocytes are long-lived cells with lifespans up to several years. In contrast, neutrophils are extremely short-lived cells, with lifespans of 1–2 days. It is important to take the extra effort to separate these two cell types prior to measuring DNA adducts. The use of white blood cells in such studies is clearly inferior to that of lymphocytes.

Experimental data can aid in the interpretation of epidemiological studies

Just as experimental studies can assist in the design of epidemiological studies for such issues as surrogate tissue selection and the development of ultrasensitive analytical methods, they can also provide valuable data related to interpretation of epidemiological data. A recent example of this involves studies on vinyl chloride. Although there is clear evidence for the induction of hepatic angiosarcomas in humans and experimental animals, there has been a long-standing controversy regarding the role of vinyl chloride in the induction of brain tumours. In many of the early epidemiological reports, a positive association was found between occupational exposure of workers to vinyl chloride and the incidence of brain tumours (Infante, 1981). As the studies became larger and more comprehensive in design, this evidence weakened. There was no relationship between exposure or length of employment and the number of brain tumours (Simonato et al., 1991). Finally, the latest evaluation of European vinyl chloride workers failed to find any relationship between brain tumours and exposure to vinyl chloride (Ward et al., 2001). However, uncertainty still remains due to the earlier associations. We have examined this issue in rats exposed to vinyl chloride (Morinello et al., 2002a). Although there were large exposure-related concentrations of DNA adducts in liver DNA, there was no increase in brain DNA adducts in the same animals. Since identical DNA adducts are induced endogenously by lipid peroxidation, it was not possible to say that there were no DNA adducts present in brain. To clarify this issue, we exposed rats to [$^{13}C_2$]vinyl chloride

and analysed N^2,3-ethenoguanine and 7-oxoethyl-guanine using mass spectrometry. This approach makes it possible to distinguish the endogenous adducts from the exogenous adducts, because of the difference in mass. These studies clearly demonstrated that endogenous adducts were present in brain and liver, but that exogenous vinyl chloride-induced adducts were present in liver, but not in brain DNA. We can conclude from this that the ultimate carcinogen of vinyl chloride is neither formed in brain nor transported to brain, even when exposures were to 1100 ppm for up to 4 weeks. These data strongly support the more comprehensive epidemiological studies that found no association between exposure to vinyl chloride and brain tumours in workers.

Endogenous DNA adducts

Improved analytical tools have also advanced our knowledge of endogenous DNA adducts. Oxidative DNA damage arises from free radical attack on the bases and deoxyribose, leading to the formation of DNA adducts, AP sites and DNA strand breaks. The most commonly studied oxidative DNA adduct is 8-oxodeoxyguanosine (8-OHdG). This adduct is present in virtually all tissues of the body and clearly induces mutations when DNA polymerase uses it as its template. Recently, it has been recognized that oxidative DNA damage, including 8-OHdG, is also easily induced as an artefact during isolation of DNA and work-up. The literature is replete with reports of 8-OHdG residues at the level of two per 10^5 guanines; however, these values must now be viewed with great scepticism. Fresh calf thymus DNA isolated with free radical trapping agents or antioxidants typically has about one 8-OHdG per 10^7 guanines and adult rat liver has 4–20 8-OHdG per 10^7 guanines. These values have been reproduced in several laboratories and are probably the true values for this adduct. It is critical that new molecular epidemiological studies also incorporate strategies for minimizing artefact.

Many additional endogenous DNA adducts are formed from lipid peroxidation products. These include etheno, propano and malondialdehyde adducts and their substituted entities. Most of these are promutagenic DNA adducts that actively cause mispairing during DNA synthesis. Such endogenous DNA adducts need to be evaluated in molecular epidemiological studies, as they are likely to be influenced by diet and lifestyle and may represent important causal factors in human disease.

Finally, endogenous alkylating agents are also formed in the human body, including methylating and hydroxyethylating agents that produce endogenous 7-methylguanine and 7-hydroxyethylguanine. Several of the endogenous DNA adducts are also formed by industrial chemicals. Examples include the etheno adducts induced by vinyl chloride and 7-hydroxyethylguanine formed by ethylene oxide. It becomes very difficult to examine DNA repair of such adducts because the endogenous adducts are continually formed. Mass spectrometry with stable isotopes is one of the few methods available. Recent studies on rats exposed to $[^{13}C_2]$vinyl chloride were able to show that exposure to 10 mg/L vinyl chloride for 4 weeks resulted in a 50% increase in N^2,3-ethenoguanine in hepatocyte DNA. Extrapolation of these data suggests that current occupational exposures to 0.1 and 1 mg/L would cause 0.5 and 5% increases over the level of endogenous adducts (Morinello et al., 2002b).

Molecular dosimetry and implications for metabolism

With these caveats in mind, DNA adducts can provide very valuable information regarding exposure, metabolism, target organ and surrogate tissue responses, as well as the biology of the adduct. Dose–response studies have been conducted in experimental animals on nearly all classes of genotoxic carcinogens. Examples of linear, sublinear and supralinear dose–responses for DNA adducts are well established and understood. These include single administration studies, as well as continuous exposures. The study of O^6- and $N7$-methylguanine (O^6-MG and $N7$-MG, respectively) in rats exposed orally to single doses of NDMA covering a dose range from 0.001 to 20 mg/kg clearly demonstrated that differences in the shape of the dose–response were evident between the two types of adducts (Figure 1) (Pegg & Hui, 1978). Whereas $N7$-MG was linear over doses covering five orders of

magnitude, O^6-MG was sublinear, with the increase in slope occurring at the point that DNA repair became saturated. On the other hand, studies by Belinsky et al. (1986) on 4-(methylnitrosamino)-1-(3-pyridyl)-1-butanone (NNK) demonstrated that the molecular dose of O^6-MG was supralinear in rat lung, owing to saturation of metabolic activation (Figure 2). DNA–protein cross-links induced in rat nasal tissue by formaldehyde were sublinear owing to saturation of detoxication (Figure 3) (Casanova et al., 1989).

There have been few studies in humans that have demonstrated dose–response relationships between chemical-specific adducts and exposure. A study by Kogevinas (2000) demonstrated a supralinear dose–response for PAH–DNA adducts and air pollution that paralleled a similar response for lung and bladder cancer versus the number of cigarettes. Such a dose–response is most likely the result of saturation of metabolic activation. Bartsch (1996) found that lung cancer patients had greater CYP1A1 activity and higher numbers of bulky aromatic DNA adducts than non-cancer patients.

Genetic polymorphisms affect metabolism and DNA repair

Genetic polymorphisms can affect metabolic activation, detoxication and DNA repair and result in different susceptibilities to adduct formation and repair (Kaderlik & Kadlubar, 1995; Rundle et al., 2000). Some of these effects can now be reproduced in transgenic mice. A strong association was found between DNA adducts in white blood cells of bladder cancer patients and N-acetyltransferase (NAT2) (Peluso et al., 1998). The NAT2 genotype is associated with slower detoxication of aromatic amines, leading to greater numbers of DNA adducts. Similarly, higher numbers of PAH–DNA adducts were found in breast cancer patients who were GSTM1 null. Kelsey et al. (1995) demonstrated a significant increase in sister chromatid exchanges in lymphocytes from GSTT1-null individuals who were exposed in vitro to 1,3-butadiene diepoxide. When haemoglobin adducts, sister chromatid exchanges and chromosomal aberrations were examined in workers exposed to 1,3-butadiene, there was no effect of GSTT1, yet the lymphocytes of the same workers did show an

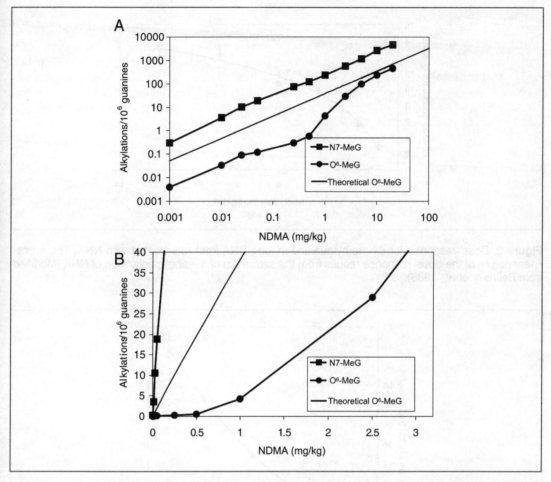

Figure 1. Dose–response relationship for *N7*-methylguanine and *O⁶*-methylguanine following a single oral dose of *N*-nitrosodimethylamine (NDMA). Plot A demonstrates the actual versus the theoretical amounts of adducts for doses covering several orders of magnitude. Plot B demonstrates the sublinear nature of the dose–response in the region where the repair of *O⁶*-methylguanine becomes saturated. Note that the number of *O⁶*-methylguanine adducts is lower than expected at doses below the point of saturation for *O⁶*-methylguanine repair. Such a relationship can exist when DNA repair/loss occurs by different mechanisms, as is the case for *N7*-methylguanine and *O⁶*-methylguanine (Data modified from Pegg & Hui, 1978).

increase in sister chromatid exchanges when exposed *in vitro* (Hayes *et al.*, 2000). The likely explanation for such observations is that 1,3-buta-diene diepoxide formation was low enough in the GSTT1-null workers that other detoxication pathways were able to eliminate most of the diepoxide. In contrast, the in-vitro exposures were much higher and saturated the detoxication pathways available in the cultured cells.

Acknowledgements

Ms Patricia Upton is thanked for her editorial assistance. This work was supported in part by grants CA 83369, P30-CA16086, P42-ES05948, P30-ES10126 and R42-ES11746 from the National Institutes of Health.

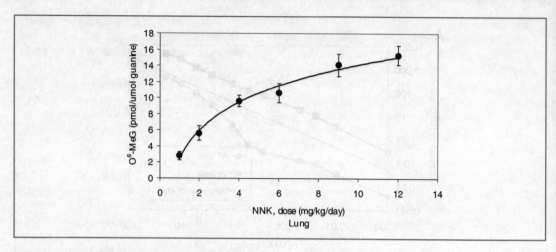

Figure 2. Dose–response for O^6-methylguanine in lung DNA from rats treated with NNK. The supralinear nature of the dose–response results from the saturation of metabolic activation of NNK (Modified from Belinsky *et al.*, 1986).

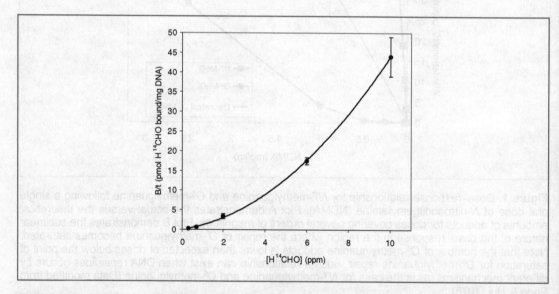

Figure 3. Dose–response for DNA–protein cross-links in nasal mucosa of rats and monkeys exposed to [^{14}C]formaldehyde by inhalation. The sublinear dose–response is the result of saturation of detoxication of formaldehyde (Modified from Casanova *et al.*, 1989).

References

Asakura, S., Nakamura, J. & Swenberg, J.A. (2002) Apurinic/apyrimidinic (AP) sites, intermediates in base excision repair, are not increased by ethylene oxide inhalation in rats (Abstract No. 1487). *Toxicol. Sci.*, **66** (Suppl. 1-S), 303

Bartsch, H. (1996) DNA adducts in human carcinogenesis: etiological relevance and structure–activity relationship. *Mutat. Res.*, **340**, 67–79

Belinsky, S.A., White, C.M., Boucheron, J.A., Richardson, F.C., Swenberg, J.A. & Anderson, M. (1986) Accumulation and persistence of DNA adducts in respiratory tissue of rats following multiple administrations of the tobacco specific carcinogen 4-(N-methyl-N-nitrosamino)-1-(3-pyridyl)-1-butanone. *Cancer Res.*, **46**, 1280–1284

Carthew, P., Rich, K.J., Martin, E.A., De Matteis, F., Lim, C.K., Manson, M.M., Festing, M.F.W., White, I.N.H. & Smith, L.L. (1995) DNA damage as assessed by ^{32}P-postlabelling in three rat strains exposed to dietary tamoxifen: the relationship between cell proliferation and liver tumour formation. *Carcinogenesis*, **16**, 1299–1304

Casanova, M., Deyo, D.F. & Heck, H.D. (1989) Covalent binding of inhaled formaldehyde to DNA in the nasal mucosa of Fischer 344 rats: analysis of formaldehyde and DNA by high-performance liquid chromatography and provisional pharmacokinetic interpretation. *Fundam. appl. Toxicol.*, **12**, 397–417

van Delft, J.H., Baan, R.A. & Roza, L. (1998) Biological effect markers for exposure to carcinogenic compound and their relevance for risk assessment. *Crit. Rev. Toxicol.*, **28**, 477–510

Denissenko, M.F., Pao, A., Tang, M. & Pfeifer, G.P. (1996) Preferential formation of benzo[a]pyrene adducts at lung cancer mutational hotspots in P53. *Science*, **274**, 430–432

Groopman, J.D. & Kensler, T.W. (1999) The light at the end of the tunnel for chemical-specific biomarkers: daylight or headlight? *Carcinogenesis*, **20**, 1–11

Hayes, R.B., Zhang, L., Yin, S., Swenberg, J.A., Xi, L., Wiencke, J., Bechtold, W.E., Yao, M., Rothman, N., Haas, R., O'Neill, J.P., Zhang, D., Wiemels, J., Dosemeci, M., Li, G. & Smith, M.T. (2000) Genotoxic markers among butadiene polymer workers in China. *Carcinogenesis*, **21**, 55–62

Hemminki, K., Rajaniemi, H., Lindahl, B. & Moberger, B. (1996) Tamoxifen-induced DNA adducts in endometrial samples from breast cancer patients. *Cancer Res.*, **56**, 4374–4377

Infante, P.F. (1981) Observations of the site-specific carcinogenicity of vinyl chloride to humans. *Environ. Health Perspect.*, **41**, 89–94

Kaderlik, K.R. & Kadlubar, F.F. (1995) Metabolic polymorphisms and carcinogen–DNA adduct formation in human populations. *Pharmacogenetics*, **5**, S108–S117

Kelsey, K.T., Wiencke, J.K., Ward, J., Bechtold, W. & Fajen, J. (1995) Sister-chromatid exchanges, gluta-

thione S-transferase theta deletion and cytogenetic sensitivity to diepoxybutane in lymphocytes from butadiene monomer production workers. *Mutat. Res.*, **335**, 267–273

Koc, H., Tretyakova, N.Y., Walker, V.E., Henderson, R.F. & Swenberg, J.A. (1999) Molecular dosimetry of N-7 guanine adduct formation in mice and rats exposed to 1,3-butadiene. *Chem. Res. Toxicol.*, **12**, 566–574

Kogevinas, M. (2000) Studies of cancer in humans. *Food Addit. Contam.*, **17**, 317–324

La, D.K. & Swenberg, J.A. (1997) Carcinogenic alkylating agents. In: Sipes, I.G., McQueen, C.A. & Gandolfi, A.J., eds, *Comprehensive Toxicology*, Vol. 12, *Chemical Carcinogens and Anticarcinogens*, Oxford, Elsevier Science, pp. 111–140

Morinello, E.J., Koc, H., Ranasinghe, A. & Swenberg, J.A. (2002a) Differential induction of N^2, 3-ethenoguanine in rat brain and liver after exposure to vinyl chloride. *Cancer Res.*, **62**, 5183–5188

Morinello, E.J., Ham, A.-J.L., Ranasinghe, A., Nakamura, J., Upton, P.B. & Swenberg, J.A. (2002b) Molecular dosimetry and repair of N^2,3-ethenoguanine in rats exposed to vinyl chloride. *Cancer Res.*, **62**, 5189–5195

Nakamura, J., La, D.K. & Swenberg, J.A. (2000) 5'-Nicked apurinic/apyrimidinic sites are resistant to β-elimination by β-polymerase and are persistent in human cultured cells after oxidative stress. *J. biol. Chem.*, **275**, 5323–5328

Nakamura, J. & Swenberg, J.A. (1999) Endogenous apurinic/apyrimidinic sites in genomic DNA of mammalian tissues. *Cancer Res.*, **59**, 2522–2526

Pegg, A.E. & Hui, G. (1978) Formation and subsequent removal of O^6-methylguanine from deoxyribonucleic acid in rat liver and kidney after small doses of dimethylnitrosamine. *Biochem. J.*, **173**, 739–748

Peluso, M., Airoldi, L., Armelle, M., Martone, T., Coda, R., Malaveille, C., Giacomelli, G., Terrone, C., Casetta, G. & Vineis, P. (1998) White blood cell DNA adducts, smoking, and NAT2 and GSTM1 genotypes in bladder cancer: a case–control study. *Cancer Epidemiol. Biomarkers Prev.*, **7**, 341–346

Ríos-Blanco, M.N., Faller, T.H., Nakamura, J., Kessler, W., Kreuzer, P.E., Ranasinghe, A., Filser, J.G. & Swenberg, J.A. (2000) Quantitation of DNA and hemoglobin adducts and apurinic/apyrimidinic sites in tissues of F344 rats exposed to propylene oxide by inhalation. *Carcinogenesis*, **21**, 2011–2018

Rundle, A., Tang, D., Zhou, J., Cho, S. & Perera, F. (2000) The association between glutathione *S*-transferase M1 genotype and polycyclic aromatic hydrocarbon–DNA adducts in breast tissue. *Cancer Epidemiol. Biomarkers Prev.*, **9**, 1079–1085

Shibutani, S., Ravindernath, A., Suzuki, N., Terashima, I., Sugarman, S.M., Grollman, A.P. & Pearl, M.L. (2000) Identification of tamoxifen–DNA adducts in the endometrium of women treated with tamoxifen. *Carcinogenesis*, **21**, 1461–1467

Simonato, L., L'Abbe, K.A., Andersen, A., Belli, S., Comba, P., Engholm, G., Ferro, G., Hagmar, L., Langard, S., Lundberg, I., Piratsu, R., Thomas, P., Winklemann, R. & Saracci, R. (1991) A collaborative study of cancer incidence and mortality among vinyl chloride workers. *Scand. J. Work Environ. Health*, **17**, 159–169

Singer, B. & Grunberger, D. (1983) *Molecular Biology of Mutagenesis and Carcinogenesis*, New York, Plenum Press

Souliotis, V.L., Chhabra, S., Anderson, L.M. & Kyrtopoulos, S.A. (1995) Dosimetry of O^6-methylguanine in rat DNA after low-dose, chronic exposure to *N*-nitrosodimethylamine (NDMA). Implications for the mechanism of NDMA hepatocarcinogenesis. *Carcinogenesis*, **16**, 2381–2387

Vainio, H. (1998) Use of biomarkers – new frontiers in occupational toxicology and epidemiology. *Toxicol. Lett.*, **102–103**, 581–589

Ward, E., Boffetta, P., Andersen, A., Colin, D., Comba, P., Deddens, J.A., De Santis, M., Engholm, G., Hagmar, L., Langård, S., Lundberg, I., McElvenny, D., Piratsu, R., Sali, D. & Simonato, L. (2001) Update of the follow-up of mortality and cancer incidence among European workers employed in the vinyl chloride industry. *Epidemiology*, **12**, 710–718

White, I.N., De Matteis, F., Davies, A., Smith, L.L., Crofton-Sleigh, C., Venitt, S., Hewer, A. & Phillips, D.H. (1992) Genotoxic potential of tamoxifen and analogues in female Fischer F344/N rats, DBA/2 and C57BL/6 mice and in human MCL-5 cells. *Carcinogenesis*, **13**, 2197–2203

Wu, K.Y., Ranasinghe, A., Upton, P.B., Walker, V.E. & Swenberg, J.A. (1999) Molecular dosimetry of endogenous and ethylene oxide-induced N7-(2-hydroxyethyl) guanine formation in tissues of rodents. *Carcinogenesis*, **20**, 1787–1792

Corresponding author:
James A. Swenberg
School of Medicine, CB 7400,
University of North Carolina,
Rosenau Hall, Room 357,
Chapel Hill, NC 27599-7525,
USA
jswenber@sph.unc.edu

Mechanisms of Carcinogenesis: Contributions of Molecular Epidemiology
Patricia Buffler, Jerry Rice, Robert Baan, Michael Bird and Paolo Boffetta, eds
IARC Scientific Publications No. 157
International Agency for Research on Cancer, Lyon, 2004

TP53 Mutation Spectra and Load: A Tool for Generating Hypotheses on the Etiology of Cancer

Magali Olivier, S. Perwez Hussain, Claude Caron de Fromentel, Pierre Hainaut and Curtis C. Harris

Summary

Among genetic alterations, the activation of proto-oncogenes and inactivation of tumour suppressor genes in affected cells are considered to be the core molecular events that provide a selective growth advantage and clonal expansion during the multistep process of carcinogenesis. The TP53 tumour suppressor gene is mutated in about half of all human cancer cases. The p53 protein modulates multiple cellular functions, such as gene transcription, DNA synthesis and repair, cell cycle arrest, senescence and apoptosis. Mutations in the TP53 gene can abrogate these functions, leading to genetic instability and progression to cancer. The molecular archaeology of the TP53 mutation spectrum generates hypotheses concerning the etiology and molecular pathogenesis of each type of cancer. The spectrum of somatic mutations in the TP53 gene, of which 75% are missense mutations, implicates environmental carcinogens and endogenous processes in the etiology of human cancer. The presence of a characteristic TP53 mutation can also manifest a molecular link between exposure to a particular carcinogen and a specific type of human cancer, e.g. exposure to aflatoxin B_1 (AFB_1) and codon 249 mutations in hepatocellular carcinoma; exposure to ultraviolet (UV) light and C:C→T:T tandem mutations in skin cancer; and cigarette smoking and the prevalence of G→T transversions in lung cancer. Although exogenous carcinogens have been shown to target p53 selectively, evidence supporting the endogenous insult of TP53 from oxyradicals and nitrogen-oxyradicals is also accumulating. TP53 mutations can

be a biomarker of carcinogen effect. Determining the characteristic TP53 mutation load in non-tumorous tissue, using a highly sensitive mutation assay, can indicate exposure to a specific carcinogen and may also help in identifying individuals at an increased risk of cancer.

Introduction

Carcinogenesis is a multistep process driven by carcinogen-induced genetic and epigenetic damage in susceptible cells that gain a selective growth advantage and undergo clonal expansion as a result of the activation of proto-oncogenes or the inactivation of tumour suppressor genes. The traditional view of carcinogenesis (Figure 1) is derived primarily from studies of animal models (Harris, 1991; Hanahan & Weinberg, 2000). The first stage of the carcinogenesis process, tumour initiation, involves the exposure of normal cells to a chemical, physical or microbial carcinogen that causes a genetic change or changes. This not only provides the initiated cells with an altered responsiveness to their microenvironment, but also exerts a selective clonal expansion advantage over surrounding normal cells. The initiated cells may have decreased responsiveness to the inter- and intracellular signals that maintain normal tissue architecture and regulate the homeostatic growth and maturation of cells. For example, initiated cells may be less responsive to negative growth factors, promoters of terminal cell differentiation or programmed cell death. Tumour promotion results in the superior survival or proliferation of the initiated cells compared with normal cells, and enhances the probability of additional genetic

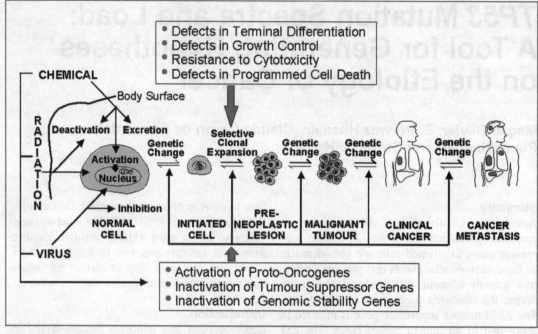

Figure 1. Molecular pathogenesis of human lung cancer

damage including endogenous mutations accumulating in the expanding population of these cells. The probability of a subpopulation of initiated cells converting to malignancy can be substantially increased by their further exposure to DNA-damaging agents that may activate proto-oncogenes or inactivate tumour suppressor genes. Malignant cells continue to exhibit progressive phenotypic changes during tumour progression and may exhibit intrinsic genomic instability that is manifested by the abnormal number (aneuploidy) and structure of chromosomes, gene amplification and altered gene expression.

Proto-oncogenes and tumour suppressor genes are critical DNA targets in the carcinogenic process. Somatic alterations of proto-oncogenes or tumour suppressor genes can be the result of endogenous processes, such as replication errors or attack by free radicals generated by cellular metabolism. Another source of DNA damage resides in exogenous genotoxic agents, such as ionizing radiation, UV radiation or chemical carcinogens. The cell possesses efficient machinery to detect and to repair all the lesions present

in the genome. Nevertheless, in some cases, errors are not repaired and permanent mutations are introduced (Hoffmann & Cazaux, 1998; Bertram, 2000).

The pattern of these mutations can be regarded as a source of information on the natural history of cancers. The factors that influence the formation of a specific mutation pattern can be seen as a succession of 'filters' that select for particular mutations (Hainaut & Hollstein, 2000).

- First, the capacity of exposed cells and tissues to metabolize carcinogens determines the capacity of a given mutagen to induce DNA damage.
- Second, the type of damage caused by a mutagen can be specific in its nature and DNA-sequence context.
- Third, the inherent capacity of cells to repair DNA corrects for most alterations and only those that escape repair will result in fixed mutations.
- Fourth, selective biological mechanisms favour cells that have acquired a proliferative advantage as a consequence of the mutation.

Weighting the contribution of these successive filters in shaping a tumour-specific mutation pattern provides interesting clues on the molecular mechanisms involved in the etiology and pathogenesis of human cancers.

Despite the multiplicity of genes involved in carcinogenesis, only a few show mutation patterns suitable as a source of information on mutagenic processes. These genes share several characteristics. They are altered in a wide range of different cancer types. They frequently show point mutations distributed within defined, short areas of the gene (less than 1–2 kb). These point mutations differ by their position and chemical nature. Table 1 summarizes the characteristics of frequently altered cancer genes that meet these requirements.

The *RAS* gene family comprises three members, Kirstein (K)-*RAS*, Harvey (H)-*RAS* and neuroblastoma (N)-*RAS*. The proteins encoded by these genes are tightly regulated enzymes involved in the intracellular transmission of signals generated by receptors at the cell membrane. Missense mutations at a very small number of codons (essentially codons 12, 13 and 61) result in the constitutive activation of these enzymes, leading to permanent stimulation of cell proliferation and inhibition of apoptosis (Crespo & Leon, 2000; Hernandez-Alcoceba *et al.*, 2000).

The three other genes, *CDKN2A* (*TP16*), *TP53* and *APC*, belong to the family of tumour suppressors. Mutation of these genes results in loss of activity, either through loss of protein expression or through expression of an abnormal, dysfunctional protein.

CDKN2A encodes the p16 protein, which is part of the cell-cycle control machinery and acts as a 'brake' to prevent untimely DNA replication (Foulkes *et al.*, 1997). This gene is frequently altered in most types of cancers by diverse mechanisms, including deletions, frameshift mutations and hypermethylation, resulting in transcriptional silencing or missense mutations (Rocco & Sidransky, 2001). The latter, however, represents a relatively infrequent mode of inactivation for this gene.

APC encodes a cytoplasmic protein which is involved in growth and cell adhesion signalling

pathways. Inherited mutations of this gene are the molecular basis of familial polyposis, a syndrome that predisposes to colorectal cancer (Groden *et al.*, 1991). Somatic mutations are detectable in non-familial colon cancer as well as in several other epithelial tumours (Sieber *et al.*, 2000; van Es *et al.*, 2001).

TP53 encodes p53, a transcription factor which controls the synthesis of several families of proteins involved in the control of the cell cycle, DNA repair, apoptosis and differentiation. It plays a central role in inhibiting the growth of cells exposed to chemical or physical stress, including cancer cells. Thus, loss of p53 functions promotes the growth of cells under stress conditions which suppress the proliferation of normal cells (Levine, 1997). Most *TP53* mutations are single-base substitutions affecting residues in the DNA-binding domain of the protein. Over 16 000 mutations have been reported to date, with mutation prevalences that vary from one type of cancer to another (Figure 2). Because of this high prevalence of very diverse mutations, *TP53* is thus particularly well suited for the analysis of cancer-specific mutation patterns.

TP53: a key gene in carcinogenesis

TP53 is located on chromosome 17 p13. It contains 11 exons spanning 20 kb and encodes a (mostly) nuclear phosphoprotein of 53 kDa. This gene belongs to a family of highly conserved genes that contains at least two other members, *TP63* and *TP73* (Kaghad *et al.*, 1997; Matsuura *et al.*, 1998; Yang *et al.*, 1998). The p53 protein appears to differ from its cousins by its unique role in tumour suppression, as illustrated by p53-deficient mice, which are developmentally normal but show a very high incidence of multiple, early tumours (Donehower *et al.*, 1992; Fronza *et al.*, 2000). In humans, inheritance of a *TP53* mutant allele results in a rare familial syndrome of multiple, early cancers, the Li–Fraumeni syndrome (Malkin *et al.*, 1990).

The p53 protein contains three main functional domains: an acidic N-terminus with a transactivating activity, a hydrophobic central core that binds to specific DNA sequences and a basic C-terminus carrying oligomerization and regulatory

Table 1. Alterations of four cancer-related genes in human cancers

Name	Type	Database[a]	Alterations	Frequency	Tumour type[b]
RAS *family*					
K-*RAS*	Oncogene	–	Missense mutation, amplification	30–60%	Lung, colon and pancreatic adenocarcinomas
H-*RAS*	Oncogene	–	Missense mutation, amplification	10–20%	Thyroid, kidney and liver cancers
N-*RAS*	Oncogene	–	Missense mutation	13–30%	AML[c], melanoma, thyroid and liver cancers
CDKN2A (*TP16*)	Tumour suppressor gene	http://pcdnr83.uio.no/	Nonsense point mutation	5–15%	Melanoma, glioblastoma and pancreatic carcinoma
			Deletion	20–60%	Melanoma, head and neck cancers and lung cancer
			Hypermethylation	10–40%	Many cancers
APC	Tumour suppressor gene	http://www.umd.necker.fr:2008/	Deletion, nonsense mutation		Colon, thyroid and stomach carcinomas
TP53	Tumour suppressor gene	http://www.iarc.fr/p53 http://www.umd.necker.fr:2001/	Point mutation	5–50%	Many cancers
			Deletion	> 50%	Many cancers
			Sequestration by mdm2	15–30%	Osteosarcoma and soft-tissue sarcoma
			Sequestration by viral protein	50%	Cervical cancer

[a] The web addresses of sites providing compilation of mutation data are indicated.
[b] Non-exhaustive list of cancers where this alteration is frequent.
[c] Acute myeloid leukaemia

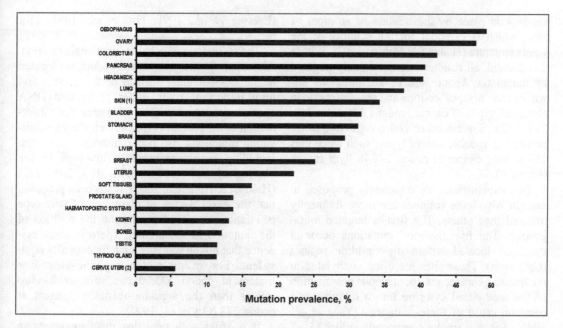

Figure 2. Prevalence of *TP53* mutations in cancers arising in various organs (data from the R5 version of the IARC *TP53* Database, 2001). (1) Includes all non-melanoma skin neoplasms. (2) In cancer of the cervix, p53 is inactivated by human papillomavirus (HPV) proteins.

functions (see May & May, 1999). Figure 3 provides a synthetic view of the p53 pathway. The p53 protein is expressed in almost all tissues as a constitutively repressed protein. Several classes of signals can lead to the de-repression of p53 and its accumulation by post-translational modifications. These signals include DNA-damaging agents

(genotoxic stress), constitutive activation of growth signalling cascades (oncogenic stress) and other types of stress such as depletion in ribonucleotides or hypoxia (Vogelstein *et al.*, 2000). Thus, p53 lies at the point of convergence of several distinct stress–response pathways (Ljungman, 2000). Once activated, p53 regulates the expression of several classes of genes and mediates coordinated anti-proliferative effects, including induction of cell cycle arrest, enhancement of DNA repair, initiation of apoptosis and inhibition of angiogenesis (Agarwal *et al.*, 1998).

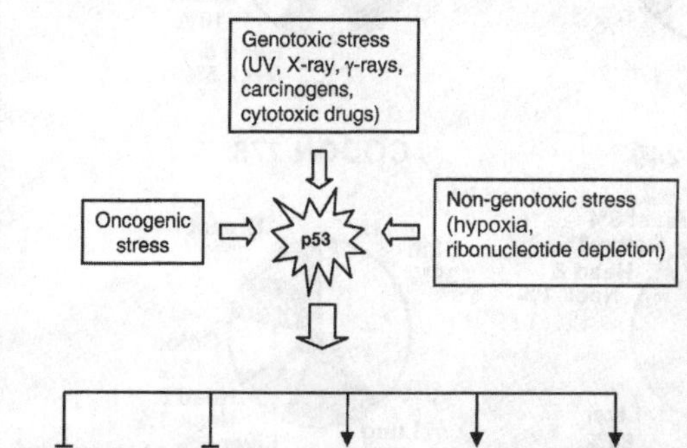

Diversity of TP53 *mutations in cancer*

Over 75% of all *TP53* mutations are missense, resulting in the substitution of a single amino-acid with another (IARC *TP53* Database, http://www.iarc.fr/P53/). Mutations are distributed in all coding exons, with a strong predominance in exons 4–9, encoding the DNA-binding domain of the protein (Hainaut & Hollstein, 2000). This domain has a complex structure made of two β-sheets (forming a sandwich) bridged by sets of loops and helixes (Cho *et al.*, 1994). These loops

Figure 3. Biological effects mediated by p53 in response to different classes of stress signals.

are kept in place by the binding of an atom of zinc, which is essential for the stability of the whole structure (Hainaut & Milner, 1993). Within this domain, all residues are not equally targeted by mutations. About 30% of all mutations fall within five 'hotspot' codons and are detectable in almost all types of cancer (codons 175, 245, 248, 273, 282). Several other codons are frequently mutated in specific cancer types, such as codons 157 in lung cancer or codon 249 in liver cancer (Figure 4).

Two explanations are commonly proposed to explain why some residues are more frequently mutated than others. The first is targeted mutagenesis. The five 'hotspot' mutations occur at cytosines located within dipyrimidine repeats (CpG sites). These sites are often methylated in the human genome, and spontaneous deamination of the methylated cytosine into a thymine is a common cause of these mutations (Yang et al., 1996). Tobacco smoke compounds induce G→T transversions at codons 157, 158, 248 and 273 in lung cancer (Hainaut & Pfeifer, 2001), and aflatoxin B_1, a carcinogenic mycotoxin, induces G→T transversions at codon 249 in liver cancer

(Bressac et al., 1991; Hsu et al., 1991) (see below).

The second explanation is functional selection. Almost all frequently mutated codons are located at the DNA-binding surface of the protein and play important roles either in protein–DNA contacts (codons 245, 248, 273) or in the conformation of the protein (175, 282). However, inactivating mutations also occur at many other sites, including particular residues involved in the binding of zinc (codons 176, 179, 238, 242) (Hainaut & Hollstein, 2000). It has been proposed that the exact degree of disruption of wild-type p53 functions may depend upon the position of the mutation in the protein. There is some evidence that not all mutations are functionally equivalent. For example, the arginine→histidine mutant at codon 175 shows stronger in-vitro effects than the arginine→histidine mutant at codon 273 (Ory et al., 1994).

It is striking to note that most mutations in TP53 do not result in the loss of the protein. Quite the opposite: most cancer cells accumulate the mutant p53 protein, and even retain high protein levels in distant metastases. These high levels are

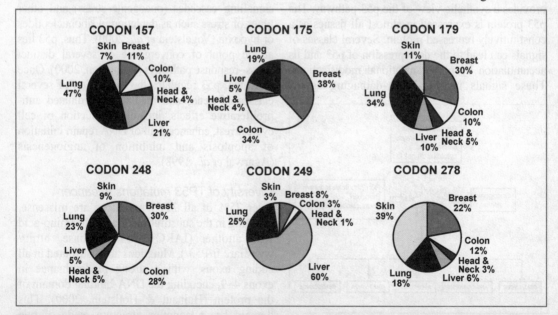

Figure 4. p53 Mutational hotspots in human cancers. Most types of human cancer show the domination of specific p53 mutations at particular mutational hotspots. The characteristic patterns suggest molecular linkage between a particular cancer and a specific exogenous or endogenous carcinogen

due to the fact that mutant p53 is more stable than the wild type, leading to protein accumulation. Thus, cancer cells behave as if they were selectively retaining the mutant p53 protein. Inactivation of the protein function is probably only one of the effects of missense mutation. It was postulated more than 10 years ago that the mutant p53 protein could exert some pro-oncogenic effect, and that mutation was in fact turning this tumour suppressor into some kind of oncogene (Michalovitz *et al.*, 1991). The molecular basis of this possible 'gain of function' is not fully elucidated (Sigal & Rotter, 2000). Recent studies have shown that some p53 mutants can interact with p63 and p73, two other members of the p53 family, and inhibit some of their functions (Di Como *et al.*, 1999; Strano *et al.*, 2000). Inactivation of the p63 and p73 pathways could explain a 'gain of function' of some p53 mutants.

Why TP53 *is often mutated in human cancers*

There is no evidence that *TP53* lies in a hypermutable region of the genome. Rather, cells that have lost p53 function may be selected during cancer development. In cancer cells with normal *TP53* alleles, the expression of the protein or its activity are often altered by, for example, overexpression of the mdm2 protein or of viral oncogenes (Scheffner *et al.*, 1990; Oliner *et al.*, 1992). Thus, one can postulate that cells should have at least some degree of p53 dysfunction to progress towards full neoplastic phenotype. This implies that activation of p53 functions occurs as part of the normal mechanisms of defence against neoplastic transformation.

At the molecular level, the focal point of these mechanisms is the interaction between p53 and mdm2, a protein that induces p53 degradation and prevents its accumulation in normal cells (Kirk *et al.*, 2000; Momand *et al.*, 2000). This interaction can be broken down by several classes of signals (Figure 5) (Oren, 1999). The first is DNA damage (Appella & Anderson, 2000; Yang *et al.*, 2000). The occurence of multiple forms of DNA damage (strand breaks, bulky adducts, oxidation damage) can trigger a cascade of kinase activation, which phosphorylate p53 at multiple sites

and thus block the interaction between p53 and mdm2 (Banin *et al.*, 1998; Appella & Anderson, 2000). This DNA damage pathway was the first p53 regulatory pathway to be identified.

The second class of signals involves as a main effector the p14^{ARF} protein. p14^{ARF} is an alternative product of the *CDKN2A* locus, which also encodes the cyclin kinase inhibitor p16 (Sherr & Weber, 2000). p14^{ARF} binds mdm2 and neutralizes its capacity to repress p53 (Kamijo *et al.*, 1998; Pomerantz *et al.*, 1998; Honda & Yasuda, 1999; Tanière *et al.*, 2000). During neoplastic transformation, deregulation of pathways such as the ras/E2F pathway, or the β-catenin/c-myc pathway, can lead to activation of p14^{ARF} (Lowe, 1999) and, consequently, to p53-dependent growth suppression. Therefore, only cells that are capable of by-passing this p53-dependent suppression can progress toward full neoplasia.

The third class of signals is less well understood. Recently, we have shown that a radioprotective drug, amifostine, could activate p53 by a pathway that is independent of DNA damage but requires the Jun–N-terminal kinase (JNK) (Pluquet *et al.*, 2003). Like mdm2, JNK regulates the degradation of p53 (Milne *et al.*, 1992; Fuchs *et al.*, 1998). This pathway may control p53 activation in response to a broad variety of stress signals. There is also evidence that hypoxia can induce a long-lasting induction of p53 by a mechanism that is different from DNA damage signalling (Alarcon *et al.*, 1999).

The process of cancer is characterized by the constitutive activation of these three classes of signals. DNA damage occurs as a consequence of exposure to environmental mutagens but can also occur through endogenous mechanisms, such as polymerase errors or defects in DNA repair processes. Constitutive activation of growth signalling pathways is a common denominator of all primary cancer lesions. Hypoxia is a very frequent phenomenon at various stages of the progression of solid tumours. Thus, during cancer initiation and progression, many different selection pressures will converge on p53 through these three mechanisms, acting either separately or in combination.

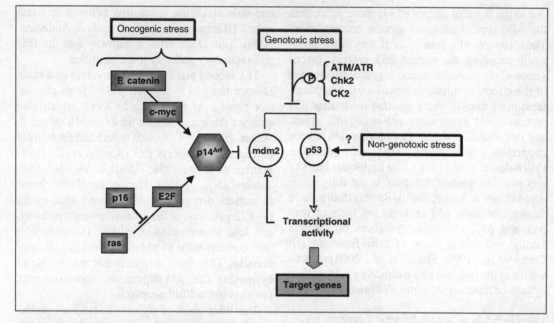

Figure 5. Classes of signals that lead to p53 activation. The feedback regulatory loop between p53 and mdm2 proteins is represented in the centre of the figure. Three classes of signals are illustrated that can break down this loop. The breakdown of the loop results in p53 accumulation and activation as a transcription factor

TP53 *mutations in cancer progression: 'late' or 'early' event?*

Although *TP53* is often mutated in many types of cancers, the timing of occurrence of the mutation during cancer progression is extremely variable from one cancer to another. In the now classical model of stepwise progression of colorectal cancers, Fearon and Vogelstein (1990) demonstrated that *TP53* mutation and loss of alleles preferentially occur at the transition between late adenoma and carcinoma *in situ*, that is, at a relatively late stage in the histopathological development of these lesions. Similar findings are reported in many common cancers, including breast and prostate cancers. In contrast, *TP53* mutation seems to occur at an early stage in many types of cancer that are caused directly by exogenous carcinogens. As discussed below, this is the case for lung cancers of smokers, non-melanoma skin cancers after exposure to UV irradiation and esophageal cancers. In these cancers, *TP53* mutations are often detectable in hyperplastic and dysplastic lesions, as well as in non-involved, apparently

normal tissues surrounding the tumour (Mandard *et al.*, 2000; Hussain *et al.*, 2001).

Moreover, the position of *TP53* mutation in the temporal sequence of events leading to cancer is not always constant. For example, in hepatocellular carcinoma (HCC), *TP53* mutations are late events in most cancers occurring in western populations, but are very early events in most of the cases in West Africa and in South-east Asia (Montesano *et al.*, 1997). In these regions, HCC occurs as a consequence of exposure to aflatoxins. This potent hepatocarcinogen contaminates the traditional diet and acts synergistically with chronic carriage of hepatitis virus B (see below). In individuals exposed to aflatoxin, *TP53* mutations are detectable in cirrhotic liver before the onset of cancer (Livni *et al.*, 1995). Another example is colon carcinoma. Apart from the well-characterized 'late' involvement of *TP53* described by Fearon and Vogelstein (1990) in polypoid carcinomas, there is evidence that *TP53* mutation can occur at an early stage in serrated carcinoma (Hawkins *et al.*, 2000). *TP53* mutations have also been found in non-

.

tumorous colonic tissue from inflamed regions in patients with ulcerative colitis (Hussain *et al.*, 2000a). In this case, they may result from an endogenous carcinogenic stress (reactive oxygen species and nitrogen species produced by the inflammatory micro-environment due to ulcerative colitis).

We suggest that the place of *TP53* mutation in the sequence of cancer progression reflects the nature of the mechanisms responsible for the activation of p53 function. In tissues heavily exposed to carcinogens (such as lung in smokers, liver in individuals exposed to aflatoxins and colon in individuals with ulcerative colitis), the p53 protein is induced as part of the normal response to DNA damage. This induction results in the suppression of damaged cells. Occurrence of a mutation in a normal, exposed cell may thus provide a selective advantage for clonal expansion. In other cancers, many genetic changes may occur before *TP53* mutation, which generate an oncogenic stress through the p14[ARF] pathway. At some point during cancer development, the presence of wild-type p53 would thus become a limiting factor for progression, and only cells that have lost p53 function will be able to progress to invasive cancer. It is clear that this concept can be expanded to explain the occurrence of *TP53* mutations at almost any stage of cancer progression.

The *TP53* database as a tool for analysing the pattern of *TP53* mutations

After the identification of frequent *TP53* mutations in cancer in 1989, it rapidly became evident that mutation patterns could significantly differ from one cancer to another (Hollstein *et al.*, 1991a; Caron de Fromentel & Soussi, 1992). These observations led to the development of computerized lists of mutations that have now evolved into complex databases. The *TP53* database, maintained and developed at the International Agency for Research on Cancer (IARC *TP53* Database, http://www.iarc.fr/P53/), includes somatic and inherited mutations, as well as polymorphisms that have been reported in the literature since 1989. The current release of the database (R6, updated in January 2002) contains 16 371 somatic mutations and 214 germline muta-

tions (Olivier *et al.*, 2002). This dataset is the largest available on variations of any human gene.

The information compiled in the database includes a detailed description of the tumour sample and of the mutation. When available, information on individual risk factors, exposures and clinical parameters are also included. It is thus possible to perform global analyses of mutation patterns by cancer type and to search for associations between a type of mutation and a specific exposure or risk factor. However, the database is affected by several biases.

- First, most of the data included are from retrospective studies, where tumour cases were selected on the basis of relevance to pathological or clinical questions. Only a minority of publications describe molecular epidemiological studies with adequate controls and exposure groups.
- Second, as the database is exclusively based on peer-reviewed literature, it reflects changing trends in reporting and publishing of mutations. Other biases may stem from the difference in specificity and sensitivity of the method used for mutation detection. Nonetheless, the database is a useful tool for analysing large sets of data easily and generating hypotheses about the mechanisms that might have caused the mutation.

TP53 mutations as fingerprints for carcinogens in human cancers

The most striking characteristic of *TP53* mutation patterns for the non-educated observer is that they look extremely similar from one cancer to the other. This similarity results from the fact that many mutations, in particular transitions at CpG sites, are common in all cancers. Nevertheless, several cancers show distinct patterns that may indicate the presence of mutations induced by exogenous carcinogens. An 'induced' mutation profile is suspected when the following features appear:

- tumour-type or exposure-group-specific 'hotspot' mutations
- unusual predominance of a particular type of base substitution

• a preferential accumulation of the mutation on the non-transcribed strand of DNA (strand bias). Strand bias is the consequence of the preferential repair of DNA adducts on the transcribed strand by transcription-coupled repair systems (Scicchitano & Hanawalt, 1992). This phenomenon results in the preferential accumulation of certain types of mutation on the non-transcribed strand as, for example, in the case of G→T transversions in lung cancer (Hainaut & Pfeifer, 2001) (see below and Figure 6).

There are only a few well-documented examples of mutation patterns caused by exogenous carcinogens in human cancers. These include HCC, lung cancer and non-melanoma skin cancer. However, in a number of other cancers, variations in the mutation profiles have been observed, which may help to generate new hypotheses on the nature of the mutagenic processes involved. This is the case in bladder, breast and esophageal cancers.

Lung cancer: tobacco smoking

Over 1700 *TP53* mutations in lung cancers are included in the *TP53* mutation database. Mutations are detected in 25–80% of tumours in all histological subtypes of lung cancers from smokers (the lowest prevalence is 25% in adeno-carcinoma). One-third of these mutations are G→T transversions, a type of mutation that represents only 14% of mutations in nonsmokers and 13% of mutations in all other cancers grouped together (Figure 7). These substitutions show a strong strand bias (90% are on the non-transcribed strand, see Figure 6) and are relatively uncommon in cancers other than of the lung. Codon 157 is a 'hotspot' in lung cancers but is rarely mutated in other cancers (see Figure 4). Codons 248 and 273 are often mutated in lung as well as in other cancers. However, the nature of the base substitution is different. In lung cancer, about 50% of the mutations are G→T transversions. In cancers other than of the lung, 92% of the mutations at codons 248 and 273 are C→T transitions within the CpG sites (reviewed in Hainaut & Pfeifer, 2001).

Experimental studies using cultured primary bronchial cells have shown that mutated bases correspond to sites where metabolites of benzo[*a*]-pyrene, a major component of tobacco smoke, form adducts *in vitro* (Denissenko *et al.*, 1996). Specific targeting of codons 248 and 273 is explained by the observation that metabolites of benzo[*a*]pyrene preferentially bind to guanines

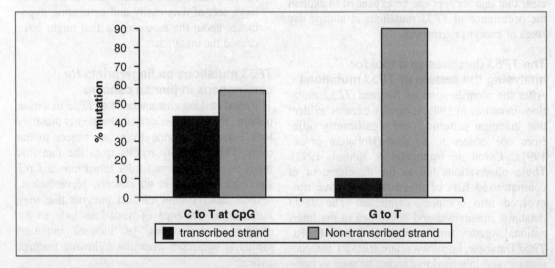

Figure 6. The proportion of C→T transitions at CpG sites and G→T transversions on each strand of DNA are represented. There is no strand bias for transitions at CpG sites, whereas there is a strong strand bias for G→T transversions (90% occur on the non-transcribed strand). This difference indicates that G→T transversions are due to a mechanism that may involve the formation of bulky DNA adducts preferentially repaired by transcription-coupled repair

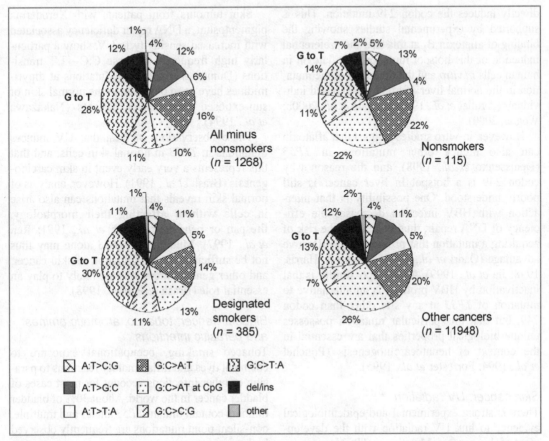

Figure 7. *TP53* mutation pattern in lung cancers (Data from the R5 version of the IARC *TP53* Database, 2001).

next to a methylated cytosine (Denissenko *et al.*, 1997; Yoon *et al.*, 2001). Furthermore, a recent study has shown that benzo[*a*]pyrene can induce mutation at codon 157 *in vitro*, and that this mutation can be detected in the non-involved tissue adjacent to lung cancer in smokers (Hussain *et al.*, 2001). Although benzo[*a*]pyrene is not the only mutagen in tobacco smoke that can induce G→T transversions, the molecular evidence from *TP53* mutations suggests that this agent is a major *TP53* mutagen in lung cancers of smokers.

Hepatocellular carcinoma: hepatitis B virus (HBV) and mycotoxins

Different *TP53* mutation patterns are observed in regions of high and low incidence of HCC. In regions of high incidence (age-standardized

incidence rate > 25/100 000/year), such as sub-Saharan Africa and South-east Asia, the *TP53* mutation profile is dominated by a single codon, codon 249 (AGG→AGT, Arg→Ser). This mutation is very rare in HCC from western Europe or North America, where the mutation pattern is much more heterogeneous (Montesano *et al.*, 1997). In regions of high incidence, mutation at codon 249 represents up to 90% of all *TP53* mutations in HCC, and approximately half of the HCC carry a mutant *TP53* (Bressac *et al.*, 1991; Hsu *et al.*, 1991; Ozturk, 1991). In these populations, the two most important and synergistically interacting risk factors are chronic HBV infection and ingestion of aflatoxins, mycotoxins that contaminate most of the traditional diet. The most plausible interpretation of this mutation profile is that the mycotoxin directly induces the codon 249 mutation. This is supported by experimental studies showing the binding of aflatoxin B_1 at this site, the preferential induction of this hotspot mutation by aflatoxin in human cells *in vitro* and the detection of the mutation in the normal liver of aflatoxin-exposed individuals (Aguilar *et al.*, 1993; Hussain *et al.*, 2000b; Wogan, 2000).

However, in-vitro studies suggest that aflatoxin can also induce other mutations in *TP53* (Denissenko *et al.*, 1998), and the reason why codon 249 is a hotspot in liver cancer is still poorly understood. One possibility is that interaction with HBV infection decreases the efficiency of DNA repair, thus increasing the risk of acquiring a mutation that provides a proliferative advantage (Qadri *et al.*, 1996; Elmore & Harris, 1998; Jia *et al.*, 1999). Another possibility is that inactivation by HBV proteins is an alternative to mutation of *TP53* at any site other than codon 249, but that this particular mutation possesses unique biological properties that are essential in the context of hepatocarcinogenesis (Ponchel *et al.*, 1994; Forrester *et al.*, 1995).

Skin cancer: UV radiation

There is strong experimental and epidemiological evidence to link UV radiation with the development of skin cancers. Mutation in *TP53* is common in all skin cancers except melanoma, in which p53 appears to be inactivated by alternative mechanisms such as mutation in p16/p14^{ARF} (Rocco & Sidransky, 2001). The *TP53* mutation spectrum in non-melanoma skin cancers shows a high frequency of C→T transitions (61%), including tandem C:C→T:T transitions (17% of all mutations) (Brash *et al.*, 1991). Such tandem transitions are extremely uncommon in any other tumour type. Tandem C:C→T:T mutations are formed as a result of inefficient repair of a common photoproduct, the cyclobutane pyrimidine dimers, induced by UV radiation (Tornaletti *et al.*, 1993). Half of the C:C→T:T transitions are within CpG sequences and recent evidence indicates that absorption of near-UV by 5-methylcytosine is up to 15-fold higher than that by cytosine, suggesting that solar UV light could preferentially affect cytosine at CpG sites (Tommasi *et al.*, 1997).

Skin tumours from patients with Xeroderma pigmentosum, a DNA repair deficiency associated with increased sensitivity to UV, show a particularly high frequency of these C:C→T:T transitions (Dumaz *et al.*, 1993). Mutations at dipyrimidines have been observed in the normal skin of sun-exposed skin cancer patients (Nakazawa *et al.*, 1994).

These observations suggest that UV induces mutations in *TP53* in normal skin cells, and that this represents a very early event in skin carcinogenesis (Brash *et al.*, 1991). However, analysis of normal skin reveals that mutations can also arise in cells without affecting their morphology, lifespan or behaviour (Brash *et al.*, 1991; Ren *et al.*, 1997). Mutation of *TP53* alone may thus not be sufficient for the initiation of skin cancer, and other genetic alterations are likely to play an essential role (Brash & Ponten, 1998).

Bladder cancer: tobacco, aromatic amines and parasitic infections

Tobacco smoking, occupational exposure to chemical dyes and inflammatory reactions to parasitic or other infections account for most cases of bladder cancer in the world. About 30% of bladder tumours contain mutant *TP53* alleles and multiple, non-silent point mutations are frequently observed in the same tumour.

Aromatic amines are mutagenic for bladder epithelial cells and are present in both tobacco smoke and compounds used in the dye industry (IARC, 1972–2002). It is therefore not surprising that the pattern of mutations in bladder cancers of smokers shows similarities with the pattern in occupationally exposed workers (Taylor *et al.*, 1996; Sorlie *et al.*, 1998). It should also be noted that smoking is a confounding factor in the cohorts of chemical dye workers that have been examined for *TP53* mutations, and that most of these cohorts were relatively small (Esteve *et al.*, 1995; Taylor *et al.*, 1996; Yasunaga *et al.*, 1997; Sorlie *et al.*, 1998). Aromatic amines can induce a number of DNA lesions, including transversions and transitions on G bases (Essigmann & Wood, 1993).

The distribution of the 551 bladder cancer *TP53* mutations compiled in the IARC database

(R5 version) shows an unusual cluster of mutations between codons 271 and 285, with a particularly high prevalence for codons 280 and 285 (4.3% and 4.9% of all mutations, respectively). Interestingly, these two codons are in the same DNA sequence context (A*GA*G for codon 280 and A*GA*G for codon 285). This suggests that this sequence may represent a preferential target for specific carcinogens, such as aromatic amines (Verghis *et al.*, 1997). Bladder tumours from regions of endemic parasitic infections show a different pattern of mutations, with a high prevalence of C→T transitions at CpG sites (Warren *et al.*, 1995). This high prevalence is in agreement with the effect of nitric oxide (NO), a common mediator of inflammation, on the rate of deamination of 5-methylcytosine (see below).

These data indicate that *TP53* mutation patterns in bladder cancers show fingerprints of exogenous exposures. Since the risk factors for bladder cancer are well characterized, it will be particularly informative to examine patients without smoking history or occupational exposure in order to distinguish between induced and spontaneous mutation signatures.

Esophageal cancer: multiple environmental risk factors

In esophageal cancers, *TP53* is mutated in 50% of in-situ or invasive carcinomas, and mutations are detectable in dysplasia as well as in precancer tissues. In adenocarcinoma, mutations have been found in the Barrett metaplasia that precedes cancer (Neshat *et al.*, 1994; Barrett *et al.*, 1999). In squamous-cell carcinoma, mutations have been observed in the mucosa of individuals with chronic esophagitis in a region of high incidence (Normandy) (Mandard *et al.*, 2000). These observations indicate that loss of p53 function is a very early, if not the earliest, genetic event detected in esophageal cancers.

The pattern of mutations differs between the two types of esophageal cancer (Montesano *et al.*, 1996). In adenocarcinoma, half of the mutations are transitions at CpG sites (Figure 8). These mutations are consistent with a role of chronic inflammatory stress (generating NO) in enhancing the rate of spontaneous deamination of methylated

cytosine. Indeed, the main risk factor for Barrett metaplasia is chronic gastro-esophageal reflux, a condition that leads to acute, chemical and inflammatory stress. Thus, in the Barrett mucosa, this stress, by generating NO, could increase the risk for formation of a CpG transition in *TP53* (Goldstein *et al.*, 1997).

Squamous-cell carcinoma shows striking geographical variations in incidence rates, and both the prevalence and profile of mutations show variations between areas of high and low incidence (Hollstein *et al.*, 1991b; Taniere *et al.*, 2000; Biramijamal *et al.*, 2001; Sepehr *et al.*, 2001). As there is little evidence for ethnic or genetic predisposition to esophageal cancer, these variations suggest the involvement of distinct environmental mutagens. However, these patterns are complex and cannot be assigned to a single causative agent or mechanism. The mutation patterns shown in Figure 8 are consistent with a role of dietary nitrosamines in high-incidence areas of China (50% are mutations at G:C base pairs at non-CpG sites) and of metabolites of alcohol in high-incidence areas of Europe (47% are mutations at A:T base pairs). Further analyses are needed to determine whether these mutational patterns can be assigned to specific environmental carcinogens.

Breast cancer: searching for clues

About 1400 mutations in breast cancers are listed in the *TP53* mutation database. They are generally associated with the most aggressive tumour types, but there are no clear data to indicate that mutations are restricted to a subtype of breast cancer. The prevalence of mutations is relatively low (20–30%), as compared with other frequent tumours such as lung or colon cancer. However, p53 protein levels are elevated in most of the cancer cases examined, leading to the hypothesis that p53 protein function could be inactivated or otherwise deregulated by mechanisms other than mutation (Midgley *et al.*, 1992; Vojtesek & Lane, 1993).

Overall, the pattern of *TP53* mutations in breast cancer does not show any striking characteristics. The most frequent type of mutation is G:C→A:T transitions (42%), and they affect CpG

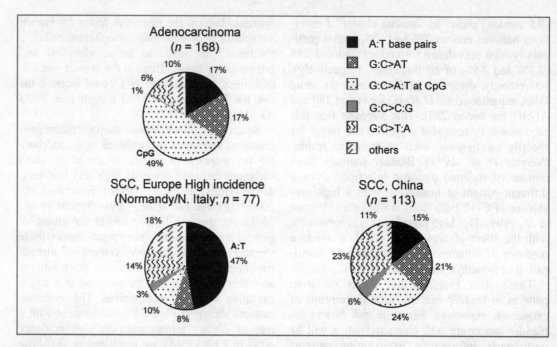

Figure 8. *TP53* mutation pattern in esophageal cancers (Data from the R5 version of the IARC *TP53* Database, 2001). SCC, squamous-cell carcinoma

and non-CpG sites equally. However, comparison between cohorts reveals differences in the nature, localization and frequency of the mutations. In particular, tumours from Europe show a greater proportion of G→T transversions than those from Japan (12% versus 5%). In contrast, deletions are more frequent in tumours from Japan than in tumours from western countries (18% versus 11%). The relatively high prevalence of G→T transversions in tumours from Europe suggests the possible involvement of unidentified, exogenous carcinogens (Olivier & Hainaut, 2001).

In breast tumours of *BRCA1* and *BRCA2* germline mutation carriers, the prevalence of *TP53* mutations is higher than that in sporadic tumours (54% versus 20%). This observation suggests that different mechanisms may be involved in the acquisition of *TP53* mutations in carriers of *BRCA1* and *BRCA2*, compared with patients without known genetic susceptibility. This hypothesis is in agreement with the notion that *BRCA1* and *BRCA2* may play specific roles in DNA repair (Moynahan *et al.*, 1999).

Overall, these data show that, although most of the mutations found in breast cancer might have a spontaneous origin, a small proportion of them bear signatures that suggest the involvement of specific mutagenic processes.

Nitric oxide as a candidate endogenous carcinogen

Aside from exogenous carcinogens, oxyradicals that are generated endogenously during various processes are a major source of mutagens in human cancer. One of these radicals is NO, an important bioregulatory and signalling molecule that may play a role in carcinogenesis (Moncada *et al.*, 1991; Bredt & Snyder, 1994; Nathan & Xie, 1994; Hentze & Kuhn, 1996; Tamir & Tannenbaum, 1996; Ambs *et al.*, 1997). NO formation is catalysed by a family of enzymes known as nitric oxide synthases (NOS) (Marletta, 1993; Forstermann & Kleinert, 1995). Of the three isoforms of NOS, two are Ca^{2+}-dependent (NOS1 and 3) and are generally found to be expressed constitutively, whereas the Ca^{2+}-independent isoform (iNOS or NOS2) requires induction (Chartrain *et al.*, 1994).

However, NOS1 and 3 can also be induced (Forstermann & Kleinert, 1995). An increased level of constitutive and inducible NOS expression or activity was observed in a variety of human cancers (Thomsen *et al.*, 1994; Cobbs *et al.*, 1995; Thomsen *et al.*, 1995; Koh *et al.*, 1999). Moreover, nitrotyrosine accumulation in the inflamed mucosa of patients with ulcerative colitis (Singer *et al.*, 1996), in the stomach of patients with a *Helicobacter pylori* gastritis (Mannick *et al.*, 1996) and in the esophagus of individuals with chronic esophagitis (Sepehr *et al.*, 2001) indicates that NO production and peroxynitrite formation also are involved in the pathogenesis of these diseases, and thus predispose individuals to cancer (Ohshima & Bartsch, 1994). Because cytokines and hypoxia induce NOS2 expression in stromal macrophages synergistically (Melillo *et al.*, 1995), the microenvironmental changes in premalignant and malignant tumour tissue may establish sustained and high NO production, thereby supporting clonal selection of preneoplastic cells and tumour growth.

A high level of NO production may modify DNA directly (Zhuang *et al.*, 1998; Tretyakova *et al.*, 2000; Zhuang *et al.*, 2000) or may inhibit DNA-repair activities (Wink *et al.*, 1996), such as human thymine–DNA glycosylase, which has been shown to repair G:T mismatches at CpG sites (Sibghat-Ullah *et al.*, 1996). Because NO production induces p53 accumulation and post-translational modification (Forrester *et al.*, 1996; Messmer & Brune, 1996), the resulting growth inhibition can provide an additional strong selection pressure for the clonal expansion of cells with mutant p53. There is good evidence that NO generated by NOS2 mutates *TP53* during human colon carcinogenesis (Ambs *et al.*, 1999). Tumours of the colon often show high levels of NOS2 expression, and there is a significant correlation between increased NOS2 activity and the presence of transition mutations at CpG sites in *TP53*. This type of transition is consistent with a role of NO in mutagenesis, since NO enhances the rate of spontaneous deamination of methylated cytosine (which occurs frequently at CpG sites) into thymine. These transitions are also common in cancers of lymphoid tissues, head and neck, stomach, esophagus, brain and breast. Increased

NOS2 expression has been demonstrated in several of these cancers, indicating that endogenous NO products can play a broad role as a human carcinogen.

Recent results indicate that NO regulates expression of vascular endothelial growth factor and neovascularization (Ambs *et al.*, 1998). Therefore, NO may also promote cancer progression by providing an angiogenic stimulus.

TP53 mutation load and cancer-prone oxyradical overload disease

An oxyradical overload disease develops from conditions with chronic inflammation and can have an etiology that is inherited (e.g. haemochromatosis, Wilson disease), acquired (e.g. hepatitis B or C virus, *Helicobacter pylori*) or chemically induced (e.g. acid reflux in Barrett esophagus). There also are a few oxyradical overload diseases with unknown etiology (e.g. ulcerative colitis, Crohn disease). Cancer-proneness is frequently a pathological consequence of extensive oxyradical damage that leads to a cycle of cell death and regeneration, and causes mutations in cancer-related genes.

We used a highly sensitive mutation assay to test the hypothesis that people with cancer-prone oxyradical overload diseases contain a high p53 mutation load. Analysis of non-tumorous colon from ulcerative colitis cases showed a higher frequency of G:C→A:T transitions at codon 248 of p53 in an inflamed lesional area compared with a non-lesional region (Linder *et al.*, 1998; Hussain *et al.*, 2000a). Furthermore, a higher frequency of G:C→T:A transversions at codon 249 was observed in the non-tumorous liver from people with haemochromatosis and Wilson disease compared with normal individuals (Hussain *et al.*, 2000b). People with Wilson disease also showed a higher frequency of G:C→T:A transversions and C:G→A:T transitions at codon 250 of p53. Cases of ulcerative colitis, haemochromatosis and Wilson disease with a high p53 mutational load also showed an increase in NOS2 activity or expression in the tissues at increased risk of cancer. These findings are consistent with the hypothesis that the generation of reactive species and aldehydes induces a high frequency of p53 mutations in oxyradical overload diseases that may contribute to the increased risk of cancer.

Perspectives: analysis of *TP53* mutations in molecular epidemiology

The examples discussed above show the usefulness of the analysis of *TP53* mutations in searching for clues to the nature of the mechanisms that lead to mutations in human cancers. However, most of the data available to date have been generated in small-scale, retrospective studies, and the application of *TP53* mutations as a biomarker in molecular epidemiology is still facing a number of technical and practical limitations. The first is the possibility of collecting suitable, well-characterized cancer tissues in population-based studies. The best source of material for *TP53* mutation analysis is tumour specimens obtained by surgery (fixed or frozen) or by biopsy. However, biopsies do not always provide a good representation of the tumour as a whole.

Analysis of the circulating DNA fragments in plasma and serum of cancer patients have shown alterations in oncogenes and tumour suppressor genes (Kirk *et al.*, 2000; Kopreski *et al.*, 2000). This approach opens a new door to cancer risk assessment. However, the success of this approach will depend on the sensitivity and reproducibility of the assay in detecting the specific gene alterations in individuals without clinically evident cancer. In the recent past, conventional methods have been used successfully in the analysis of plasma or serum DNA in cancer cases. Currently, we are working to develop this approach one step further by using our highly sensitive assay to detect altered gene fragments that occur with extremely low frequency in individuals from high-risk groups. This assay will allow us to determine the p53 mutation load in these individuals in contrast to existing methods that determine only the presence or absence of this alteration. If successful, this approach will be a better non-invasive way of identifying individuals at increased cancer risk.

The second obstacle to using *TP53* as a marker in molecular epidemiology is the absence of validated, high-throughput technology for large-scale studies. Mutation analysis still relies on the

sequencing of portions of the *TP53* gene to determine the exact nature and position of the mutation. Tumour DNA always contains a proportion of wild-type material due to the presence of wild-type alleles in cancer cells, or of non-cancer cells in the original tissue specimens. Therefore, DNA sequencing needs to be highly sensitive in order to detect mutant DNA against a background of wild-type material. Such sensitivity is not always achieved by standard, automated direct sequencing methods. Thus, *TP53* mutation analysis remains an expensive and labour-intensive process. The most common techniques used for *p53* mutation analysis include PCR-based assays such as single-strand conformational polymorphism (SSCP), denaturing gradient gel electrophoresis (DGGE), and DNA sequencing. Another method based on yeast functional assays was developed to detect p53 mutations (Scharer & Iggo, 1992; Ishioka *et al.*, 1995; Moshinsky & Wogan, 1997). In this assay, the loss of DNA binding and transcriptional–transactivation function in mutant p53 is detected by the colony colour of yeast. A very elegant and reliable assay, the short oligonucleotide mass assay (SOMA), has also been developed that involves PCR and mass spectrometry (Laken *et al.*, 1998). This assay enables simultaneous analysis of both strands of the gene. Recent publications have also described microarray-based methods for rapid screening of *TP53* mutations. The microarray developed by Affymetrix (Santa Clara, CA) is based on direct hybridization of *TP53* DNA fragments on immobilized oligonucleotides. This array shows good specificity but its sensitivity is still limited and its application in large-scale studies needs to be evaluated further (Ahrendt *et al.*, 1999; Wikman *et al.*, 2000). Another, commercial array is currently developed by Asper technologies (Tartu, Estonia). This assay is based on the use of immobilized oligonucleotides to perform a primer-extension reaction incorporating fluorescent nucleotides (APEX technology). This method is currently being evaluated for scaling-up (Tonisson *et al.*, 2002).

Beyond technical considerations, one of the main challenges for the exploitation of mutation analysis in molecular epidemiology lies in the correct assessment of individual exposures. So far, there are only a handful of studies in which the individual exposure to suspected risk factors has been evaluated, mostly using questionnaires (Sorlie *et al.*, 1998; Vahakangas *et al.*, 2001). In the future, it will be essential to combine mutation analysis with detailed assessment of individual exposures using reliable biomarkers. It should be noted that, in several instances, the prevalence of certain types of *TP53* mutations is correlated with the intensity of exposure to the suspected factor of risk. For example, the prevalence of G→T transversions in *TP53* is close to 50% in individuals reported to be heavy smokers, compared with 30% in those reported to be smokers and 10% in those reported to be nonsmokers (Vahakangas *et al.*, 2001).

Finally, the correct interpretation of mutation patterns will require the influence of genetic susceptibility to be taken into account. The data presented above on mutations in breast cancers of *BRCA1* and *BRCA2* mutation carriers and in skin cancers of patients with xeroderma pigmentosum clearly show that genetic make-up can influence the frequency and type of somatic mutations in *TP53*. These two examples relate to high-penetrance, low-frequency genetic alterations, but there is growing evidence that low-penetrance genetic variations, such as polymorphisms in carcinogen-metabolizing enzymes or in DNA-repair genes, can also influence the mutation pattern (Hussain & Harris, 1998). Thus, in the future, it will be important to develop batteries of genetic tests to identify the presence of such polymorphisms, in relation to the acquisition of specific types of *TP53* mutations. The methods described above for detecting point mutations are not sensitive enough to be used for analysis of non-tumorous tissue, which may contain very few mutant cells. The development of a highly sensitive genotypic assay by Cerutti and coworkers has allowed the detection of low-frequency mutations in normal-appearing human tissues, as well as in cells exposed to an environmental carcinogen (Aguilar *et al.*, 1993, 1994; Hussain *et al.*, 1994a,b, 1997). Furthermore, we have modified this assay for the analysis of codon 157 of p53, which is a unique hotspot for mutation in lung cancers among smokers (Hussain

et al., 2001). The detection of a particular mutation in normal-appearing tissue provides further support for the involvement of a specific carcinogen in a particular human cancer and may help identify individuals at increased cancer risk who are exposed to a particular carcinogen in the environment.

In the future, studies on *TP53* mutations will need to include large numbers of well-characterized cancer cases, with adequate exposure assessment and analysis of multiple genetic polymorphisms. The presence of mutations in non-tumorous tissue of exposed individuals will also need to be investigated. The interpretation of the data generated by such studies will largely rely on the availability of public databases to compile, retrieve and sort mutation data. In its 10 years of existence, the IARC *TP53* mutation database has developed from a simple, tabular list into a complex relational database, and considerable efforts have been devoted to the improvement and standardization of annotations to the database (Olivier *et al.*, 2002). Much of the biology of tomorrow will depend upon discoveries made by proper analysis of the information contained in databases accessible to the scientific community. Management of such large data sets is therefore becoming a central issue in *TP53* mutation analysis, given the interest of *TP53* mutation profiles for both molecular epidemiology and molecular pathology.

Acknowledgements
We thank Ms Dorothea Dudek for editorial and graphic assistance. We also thank Mr Mohammed Khan for help in the analysis of the *TP53*-mutation data.

The development of IARC *TP53* database is partially supported by a BIOMED program of the European Community (QLG-1999–00273). C. Caron de Fromentel is Chargé de Recherche 1 of the French National Institute of Medical Research (INSERM) and is a Visiting Scientist at IARC.

References
Agarwal, M.L., Taylor, W.R., Chernov, M.V., Chernova, O.B. & Stark, G.R. (1998) The p53 network. *J. biol. Chem.*, **273**, 1–4

Aguilar, F., Hussain, S.P. & Cerutti, P. (1993) Aflatoxin B1 induces the transversion of G→T in codon 249 of the p53 tumor suppressor gene in human hepatocytes. *Proc. natl Acad. Sci. USA*, **90**, 8586–8590

Aguilar, F., Harris, C.C., Sun, T., Hollstein, M. & Cerutti, P. (1994) Geographic variation of p53 mutational profile in nonmalignant human liver. *Science*, **264**, 1317–1319

Ahrendt, S.A., Halachmi, S., Chow, J.T., Wu, L., Halachmi, N., Yang, S.C., Wehage, S., Jen, J. & Sidransky, D. (1999) Rapid p53 sequence analysis in primary lung cancer using an oligonucleotide probe array. *Proc. natl Acad. Sci. USA*, **96**, 7382–7387

Alarcon, R., Koumenis, C., Geyer, R.K., Maki, C.G. & Giaccia, A.J. (1999) Hypoxia induces p53 accumulation through MDM2 down-regulation and inhibition of E6-mediated degradation. *Cancer Res.*, **59**, 6046–6051

Ambs, S., Hussain, S.P. & Harris, C.C. (1997) Interactive effects of nitric oxide and the p53 tumor suppressor gene in carcinogenesis and tumor progression. *FASEB J.*, **11**, 443–448

Ambs, S., Merriam, W.G., Ogunfusika, M.O., Bennett, W.P., Ishibe, N., Hussain, S.P., Tzeng, E.E., Geller, D.A., Billiar, T.R. & Harris, C.C. (1998) p53 and vascular endothelial growth factor regulate tumor growth of NOS2-expressing human carcinoma cells. *Nature Med.*, **4**, 1371–1376

Ambs, S., Bennett, W.P., Merriam, W.G., Ogunfusika, M.O., Oser, S.M., Harrington, A.M., Shields, P.G., Felley-Bosco, E., Hussain, S.P. & Harris, C.C. (1999) Relationship between p53 mutations and inducible nitric oxide synthase expression in human colorectal cancer. *J. natl Cancer Inst.*, **91**, 86–88

Appella, E. & Anderson, C.W. (2000) Signaling to p53: breaking the posttranslational modification code. *Pathol. Biol. (Paris)*, **48**, 227–245

Banin, S., Moyal, L., Shieh, S., Taya, Y., Anderson, C.W., Chessa, L., Smorodinsky, N.I., Prives, C., Reiss, Y., Shiloh, Y. & Ziv, Y. (1998) Enhanced phosphorylation of p53 by ATM in response to DNA damage. *Science*, **281**, 1674–1677

Barrett, M.T., Sanchez, C.A., Prevo, L.J., Wong, D.J., Galipeau, P.C., Paulson, T.G., Rabinovitch, P.S. & Reid, B.J. (1999) Evolution of neoplastic cell

lineages in Barrett oesophagus. *Nature Genet.*, **22**, 106–109

Bertram, J.S. (2000) The molecular biology of cancer. *Mol. Aspects Med.*, **21**, 167–223

Biramijamal, F., Allameh, A., Mirbod, P., Groene, H.J., Koomagi, R. & Hollstein, M. (2001) Unusual profile and high prevalence of p53 mutations in esophageal squamous cell carcinomas from northern Iran. *Cancer Res.*, **61**, 3119–3123

Brash, D.E. & Ponten, J. (1998) Skin precancer. *Cancer Surv.*, **32**, 69–113

Brash, D.E., Rudolph, J.A., Simon, J.A., Lin, A., McKenna, G.J., Baden, H.P., Halperin, A.J. & Ponten, J. (1991) A role for sunlight in skin cancer: UV-induced p53 mutations in squamous cell carcinoma. *Proc. natl Acad. Sci. USA*, **88**, 10124–10128

Bredt, D.S. & Snyder, S.H. (1994) Nitric oxide: a physiologic messenger molecule. *Annu. Rev. Biochem.*, **63**, 175–195

Bressac, B., Kew, M., Wands, J. & Ozturk, M. (1991) Selective G to T mutations of p53 gene in hepatocellular carcinoma from southern Africa. *Nature*, **350**, 429–431

Caron de Fromentel, C. & Soussi, T. (1992) TP53 tumor suppressor gene: a model for investigating human mutagenesis. *Genes Chromosomes Cancer*, **4**, 1–15

Chartrain, N.A., Geller, D.A., Koty, P.P., Sitrin, N.F., Nussler, A.K., Hoffman, E.P., Billiar, T.R., Hutchinson, N.I. & Mudgett, J.S. (1994) Molecular cloning, structure, and chromosomal localization of the human inducible nitric oxide synthase gene. *J. biol. Chem.*, **269**, 6765–6772

Cho, Y., Gorina, S., Jeffrey, P.D. & Pavletich, N.P. (1994) Crystal structure of a p53 tumor suppressor-DNA complex: understanding tumorigenic mutations. *Science*, **265**, 346–355

Cobbs, C.S., Brenman, J.E., Aldape, K.D., Bredt, D.S. & Israel, M.A. (1995) Expression of nitric oxide synthase in human central nervous system tumors. *Cancer Res.*, **55**, 727–730

Crespo, P. & Leon, J. (2000) Ras proteins in the control of the cell cycle and cell differentiation. *Cell. mol. Life Sci.*, **57**, 1613–1636

Denissenko, M.F., Pao, A., Tang, M. & Pfeifer, G.P. (1996) Preferential formation of benzo[*a*]pyrene adducts at lung cancer mutational hotspots in P53. *Science*, **274**, 430–432

Denissenko, M.F., Chen, J.X., Tang, M.S. & Pfeifer, G.P. (1997) Cytosine methylation determines hot spots of DNA damage in the human P53 gene. *Proc. natl Acad. Sci. USA*, **94**, 3893–3898

Denissenko, M.F., Koudriakova, T.B., Smith, L., O'Connor, T.R., Riggs, A.D. & Pfeifer, G.P. (1998) The p53 codon 249 mutational hotspot in hepatocellular carcinoma is not related to selective formation or persistence of aflatoxin B1 adducts. *Oncogene*, **17**, 3007–3014

Di Como, C.J., Gaiddon, C. & Prives, C. (1999) p73 function is inhibited by tumor-derived p53 mutants in mammalian cells. *Mol. cell. Biol.*, **19**, 1438–1449

Donehower, L.A., Harvey, M., Slagle, B.L., McArthur, M.J., Montgomery, C.A., Jr, Butel, J.S. & Bradley, A. (1992) Mice deficient for p53 are developmentally normal but susceptible to spontaneous tumours. *Nature*, **356**, 215–221

Dumaz, N., Drougard, C., Sarasin, A. & Daya-Grosjean, L. (1993) Specific UV-induced mutation spectrum in the p53 gene of skin tumors from DNA-repair-deficient xeroderma pigmentosum patients. *Proc. natl Acad. Sci. USA*, **90**, 10529–10533

Elmore, L.W. & Harris, C.C. (1998) Hepatocellular carcinoma. In: Vogelstein, B. & Kinzler, K.W., eds, *The Genetic Basis of Human Cancer*, McGraw-Hill, New York, pp. 681–689

van Es, J.H., Giles, R.H. & Clevers, H.C. (2001) The many faces of the tumor suppressor gene APC. *Exp. Cell Res.*, **264**, 126–134

Essigmann, J.M. & Wood, M.L. (1993) The relationship between the chemical structures and mutagenic specificities of the DNA lesions formed by chemical and physical mutagens. *Toxicol. Lett.*, **67**, 29–39

Esteve, A., Sorlie, T., Martel-Planche, G., Hollstein, M., Kusters, I., Lewalter, J., Vineis, P., Stephan-Odenthal, M. & Montesano, R. (1995) Screening for p53 gene mutations in archived tumors of workers occupationally exposed to carcinogens: examples from analysis of bladder tumors. *J. occup. environ. Med.*, **37**, 59–68

Fearon, E.R. & Vogelstein, B. (1990) A genetic model for colorectal tumorigenesis. *Cell*, **61**, 759–767

Forrester, K., Lupold, S.E., Ott, V.L., Chay, C.H., Band, V., Wang, X.W. & Harris, C.C. (1995) Effects of p53 mutants on wild-type p53-mediated transactivation are cell type dependent. *Oncogene*, **10**, 2103–2111

Forrester, K., Ambs, S., Lupold, S.E., Kapust, R.B., Spillare, E.A., Weinberg, W.C., Felley-Bosco, E., Wang, X.W., Geller, D.A., Tzeng, E., Billiar, T.R. & Harris, C.C. (1996) Nitric oxide-induced p53 accumulation and regulation of inducible nitric oxide synthase expression by wild-type p53. *Proc. natl Acad. Sci. USA*, **93**, 2442–2447

Forstermann, U. & Kleinert, H. (1995) Nitric oxide synthase: expression and expressional control of the three isoforms. *Naunyn Schmiedeberg's Arch. Pharmacol.*, **352**, 351–364

Foulkes, W.D., Flanders, T.Y., Pollock, P.M. & Hayward, N.K. (1997) The CDKN2A (p16) gene and human cancer. *Mol. Med.*, **3**, 5–20

Fronza, G., Inga, A., Monti, P., Scott, G., Campomenosi, P., Menichini, P., Ottaggio, L., Viaggi, S., Burns, P.A., Gold, B. & Abbondandolo, A. (2000) The yeast p53 functional assay: a new tool for molecular epidemiology. Hopes and facts. *Mutat. Res.*, **462**, 293–301

Fuchs, S.Y., Adler, V., Buschmann, T., Yin, Z., Wu, X., Jones, S.N. & Ronai, Z. (1998) JNK targets p53 ubiquitination and degradation in nonstressed cells. *Genes Dev.*, **12**, 2658–2663

Goldstein, S.R., Yang, G.Y., Curtis, S.K., Reuhl, K.R., Liu, B.C., Mirvish, S.S., Newmark, H.L. & Yang, C.S. (1997) Development of esophageal metaplasia and adenocarcinoma in a rat surgical model without the use of a carcinogen. *Carcinogenesis*, **18**, 2265–2270

Groden, J., Thliveris, A., Samowitz, W., Carlson, M., Gelbert, L., Albertsen, H., Joslyn, G., Stevens, J., Spirio, L., Robertson, M., Sargeant, L., Krapcho, K., Wolff, E., Burt, R., Hughes, J.P., Warrington, J., McPherson, J., Wasmuth, J., Le Paslier, D., Abderrahim, H., Cohen, D., Leppert, M. & White, R. (1991) Identification and characterization of the familial adenomatous polyposis coli gene. *Cell*, **66**, 589–600

Hainaut, P. & Hollstein, M. (2000) p53 and human cancer: the first ten thousand mutations. *Adv. Cancer Res.*, **77**, 81–137

Hainaut, P. & Milner, J. (1993) A structural role for metal ions in the 'wild-type' conformation of the tumor suppressor protein p53. *Cancer Res.*, **53**, 1739–1742

Hainaut, P. & Pfeifer, G.P. (2001) Patterns of p53 G→T transversions in lung cancers reflect the primary mutagenic signature of DNA-damage by tobacco smoke. *Carcinogenesis*, **22**, 367–374

Hanahan, D. & Weinberg, R.A. (2000) The hallmarks of cancer. *Cell*, **100**, 57–70

Harris, C.C. (1991) Chemical and physical carcinogenesis: advances and perspectives for the 1990s. *Cancer Res.*, **51** (Suppl. 18), 5023S–5044S

Hawkins, N.J., Gorman, P., Tomlinson, I.P., Bullpitt, P. & Ward, R.L. (2000) Colorectal carcinomas arising in the hyperplastic polyposis syndrome progress through the chromosomal instability pathway. *Am. J. Pathol.*, **157**, 385–392

Hentze, M.W. & Kuhn, L.C. (1996) Molecular control of vertebrate iron metabolism: mRNA-based regulatory circuits operated by iron, nitric oxide, and oxidative stress. *Proc. natl Acad. Sci. USA*, **93**, 8175–8182

Hernandez-Alcoceba, R., del Peso, L. & Lacal, J.C. (2000) The Ras family of GTPases in cancer cell invasion. *Cell. mol. Life Sci.*, **57**, 65–76

Hoffmann, J.S. & Cazaux, C. (1998) DNA synthesis, mismatch repair and cancer. *Int. J. Oncol.*, **12**, 377–382

Hollstein, M., Sidransky, D., Vogelstein, B. & Harris, C.C. (1991a) p53 Mutations in human cancers. *Science*, **253**, 49–53

Hollstein, M.C., Peri, L., Mandard, A.M., Welsh, J.A., Montesano, R., Metcalf, R.A., Bak, M. & Harris, C.C. (1991b) Genetic analysis of human esophageal tumors from two high incidence geographic areas: frequent p53 base substitutions and absence of ras mutations. *Cancer Res.*, **51**, 4102–4106

Honda, R. & Yasuda, H. (1999) Association of p19(ARF) with Mdm2 inhibits ubiquitin ligase activity of Mdm2 for tumor suppressor p53. *EMBO J.*, **18**, 22–27

Hsu, I.C., Metcalf, R.A., Sun, T., Welsh, J.A., Wang, N.J. & Harris, C.C. (1991) Mutational hotspot in the p53 gene in human hepatocellular carcinomas. *Nature*, **350**, 427–428

Hussain, S.P. & Harris, C.C. (1998) Molecular epidemiology of human cancer: contribution of mutation spectra studies of tumor suppressor genes. *Cancer Res.*, **58**, 4023–4037

Hussain, S.P., Aguilar, F., Amstad, P. & Cerutti, P. (1994a) Oxy-radical induced mutagenesis of hotspot codons 248 and 249 of the human p53 gene. *Oncogene*, **9**, 2277–2281

Hussain, S.P., Aguilar, F. & Cerutti, P. (1994b) Mutagenesis of codon 248 of the human p53 tumor suppressor gene by *N*-ethyl-*N*-nitrosourea. *Oncogene*, **9**, 13–18

Hussain, S.P., Kennedy, C.H., Amstad, P., Lui, H., Lechner, J.F. & Harris, C.C. (1997) Radon and lung carcinogenesis: mutability of p53 codons 249 and 250 to 238Pu alpha-particles in human bronchial epithelial cells. *Carcinogenesis*, **18**, 121–125

Hussain, S.P., Amstad, P., Raja, K., Ambs, S., Nagashima, M., Bennett, W.P., Shields, P.G., Ham, A.J., Swenberg, J.A., Marrogi, A.J. & Harris, C.C. (2000a) Increased p53 mutation load in noncancerous colon tissue from ulcerative colitis: a cancer-prone chronic inflammatory disease. *Cancer Res.*, **60**, 3333–3337

Hussain, S.P., Raja, K., Amstad, P.A., Sawyer, M., Trudel, L.J., Wogan, G.N., Hofseth, L.J., Shields, P.G., Billiar, T.R., Trautwein, C., Hohler, T., Galle, P.R., Phillips, D.H., Markin, R., Marrogi, A.J. & Harris, C.C. (2000b) Increased p53 mutation load in nontumorous human liver of wilson disease and hemochromatosis: oxyradical overload diseases. *Proc. natl Acad. Sci. USA*, **97**, 12770–12775

Hussain, S.P., Amstad, P., Raja, K., Sawyer, M., Hofseth, L., Shields, P.G., Hewer, A., Phillips, D.H., Ryberg, D., Haugen, A. & Harris, C.C. (2001) Mutability of p53 hotspot codons to benzo(*a*)pyrene diol epoxide (BPDE) and the frequency of p53 mutations in nontumorous human lung. *Cancer Res.*, **61**, 6350–6355

IARC (1972–2002) *IARC Monographs on the Evaluation of Carcinogenic Risks to Humans*, Vols 1 to 81, Lyon, IARCPress

Ishioka, C., Englert, C., Winge, P., Yan, Y.X., Engelstein, M. & Friend, S.H. (1995) Mutational analysis of the carboxy-terminal portion of p53 using both yeast and mammalian cell assays in vivo. *Oncogene*, **10**, 1485–1492

Jia, L., Wang, X.W. & Harris, C.C. (1999) Hepatitis B virus X protein inhibits nucleotide excision repair. *Int. J. Cancer*, **80**, 875–879

Kaghad, M., Bonnet, H., Yang, A., Creancier, L., Biscan, J.C., Valent, A., Minty, A., Chalon, P., Lelias, J.M., Dumont, X., Ferrara, P., McKeon, F. & Caput, D. (1997) Monoallelically expressed gene related to p53 at 1p36, a region frequently deleted in neuroblastoma and other human cancers. *Cell*, **90**, 809–819

Kamijo, T., Weber, J.D., Zambetti, G., Zindy, F., Roussel, M.F. & Sherr, C.J. (1998) Functional and physical interactions of the ARF tumor suppressor with p53 and Mdm2. *Proc. natl Acad. Sci. USA*, **95**, 8292–8297

Kirk, G.D., Camus-Randon, A.M., Mendy, M., Goedert, J.J., Merle, P., Trepo, C., Brechot, C., Hainaut, P. & Montesano, R. (2000) Ser-249 p53 mutations in plasma DNA of patients with hepatocellular carcinoma from The Gambia. *J. natl Cancer Inst.*, **92**, 148–153

Koh, E., Noh, S.H., Lee, Y.D., Lee, H.Y., Han, J.W., Lee, H.W. & Hong, S. (1999) Differential expression of nitric oxide synthase in human stomach cancer. *Cancer Lett.*, **146**, 173–180

Kopreski, M.S., Benko, F.A., Borys, D.J., Khan, A., McGarrity, T.J. & Gocke, C.D. (2000) Somatic mutation screening: identification of individuals harboring K-ras mutations with the use of plasma DNA. *J. natl Cancer Inst.*, **92**, 918–923

Laken, S.J., Jackson, P.E., Kinzler, K.W., Vogelstein, B., Strickland, P.T., Groopman, J.D. & Friesen, M.D. (1998) Genotyping by mass spectrometric analysis of short DNA fragments. *Nature Biotechnol.*, **16**, 1352–1356

Levine, A.J. (1997) p53, The cellular gatekeeper for growth and division. *Cell*, **88**, 323–331

Linder, C., Linder, S., Munck-Wikland, E. & Strander, H. (1998) Independent expression of serum vascular endothelial growth factor (VEGF) and basic fibroblast growth factor (bFGF) in patients with carcinoma and sarcoma. *Anticancer Res.*, **18**, 2063–2068

Livni, N., Eid, A., Ilan, Y., Rivkind, A., Rosenmann, E., Blendis, L.M., Shouval, D. & Galun, E. (1995) p53 Expression in patients with cirrhosis with and without hepatocellular carcinoma. *Cancer*, **75**, 2420–2426

Ljungman, M. (2000) Dial 9–1–1 for p53: mechanisms of p53 activation by cellular stress. *Neoplasia*, **2**, 208–225

Lowe, S.W. (1999) Activation of p53 by oncogenes. *Endocr. relat. Cancer*, **6**, 45–48

Malkin, D., Li, F.P., Strong, L.C., Fraumeni, J.F., Jr, Nelson, C.E., Kim, D.H., Kassel, J., Gryka, M.A., Bischoff, F.Z., Tainsky, M.A. & Friend, S.H. (1990) Germ line p53 mutations in a familial syndrome of breast cancer, sarcomas, and other neoplasms. *Science*, **250**, 1233–1238

Mandard, A.M., Hainaut, P. & Hollstein, M. (2000) Genetic steps in the development of squamous cell carcinoma of the esophagus. *Mutat. Res.*, **462**, 335–342

Mannick, E.E., Bravo, L.E., Zarama, G., Realpe, J.L., Zhang, X.J., Ruiz, B., Fontham, E.T., Mera, R., Miller, M.J. & Correa, P. (1996) Inducible nitric oxide synthase, nitrotyrosine, and apoptosis in *Helicobacter pylori* gastritis: effect of antibiotics and antioxidants. *Cancer Res.*, **56**, 3238–3243

Marletta, M.A. (1993) Nitric oxide synthase structure and mechanism. *J. biol. Chem.*, **268**, 12231–12234

Matsuura, S., Tauchi, H., Nakamura, A., Kondo, N., Sakamoto, S., Endo, S., Smeets, D., Solder, B., Belohradsky, B.H., Der Kaloustian, V.M., Oshimura, M., Isomura, M., Nakamura, Y. & Komatsu, K. (1998) Positional cloning of the gene for Nijmegen breakage syndrome. *Nature Genet.*, **19**, 179–181

May, P. & May, E. (1999) Twenty years of p53 research: structural and functional aspects of the p53 protein. *Oncogene*, **18**, 7621–7636

Melillo, G., Musso, T., Sica, A., Taylor, L.S., Cox, G.W. & Varesio, L. (1995) A hypoxia-responsive element mediates a novel pathway of activation of the inducible nitric oxide synthase promoter. *J. exp. Med.*, **182**, 1683–1693

Messmer, U.K. & Brune, B. (1996) Nitric oxide-induced apoptosis: p53-dependent and p53-independent signalling pathways. *Biochem. J.*, **319**, 299–305

Michalovitz, D., Halevy, O. & Oren, M. (1991) p53 mutations: gains or losses? *J. Cell Biochem.*, **45**, 22–29

Midgley, C.A., Fisher, C.J., Bartek, J., Vojtesek, B., Lane, D. & Barnes, D.M. (1992) Analysis of p53 expression in human tumours: an antibody raised against human p53 expressed in *Escherichia coli*. *J. Cell Sci.*, **101**, 183–189

Milne, D.M., Palmer, R.H., Campbell, D.G. & Meek, D.W. (1992) Phosphorylation of the p53 tumour-suppressor protein at three N-terminal sites by a novel casein kinase I-like enzyme. *Oncogene*, **7**, 1361–1369

Momand, J., Wu, H.H. & Dasgupta, G. (2000) MDM2–master regulator of the p53 tumor suppressor protein. *Gene*, **242**, 15–29

Moncada, S., Palmer, R.M. & Higgs, E.A. (1991) Nitric oxide: physiology, pathophysiology, and pharmacology. *Pharmacol. Rev.*, **43**, 109–142

Montesano, R., Hollstein, M. & Hainaut, P. (1996) Genetic alterations in esophageal cancer and their relevance to etiology and pathogenesis: a review. *Int. J. Cancer*, **69**, 225–235

Montesano, R., Hainaut, P. & Wild, C.P. (1997) Hepatocellular carcinoma: from gene to public health. *J. natl Cancer Inst.*, **89**, 1844–1851

Moshinsky, D.J. & Wogan, G.N. (1997) UV-induced mutagenesis of human p53 in a vector replicated in *Saccharomyces cerevisiae*. *Proc. natl Acad. Sci. USA*, **94**, 2266–2271

Moynahan, M.E., Chiu, J.W., Koller, B.H. & Jasin, M. (1999) Brca1 controls homology-directed DNA repair. *Mol. Cell*, **4**, 511–518

Nakazawa, H., English, D., Randell, P.L., Nakazawa, K., Martel, N., Armstrong, B.K. & Yamasaki, H. (1994) UV and skin cancer: specific p53 gene mutation in normal skin as a biologically relevant exposure measurement. *Proc. natl Acad. Sci. USA*, **91**, 360–364

Nathan, C. & Xie, Q.W. (1994) Nitric oxide synthases: roles, tolls, and controls. *Cell*, **78**, 915–918

Neshat, K., Sanchez, C.A., Galipeau, P.C., Blount, P.L., Levine, D.S., Joslyn, G. & Reid, B.J. (1994) p53 mutations in Barrett's adenocarcinoma and high-grade dysplasia. *Gastroenterology*, **106**, 1589–1595

Ohshima, H. & Bartsch, H. (1994) Chronic infections and inflammatory processes as cancer risk factors: possible role of nitric oxide in carcinogenesis. *Mutat. Res.*, **305**, 253–264

Oliner, J.D., Kinzler, K.W., Meltzer, P.S., George, D.L. & Vogelstein, B. (1992) Amplification of a gene encoding a p53-associated protein in human sarcomas. *Nature*, **358**, 80–83

Olivier, M. & Hainaut, P. (2001) TP53 mutation patterns in breast cancers: searching for clues of environmental carcinogenesis. *Semin. Cancer Biol.*, **11**, 353–360

Olivier, M., Eeles, R., Hollstein, M., Khan, M.A., Harris, C.C. & Hainaut, P. (2002) The IARC TP53 database: new online mutation analysis and recommendations to users. *Hum. Mutat.*, **19**, 607–614

Oren, M. (1999) Regulation of the p53 tumor suppressor protein. *J. biol. Chem.*, **274**, 36031–36034

Ory, K., Legros, Y., Auguin, C. & Soussi, T. (1994) Analysis of the most representative tumour-derived p53 mutants reveals that changes in protein conformation are not correlated with loss of trans-activation or inhibition of cell proliferation. *EMBO J.*, **13**, 3496–3504

Ozturk, M. (1991) p53 Mutation in hepatocellular carcinoma after aflatoxin exposure. *Lancet*, **338**, 1356–1359

Pluquet, O., North, S., Bhoumik, A., Dimas, K., Ronai, Z. & Hainaut P. (2003) The cytoprotective amino-thiol WR1065 activates p53 through a non-genotoxic signaling pathway involving c-Jun N-terminal kinase. *J. biol. Chem.*, **278**, 11879–11887

Pomerantz, J., Schreiber-Agus, N., Liegeois, N.J., Silverman, A., Alland, L., Chin, L., Potes, J., Chen, K., Orlow, I., Lee, H.W., Cordon-Cardo, C. & DePinho, R.A. (1998) The Ink4a tumor suppressor gene product, p19Arf, interacts with MDM2 and neutralizes MDM2's inhibition of p53. *Cell*, **92**, 713–723

Ponchel, F., Puisieux, A., Tabone, E., Michot, J.P., Froschl, G., Morel, A.P., Frebourg, T., Fontaniere, B., Oberhammer, F. & Ozturk, M. (1994) Hepatocarcinoma-specific mutant p53–249ser induces mitotic activity but has no effect on transforming growth factor beta 1-mediated apoptosis. *Cancer Res.*, **54**, 2064–2068

Qadri, I., Conaway, J.W., Conaway, R.C., Schaack, J. & Siddiqui, A. (1996) Hepatitis B virus trans-activator protein, HBx, associates with the components of TFIIH and stimulates the DNA helicase activity of TFIIH. *Proc. natl Acad. Sci. USA*, **93**, 10578–10583

Ren, Z.P., Ahmadian, A., Ponten, F., Nister, M., Berg, C., Lundeberg, J., Uhlen, M. & Ponten, J. (1997) Benign clonal keratinocyte patches with p53 mutations show no genetic link to synchronous squamous cell precancer or cancer in human skin. *Am. J. Pathol.*, **150**, 1791–1803

Rocco, J.W. & Sidransky, D. (2001) p16(MTS-1/CDKN2/INK4a) in cancer progression. *Exp. Cell Res.*, **264**, 42–55

Scharer, E. & Iggo, R. (1992) Mammalian p53 can function as a transcription factor in yeast. *Nucleic Acids Res.*, **20**, 1539–1545

Scheffner, M., Werness, B.A., Huibregtse, J.M., Levine, A.J. & Howley, P.M. (1990) The E6 oncoprotein encoded by human papillomavirus types 16 and 18 promotes the degradation of p53. *Cell*, **63**, 1129–1136

Scicchitano, D.A. & Hanawalt, P.C. (1992) Intragenomic repair heterogeneity of DNA damage. *Environ. Health Perspect.*, **98**, 45–51

Sepehr, A., Taniere, P., Martel-Planche, G., Zia'ee, A.A., Rastgar-Jazii, F., Yazdanbod, M., Etemad-Moghadam, G., Kamangar, F., Saidi, F. & Hainaut, P. (2001) Distinct pattern of TP53 mutations in squamous cell carcinoma of the esophagus in Iran. *Oncogene*, **20**, 7368–7374

Sherr, C.J. & Weber, J.D. (2000) The ARF/p53 pathway. *Curr. Opin. genet. Dev.*, **10**, 94–99

Sibghat-Ullah, Gallinari, P., Xu, Y.Z., Goodman, M.F., Bloom, L.B., Jiricny, J. & Day, R.S., III (1996) Base analog and neighboring base effects on substrate specificity of recombinant human G:T mismatch-specific thymine DNA-glycosylase. *Biochemistry*, **35**, 12926–12932

Sieber, O.M., Tomlinson, I.P. & Lamlum, H. (2000) The adenomatous polyposis coli (APC) tumour suppressor–genetics, function and disease. *Mol. Med. Today*, **6**, 462–469

Sigal, A. & Rotter, V. (2000) Oncogenic mutations of the p53 tumor suppressor: the demons of the guardian of the genome. *Cancer Res.*, **60**, 6788–6793

Singer, I.I., Kawka, D.W., Scott, S., Weidner, J.R., Mumford, R.A., Riehl, T.E. & Stenson, W.F. (1996) Expression of inducible nitric oxide synthase and nitrotyrosine in colonic epithelium in inflammatory bowel disease. *Gastroenterology*, **111**, 871–885

Sorlie, T., Martel-Planche, G., Hainaut, P., Lewalter, J., Holm, R., Borresen-Dale, A.L. & Montesano, R. (1998) Analysis of p53, p16MTS, p21WAF1 and H-ras in archived bladder tumours from workers exposed to aromatic amines. *Br. J. Cancer*, **77**, 1573–1579

Strano, S., Munarriz, E., Rossi, M., Cristofanelli, B., Shaul, Y., Castagnoli, L., Levine, A.J., Sacchi, A., Cesareni, G., Oren, M. & Blandino, G. (2000) Physical and functional interaction between p53 mutants and different isoforms of p73. *J. biol. Chem.*, **275**, 29503–29512

Tamir, S. & Tannenbaum, S.R. (1996) The role of nitric oxide (NO) in the carcinogenic process. *Biochim. biophys. Acta*, **1288**, F31–F36

Taniere, P., Martel-Planche, G., Puttawibul, P., Casson, A., Montesano, R., Chanvitan, A. & Hainaut, P. (2000) TP53 mutations and MDM2 gene amplification in squamous-cell carcinomas of the esophagus in south Thailand. *Int. J. Cancer*, **88**, 223–227

Taylor, J.A., Li, Y., He, M., Mason, T., Mettlin, C., Vogler, W.J., Maygarde, S. & Liu, E. (1996) p53 mutations in bladder tumors from arylamine-exposed workers. *Cancer Res.*, **56**, 294–298

Thomsen, L.L., Lawton, F.G., Knowles, R.G., Beesley, J.E., Riveros-Moreno, V. & Moncada, S. (1994) Nitric oxide synthase activity in human gynecological cancer. *Cancer Res.*, **54**, 1352–1354

Thomsen, L.L., Miles, D.W., Happerfield, L., Bobrow, L.G., Knowles, R.G. & Moncada, S. (1995) Nitric oxide synthase activity in human breast cancer. *Br. J. Cancer*, **72**, 41–44

Tommasi, S., Denissenko, M.F. & Pfeifer, G.P. (1997) Sunlight induces pyrimidine dimers preferentially at 5-methylcytosine bases. *Cancer Res.*, **57**, 4727–4730

Tonisson, N., Zernant, J., Kurg, A., Pavel, H., Slavin, G., Roomere, H., Meiel, A., Hainaut, P. & Metspalu, A. (2002) Evaluating the arrayed primer extension ressequencing assay of TP53 tumor suppressor gene. *Proc. natl Acad. Sci. USA*, **99**, 5503–5508

Tornaletti, S., Rozek, D. & Pfeifer, G.P. (1993) The distribution of UV photoproducts along the human p53 gene and its relation to mutations in skin cancer. *Oncogene*, **8**, 2051–2057

Tretyakova, N.Y., Burney, S., Pamir, B., Wishnok, J.S., Dedon, P.C., Wogan, G.N. & Tannenbaum, S.R. (2000) Peroxynitrite-induced DNA damage in the supF gene: correlation with the mutational spectrum. *Mutat. Res.*, **447**, 287–303

Vahakangas, K.H., Bennett, W.P., Castren, K., Welsh, J.A., Khan, M.A., Blomeke, B., Alavanja, M.C. & Harris, C.C. (2001) p53 and K-ras mutations in lung cancers from former and never-smoking women. *Cancer Res.*, **61**, 4350–4356

Verghis, S.B., Essigmann, J.M., Kadlubar, F.F., Morningstar, M.L. & Lasko, D.D. (1997) Specificity of mutagenesis by 4-aminobiphenyl: mutations at G residues in bacteriophage M13 DNA and G→C transversions at a unique dG(8-ABP) lesion in single-stranded DNA. *Carcinogenesis*, **18**, 2403–2414

Vogelstein, B., Lane, D. & Levine, A.J. (2000) Surfing the p53 network. *Nature*, **408**, 307–310

Vojtesek, B. & Lane, D.P. (1993) Regulation of p53 protein expression in human breast cancer cell lines. *J. Cell Sci.*, **105**, 607–612

Warren, W., Biggs, P.J., el-Baz, M., Ghoneim, M.A., Stratton, M.R. & Venitt, S. (1995) Mutations in the p53 gene in schistosomal bladder cancer: a study of 92 tumours from Egyptian patients and a comparison between mutational spectra from schistosomal and non-schistosomal urothelial tumours. *Carcinogenesis*, **16**, 1181–1189

Wikman, F.P., Lu, M.L., Thykjaer, T., Olesen, S.H., Andersen, L.D., Cordon-Cardo, C. & Orntoft, T.F. (2000) Evaluation of the performance of a p53 sequencing microarray chip using 140 previously sequenced bladder tumor samples. *Clin. Chem.*, **46**, 1555–1561

Wink, D.A., Hanbauer, I., Grisham, M.B., Laval, F., Nims, R.W., Laval, J., Cook, J., Pacelli, R., Liebmann, J., Krishna, M., Ford, P.C. & Mitchell, J.B. (1996) Chemical biology of nitric oxide: regulation and protective and toxic mechanisms. *Curr. Top. Cell Regul.*, **34**, 159–187

Wogan, G.N. (2000) Impacts of chemicals on liver cancer risk. *Semin. Cancer Biol.*, **10**, 201–210

Yang, A.S., Gonzalgo, M.L., Zingg, J.M., Millar, R.P., Buckley, J.D. & Jones, P.A. (1996) The rate of CpG mutation in Alu repetitive elements within the p53 tumor suppressor gene in the primate germline. *J. mol. Biol.*, **258**, 240–250

Yang, A., Kaghad, M., Wang, Y., Gillett, E., Fleming, M.D., Dotsch, V., Andrews, N.C., Caput, D. & McKeon, F. (1998) p63, A p53 homolog at 3q27–29, encodes multiple products with trans-

activating, death-inducing, and dominant-negative activities. *Mol. Cell*, **2**, 305–316

Yang, A., Walker, N., Bronson, R., Kaghad, M., Oosterwegel, M., Bonnin, J., Vagner, C., Bonnet, H., Dikkes, P., Sharpe, A., McKeon, F. & Caput, D. (2000) p73-Deficient mice have neurological, pheromonal and inflammatory defects but lack spontaneous tumours. *Nature*, **404**, 99–103

Yasunaga, Y., Nakanishi, H., Naka, N., Miki, T., Tsujimura, T., Itatani, H., Okuyama, A. & Aozasa, K. (1997) Alterations of the p53 gene in occupational bladder cancer in workers exposed to aromatic amines. *Lab. Invest.*, **77**, 677–684

Yoon, J.H., Smith, L.E., Feng, Z., Tang, M., Lee, C.S. & Pfeifer, G.P. (2001) Methylated CpG dinucleotides are the preferential targets for G-to-T transversion mutations induced by benzo[*a*]pyrene diol epoxide in mammalian cells: similarities with the p53 mutation spectrum in smoking-associated lung cancers. *Cancer Res.*, **61**, 7110–7117

Zhuang, J.C., Lin, C., Lin, D. & Wogan, G.N. (1998) Mutagenesis associated with nitric oxide production in macrophages. *Proc. natl Acad. Sci. USA*, **95**, 8286–8291

Zhuang, J.C., Wright, T.L., deRojas-Walker, T., Tannenbaum, S.R. & Wogan, G.N. (2000) Nitric oxide-induced mutations in the HPRT gene of human lymphoblastoid TK6 cells and in *Salmonella typhimurium*. *Environ. mol. Mutag.*, **35**, 39–47

Corresponding author:

Pierre Hainaut
Molecular Carcinogenesis Group,
International Agency for Research on Cancer,
150, cours Albert Thomas,
69372 Lyon Cedex 08, France
hainaut@iarc.fr

Mechanisms of Carcinogenesis: Contributions of Molecular Epidemiology
Patricia Buffler, Jerry Rice, Robert Baan, Michael Bird and Paolo Boffetta, eds
IARC Scientific Publications No. 157
International Agency for Research on Cancer, Lyon, 2004

Identification and Characterization of Potential Human Carcinogens using B6.129tm1 *Trp53* Heterozygous Null Mice and Loss of Heterozygosity at the *Trp53* Locus

John E. French

Summary

Rodent models are often used as surrogates for humans in toxicology and cancer research. Transgenic mice have been useful for studying gene function by loss of function or gain of function through mutation or overexpression. Thus, transgenic or genetically altered mouse models could play an important role in understanding environment–gene interactions. Wild-type Trp53 protein is critical for cell function and maintaining integrity of the genome, which suppresses cancer in humans and rodents. Mice heterozygous for a *Trp53* null and a wild-type allele are p53 haplo-insufficient. This reduction in p53 protein results in deficiencies in cell cycle check-point control and induction of apoptosis. p53 Haplo-insufficient mice do not immediately develop neoplasia as a result of this signalling dysregulation. However, exposure to mutagenic carcinogens induces neoplasia during the period in which unexposed, co-isogenic haplo-insufficient and homozygous wild-type mice are free from neoplasia. These observations provide a basis for evaluation of p53 haplo-insufficient mice for mechanism-based identification of carcinogens. Maximum tolerated doses (MTD) determined and used for 2-year NCI/NTP cancer bioassays and/or by 28-day toxicokinetic studies to predict MTD for subchronic studies were, generally, effective in inducing neoplasia with reduced latency in 26-week exposure studies in p53 haplo-insufficient mice. The latency of tumour development may be shortened by requiring only an additional genetic

alteration (or alterations) in p53 (mutation or loss of heterozygosity (LOH) involving the *Trp*53 locus) or in other tumour-suppressor genes by mutation or inactivation. LOH is a loss of genetic loci through chromosomal aberrations and reduction to homozygosity that often results in loss of tumour-suppressor genes. Interspecies extrapolation between rodents and humans is difficult owing to the possibility of species differences, but demonstration of an operational mechanism, such as mutation or loss of p53 function through LOH, may help in reducing uncertainty and, thus, lead to identification of carcinogens of presumed risk to humans.

Introduction

Prospective identification of agents that may be of presumptive risk to humans exposed to them is clearly in the best interest of public health. Carcinogenicity in experimental animals is often used as a surrogate for human exposure, and is one of the primary tools used in toxicology for the identification of potentially harmful agents. This chapter contains a review of the current status of evaluation of one genetically altered mouse model, the B6.129-*Trp53*tm1Brd (p53-deficient) mouse model, used to test carcinogens identified or classified by the International Agency for Research on Cancer (IARC) or the US National Toxicology Program Report on Carcinogens (US NTP ROC).

The wild-type p53 protein suppresses cancer in humans and rodents. As a transcription factor, p53 regulates the activity of a variety of genes involved in cell-cycle arrest, apoptosis, anti-angiogenesis, differentiation, repair and genomic stability (el-Deiry, 1998; Prives & Hall, 1999). *Trp*53 homozygous null allele (–/–) mice that are completely deficient in p53 protein develop tumours, mostly lymphomas and sarcomas, that arise spontaneously in the first 3–6 months of life (Donehower *et al.*, 1992). The *Trp*53 heterozygous null allele (+/–) mouse model has one copy of the wild-type allele of the p53 tumour-suppressor gene and one copy of a null allele that is not transcribed or translated (Donehower *et al.*, 1992; Harvey *et al.*, 1993a,b). The p53 heterozygotes (+/–) have a low spontaneous tumour incidence up to 9 months of age, but have increased spontaneous tumour rates thereafter with approximately 50% survival at 18 months. Thus, mice exposed to positive-control and test agents between 7 and 33 weeks of age are relatively free from the development of sporadic tumours. This allows a clear distinction between induced tumours and sporadically arising tumours that may confound long-term chronic cancer bioassays (Haseman & Elwell, 1996; Karstadt & Haseman, 1997).

In human cancers, where mutations have been found in up to 50% of all tumours (Hollstein *et al.*, 1991; Greenblatt *et al.*, 1994), point mutations or deletions in one allele of the *p53* gene that create a heterozygous allelic state are usually accompanied by loss of the normal allele (or LOH) (Weinberg, 1991). Since p53 (+/–) mice already carry one of these two possible mutational events in all cells (germline), these mice were expected, according to the Knudson *et al.* two-hit hypothesis (Knudson *et al.*, 1975; Knudson, 1996), to show a shorter latency period for tumours induced by genotoxic agents. Alternatively, there is evidence that the acceleration of tumorigenesis in p53 (+/–) mice may be due to a gene dosage effect and a haplo-insufficient phenotype such that a second (p53 LOH) event is not required (Venkatachalam & Donehower, 1998; Venkatachalam *et al.*, 1998; French *et al.*, 2001a).

The heterozygous *Trp*53 allele mouse (B6.129-*Trp*53^{tm1Brd}) is a candidate model for the identifi-

cation of mutagenic carcinogens (Donehower *et al.*, 1992; Harvey *et al.*, 1993b; Tennant *et al.*, 1995, 1996). Initial studies with several genotoxic and non-genotoxic chemicals using this mouse indicated induction of neoplasia by mutagenic carcinogens with a decrease in tumour latency. This result suggests that this model might have utility as a short-term in-vivo test for this class of carcinogens (Donehower *et al.*, 1992; Harvey *et al.*, 1993b; Kemp *et al.*, 1993, 1994; Tennant *et al.*, 1995, 1996; Eastin *et al.*, 1998). The purpose here is to determine the utility of this model to identify potential mutagenic carcinogens, the class of carcinogens presumed to be of greatest potential risk to the human population.

An effective rodent model (e.g. the heterozygous p53-deficient mouse model) used as a surrogate for human exposure should test positive for 'known', 'probable' or 'possible' human carcinogens (i.e. IARC Groups 1, 2A or 2B). However, peer-reviewed IARC Group 3 agents might be expected to test negative, since they are the agents that are least likely to cause cancer in humans. Group 3 includes those agents (mixtures or exposure circumstances) that are 'not classifiable as to [their] carcinogenicity to humans'. Many Group 3 agents lack human exposure data and/or animal studies that conclusively demonstrate carcinogenicity. Of course, as new evidence becomes available and new peer reviews of the evidence are conducted, Group 3 agents may be reclassified. Thus, there is less certainty whether the response in the heterozygous p53-deficient mouse model should be positive or negative for agents from IARC Group 3. On the basis of initial published research, the p53-deficient mouse model should be susceptible to mutagenic carcinogens. We do not expect the p53-deficient mouse model to be overtly sensitive and test positive for potential genotoxic or non-genotoxic carcinogens listed in IARC Group 3. There are many agents in IARC Group 3 that may have been positive in only one or more of the four groups (for each sex of the two species tested) in a 2-year rodent bioassay. In general, the IARC Group 3 agents do not meet the 'weight of evidence' that is required for peer-reviewed classification as 'known', 'probable' or 'possible' human carcinogens.

Methods

Data collection

Results from published independent laboratory research and personal communication (where appropriate) for unpublished results and the NCI/NTP results for 2-year studies of toxicology and carcinogenesis in rodents on 59 chemical carcinogens were compiled. Twelve were classified as IARC Group 1 (known human carcinogen) and/or NTP ROC 'known' carcinogens (Table 1). Nineteen were classified as IARC Groups 2A and 2B (probable/possible human carcinogens) and/or ROC 'reasonably anticipated' to be human carcinogens (Table 2). Finally, 28 were chemicals with no evidence or inadequate evidence of carcinogenicity that were classified as IARC Group 3 and/or were 'not listed' in ROC (Table 3). Results on LOH at the *Trp53* locus in tumours from heterozygous p53 mice were also included for comparison where available and to provide mechanistic data for rapid induction of neoplasia.

Analysis of the model for identification of carcinogens

Using a database of 59 chemicals (Tables 1–3), this model was analysed to determine how well it could distinguish known or suspected human carcinogens (consensus-derived IARC Group 1 or 2A/2B chemicals) from IARC Group 3 chemicals, which (for the purposes of this analysis) are considered to present the lowest risk for potential human carcinogenicity on the basis of currently available data. For comparison, results from NCI/NTP standard 2-year, two-species rodent cancer bioassays were used in conjunction with results from genotoxicity assays (operationally defined by results from in-vitro *Salmonella* and/or in-vivo micronuclei assays). In order to apply the results in a consistent manner, no additional review (individual studies of positive and negative findings) was performed beyond the peer-reviewed conclusions already published.

Results

IARC Group 1/ROC 'known' human carcinogens

Of 12 human carcinogens, 10 were identified as positive in the p53-deficient mouse model (Table 1). Two non-mutagenic human carcinogens, estradiol-17β and 2,3,7,8-tetrachlorodibenzo-*para*-dioxin, were negative. All six of the mutagenic human carcinogens were positive in the short-term cancer bioassay in this model and all four of these that were examined induced significant levels of LOH involving the *Trp53* wild-type allele, including melphalan (see Figure 1 for representative data). Four of five of the human carcinogens were positive in the conventional 2-year rodent cancer bioassay. Under the conditions of the inhalation studies conducted in rats and mice, asbestos fibres were negative.

IARC Group 2 (A or B) 'probable' or 'possible'/ROC 'reasonable' human carcinogens

Both IARC Group 2A and Group 2B classifications are based on peer-reviewed data from exposures that are considered to provide 'limited' or 'inadequate' evidence for cancer in humans. For most Group A and Group B agents there are positive bioassay data that are considered to be 'sufficient' evidence for carcinogenicity in animals. Of 19 'probable or reasonably anticipated to be' human carcinogens, the results in the short-term cancer bioassay in this model were 10/19 overall and 11/14 for those compounds identified as mutagens (Table 2). Correlation increased when Group 2A and Group 2B chemical carcinogens were distinguished. Five of eight IARC Group 2A compounds showed a positive result, which increased to 5/6 when non-mutagenic chemicals were excluded. Of chemicals in Group 2B, 5/10 were positive in the p53-deficient mouse model whereas 5/7 of the mutagenic compounds were positive. Each class showed 4/4 tumour sets that demonstrated LOH of the *Trp53* wild-type allele (8/8 overall). LOH results were 9/9 when 7,12-dimethylbenz[*a*]anthracene was included in the analysis. Ten of 10 IARC Group B carcinogens were positive in 2-year rodent cancer bioassays.

IARC Group 3 (no data or insufficient evidence)/ROC (not listed) chemical agents

Only one of 28 agents in Group 3 (foreign body, i.e. microchip transponder) was positive in the p53-deficient mouse model, whereas nine of 28

Table 1. Results from B6.129 N5 mice heterozygous for a *Trp53* wild-type and null allele exposed[a] to human carcinogens (IARC Group 1 carcinogens) for 24–26 weeks compared (where available) with 2-year or lifetime cancer bioassays in rats and mice

Agent	CAS No.	IARC[b]	NTP ROC[c]	NCI/NTP bioassays[e]	Rapid bioassay	LOH[f]
Benzene	71-43-2	1	Known	+; +; +; + g[g] (NTP, 1986)	+ g; + g (French et al., 2001a; Storer et al., 2001)	+++ French et al. (2001a)
Cyclophosphamide	6055-19-2	1	Known	+; +; + (Weisburger, 1977)	+ g (Eastin et al., 1998; Storer et al., 2001)	NT
Melphalan	148-82-3	1	Known	+; +; + ip (Weisburger, 1977)	+ ip; + ip (Eastin et al., 1998; Storer et al., 2001)	++++ (Fig. 1)
Cyclosporin A	79217-60-0	1	Known	NT	– g; + f; f (Eastin et al., 1998; Storer et al., 2001)	NT
Diethylstilbestrol	56-53-1	1	Known	NT	– sc; + f (Eastin et al., 1998; Storer et al., 2001)	NT
Estradiol-17β	50-28-2	1	Reasonable	NT	± g; – g (Storer et al., 2001)	NT
TCDD	1746-01-6	1	Known	+; +; +; + f (NCI/NTP, 1982c)	– g (Eastin et al., 1998)	NT
UVR (312–450 nm)	NA	1	Known	NT	+ d (Jiang et al., 1999)	+++ Jiang et al., 1999)
Asbestos fibres	1332-21-4	1	Known	–; –; NT; NT d (NTP, 1988a)	+ ip[h] (Marsella et al., 1997)	NT
Beryllium	7440-41-7	1	Reasonable	NT	+ i (Finch et al., 1998)	NT

Table 1 (contd)

Agent	CAS No.	IARC[b]	NTP ROC[c]	NCI/NTP bioassays[a]	Rapid bioassay	LOH[f]
Plutonium-239[i]	NA	1	Known	NT	+ i (Finch et al., 1998)	NT
Cobalt-60 (LET)	NA	1	Known	NT	+ wb (Kemp et al., 1994)	+++ (Kemp et al., 1994)

[a] Maximum tolerated dose (MTD) or proportional fractions of MTD as determined by toxicokinetic and range-finding studies in the test strain using positive- and negative-control groups and non-genetically altered co-isogenic reference controls

[b] IARC Group 1: The agent (mixture) is carcinogenic to humans. The exposure circumstance entails exposures that are carcinogenic to humans.

[c] NTP: Known to be a human carcinogen (9th Report on Carcinogens, revised January 2001)

[d] Salmonella (Ames) assay; in-vivo micronuclei assay results as reported by IARC (http://193.51.164.11/default.html) or the US NTP [e] (http://ntp-server.niehs.nih.gov/cgi/iH_Indexes/ALL_SRCH/iH_ALL_SRCH_Frames.html)

[e] Standard National Cancer Institute NTP 2-year or lifetime cancer bioassay

[f] LOH was quantified for the p53 locus from mouse chromosome 11. LOH is expressed from ++++ (100% LOH) to + (25% or less) of the number of tumours showing significant signal reduction by image analysis of Southern blots of BamH1-restricted genomic DNA probed with p53 exon 2-6 (LR-10) courtesy of L. Donehower.

[g] Peer-reviewed conclusions for male Fischer 344 rat, female Fischer 344 rat, male B6C3F1 mouse or female B6C3F1 mouse, respectively.

[h] Crocidolite fibres

[i] Single inhalation exposure to 100 or 500 Beq plutonium-239 and held for lifetime. Positive result based on significant decrease in time to tumour development for pulmonary neoplasms relative to p53 wild-type control mice.

Abbreviations: +, positive; −, negative; ±, equivocal; f, feed; g, gavage, d, dermal; i, inhalation; ip, intraperitoneal injection; LOH, loss of heterozygosity; NT, not tested or no published record; sc, subcutaneous; TCDD, 2,3,7,8-tetrachlorodibenzo-para-dioxin; wb, whole body exposure

Table 2. Results from B6.129 N5 mice heterozygous for a *Trp53* wild-type allele exposed to 19 rodent (reasonably anticipated to be human) carcinogens exposed[a] for 24–26 weeks compared (where available) with 2-year or lifetime cancer bioassays in rats and mice

Agent	CAS No.	IARC[b]	NTP ROC[c]	Geno-toxicity[d]	NCI/NTP bioassay[e]	Rapid bioassay	LOH[f]
para-Cresidine	120-71-8	2B	Reasonable	+; –	+; +; +; + f (NTP, 1979)	+ f; + g (Tennant et al., 1995; Storer et al., 2001)	+(French et al., 2001a)
Glycidol	556-52-5	2A	Reasonable	+; +	+; +; +; + g (NTP, 1990b)	– g (Tennant et al., 1999)	NT
Phenolphthalein	77-09-8	2B	Reasonable	–; +	+; +; +; + f (NTP, 1995b)	+ f; + f (Dunnick et al., 1997)	+++ (French et al., 2001a)
4-Vinyl-1-cyclohexene diepoxide	106-87-6	2B	Reasonable	+; +	+; +; +; + d (NTP, 1989a)	+ d (Tennant et al., 1995)	+++ (French, J. personal communication)
2,4-Diaminotoluene	95-80-7	2B	Reasonable	+; –	+; +; –; + f (NCI/NTP, 1979a)	± f (Eastin et al., 1998)	NT
Chloroprene	126-99-8	2B	Reasonable	–; –	+; +; +; + i (NTP, 1998b)	– i (French, J. personal communication)	NT
Pentachlorophenol	87-86-5	2B	Not listed	–; –	+; h–; +; + f (NTP, 1999e)	– f (Spalding et al., 2000)	NT
Phenacetin	62-44-2	2A	Reasonable	–; NT	NT	–f; – g (Storer et al., 2001)	NT
Phenobarbital	50-06-6	2B	Not listed	wk+; NT	NT	– f; – f (Sagartz et al., 1998; Storer et al., 2001)	NT
Chloroform	67-66-3	2B	Reasonable	–; +	+; –; +; + w (Griesemer et al., 1980)	± g (Storer et al., 2001)	NT
Benzo[a]pyrene	50-32-8	2A	Reasonable	+; NT	NT	+ d,g (Martin et al., 2001)	+++ (Martín et al., 2001)
N-Nitrosodimethylamine	62-75-9	2A	Not listed	+; NT	NT	+ w (Harvey et al., 1993b)	+++ (Harvey et al., 1993b)

Table 2 (contd)

Agent	CAS No.	IARC[b]	NTP ROC[c]	Geno-toxicity[d]	NCI/NTP bioassay[e]	Rapid bioassay	LOH[f]
7,12-Dimethylbenz[a]-anthracene	57-97-6	NE	Not listed	+; +	NT; NT; +; + d, ip (NTP, 1996)	+ d (Kemp et al., 1993)	+++ (Kemp et al., 1993)
N-Ethyl-N-nitrosourea	759-73-9	2A	Not listed	+; +	NT	+ ip (Mitsumori et al., 2000)	+++ (Mitsumori et al., 2000)
2-Amino-3-methylimidazo-[4,5-f]quinoline	76180-96-6	2A	Not listed	+; +	NT	+ g (Nagao, 1999)	NT
N-Butyl-N-(4-hydroxy-butyl) nitrosamine	64091-91-4	2B	Not listed	NT; −	NT	+ w (Ozaki et al., 1998)	+ (Ozaki et al., 1998)
N-Methyl-N-nitrosourea	684-93-5	2A	Not listed	NT; +	NT	+ ip (Yamamoto et al., 2000)	+++ (Yamamoto et al., 2000)
Urethane	51-79-6 5	2B	Reasonable	+; +	NT	+ ip (Carmichael et al., 2000)	NT
Oxymetholone	434-07-1	2A	Reasonable	−; −	±; +; NT; NT (NTP, 1999d)	− g (Stoll et al., 1999)	NT

[a] Maximum tolerated dose (MTD) or proportional fractions of MTD as determined by toxicokinetic and range-finding studies in the test strain using positive- and negative-control groups and non-genetically altered co-isogenic reference controls

[b] IARC: Group 2A: The agent (mixture) is probably carcinogenic to humans. The exposure circumstance entails exposures that are probably carcinogenic to humans. Group 2B: The agent (mixture) is possibly carcinogenic to humans. The exposure circumstance entails exposures that are possibly carcinogenic to humans.

[c] NTP: Reasonably anticipated to be a human carcinogen (9th Report on Carcinogens, revised January 2001).

[d] Salmonella (Ames) assay; in-vivo micronuclei assay results as reported by IARC (http://193.51.164.11/default.html) or the US NTP (http://ntp-server.niehs.nih.gov/cgi/iH_Indexes/ALL_SRCH/iH_ALL_SRCH_Frames.html)

[e] National Cancer Institute; National Toxicology Program cancer bioassay

[f] LOH was quantified for the p53 locus from mouse chromosome 11. LOH is expressed from ++++ (100% LOH) to + (25% or less) of the number of tumours showing significant signal reduction by image analysis of Southern blots of BamH1-restricted genomic DNA probed with p53 exon 2–6 (LR-10) courtesy of L. Donehower.

[g] Peer-reviewed conclusions for male Fischer 344 rat, female Fischer 344 rat, male B6C3F1 mouse or female B6C3F1 mouse

[h] Positive in 1000 ppm−1 year exposure stop study but not with 2-year exposure to technical-grade pentachlorophenol (technical-grade, TR349; purified, TR483).

Abbreviations: +, positive; −, negative; ±, equivocal; f, feed; g, gavage; d, dermal; ip, intraperitoneal injection; i, inhalation; LOH, loss of heterozygosity; NT, not tested or no published record; sc, subcutaneous; wb, whole body exposure

Table 3. Results from carcinogenicity studies in B6.129 N5 mice heterozygous for a *Trp53* wild-type and null allele exposed[a] for 24–26 weeks to 28 agents for which there is no or insufficient evidence of human carcinogenicity compared (where available) with 2-year or lifetime cancer bioassays in rats and mice

Agent	CAS No.	IARC[b]	NTP ROC[c]	Geno-toxicity[d]	NCI/NTP bioassay[e]	Trp53[+/-]	LOH[f]
para-Anisidine	90-04-0	3	Not listed	+; –	±; –; –; – f (NCI/NTP, 1978a)	– f (Tennant et al., 1995)	NEG
1-Chloro-2-propanol	127-00-4	NE	Not listed	+; NT	–; –; –; – w (NTP, 1998a)	– g (Tennant et al., 1999)	NT
2,6-Diaminotoluene	820-40-5	NE	Not listed	+; –	–; –; –; – f (Battershill & Fielder, 1998)	– f (Eastin et al., 1998)	NT
8-Hydroxyquinoline	148-24-3	3	Not listed	+; –	–; –; –; – f (NTP, 1985)	– f (Eastin et al., 1998)	NT
Coconut oil diethanolamine	68603-42-9	NE	Not listed	–; +	–; ±; +; + d (NTP, 2001)	– d (Spalding et al., 2000)	NT
Lauric acid diethanolamine	120-40-1	NE	Not listed	–; –	–; –; +; + d (NTP, 1999a)	– f (Spalding et al., 2000)	NT
N-Methylolacrylamide	924-42-5	3	Not listed	–; –	–; –; +; + g (NTP, 1989b)	– g (Tennant et al., 1995)	NEG
Methylphenidate	298-59-9	NE	Not listed	–; NT	–; –; ±; + f (NTP, 1995a)	– f (Tennant et al., 1999)	NEG
Pyridine	110-86-1	3	Not listed	–; –	+; ±; +; + w (NTP, 2000)	– g (Spalding et al., 2000)	NT
Reserpine	50-55-5	3	Reasonable	–; –	+; –; +; + f (NCI/NTP, 1982b)	– f (Tennant et al., 1995)	NEG
Rotenone	83-79-4	NE	Not listed	–; NT	±; –; –; – f (NTP, 1988b)	– f (Eastin et al., 1998)	NT
Resorcinol	108-46-3	3	Not listed	–; +	–; –; –; – g (NTP, 1992)	– g (Eastin et al., 1998)	NT
Oleic acid diethanolamide	93-83-4	NE	Not listed	–; NT	–; –; –; – d (NTP, 1999c)	– d (Spalding et al., 2000)	NT
Clofibrate	637-07-0	3	Not listed	–; –	NT	g; – g (Storer et al., 2001)	NT
Dieldrin	60-57-1	3	Not listed	–; NT	–; –; ±; – f (NCI/NTP, 1978b)	– f (Storer et al., 2001)	NT
Methapyrilene HCl	135-23-9	NE	Not listed	–; –	+; +; NT; NT f (Lijinsky et al., 1980)	g; – f (Storer et al., 2001)	NT
Haloperidol	52-86-8	NE	Not listed	NT; NT	NT	– g (Storer et al., 2001)	NT
Chlorpromazine HCl	69-09-0	NE	Not listed	–; NT	NT	g; – g (Storer et al., 2001)	NT
Metaproterenol	586-06-1	NE	Not listed	NT; NT	NT	f; – f (Storer et al., 2001)	NT
WY-14643	50892-23-4	NE	Not listed	NT; NT	NT	– f (Storer et al., 2001)	NT
Di(2-ethylhexyl)phthalate	117-81-7	3	Reasonable	–; –	+; +; +; + f (NTP, 1982)	± f (Storer et al., 2001)	NT
Sulfamethoxazole	723-46-6	3	Not listed	–; NT	NT	– f (Storer et al., 2001)	NT
Sulfisoxazole	127-69-5	3	Not listed	–; NT	–; –; –; – f (NCI/NTP, 1979b)	– f (Storer et al., 2001)	NT
Ampicillin	7177-48-2	3	Not listed	–; NT	±; –; –; – f (NTP, 1987)	– g (Storer et al., 2001)	NT

Table 3 (contd)

Agent	CAS No.	IARC[b]	NTP ROC[c]	Geno-toxicity[d]	NCI/NTP bioassay[e]	Trp53[+/-]	LOH[f]
D-Mannitol	69-65-8	NE	Not listed	–; –	–; –; –; – f (NCI/NTP, 1982a)	– f (Storer et al., 2001)	NT
d-Limonene	5989-27-5	3	Not listed	–; NT	+; –; –; – f (NTP, 1990a)	– g (Carmichael et al., 2000)	NT
Foreign body (transponder)	NA	NE	Not listed	–; –	NT	+ sc (Blanchard et al., 1999)	+++ (Blanchard et al., 1999)
Magnetic fields (60 MHz)	NA	NE	Not listed	–; –	– (NTP, 1999b)	– wb (McCormick et al., 1998)	NT

[a] Maximum tolerated dose (MTD) or proportional fractions of MTD as determined by toxicokinetic and range-finding studies in the test strain using positive- and negative-control groups and non-genetically altered co-isogenic reference controls

[b] IARC: Group 3: The agent (mixture or exposure circumstance) is not classifiable as to its carcinogenicity to humans.

[c] NTP: Not listed (9th Report on Carcinogens, revised January 2001)

[d] Salmonella (Ames) assay; in-vivo micronuclei assay results as reported by IARC (http://193.51.164.11/default.html) or the US NTP

[e] National Cancer Institute/National Toxicology Program cancer bioassay

[f] LOH was quantified for the p53 locus from mouse chromosome 11. LOH is expressed from ++++ (100% LOH) to + (25% or less) of the number of tumours showing significant signal reduction by image analysis of Southern blots of BamH1-restricted genomic DNA probed with p53 exon 2–6 (LR-10) courtesy of L. Donehower.

Abbreviations: +, positive; –, negative; ±, equivocal; inc, incomplete; f, feed; g, gavage; d, dermal; ip, intraperitoneal injection; i, inhalation; LOH, loss of heterozygosity; NEG, negative (no detectable LOH at the Trp53 locus observed); NT, not tested or no published record; sc, subcutaneous; wb, whole body exposure

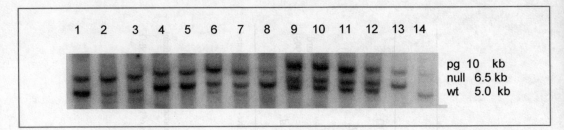

Figure 1. Loss of heterozygosity at the Trp53 locus observed by Southern blot analysis of genomic DNA from melphalan-induced thymic lymphomas or normal thymic tissue (untreated controls) using ³²P-radiolabelled probe spanning exons 2–6 (LR10, courtesy of L. Donehower). Lanes 1–8, thymic lymphoma; lanes 9–12, normal thymus; lane 13, control homozygous for the null allele; lane 14, control homozygous for the wild-type allele

were positive to some extent in a conventional 2-year rodent cancer bioassay (Table 3). Out of six categories examined, only the tumours induced by foreign bodies showed LOH at the *Trp53* wild-type allele locus. Six of 28 compounds were positive in either the Ames (*Salmonella*) assay for mutagenicity or the in-vivo assay for micronuclei, or both.

Overall accuracy

Under the conditions of the short-term carcinogenicity bioassay in p53-deficient mice (24–26-week exposures based on variable dose-setting standards), the model showed an accuracy of 80% for prediction on all test compounds on the basis of this scheme of comparison (Table 4). Accuracy for the short-term cancer bioassay model improves to 88% if comparison is restricted to genotoxic Group 1 and Group 2A or 2B carcinogens. Overall, the conventional 2-year cancer bioassay showed 72% accuracy with this set of agents used for comparison (Table 4). Interestingly, if the test compounds were further sorted by classification and compared, accuracy appears to decline as the strength of evidence used for classification decreases (Table 5).

Discussion

The correlation between outcome in the retrospective analysis of this mouse model exposed to 'known' and 'probable/possible' (IARC Groups 1 and 2A/2B) carcinogens versus those compounds least likely to be human carcinogens (IARC

Group 3 agents) was 80% (47/59). When only genotoxic carcinogens (operationally defined as genotoxic by positive outcome in either an in-vitro *Salmonella* or an in-vivo micronuclei assay) were compared, the correlation increased to 88% (23/26). This model has been proposed to be susceptible to mutagenic carcinogens (Tennant *et al.*, 1995, 1996; French *et al.*, 2001a,b). The conventional 2-year cancer bioassay in rats and mice showed a correlation of 72% (26/36) using this method of comparison without factoring in genotoxicity. In the conventional assay, factoring genotoxicity increased the correlation to 100%, as previous reports have predicted (Ashby & Tennant, 1991; Tennant & Zeiger, 1993). Interestingly, as certainty of the carcinogenic response decreased from Group 1 to Group 2A to Group 2B through to Group 3 agents, the correlation decreased. Only IARC-classified chemicals with data available on both short-term and conventional rodent cancer bioassays were considered in this context. Under the stringent conditions of these short-term (24–26-week exposure) protocols, the false positives (potential rodent but not human carcinogens) were reduced (if not eliminated), but potential false-negative results were not. Additional studies will be required to determine the optimal protocol parameters (including exposure period) for individual short-term genetically altered mouse models for carcinogen identification.

A major confounding character of the 2-year cancer bioassay studies is the occurrence of

Table 4. Performance of the p53 heterozygous mouse model in rapid (26-week) and the conventional 2-year cancer bioassay comparing 'known, probable and possible' human carcinogens (IARC Groups 1, 2A and 2B) with chemicals that are least likely to be human carcinogens (IARC Group 3)

Strategy	True positive	True negative	False positive	False negative	Overall
Trp53+/- (all)	20/31	27/28	1/28	11/31	47/59 (80%)
Trp53+/- (genotoxic)	17/20	6/6	0/6	3/20	23/26 (88%)
Trp53+/- (genotoxic and induces LOH)	12/12	5/5	0/12	0/5	17/17 (100%)
Rodent 2-year bioassay (all)	14/15	12/21	9/21	1/15	26/36 (72%)
Rodent 2-year bioassay (genotoxic)	10/10	6/6	0/6	0/10	16/16 (100%)

Table 5. Performance of the p53 heterozygous mouse model in rapid (26-week) and conventional 2-year cancer bioassays comparing results by classification (weight of evidence for human carcinogenicity)

IARC Group	1	2A	2B	3
Trp53+/- (all)	10/12 (83%)	5/8 (63%)	5/10 (50%)	1/28 (4%)
Trp53+/- (genotoxic)	6/6 (100%)	5/6 (83%)[a]	5/8 (63%)[b]	0/5 (0%)
Rat and mouse bioassay	4/5 (80%)	1/2 (50%)[c]	9/9 (100%)	8/28 (29%)

[a] Glycidol

[b] Chloroform, 2,4-diaminotoluene, phenobarbital;

[c] Oxymetholone

sporadic tumours associated with genetic background, and determining the strength of the association between exposure to the test agent and induction of tumours (independent of the sporadically occurring tumours) in ageing rodents. This may be the greatest source of variability in the conventional 2-year rodent cancer bioassay and may be a source of potential false-positive results (9/21 of the expected negative results). The range of tumour phenotypes expressed in the B6.129 (N5) p53 haplo-insufficient mouse is broad, including both sporadic (at ≥ 12 months of age) and carcinogen-induced tumours, as indicated by Donehower's group (Donehower et al., 1992; Donehower & Bradley, 1993; Harvey et al., 1993a,b; Donehower et al., 1996) and by other research groups (Tennant et al., 1995, 1996, 1999; French et al., 2001a). Sporadic tumour incidence in

the B6.129 (N5) p53 haplo-insufficient mouse requires more investigation, but initial studies under defined conditions for studies of toxicology and carcinogenesis indicate that both survival and sporadic incidence were not likely to be confounding factors during the prescribed 26–36-week exposure protocols (Mahler et al., 1998; Mahler, 2000; Storer et al., 2001). Nevertheless, understanding the influence of genotype on the phenotype of a strain or stains of rodents used in generation of the model and the outcome in studies of chemical carcinogenesis is critical. Inbred mouse strains are known to demonstrate a broad variation in tissue susceptibility to the development of both sporadic and induced cancers. For example, naturally occurring or sporadic intestinal (C57BL/6 >> CBA or DBA/2 > AKR), liver (DBA ≥ C3H/HeJ > B6C3F$_1$ > C57BL/6 ≥ A ≥ BALB/c), lung (A/J >> C57BL/6 ≥ B6C3F₁ > C3H/He or DBA/2) and skin (SENCAR >> DBA/2 or FVB > C3H/He > B6C3F₁ >> C57BL/6) cancers vary dramatically from one strain to another (see Bult *et al.*, 2000). These same relative susceptibilities are observed for tumours at these sites that are induced by carcinogens. Note that the C57BL/6 strain (dominant portion of the genome in the model under discussion) ranges from resistant (liver, lung, skin) to susceptible (intestinal, lymphohematopoietic) depending on tumour site. Thus, inherent susceptibilities may influence either sporadic tumour development in ageing mice or carcinogen-induced neoplasia unless the carcinogen has a particular affinity (organotropy) for a specific tissue. This affinity may be based on the carcinogen's pattern of systemic absorption and distribution, and sites or products of its toxicity or metabolism that increase its potency and penetrance. For example, *para*-cresidine, an aromatic amine, is highly specific for the induction of bladder and liver tumours (French *et al.*, 2001a), for which the C57BL/6 strain shows no sporadic incidence or is resistant. The short tumour latency in susceptible tissues may preclude observation at other less susceptible tissue sites due to tissue resistance, as reflected by increased tumour latency. The outcome or carcinogen-specific tumour phenotype of rapid cancer bioassays will thus always be influenced by strain (tissue susceptibility) as reflected by its sporadic tumour phenotype, the dose and dose–rate, and the specific susceptibility of the line due to specific incorporated genetic alterations (e.g. intrinsic to the signalling pathways of cell cycle control, proliferation, apoptosis). Together, these factors influence the penetrance of the observable phenotype. Whether these inbred mouse strain susceptibilities (allelic conservation) reflect the same or similar inherited susceptibilities in humans is an open question. If so, the application of genetically altered mouse models for investigation of human carcinogens might be used to determine useful biomarkers of exposure and to define potential mechanisms of carcinogen induction.

Additional research on those potential human carcinogens (IARC Groups 2A/2B) identified as potential false negatives (e.g. glycidol, phena-cetin, 2,4-diaminotoluene, phenobarbital, chloroform) will require further investigation to confirm the negative test results reported. With the exception of glycidol, the latter compounds were positive in the *Salmonella* assay only at high doses. Interestingly, phenacetin, a component of the known human carcinogen, analgesic mixtures (aspirin, phenacetin and caffeine), has been reported to be negative for tumour induction (under the assay conditions) in a number of other transgenic mouse models — Tg.AC (Eastin *et al.*, 2001), XPA- or XPA-p53-deficient (van Kreijl *et al.*, 2001) and the neonatal mouse (McClain *et al.*, 2001). However, it was reported to be positive in the RasH2 mouse model (Usui *et al.*, 2001). Finally, the one positive result in the p53-deficient mouse from the presumed IARC Group 3 agents (inferred from analysis of medical devices and implants) was the transponder (microchip used for animal identification). Tumours associated with the site of implantation may be associated with inflammation and oxidative stress due to repetitive injury from handling. Further investigation of this observation in relation to strain susceptibility, oxidative stress and LOH is required to place this result in the proper context.

Application of data demonstrating a potential mechanistic basis for tumour induction or progression with a reduced latency of expression would help to remove some of the uncertainty. Malignancies induced by mutagenic carcinogens (12/12 examined) in heterozygous p53-deficient mice, but not target tissues from non-mutagenic carcinogen-exposed p53-deficient mice, showed LOH at the *Trp53* locus by Southern blot analysis. Histologically, normal target tissues from p53 wild-type co-isogenic controls exposed to mutagenic carcinogens also did not show LOH under the conditions and length of exposure of the assay. The LOH observed often varied in frequency and according to the target tissue of the carcinogen (French *et al.*, 2001a). Two potent mutagenic aromatic amines, *para*-cresidine and *N*-butyl-*N*-(4-hydroxybutyl)nitrosamine, induced a low level of LOH without a significant number of observable mutations in the *Trp53* wild-type allele from the urinary bladder, suggesting mutation or inactivation of other tumour-suppressor genes. Using allelotype analysis with simple sequence length repeat sequences on chromosome 11, the primary source of LOH may be due to mis-segregation (non-disjunction) events leading to the loss of chromosome 11 bearing the wild-type *Trp53* allele (Hulla *et al.*, 2001a,b). LOH of the wild-type *Trp53* allele may also be due to recombination events induced by double-stranded breaks between homologous chromosomes 11 (Boley *et al.*, 2000). The basis for LOH in the *Trp53* haplo-insufficient mouse may be in part due to the predisposition for LOH attributed to the genetic background (Shoemaker *et al.*, 1998; French *et al.*, 2001b) in addition to the consequence of *Trp53* haplo-insufficiency and response to genotoxic damage (Venkatachalam *et al.*, 1998, 2001). The correlation between induction of tumours with LOH at the *Trp53* locus by mutagenic carcinogens in Groups 1, 2A and 2B is high, and aids in the elimination of uncertainty arising from extrapolation from rodents to humans. These results, in general, support the use of the B6.129[tm1]*Trp53* N5 or N12 generation mouse heterozygous for a *Trp53*-null allele as a model for identification of presumptive human carcinogens. LOH induced in mouse models derived from C57BL/6 backcrossing may be a highly penetrant event, as described above (Shoemaker *et al.*, 1998). Providing a mechanistic basis, albeit limited, may help to decrease uncertainty in the extrapolation of results for carcinogen identification from rodents to humans.

References

Ashby, J. & Tennant, R.W. (1991) Definitive relationships among chemical structure, carcinogenicity and mutagenicity for 301 chemicals tested by the U.S. NTP. *Mutat. Res.*, **257**, 229–306

Battershill, J.M. & Fielder, R.J. (1998) Mouse-specific carcinogens: an assessment of hazard and significance for validation of short-term carcinogenicity bioassays in transgenic mice. *Hum. exp. Toxicol.*, **17**, 193–205

Blanchard, K.T., Barthel, C., French, J.E., Holden, H.E., Moretz, R., Pack, F.D., Tennant, R.W. & Stoll, R.E. (1999) Transponder-induced sarcoma in the heterozygous p53+/− mouse. *Toxicol. Pathol.*, **27**, 519–527

Boley, S.E., Anderson, E.E., French, J.E., Donehower, L.A., Walker, D.B. & Recio, L. (2000) Loss of p53 in benzene-induced thymic lymphomas in p53+/− mice: evidence of homologous recombination. *Cancer Res.*, **60**, 2831–2835

Bult, C.J., Krupke, D.M., Sundberg, J.P. & Eppig, J.T. (2000) Mouse tumor biology database (MTB): enhancements and current status. *Nucleic Acids Res.*, **28**, 112–114

Carmichael, N.G., Debruyne, E.L. & Bigot-Lasserre, D. (2000) The p53 heterozygous knockout mouse as a model for chemical carcinogenesis in vascular tissue. *Environ. Health Perspect.*, **108**, 61–65

Donehower, L.A. & Bradley, A. (1993) The tumor suppressor p53. *Biochim. biophys. Acta*, **1155**, 181–205

Donehower, L.A., Godley, L.A., Aldaz, C.M., Pyle, R., Shi, Y.P., Pinkel, D., Gray, J., Bradley, A., Medina, D. & Varmus, H.E. (1996) The role of p53 loss in genomic instability and tumor progression in a murine mammary cancer model. *Progr. clin. biol. Res.*, **395**, 1–11

Donehower, L.A., Harvey, M., Slagle, B.L., McArthur, M.J., Montgomery, C.A., Jr, Butel, J.S. & Bradley, A. (1992) Mice deficient for p53 are developmentally normal but susceptible to spontaneous tumors. *Nature*, **356**, 215–221

Dunnick, J.K., Hardisty, J.F., Herbert, R.A., Seely, J.C., Furedi-Machacek, E.M., Foley, J.F., Lacks, G.D., Stasiewicz, S. & French, J.E. (1997) Phenolphthalein induces thymic lymphomas accompanied by loss of the p53 wild type allele in heterozygous p53-deficient (+/−) mice. *Toxicol. Pathol.*, **25**, 533–540

Eastin, W.C., Haseman, J.K., Mahler, J.F. & Bucher, J.R. (1998) The National Toxicology Program evaluation of genetically altered mice as predictive models for identifying carcinogens. *Toxicol. Pathol.*, **26**, 461–473

Eastin, W.C., Mennear, J.H., Tennant, R.W., Stoll, R.E., Branstetter, D.G., Bucher, J.R., McCullough, B., Binder, R.L., Spalding, J.W. & Mahler, J.F. (2001) Tg.AC genetically altered mouse: assay working group overview of available data. *Toxicol. Pathol.*, **29** (Suppl.), 60–80

el-Deiry, W.S. (1998) Regulation of p53 downstream genes. *Semin. Cancer Biol.*, **8**, 345–357

Finch, G.L., March, T.H., Hahn, F.F., Barr, E.B., Belinsky, S.A., Hoover, M.D., Lechner, J.F., Nikula, K.J. & Hobbs, C.H. (1998) Carcinogenic responses of transgenic heterozygous p53 knockout mice to inhaled $^{239}PuO_2$ or metallic beryllium. *Toxicol. Pathol.*, **26**, 484–491

French, J.E., Lacks, G.D., Trempus, C., Dunnick, J.K., Mahler, J., Tice, R.R. & Tennant, R.W. (2001a) Loss of heterozygosity frequency at the Trp53 locus in p53-deficient (+/–) mouse tumors is carcinogen and tissue dependent. *Carcinogenesis*, **22**, 99–106

French, J., Storer, R.D. & Donehower, L.A. (2001b) The nature of the heterozygous Trp53 knockout model for identification of mutagenic carcinogens. *Toxicol. Pathol.*, **29** (Suppl.), 24–29

Greenblatt, M.S., Bennett, W.P., Hollstein, M. & Harris, C.C. (1994) Mutations in the p53 tumor suppressor gene: clues to cancer etiology and molecular pathogenesis. *Cancer Res.*, **54**, 4855–4878

Griesemer, R.A. & Cueto, C., Jr (1980) Toward a classification scheme for degrees of experimental evidence for the carcinogenicity of chemicals for animals. In: Montesano, R., Bartsch, H. & Tomatis, L., eds, *Molecular and Cellular Aspects of Carcinogen Screening Tests* (IARC Scientific Publications No. 27), Lyon, IARC*Press*, pp. 259–281

Harvey, M., McArthur, M.J., Montgomery, C.A., Jr, Bradley, A. & Donehower, L.A. (1993a) Genetic background alters the spectrum of tumors that develop in p53-deficient mice. *FASEB J.*, **7**, 938–943

Harvey, M., McArthur, M.J., Montgomery, C.A., Jr, Butel, J.S., Bradley, A. & Donehower, L.A. (1993b) Spontaneous and carcinogen-induced tumorigenesis in p53-deficient mice. *Nature Genet.*, **5**, 225–229

Haseman, J.K. & Elwell, M.R. (1996) Evaluation of false positive and false negative outcomes in NTP long-term rodent carcinogenicity studies. *Risk Anal.*, **16**, 813–820

Hollstein, M., Sidransky, D., Vogelstein, B. & Harris, C.C. (1991) p53 Mutations in human cancers. *Science*, **253**, 49–53

Hulla, J.E., French, J.E. & Dunnick, J. (2001a) Chromosome 11 allelotypes reflect mechanism of chemical carcinogenesis in heterozygous p53-deficient mice. *Carcinogenesis*, **22**, 89–98

Hulla, J.E., French, J.E. & Dunnick, J.K. (2001b) Chromosome 11 loss from thymic lymphomas induced in heterozygous Trp53 mice by phenolphthalein. *Toxicol. Sci.*, **60**, 264–270

Jiang, W., Ananthaswamy, H.N., Muller, H.K. & Kripke, M.L. (1999) p53 Protects against skin cancer induction by UV-B radiation. *Oncogene*, **18**, 4247–4253

Karstadt, M. & Haseman, J.K. (1997) Effect of discounting certain tumor types/sites on evaluations of carcinogenicity in laboratory animals. *Am. J. ind. Med.*, **31**, 485–494

Kemp, C.J., Donehower, L.A., Bradley, A. & Balmain, A. (1993) Reduction of p53 gene dosage does not increase intitiation or promotion but enhances malignant progression of chemically induced skin tumors. *Cell*, **74**, 813–822

Kemp, C.J., Wheldon, T. & Balmain, A. (1994) p53-Deficient mice are extremely susceptible to radiation-induced tumorigenesis. *Nature Genet.*, **8**, 66–69

Knudson, A.G. (1996) Hereditary cancer: two hits revisited. *J. Cancer. Res. clin. Oncol.*, **122**, 135–140

Knudson, A.G., Jr, Hethcote, H.W. & Brown, B.W. (1975) Mutation and childhood cancer: a probabilistic model for the incidence of retinoblastoma. *Proc. natl Acad. Sci. USA*, **72**, 5116–5120

van Kreijl, C.F., McAnulty, P.A., Beems, R.B., Vynckier, A., van Steeg, H., Fransson-Steen, R., Alden, C.L., Forster, R., van der Laan, J.W. & Vandenberghe, J. (2001) Xpa and Xpa/p53+/– knockout mice: overview of available data. *Toxicol. Pathol.*, **29** (Suppl.), 117–127

Lijinsky, W., Reuber, M.D. & Blackwell, B.N. (1980) Liver tumors induced in rats by oral administration of the antihistaminic methapyrilene hydrochloride. *Science*, **209**, 817–819

Mahler, J.F. (2000) The use of genetically altered animals in toxicology. *Toxicol. Pathol.*, **28**, 447–449

Mahler, J.F., Flagler, N.D., Malarkey, D.E., Mann, P.C., Haseman, J.K. & Eastin, W. (1998) Spontaneous and chemically induced proliferative lesions in Tg.AC transgenic and p53-heterozygous mice. *Toxicol. Pathol.*, **26**, 501–511

Marsella, J.M., Liu, B.L., Vaslet, C.A. & Kane, A.B. (1997) Susceptibility of p53-deficient mice to induction of mesothelioma by crocidolite asbestos fibers. *Environ. Health Perspect.*, **105** (Suppl. 5), 1069–1072

Martin, K., Trempus, C., Saulnier, M., Kari, F.W., Barrett, J.C. & French, J.E. (2001) Dietary *N*-acetyl-L-cysteine modulates benzo[*a*]pyrene-induced skin tumors in cancer-prone p53 haplo-insufficient Tg.AC (v-Ha-ras) mice. *Carcinogenesis*, **22**, 1373–1378

McClain, R.M., Keller, D., Casciano, D., Fu P., MacDonald, J., Popp, J. & Sagartz, J. (2001) Neo-natal mouse model: review of methods and results. *Toxicol. Pathol.*, **29** (Suppl.), 128–137

McCormick, D.L., Ryan, B.M., Findlay, J.C., Gauger, J.R., Johnson, T.R., Morrissey, R.L. & Boorman, G.A. (1998) Exposure to 60 Hz magnetic fields and risk of lymphoma in PIM transgenic and TSG-p53 (p53 knockout) mice. *Carcinogenesis*, **19**, 1649–1653

Mitsumori, K., Onodera, H., Shimo, T., Yasuhara, K., Takagi, H., Koujitani, T., Hirose, M., Maruyama, C. & Wakana, S. (2000) Rapid induction of uterine tumors with p53 point mutations in heterozygous p53-deficient CBA mice given a single intraperitoneal administration of *N*-ethyl-*N*-nitrosourea. *Carcinogenesis*, **21**, 1039–1042

Nagao, M. (1999) A new approach to risk estimation of food-borne carcinogens – heterocyclic amines – based on molecular information. *Mutat. Res.*, **431**, 3–12

NCI/NTP (1978a) *Bioassay of p-Anisidine Hydrochloride for Possible Carcinogenicity (CAS No. 20265-97-8)* (Tech. Rep. Ser. No. 116; DHEW Publ. No. (NIH) 78-1371), Bethesda, MD, National Cancer Institute/National Toxicology Program

NCI/NTP (1978b) *Bioassays of Aldrin and Dieldrin for Possible Carcinogenicity (CAS No. 60-57-1)* (Tech. Rep. Ser. No. 21; DHEW Publ. No. (NIH) 78-821), Bethesda, MD, National Cancer Institute/National Toxicology Program

NCI/NTP (1979a) *Bioassay of 2,4-Diaminotoluene for Possible Carcinogenicity (CAS No. 95-80-7)*, (Tech. Rep. Ser. No. 162; DHEW Publ. No. (NIH) 79-1718), Bethesda, MD, National Cancer Institute/National Toxicology Program

NCI/NTP (1979b) *Bioassay of Sulfisoxazole for Possible Carcinogenicity (CAS No. 127-69-5)*, (Tech. Rep. Ser. No. 138; DHEW Publ. No. (NIH) 79-1393), Bethesda, MD, National Cancer Institute/National Toxicology Program

NCI/NTP (1982a) *Carcinogenesis Bioassay of D-Mannitol (CAS No. 69-65-8) in F344/N Rats and B6C3F1 Mice (Feed Study)* (Tech. Rep. Ser. No. 236), Research Triangle Park, NC, National Cancer Institute/National Toxicology Program

NCI/NTP (1982b) *Bioassay of Reserpine for Possible Carcinogenicity (CAS No. 50-55-5)* (Tech. Rep. Ser. No. 193), Bethesda, MD, National Cancer Institute/National Toxicology Program

NCI/NTP (1982c) *Carcinogenesis Bioassay of 2,3,7,8-Tetrachlorodibenzo-p-dioxin (CAS No. 1746-01-6) in Osborne-Mendel Rats and B6C3F1 Mice (Gavage Study)* (Tech. Rep. Ser. No. 198), Bethesda, MD, National Cancer Institute/National Toxicology Program

NTP (1979) *Bioassay of p-Cresidine for Possible Carcinogenicity* (Tech. Rep. Ser. No. 142; DHEW Publ. No. (NIH) 79-1397), Research Triangle Park, NC, National Toxicology Program

NTP (1982) *Carcinogenesis Bioassay of Di(2-ethylhexyl)phthalate (CAS No. 117-81-7) in F344 Rats and B6C3F1 Mice (Feed Studies)* (Tech. Rep. Ser. No. 217), Research Triangle Park, NC, National Toxicology Program

NTP (1985) *Toxicology and Carcinogenesis Studies of 8-Hydroxyquinoline (CAS No. 148-24-3) in F344/N Rats and B6C3F1 Mice (Feed Studies)* (Tech. Rep. Ser. No. 276), Research Triangle Park, NC, National Toxicology Program

NTP (1986) *Toxicology and Carcinogenesis Studies of Benzene (CAS No. 71-43-2) (Gavage Studies) in F344/N Rats and B6C3F1 Mice* (Tech. Rep. Ser. No. 289; Research Triangle Park, NC, National Toxicology Program

NTP (1987) *Toxicology and Carcinogenesis Studies of Ampicillin Trihydrate (CAS No. 7177-48-2) in F344/N Rats and B6C3F1 Mice (Gavage Studies)* (Tech. Rep. Ser. No. 318), Research Triangle Park, NC, National Toxicology Program

NTP (1988a) *Toxicology and Carcinogenesis Studies of Crocidolite Asbestos (CAS No. 12001-28-4) in F344/N Rats (Feed Studies)*, Research Triangle Park, NC, National Toxicology Program

NTP (1988b) *Toxicology and Carcinogenesis Studies of Rotenone (CAS No. 83-79-4) in F344/N Rats and B6C3F1 Mice (Feed Studies)* (Tech. Rep. Ser.

No. 320), Research Triangle Park, NC, National Toxicology Program

NTP (1989a) *Toxicology and Carcinogenesis Studies of 4-Vinyl-1-cyclohexene Diepoxide (CAS No. 106-87-6) in F344/N Rats and B6C3F1 Mice (Dermal Studies)* (Tech. Rep. Ser. No. 362), Research Triangle Park, NC, National Toxicology Program

NTP (1989b) *Toxicology and Carcinogenesis Studies of N-Methylolacrylamide (CAS No. 924-42-5) in F344/N Rats and B6C3F1 Mice (Gavage Studies)* (Tech. Rep. Ser. No. 352), Research Triangle Park, NC, National Toxicology Program

NTP (1990a) *Toxicology and Carcinogenesis Studies of d-Limonene (CAS No. 5989-27-5) in F344/N Rats and B6C3F1 Mice (Gavage Studies)* (Tech. Rep. Ser. No. 347), Research Triangle Park, NC, National Toxicology Program

NTP (1990b) *Toxicology and Carcinogenesis Studies of Glycidol (CAS No. 556-52-5) in F344/N Rats and B6C3F1 Mice (Gavage Studies)* (Tech. Rep. Ser. No. 374), Research Triangle Park, NC, National Toxicology Program

NTP (1992) *Toxicology and Carcinogenesis Studies of Resorcinol (CAS No. 108-46-3) in F344 Rats and B6C3F1 Mice (Gavage Studies)* (Tech. Rep. Ser. No. 403), Research Triangle Park, NC, National Toxicology Program

NTP (1995a) *Toxicology and Carcinogenesis Studies of Methylphenidate Hydrochloride (CAS No. 298-59-9) in F344/N Rats and B6C3F1 Mice (Feed Studies)* (Tech. Rep. Ser. No. 439), Research Triangle Park, NC, National Toxicology Program

NTP (1995b) *Toxicology and Carcinogenesis Studies of Phenolphthalein (CAS No. 77-09-08) in F344/N Rats and B6C3F1 Mice (Feed Studies)* (Tech. Rep. Ser. No. 465), Research Triangle Park, NC, National Toxicology Program

NTP (1996) *Comparative Initiation/Promotion Skin Paint Studies of B6C3F1 Mice, Swiss (CD-1®) Mice, and SENCAR Mice*, Research Triangle Park, NC, National Toxicology Program

NTP (1998a) *Toxicology and Carcinogenesis Studies of 1-Chloro-2-propanol (Technical Grade) (CAS No. 127-00-4) in F344/N Rats and B6C3F1 Mice (Drinking Water Studies)* (Tech. Rep. Ser. No. 477), Research Triangle Park, NC, National Toxicology Program

NTP (1998b) *Toxicology and Carcinogenesis Studies of Chloroprene (CAS No. 126-99-8) in F344/N Rats and B6C3F1 Mice (Inhalation Studies)* (Tech. Rep. Ser. No. 467), Research Triangle Park, NC, National Toxicology Program

NTP (1999a) *Toxicology and Carcinogenesis Studies of Lauric Acid Diethanolamine Condensate (CAS No. 120-40-1) in F344/N Rats and B6C3F1 Mice (Dermal Studies)* ((Tech. Rep. Ser. No. 480), Research Triangle Park, NC, National Toxicology Program

NTP (1999b) *Toxicology and Carcinogenesis Studies of Magnetic Field Promotion (DMBA Initiation) in Female Sprague-Dawley Rats (Whole-body Exposure/Gavage Studies)* (Tech. Rep. Ser. No. 489), Research Triangle Park, NC, National Toxicology Program

NTP (1999c) *Toxicology and Carcinogenesis Studies of Oleic Acid Diethanolamine Condensate (CAS No. 93-83-4) in F344/N Rats and B6C3F1 Mice (Dermal Studies)* (Tech. Rep. Ser. No. 481), Research Triangle Park, NC, National Toxicology Program

NTP (1999d) *Toxicology and Carcinogenesis Studies of Oxymetholone (CAS No. 434-07-1) in F344/N Rats and Toxicology Studies of Oxymetholone in B6C3F1 Mice (Gavage Studies)* (Tech. Rep. Ser. No. 485), Research Triangle Park, NC, National Toxicology Program

NTP (1999e) *Toxicology and Carcinogenesis Studies of Pentachlorophenol (CAS No. 87-86-5) in F344/N Rats (Feed Studies)* (Tech. Rep. Ser. No. 483), Research Triangle Park, NC, National Toxicology Program

NTP (2000) *Toxicology and Carcinogenesis Studies of Pyridine (CAS No. 110-86-1) in F344/N Rats, Wistar Rats, and B6C3F1 Mice (Drinking Water Studies)* (Tech. Rep. Ser. No. 470), Research Triangle Park, NC, National Toxicology Program

NTP (2001) *Toxicology and Carcinogenesis Studies of Coconut Oil Acid Diethanolamine Condensate (CAS No. 68603-42-9) in F344/N Rats And B6C3F1 Mice (Dermal Studies)*, (Tech. Rep. Ser. No. 479), Research Triangle Park, NC, National Toxicology Program

Ozaki, K., Sukata, T., Yamamoto, S., Uwagawa, S., Seki, T., Kawasaki, H., Yoshitake, A., Wanibuchi, H., Koide, A., Mori, Y. & Fukushima, S. (1998) High susceptibility of p53(+/–) knockout mice in

N-butyl-N-(4-hydroxybutyl)nitrosamine urinary bladder carcinogenesis and lack of frequent mutation in residual allele. *Cancer Res.*, **58**, 3806–3811

Prives, C. & Hall, P.A. (1999) The p53 pathway. *J. Pathol.*, **187**, 112–126

Sagartz, J.E., Curtiss, S.W., Bunch, R.T., Davila, J.C., Morris, D.L. & Alden, C.L. (1998) Phenobarbital does not promote hepatic tumorigenesis in a twenty-six-week bioassay in p53 heterozygous mice. *Toxicol. Pathol.*, **26**, 492–500

Shoemaker, A.R., Moser, A.R., Midgley, C.A., Clipson, L., Newton, M.A. & Dove, W.F. (1998) A resistant genetic background leading to incomplete penetrance of intestinal neoplasia and reduced loss of heterozygosity in ApcMin/+ mice. *Proc. natl Acad. Sci. USA*, **95**, 10826–10831

Spalding, J.W., French, J.E., Stasiewicz, S., Furedi-Machacek, M., Conner, F., Tice, R.R. & Tennant, R.W. (2000) Responses of transgenic mouse lines p53(+/–) and Tg.AC to agents tested in conventional carcinogenicity bioassays. *Toxicol. Sci.*, **53**, 213–223

Stoll, R.E., Holden, H.E., Barthel, C.H. & Blanchard, K.T. (1999) Oxymetholone: III. Evaluation in the p53+/– transgenic mouse model. *Toxicol. Pathol.*, **27**, 513–518

Storer, R.D., French, J.E., Haseman, J., Hajian, G., LeGrand, E.K., Long, G.G., Mixson, L.A., Ochoa, R., Sagartz, J.E. & Soper, K.A. (2001) p53+/– Hemizygous knockout mouse: overview of available data. *Toxicol. Pathol.*, **29** (Suppl.), 30–50

Tennant, R.W. & Zeiger, E. (1993) Genetic toxicology: current status of methods of carcinogen identification. *Environ. Health Perspect.*, **100**, 307–315

Tennant, R.W., French, J.E. & Spalding, J.W. (1995) Identifying chemical carcinogens and assessing potential risk in short-term bioassays using transgenic mouse models. *Environ. Health Perspect.*, **103**, 942–950

Tennant, R.W., Spalding, J. & French, J.E. (1996) Evaluation of transgenic mouse bioassays for identifying carcinogens and noncarcinogens. *Mutat. Res.*, **365**, 119–127

Tennant, R.W., Stasiewicz, S., Mennear, J., French, J.E. & Spalding, J.W. (1999) Genetically altered mouse models for identifying carcinogens. In: McGregor, D.B., Rice, J.M. & Venitt, S., eds, *The Use of Short- and Medium-term Tests for Carcinogens and Data on Genetic Effects in Carcinogenic Hazard Evaluation.* (IARC Scientific Publications No. 146), Lyon, IARC*Press*, pp. 123–150

Usui, T., Mutai, M., Hisada, S., Takoaka, M., Soper, K.A., McCullough, B. & Alden, C. (2001) CB6F1-rasH2 mouse: overview of available data. *Toxicol. Pathol.*, **29** (Suppl.), 90–108

Venkatachalam, S. & Donehower, L.A. (1998) Murine tumor suppressor models. *Mutat. Res.*, **400**, 391–407

Venkatachalam, S., Shi, Y.P., Jones, S.N., Vogel, H., Bradley, A., Pinkel, D. & Donehower, L.A. (1998) Retention of wild-type p53 in tumors from p53 heterozygous mice: reduction of p53 dosage can promote cancer formation. *EMBO J.*, **17**, 4657–4667

Venkatachalam, S., Tyner, S.D., Pickering, C.R., Boley, S., Recio, L., French, J.E. & Donehower, L.A. (2001) Is p53 haploinsufficient for tumor suppression? Implications for the p53+/– mouse model in carcinogenicity testing. *Toxicol. Pathol.*, **29** (Suppl.), 147–154

Weinberg, R.A. (1991) Tumor suppressor genes. *Science*, **254**, 1138–1146

Weisburger, E.K. (1977) Bioassay program for carcinogenic hazards of cancer chemotherapeutic agents. *Cancer*, **40** (Suppl. 4), 1935–1949

Yamamoto, M., Tsukamoto, T., Sakai, H., Shirai, N., Ohgaki, H., Furihata, C., Donehower, L.A., Yoshida, K. & Tatematsu, M. (2000) p53 knockout mice (–/–) are more susceptible than (+/–) or (+/+) mice to N-methyl-N-nitrosourea stomach carcinogenesis. *Carcinogenesis*, **21**, 1891–1897

Corresponding author:

John E. French
Transgenic Carcinogenesis,
Laboratory of Molecular Toxicology
National Institute of Environmental Health
Sciences, PO Box 12233, MD F1-05
Research Triangle Park, NC 27709
USA
french@niehs.nih.gov

Mechanisms of Carcinogenesis: Contributions of Molecular Epidemiology
Patricia Buffler, Jerry Rice, Robert Baan, Michael Bird and Paolo Boffetta, eds
IARC Scientific Publications No. 157
International Agency for Research on Cancer, Lyon, 2004

Multiple Primary Cancers as Clues to Environmental and Heritable Causes of Cancer and Mechanisms of Carcinogenesis

Kari Hemminki and Paolo Boffetta

Summary
Successes in cancer therapy are leading to an increasing incidence of second cancers, which may be due to the same factors that cause first cancers or to the effect of therapy for the first cancer. There are also a number of specific methodological and sampling problems that have to be controlled before informative studies can be embarked upon. The risk of a second cancer is higher than that for the first one, which may be an indication of a particular exposure, an inherited set of genes, or both. We show clustering of multiple cancers caused by tobacco, alcohol and infections. We discuss familial aggregation of cancer as one of the causes of multiple primary cancers. However, multiple primary cancers may particularly be a manifestation of polygenic susceptibility, which cannot easily be recognized as familial clustering, and multiple cancers may offer a model for understanding the complex etiology of human cancer and for generating and testing hypotheses on mechanisms of carcinogenesis.

Introduction
Multiple or second primary tumours arise because of either inherited or acquired mutations or deficiencies, and they may develop early or late after treatment of the first primary tumour. With the increasing success of modern cancer therapy in achieving long-term remissions in many patients, second primary tumours are a rapidly increasing category of disease. The increased occurrence of second primary cancers after an initial primary could result from

- intensive medical surveillance after first diagnosis
- therapy-induced exposure to chemical or physical carcinogens
- environmental and hereditary factors shared between the first and the second cancer.

All these aspects need to be considered when studies of second cancers are interpreted. In this chapter, we consider some challenges and attractions of the study of second cancers, in particular with respect to the increasing knowledge of mechanisms of carcinogenesis. Examples are taken from tumours discussed in these proceedings, using mainly data from the Swedish Family-Cancer Database (Hemminki *et al.*, 2001a). We focus on cancers of the upper aero-digestive tract (UADT), including the oral cavity, pharynx and larynx. Multiple primary cancers provide many epidemiological challenges, but this review is limited to the availability and interpretation of data; methods of analysis fall outside the scope of this presentation.

Difficulties and pitfalls
Epidemiological studies of second cancers are more difficult than those of first primaries because of many biological and clinical features of second cancers. These cancers are fewer, and some organs may be completely removed when surgery is the therapy of choice. It may be impossible to distinguish second tumours as independent primaries. Some of the uncertainty may be avoided if other (discordant) organs are studied, or in the same organ, if anatomically remote or histologically distinct tumours are

considered. For example, in the International Classification of Diseases codes, it is possible to distinguish anatomically or topologically distinct sites, assuring to some degree that the second event is independent of the first (Dong & Hemminki, 2001a). Other classifications, however, do not allow second primary tumours in the same organ or in the contralateral organ (Muir & Percy, 1991). The Swedish Cancer Registry has developed clear instructions about the reporting of multiple primary malignancies, and a re-evaluation of 209 multiple primary tumours found 98% of second malignancies to be correctly classified (Frödin et al., 1997).

Another issue is the likelihood of surveillance, lead-time bias during treatment for the first cancer and the ensuing follow-up period. Usually the risks are increased for nearby anatomical sites, and slow-growing, indolent tumours, such as carcinoids, may be particularly noted because they have reached a large size (Hemminki & Li, 2001). However, if the cancer registration system requires a histopathological or cytological verification of the tumours, diagnostic misclassification is unlikely. The consequence is that the diagnosis of second cancer may be arrived at earlier, causing an increase in incidence of second cancers during the first year of follow-up and a deficit later. Some authors try to avoid the surveillance bias by starting the follow-up for second primaries at some interval, such as 1 year after diagnosis of the first primary. In doing so, they disregard the large number of tumours that appear during the early surveillance period and bias the study towards null effects. To us, it appears recommendable to consider all histologically verified tumours at sites that can reasonably be considered independent primaries and then to divide the follow-up period into sequences that allow observation of time-dependent changes in relative risks. Such time intervals are also helpful in interpreting the effects of treatment.

Survival from many cancers is poor, and we have seen evidence that reporting of multiple primaries from fatal cancer is incomplete even in a well-functioning cancer registration system. In Sweden, for example, the median survival from esophageal and lung cancer is 1 year, and under-reporting of second primaries after these cancers is possible (Dong & Hemminki, 2001b). At these sites, it may be of interest to consider second cancers appearing after primary cancers at sites of better survival (Hemminki et al., 2001b; Hemminki & Jiang, 2002).

Therapeutic effects

The treatment of cancer has undergone constant changes, particularly since the large-scale introduction of chemotherapy in the 1960s (Boice & Shriner, 1996). The available range of antineoplastic agents and therapeutic modalities has increased, and more aggressive therapies have been introduced. For some malignancies, effective therapies have been achieved, and consequently, it has become possible to follow the long-term effects of the therapies used. The treatment for Hodgkin disease has been of particular interest in this regard (Storm & Prener, 1985; Swerdlow et al., 1997). The prognosis has improved markedly; for example, the 5-year survival from Hodgkin disease improved threefold in Sweden between 1962 and 1988 (Stenbeck et al., 1995). Hodgkin disease affects relatively young people, who undergo intense radiotherapy or chemotherapy or both, and who thus are at a risk for second cancer. Many studies have been carried out on the treatment of Hodgkin disease, and increased risks in survivors have been observed for acute leukaemia, lung, gastrointestinal, breast, thyroid, bone and connective tissue cancers, and non-Hodgkin lymphoma (Metayer et al., 2000; Swerdlow et al., 2000). The risks have been related to the age at treatment and to the modalities used. A main interest in these studies is to identify the harmful agents in order to devise therapeutic regimens in which efficacy and long-term safety are maximized (Boice & Shriner, 1996).

Many chemotherapeutic agents and radiotherapy cause DNA damage, which may be directly related to the risk of subsequent cancer. Often second cancers arise at sites that are in radiation fields, suggesting that second cancers arise because of direct damage caused by radiation. However, for tumours arising at remote sites, indirect mechanisms may be involved.

Intense therapy depresses immune function, and another mechanism may be escape of malignant cells from immune surveillance, as in patients undergoing immunosuppressive therapy for organ transplantation (Birkeland et al., 1995; IARC, 1996). Such tumours would be expected to arise shortly after therapy and they may present a typical spectrum of sites, including squamous-cell carcinoma of the skin and non-Hodgkin lymphoma.

Environmental causes

Tobacco smoking, alcohol drinking and a diet poor in fresh fruits and vegetables are the overwhelming risk factors for UADT cancers as well as other respiratory and digestive malignancies, and these cancers cluster as multiple primaries. An example is shown in Table 1, in which standardized incidence ratios (SIRs) for male esophageal cancer are shown after the first cancers listed in the left column; the data are from the Swedish Family-Cancer Database (Hemminki & Jiang, 2002). Esophageal cancer is increased after UADT, gastric and lung cancers, as would be expected because of shared risk factors. The risk during the first year after another UADT cancer is very high, suggesting also a contribution of clinical surveillance (i.e. lead time bias). On the other hand, there are no increases at the longest follow-up period, suggesting that the effects of treatment at the given sites do not affect the risk of esophageal cancer.

The contribution to multiple primaries of shared exposure to other risk factors of UADT cancers, including infection with human papilloma virus (HPV) and occupational exposures such as asbestos, is less clear, but it is likely to be much smaller than that of tobacco, alcohol and diet. One reason for this is the relatively weak carcinogenicity of these risk factors. In addition, they tend to exert their action on only part of the UADT (e.g. the oropharynx in the case of HPV infection and the larynx in the case of asbestos).

Cancers of the UADT are often multiple tumours at presentation. A frequent occurrence of multiple tumours, 'field cancerization', is common in oropharyngeal and nasopharyngeal cancers (van Oijen & Slootweg, 2000). In Table 2,

we show data on the risk of multiple primary cancers in nasal cancer patients using the Swedish Family-Cancer Database to follow second cancers after nasal cancer (Dong & Hemminki, 2001c). For confirmation of the findings, we also calculated SIRs for second primary nasal cancer in patients with an initial primary cancer of the UADT and skin (squamous-cell) and non-Hodgkin lymphoma. Our data showed that, compared with the general population, nasal cancer patients had a marked excess of second nasal cancer, with an overall SIR of 43.1. They also had an at least 2.5-fold significantly increased risk for second primary UADT, skin cancer or non-Hodgkin lymphoma. An increased SIR for second primary nasal cancer was also observed in patients with an initial UADT, skin cancer or non-Hodgkin lymphoma. Also, oral cancers after UADT tumours were remarkably increased, to an SIR of 7.9. Probably because of intensive medical surveillance, the SIRs were much higher within 1 year of the first diagnosis. Compared with the period covering years 1–9 of follow-up, the last follow-up period showed a moderate increase in the risk for second nasal cancer after nasal and skin cancer and non-Hodgkin lymphoma, suggesting a treatment-induced effect. The across-site associations confirmed in reverse order and for both sexes were unlikely to be due to chance. Although the moderate increase in risk for second primary cancer in the final follow-up period suggests a small contribution from radiotherapy, the unusual clustering of multiple primary cancers at these sites strongly suggests that nasal cancer may share some common risk factors with UADT, skin cancer, and non-Hodgkin lymphoma. It has been suggested that these common risk factors may be exposure to ultraviolet light and infection with Epstein–Barr virus in transiently immunocompromised individuals (Brennan et al., 2000; Hemminki & Dong, 2000a,b). The causal links between these exposures and cancer await molecular epidemiological proof.

Heritable causes

The phenomenon of field cancerization mentioned above may be an expression of heritable or environmental effects, or the interaction of both,

Table 1. SIR for second esophageal cancer after cancers in men

First cancer sites	Follow-up interval (years)																			
	< 1				1–10				> 10				All							
	O	E	SIR	95% CI	O	E	SIR	95% CI	O	E	SIR	95% CI	O	E	SIR	95% CI				
UADT	17	0.57	29.73	17.27	45.54	46	5.11	9.00	6.58	11.78	5	2.57	1.95	0.61	4.03	68	8.25	8.24	6.40	10.31
Esophagus	3	0.47	6.39	1.20	15.67	1	0.51	1.98	0.00	7.75	1	0.11	9.17	0.00	35.93	5	1.08	4.61	1.46	9.54
Stomach	5	1.55	3.23	1.02	6.69	8	4.35	1.84	0.79	3.33	2	1.82	1.10	0.10	3.16	15	7.71	1.95	1.09	3.05
Colon	1	2.00	0.50	0.00	1.96	13	12.48	1.04	0.55	1.69	5	4.30	1.16	0.37	2.40	19	18.78	1.01	0.61	1.52
Rectum	2	1.33	1.50	0.14	4.30	8	8.90	0.90	0.38	1.63	5	2.80	1.79	0.56	3.69	15	13.03	1.15	0.64	1.81
Larynx	1	0.27	3.72	0.00	14.57	12	3.03	3.97	2.04	6.53	4	1.45	2.77	0.72	6.14	17	4.74	3.59	2.08	5.49
Lung	6	2.94	2.04	0.73	4.00	10	4.93	2.03	0.97	3.48	3	1.32	2.28	0.43	5.58	19	9.19	2.07	1.24	3.10
Prostate	7	7.96	0.88	0.35	1.65	59	58.16	1.01	0.77	1.29	7	7.04	0.99	0.39	1.87	73	73.16	1.00	0.78	1.24
Kidney	1	0.90	1.11	0.00	4.33	5	5.25	0.95	0.30	1.97	0	2.23				6	8.39	0.72	0.26	1.40
Bladder	2	2.03	0.99	0.09	2.83	20	18.11	1.10	0.67	1.64	6	6.21	0.97	0.35	1.89	28	26.35	1.06	0.71	1.49
Melanoma	1	0.58	1.73	0.00	6.77	3	6.18	0.49	0.09	1.19	3	2.89	1.04	0.20	2.54	7	9.65	0.73	0.29	1.36
Skin	1	1.19	0.84	0.00	3.30	12	10.52	1.14	0.59	1.88	3	2.71	1.11	0.21	2.72	16	14.42	1.11	0.63	1.72
Nervous system	1	0.51	1.97	0.00	7.74	2	2.28	0.88	0.08	2.51	3	1.78	1.68	0.32	4.13	6	4.57	1.31	0.47	2.57
NHL	1	0.78	1.29	0.00	5.06	3	4.45	0.67	0.13	1.65	1	1.13	0.88	0.00	3.47	5	6.36	0.79	0.25	1.63
All	55	27.81	1.98	1.49	2.54	216	162.18	1.33	1.16	1.52	58	47.12	1.23	0.93	1.57	329	237.10	1.39	1.24	1.54

All expected numbers were calculated based on site, age, period, residence and socioeconomic level-specific incidence.
SIR, standardized incidence ratio; NHL, non-Hodgkin lymphoma; UADT, upper aerodigestive tract
Sites are included if a total of ≥ 5 cases were recorded.
In **bold**, significant SIR

Table 2. Risk of multiple primary tumours following nasal, UADT and squamous-cell skin cancer and non-Hodgkin lymphoma

First primary cancer	Second primary cancer	Follow-up interval (years)											
		<1			1-9			10-38			Total		
		O	SIR	(95% CI)	O	SIR	(95% CI)	O	SIR	(95% CI)	O	SIR	(95% CI)
Nose	Nose	3	106	(20.0-314)	4	31.0	(8.1-80.1)	2	39.0	(3.7-144)	9	43.1	(19.6-82.3)
	UADT	2	10.0	(0.9-36.9)	6	4.7	(1.7-10.2)	3	3.9	(0.7-11.5)	11	4.9	(2.4-8.7)
	Skin	1	3.5	(0.0-19.9)	9	5.1	(2.3-9.7)	5	3.5	(1.1-8.2)	15	4.3	(2.4-7.1)
	NHL				6	3.4	(1.2-7.5)	2	1.7	(0.2-6.2)	8	2.5	(1.1-4.9)
UADT	Nose	4	24.4	(6.3-63.1)	6	4.5	(1.6-9.8)				10	6.7	(3.2-12.3)
	Oral	75	28.9	(22.8-36.3)	129	6.3	(5.3-7.5)	65	6.0	(4.6-7.7)	269	7.9	(7.0-9.0)
	Skin	22	6.7	(4.2-10.1)	130	4.9	(4.1-5.8)	66	3.3	(2.6-4.3)	218	4.4	(3.8-5.0)
	NHL	6	1.9	(0.7-4.1)	31	1.2	(0.8-1.9)	20	1.3	(0.8-1.9)	57	1.3	(1.0-1.6)
Skin	Nose	4	17.3	(4.5-44.8)	6	3.3	(1.2-7.3)	3	5.2	(1.0-15.4)	13	5.0	(2.6-8.5)
	UADT	18	5.5	(3.3-8.7)	82	3.2	(2.6-4.0)	25	3.1	(2.0-4.6)	125	3.4	(2.8-4.1)
	Skin	199	25.9	(22.4-29.8)	857	15.0	(14.0-16.1)	175	9.2	(7.9-10.6)	1231	14.7	(13.9-15.5)
	NHL	10	1.8	(0.9-3.4)	73	1.8	(1.4-2.2)	18	1.3	(0.7-2.0)	101	1.6	(1.3-2.0)
NHL	Nose	2	9.7	(0.9-35.8)	3	2.4	(0.5-7.2)	2	4.9	(0.5-18.1)	7	3.8	(1.5-7.8)
	UADT	14	2.4	(1.3-4.0)	36	1.1	(0.7-1.5)	14	1.2	(0.7-2.1)	64	1.3	(1.0-1.6)
	Skin	11	2.2	(1.1-3.9)	124	4.0	(3.3-4.8)	35	3.1	(2.2-4.3)	170	3.6	(3.1-4.2)
	NHL	16	4.2	(2.4-6.9)	54	2.4	(1.8-3.1)	19	2.4	(1.5-3.8)	89	2.6	(2.1-3.2)

SIR, standardized incidence ratio; NHL, non-Hodgkin lymphoma; UADT, upper aerodigestive tract
In **bold**, significant SIR

or migration of tumour cells from an adjacent location (van Oijen & Slootweg, 2000). The high risks reported above for nasal and UADT cancers, rarely seen for any environmental or familial cause, may give important mechanistic clues as to the causation of cancer (Hemminki & Mutanen, 2001). We have systematically compared familial risks and risks for second cancers; the latter are always higher than the former, suggesting that the increased risk of second cancer is not a simple function of heritability such as can be observed in a family study (Dong & Hemminki, 2001b,d). Multiple primaries are common in individuals affected by the high-penetrance cancer suscepti-bility genes. These include colon cancer in carriers of *APC* and mismatch repair gene muta-tions (Lynch & de la Chapelle, 1999), breast cancer in *BRCA1*, *BRCA2* and *ATM*-related families (Peto *et al.*, 1999; Broeks *et al.*, 2000) and melanoma in carriers of the $P16^{INK4a}$ mutation (Aitken *et al.*, 1999). On the other hand, very few population-based studies have been conducted in order to assess the role of family history in the development of multiple primary cancers at these sites. However, we described recently familial effects in multiple primaries on breast, colorectal and skin cancer (melanoma) (Vaittinen & Hemminki, 2000; Dong & Hemminki, 2001a; Hemminki *et al.*, 2001c). At all these sites, fami-lial clustering appears to be an important cause of multiple primary cancers, but it explains only a small proportion of second primaries at these sites. Familial risks are much higher than those observed for the first primary cancer but, because they explain only a small proportion of second cancers, other causes have to be invoked. Poly-genic effects are a likely mechanism because familial risks would not be obvious but those with an unfortunate genotype would be severely affected (Hemminki & Mutanen, 2001; Pharoah *et al.*, 2002).

Experimental models of cancer and age–inci-dence relationships in human cancers suggest that most cancers are multistage diseases (Armitage & Doll, 1954, 1957; Moolgavkar & Luebeck, 1992; Herrero-Jimenez *et al.*, 1998; Hanahan & Weinberg, 2000; Herrero-Jimenez *et al.*, 2000). Cancers almost always have many causes and therefore they are complex diseases of interacting genes and environmental factors. In polygenic cancers, the individual mutant genes are not sufficient to cause the disease, and thus familial risks are weak because, for each family member, the probability of inheriting exactly the same set of genes diminishes with the number of such genes (Hemminki & Mutanen, 2001). Those indi-viduals who have inherited a harmful set of genes are, however, at high risk for multiple cancers. Progress in the understanding of polygenic cancers has been hampered by the lack of model systems for study. However, multiple primary cancers may be such a model, analogous to the way that identical twins represent two individuals with an identical genetic background (Lichten-stein *et al.*, 2000; Peto & Mack, 2000). We suggest that one of the reasons for the high risks of a second cancer compared with a first cancer is the polygenic nature of common cancers.

Mechanisms of carcinogenesis

Analysis of the occurrence of second primaries may contribute to the study of different aspects of mechanisms of carcinogenesis. An increased risk of a second primary neoplasm that persists throughout the follow-up period is suggestive of shared risk factors and mechanisms of action. A classic example is that of tobacco-related cancers from the UADT and the lung (Wu *et al.*, 1999). The observed increased risk of skin melanoma following non-Hodgkin lymphoma is an addi-tional example, which may reflect a role of immunosuppression in the pathogenesis of both neoplasms (Boffetta *et al.*, 1999).

The pattern of risk in the case of shared etio-logy or mechanism is different from that found following a carcinogenic treatment effect, in which no excess risk is usually apparent during the first few years of follow-up, as in the case of leukaemia following treatment for Hodgkin lymphoma (Felix, 1999). However, the study of treatment-related second primaries may contri-bute to the understanding of mechanisms of carci-nogenesis in humans, since it is based on the observation of humans exposed to carcinogens under semi-experimental conditions. It is there-fore possible to assess the risk of second cancer following exposure to agents active on different cellular and molecular targets. For example, the study of the risk of osteosarcoma following radiotherapy for retinoblastoma contributed to the elucidation of the two-step model in retinoblastoma mutation carriers (Draper et al., 1986). Molecular epidemiological studies, including prospective collection of samples from patients treated with chemotherapy and radiotherapy, offer great opportunities to investigate better the mechanisms of second primary carcinogenesis and to identify patients at increased risk (Califano & Sidransky, 1999).

Polygenic diseases are a particular problem to geneticists because familial patterns cannot be discerned in pedigrees (Hemminki & Mutanen, 2001; Pharoah et al., 2002). Practically the only human model in which polygenic diseases have been tackled has been the comparison of concordance between monozygotic and dizygotic twins (Lichtenstein et al., 2000; Risch, 2001; Hemminki, 2002). However, twinning is rare, and the power in twin studies has barely been enough to assess the effects in the commonest cancers. Monozygotic twins are genetically identical, and thus any polygenic effect should manifest in both twins. Typically, the concordance between monozygotic twins would exceed that between dizygotic twins by well over twofold (Risch, 2001; Hemminki, 2002). Like cancer monozygotic twins, multiple primaries arise in a single individual, i.e. in a uniform genetic background. We believe that multiple primary cancers will become a second model for polygenic effects by low-penetrance genes. Moreover, sampling of patients may be logistically easier than that of twins, which may facilitate molecular epidemiological studies.

Conclusions
The high and, at certain sites, very high risks of a second cancer compared with a first cancer call for explanation. It is unlikely that the studies on second tumours based on well-functioning cancer registries can be explained solely by therapeutic effects, surveillance bias or reporting of recurrent tumours. Instead, the individuals affected by the first cancer may be heavily exposed to environ-

mental carcinogens, they may have inherited a set of genes conveying susceptibility, or the combination of the two possibly interacting factors may make them the unfortunate victims of a second malignancy. We believe that future studies of cancer mechanism and gene–environment interactions will greatly benefit from a penetrating scrutiny of second cancers.

Acknowledgements
The work was supported by The Swedish Cancer Society and The King Gustaf V's Jubileefund.

References
Aitken, J., Welch, J., Duffy, D., Milligan, A., Green, A., Martin, N. & Hayward, N. (1999) CDKN2A variants in a population-based sample of Queensland families with melanoma. J. natl Cancer Inst., 91, 446–452

Armitage, P. & Doll, R. (1954) The age distribution of cancer and a multi-stage theory of carcinogenesis. Br. J. Cancer, 8, 1–12

Armitage, P. & Doll, R. (1957) A two-stage theory of carcinogenesis in relation to the age distribution of human cancer. Br. J. Cancer, 161–169

Birkeland, S. A., Storm, H.H, Lamm, L.U., Barlow, L., Blohme, I., Forsberg, B., Eklund, B., Fjeldborg, O., Friedberg, M., Frödin, L., Glattre, E., Halvorsen, S., Holm, N.V., Jacobsen, A., Jörgensen, H.E., Ladefoged, J., Lindholm, T., Lundgren, G. & Pukkala, E. (1995) Cancer risk after renal transplantation in the Nordic countries, 1964–1986. Int. J. Cancer, 60, 183–189

Boffetta, P., Butler, J., Maynadie, M. & Brennan, P. (1999) Lymphomas. In: Neugut, A.I., Meadows, A.T. & Robinson, E., eds, Multiple Primary Cancers, Philadelphia, Lippincott Williams & Williams, pp. 277–301

Boice, J., Jr & Shriner, D. (1996) Second malignancies after chemotherapy. In: Perry, M., ed., The Chemotherapy Source Book, Baltimore, Williams & Wilkins, pp. 559–569

Brennan, P., Coates, M., Armstrong, B., Colin, D. & Boffetta, P. (2000) Second primary neoplasms following non-Hodgkin's lymphoma in New South Wales, Australia. Br. J. Cancer, 82, 1344–1347

Broeks, A., Urbanus, J.H., Floore, A.N., Daher, E.C., Klijn, J.G, Rutgers, E.J., Devilee, P., Russell, N.S., van Leeuven, F.E. & van't Veer, L.J. (2000) ATM-heterozygous germline mutations contribute to breast cancer-susceptibility. *Am. J. hum. Genet.*, **66**, 494–500

Califano, J.A. & Sidransky, D. (1999) Molecular analysis of tumours. In: Neugut, A.I., Meadows, A.T. & Robinson, E., eds, *Multiple Primary Cancers*, Philadelphia, Lippincott Williams & Williams, pp. 225–232

Dong, C. & Hemminki, K. (2001a) Multiple primary cancers of the colon, breast and skin (melanoma) as models for polygenic cancers. *Int. J. Cancer*, **92**, 883–887

Dong, C. & Hemminki, K. (2001b) Second primary neoplasms in 633,964 cancer patients in Sweden, 1958–1996. *Int. J. Cancer*, **93**, 155–161

Dong, C. & Hemminki, K. (2001c) Risk of multiple primary cancers in nasal cancer patients. *Epidemiology*, **12**, 367–369

Dong, C. & Hemminki, K. (2001d) Modification of cancer risks in offspring by sibling and parental cancers from 2,112,616 nuclear families. *Int. J. Cancer*, **92**, 144–150

Draper, G.J., Sanders, B.M. & Kingston, J.E. (1986) Second primary neoplasms in patients with retinoblastoma. *Br. J. Cancer*, **53**, 661–671

Felix, C.A. (1999) Chemotherapy-related second cancers. In: Neugut, A.I., Meadows, A.T. & Robinson, E., eds, *Multiple Primary Cancers*, Philadelphia, Lippincott Williams & Williams, pp. 137–164

Frödin, J.-E., Ericsson, J. & Barlow, L. (1997) Multiple primary malignant tumors in a national cancer registry–reliability of reporting. *Acta oncol.*, **36**, 465–469

Hanahan, D. & Weinberg, R. (2000) The hallmarks of cancer. *Cell*, **100**, 57–70

Hemminki, K. (2002) Correspondence re: Risch, N.: Genetic epidemiology of cancer: interpreting family and twin studies and their implications for molecular genetic approaches, Cancer Epidemiol. Biomarkers Prev., 10: 733–741, 2001. *Cancer Epidemiol. Biomarkers Prev.*, **11**, 423

Hemminki, K. & Dong, C. (2000a) Letter to Editor: Primary cancers following squamous cell carcinoma of the skin suggest involvement of Epstein-Barr virus. *Epidemiology*, **11**, 94

Hemminki, K. & Dong, C. (2000b) Subsequent cancers after in situ and invasive squamous cell carcinoma of the skin. *Arch. Dermatol.*, **136**, 647–651

Hemminki, K. & Jiang, Y. (2002) Familial and second esophageal cancers: a nation-wide epidemiologic study from Sweden. *Int. J. Cancer*, **98**, 106–109

Hemminki, K. & Li, X. (2001) Familial carcinoid tumors and subsequent cancers: a nation-wide epidemiological study from Sweden. *Int. J. Cancer*, **94**, 444–448

Hemminki, K. & Mutanen, P. (2001) Genetic epidemiology of multistage carcinogenesis. *Mutat. Res.*, **473**, 11–21

Hemminki, K., Li, X., Plna, K., Granström, C. & Vaittinen, P. (2001a) The nation-wide Swedish Family-Cancer Database: updated structure and familial rates. *Acta oncol.*, **40**, 772–777

Hemminki, K., Jiang, Y. & Dong, C. (2001b) Second primary cancers after anogenital, skin, oral, esophageal and rectal cancers: etiological links? *Int. J. Cancer*, **93**, 294–298

Hemminki, K., Li, X. & Dong, C. (2001c) Second primary cancers after sporadic and familial colorectal cancer. *Cancer Epidemiol. Biomarkers Prev.*, **10**, 793–798

Herrero-Jimenez, P., Thilly, G., Southam, P., Tomita-Mitchell, A., Morgenthaler, S., Furth, E. & Thilly, W. (1998) Mutation, cell kinetics, and subpopulations at risk for colon cancer in the United States. *Mutat. Res.*, **400**, 553–578

Herrero-Jimenez, P., Tomita-Mitchell, A., Furth, E., Morgenthaler, S. & Thilly, W. (2000) Population risk and physiological rate paramenters for colon cancer. The union of an explicit model for carcinogenesis with the public health records of the United States. *Mutat. Res.*, **447**, 73–116

IARC (1996) *IARC Monographs on the Evaluation of Carcinogenic Risks to Humans*, Vol. 67, *Human Immunodeficiency Viruses and Human T-Cell Lymphotrophic Viruses*, Lyon, IARCPress

Lichtenstein, P., Holm, N.V., Verkasalo, P.K., Iliadou, A., Kaprio, J., Koskenvuo, M., Pukkala, E., Skytthe, A. & Hemminki, K. (2000) Environmental and heritable factors in the causation of cancer–analyses of cohorts of twins from Sweden, Denmark and Finland. *New Engl. J. Med.*, **343**, 78–85

Lynch, H.T. & de la Chapelle, A. (1999) Genetic susceptibility to non-polyposis colorectal cancer. *J. med. Genet.*, **36**, 801–818

Metayer, C., Lynch, C.F., Clarke, E.A., Glimelius, B., Storm, H., Pukkala, E., Joensuu, T., van Leeuwen, F.E., van't Veer, M.B., Curtis, R.E., Holowaty, E.J., Andersson, M., Wiklund, T., Gospodarowicz, M. & Travis, L.B. (2000) Second cancers among long-term survivors of Hodgkin's disease diagnosed in childhood and adolescence. *J. clin. Oncol.*, **18**, 2435–2443

Moolgavkar, S.H. & Luebeck, E.G. (1992) Multistage carcinogenesis: population-based model for colon cancer. *J. natl Cancer Inst.*, **84**, 610–618

Muir, C.S. & Percy, C. (1991) Classification and coding of neoplasms. In: Jensen, O.M., Parkin, D.M., MacLennan, R., Muir, C.S. & Skeet, R., eds, *Cancer Registration: Principles and Methods* (IARC Scientific Publications No. 95), Lyon, IARC*Press*, pp. 64–81

van Oijen, M.G. & Slootweg, P.J. (2000) Oral field cancerization: carcinogen-induced independent events or micrometastatic deposits? *Cancer Epidemiol. Biomarkers Prev.*, **9**, 249–256

Peto, J. & Mack, T.M. (2000) High constant incidence in twins and other relatives of women with breast cancer. *Nature Genet.*, **26**, 411–414

Peto, J., Collins, N., Barfoot, R., Seal, S., Warren, W., Rahman, N., Easton, D.F., Evans, C., Deacon, J. & Stratton, M.R. (1999) Prevalence of *BRCA1* and *BRCA2* gene mutations in patients with early-onset breast cancer. *J. natl Cancer Inst.*, **91**, 943–949

Pharoah, P.D., Antoniou, A., Bobrow, M., Zimmern, R.L., Easton, D.F. & Ponder, B.A. (2002) Polygenic susceptibility to breast cancer and implications for prevention. *Nature Genet.*, **31**, 33–36

Risch, N. (2001) The genetic epidemiology of cancer: interpreting family and twin studies and their implications for molecular genetic approaches. *Cancer Epidemiol. Biomarkers Prev.*, **10**, 733–741

Stenbeck, M., Rosen, M. & Holm, L.E. (1995) Cancer survival in Sweden during three decades, 1961–1991. *Acta oncol.*, **34**, 881–891

Storm, H.H. & Prener, A. (1985) Second cancer following lymphatic and hematopoietic cancers in Denmark, 1943–1980. *Natl Cancer Inst. Monogr.*, **68**, 389–409

Swerdlow, A.J., Barber, J.A., Horwich, A., Cunningham, D., Milan, S. & Omar, R.Z. (1997) Second malignancy in patients with Hodgkin's disease treated at the Royal Marsden Hospital. *Br. J. Cancer*, **75**, 116–123

Swerdlow, A.J., Barber, J.A., Hudson, G.V., Cunningham, D., Gupta, R.K., Hancock, B.W., Horwich, A., Lister, T.A. & Linch, D.C. (2000) Risk of second malignancy after Hodgkin's disease in a collaborative British cohort: the relation to age at treatment. *J. clin. Oncol.*, **18**, 498–509

Vaittinen, P. & Hemminki, K. (2000) Risk factors and age-incidence relationships for contralateral breast cancer. *Int. J. Cancer*, **88**, 998–1002

Wu, X.F., Hu, Y.H. & Lippman, S.M. (1999) Upper aerodigestive tract cancers. In: Neugut, A.I., Meadows, A.T. & Robinson, E., eds, *Multiple Primary Cancers*, Philadelphia, Lippincott Williams & Williams, pp. 319–346

Corresponding author:

Kari Hemminki
Department of Biosciences at
Novum, Karolinska Institute
Hälsovagen 7
141 57 Huddinge
Sweden
kari.hemminki@cnt.ki.se

Target Organs

Mechanisms of Carcinogenesis: Contributions of Molecular Epidemiology
Patricia Buffler, Jerry Rice, Robert Baan, Michael Bird and Paolo Boffetta, eds
IARC Scientific Publications No. 157
International Agency for Research on Cancer, Lyon, 2004

The Biological Model of Gastric Carcinogenesis

Pelayo Correa

Summary

The biological model of gastric carcinogenesis can be described as a series of sequential phases. The first consists of a chronic active inflammatory response to *Helicobacter pylori* infection. Infiltration of the gastric mucosa by mucosa-associated lymphoid tissue and polymorphonuclear neutrophils, as well as damage to the epithelial cells, characterize this phase. The second phase is dominated by alterations of the epithelial cell cycle, especially increased rates of apoptosis and cell proliferation. These changes may be responsible for the multifocal atrophy that characterizes the type of gastritis associated with an increased risk of cancer. The third, more advanced phase of the model displays nuclear and architectural abnormalities, which may represent progressive mutational events as expected in classical molecular models of carcinogenesis.

The importance of a comprehensive view of the biological model is stressed.

Introduction

There is currently considerable demand for 'molecular' models of carcinogenesis. The colon cancer model of Vogelstein *et al.* (1988) is often cited as the paradigm to follow. A sequential chain of molecular events is being sought for each major cancer. This is expected to serve the present 'molecular revolution' which is to lead to cancer cure and prevention, perhaps by designing strategies to interrupt the proposed chain of events. Despite considerable efforts, the Vogelstein model paradigm has not been found to fit other organs well. This is especially true of gastric carcinogenesis, the study of which has not led clearly to identification of molecular events amenable to preventive or curative interventions. It is tempting to speculate on causal factors behind the conundrum which contrasts proximal and distal segments of the gastrointestinal tract. Two possible explanations might contribute to the riddle:

- The molecular models address fascinating mechanistic pathways, but do not really identify the 'etiological' forces, which are equally fascinating. The considerable resources dedicated today by major funding agencies are by-passing etiology in the interests of molecular mechanistic considerations.
- The biology of the gastric precancerous process involves more than molecular abnormalities. Its study is better served by the classical approach of epidemiology, namely the interactions of agent, host and environment. The biological model of gastric carcinogenesis, described long before the molecular revolution, consists of at least three different processes (Correa *et al.*, 1975). First, there is chronic active inflammation, in this case mainly as a response to the infectious agent *H. pylori*. Second, there is the loss of gastric glands, or atrophy, which may result from a disturbance of the cell cycle: a loss of balance between apoptosis and cell proliferation (Correa, 1997). Lastly, there is a progressive loss of differentiation, leading to abnormal cellular genotypes capable of invading their neighbours in the gastric mucosa (Rugge *et al.*, 2000).

It could be argued that molecular alterations can be found in each of the three components of the biological model, but each step may have its own independent dynamics. The forces that drive the precancerous events in each component of the biological model are the backbone of the etiological model. A well-defined etiological model may be more useful than other models in lessening the human cancer burden.

In this chapter the biological model of gastric carcinogenesis will be summarized.

Chronic active inflammation

Although several viral agents have been linked to carcinogenesis (human T-cell lymphotropic virus I, Epstein-Barr virus, hepatitis B virus, hepatitis C virus, human papillomavirus), *H. pylori* is the first bacterium to be identified as a cause of cancer in humans (IARC, 1994) (Figure 1). The organism is usually acquired in early childhood or infancy (Goodman & Correa, 2000), and, once established as a persistent infection, it induces a chronic inflammatory response in the gastric mucosa that lasts for decades, often throughout the lifespan of the individual (Correa, 1995). The constant component of the inflammatory response is the attraction to the gastric mucosa of white blood cells not normally present in it: the mucosa-associated lymphoid tissue, made up of lymphocytes and plasma cells (Figure 2). These inflammatory cells infiltrate the mucosa diffusely as long as the infection persists and may remain there months after the infection is cured with antibiotics. A second, very frequent

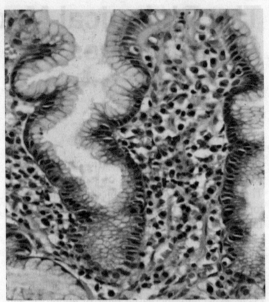

Figure 2. Gastric biopsy of patient infected with *H. pylori*. A dense infiltrate of lymphocytes and plasma cells is seen in the lamina propria of the mucosa.

component of the inflammatory responses is the polymorphonuclear leukocytes, mostly neutrophils. They tend to be present in small clusters in the stroma as well as in the epithelium, both at the surface and the gland necks. They are considered to represent recent active cell injury ('activity').

The bacteria remain outside the epithelial cells but damage them in several ways, especially by causing a partial depletion of the cytoplasmic mucus.

The inflammatory response to the infection varies considerably among individuals and populations. The great majority of infected adults in affluent societies have a very mild response to the infection without clinical manifestations or disease outcome (Correa, 1995). When the inflammatory response is more than mild, it leads to one of two nosological entities characterized by either the absence or the presence of multifocal loss of gastric glands. In the absence of gland loss, the entity is called non-atrophic gastritis (Dixon *et al.*, 1996). The inflammatory changes concentrate in the gastric antrum (antrum predominant non-atrophic gastritis) (Figure 3). This syndrome

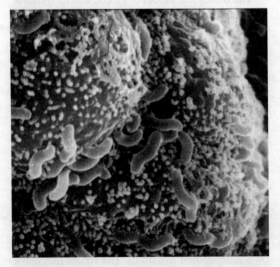

Figure 1. Scanning electron microphotograph of the gastric mucosa infected with *H. pylori*. Loosely spiralled bacteria are on the mucosal surface. They cluster around the intercellular junctions. Photograph courtesy of Dr Francisco Hernandez, University of Costa Rica.

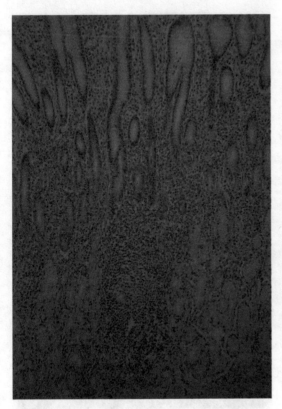

Figure 3. Antral mucosa from a patient with non-atrophic chronic gastritis. The dense mononuclear infiltrate separates but does not destroy the gastric glands.

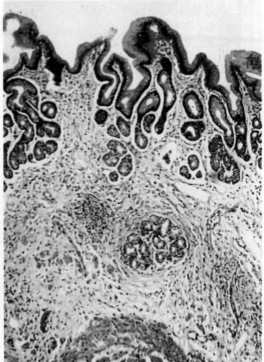

Figure 4. Gastric mucosa of a patient with MAG. Most gastric glands have disappeared. Only a small cluster of glands remains in the centre of the field.

appears mostly in young adults. It is characteristically associated with intact or exaggerated acid–pepsin secretion. Patients with duodenal ulcer consistently display this type of gastritis. Before *H. pylori* was identified as the cause of duodenal ulcer, the ulcer itself (but not the gastritis) could be treated successfully with antacid medication but the ulcer recurred when such medication was discontinued. Curing the infection results in the definitive resolution of both the gastritis and the ulcer.

Multiple foci of gland loss characterize the chronic gastritis as a multifocal atrophic gastritis (MAG) response to *H. pylori* infection. MAG occurs in populations at high risk of gastric cancer (Figure 4). The foci of gland loss first appear in the antrum–corpus junction, especially around the

incisura angularis (Figure 5). The lost glands are frequently replaced by epithelial cells with intestinal phenotype (intestinal metaplasia). Such foci increase in size and number, coalesce with each other and extend with time up and down the lesser curvature and later the anterior and posterior walls of both antrum and corpus. In most patients, the intestinalized cells are of small intestinal phenotype: absorptive enterocytes alternating with goblet cells containing sialomucins (Figure 6). In some individuals, such 'mature' metaplastic phenotypes (type I) gradually change: in addition to the sialomucins which normally characterize the small intestine, the metaplastic cells also synthesize sulfomucins, which in normal subjects are present only in the large intestine (colon and rectum). Other phenotypic characteristics of large intestine also appear in the metaplastic cells such as the loss of the multiple

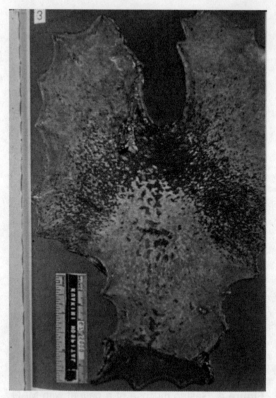

Figure 5. Gross anatomy of gastrectomy specimen stained for alkaline phosphatase. Red areas represent foci of intestinal metaplasia. The typical distribution of foci of metaplastic atrophy stand out: mostly the antrum–corpus junction, the incisura angularis, the lesser curvature. Photograph courtesy of Dr. Grant Stemmermann.

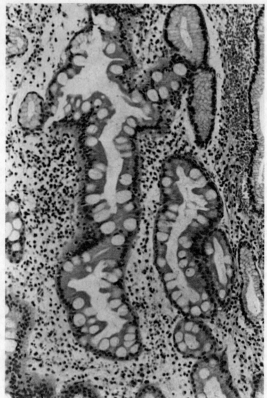

Figure 6. Complete intestinal metaplasia of gastric glands replaced by absorptive enterocytes with brush border alternating with goblet cells.

microvilli ('brush border') and the digestive enzymes of the small intestinal cells (Figure 7). When these changes are present, the intestinal crypts frequently become more irregular and nuclear replicative activity increases. Such metaplasias have been called 'colonic' or type III metaplasia. They are frequently found in stomachs with focal areas of dysplasia (Correa, 1992).

Dysplasia may be polypoid or (more frequently) flat. It represents a neoplastic transformation of epithelial cells without the capacity to break down the glandular basement membrane and invade the stroma (Figures 8 and 9).

Atrophy and hyperproliferation

As described, gland loss (atrophy) is a component of the response of the gastric mucosa to infection with *H. pylori*. The mechanism by which such an event takes place is not clear.

In the normal gastric mucosa, epithelial cell replication takes place only at the level of the glandular necks. The replicating cells migrate either towards the surface or towards the deep glands. Differentiation to the mature phenotype takes place as the migration evolves. Cell damage induced by *H. pylori* infection may lead to cell necrosis. It is not clear if the absence of atrophy in antral non-atrophic gastritis indicates that cell necrosis does not take place, or that intact repair mechanisms result in restitution of damaged glandular structures to their original state. In MAG,

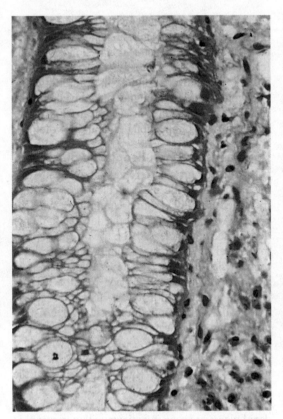

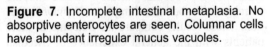

Figure 7. Incomplete intestinal metaplasia. No absorptive enterocytes are seen. Columnar cells have abundant irregular mucus vacuoles.

Figure 8. Dysplastic gland (low grade) surrounded by incomplete intestinal metaplastic glands.

there is obviously gland loss as well as inadequate repair mechanisms. It appears that repair mechanisms must be a key determinant of the outcome of *H. pylori* infection.

The integrity of the gastric mucosa in the normal individual is guaranteed by an adequate control system for the epithelial cell cycle. Two events dominate such cell cycles: apoptosis and proliferation. The first impedes and the second stimulates the replacement of gastric glands that may be lost due to *H. pylori* infection or to other 'injuries'. It has been found that (paradoxically) both apoptosis and proliferation are stimulated by *H. pylori* infection (Brenes *et al.*, 1993; Mannick *et al.*, 1996). Another unexpected finding has been that the infection increases the rate of apoptosis at the level of the gland necks, not so much

at the surface, where apoptotic cells are normally shed and are not needed to replace other cells.

The intricacies of the alterations in cell cycle regulation brought about by *H. pylori* infection have not been well clarified. A balance between apoptosis and proliferation stimuli is supposedly needed to maintain the integrity of the normal gastric mucosal architecture. Some reports indicated that the stimulus to proliferate was greater than the apoptosis stimulus in *CagA*-positive strains, tilting the balance towards an eventual proneoplastic chain of events (Peek *et al.*, 1999). Such differential signalling was not replicated in other studies of infection by *CagA*-positive strains (Moss *et al.*, 2001). Although the discrepancies are not well understood, it could be speculated that host factors are involved: the first study was

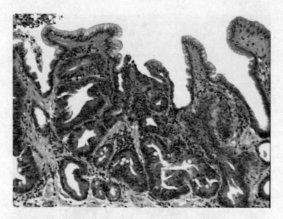

Figure 9. High grade dysplasia. Dysplastic glands with irregular lumens and nuclear atypia.

conducted in southern US whites whereas the second involved mostly immigrant hispanics. It may be that other genotypic markers of bacterial virulence, as well as CagA, may play a role.

Loss of differentiation

The more prominent cellular changes in the advanced stages of the precancerous process are mostly genetic nuclear abnormalities. They fit the 'molecular' model of carcinogenesis better. Morphologically progressive nuclear and architectural abnormalities take place, collectively known as 'dysplasia'. There have been some semantic difficulties in classifying them on histopathological grounds. Recently, an international classification was proposed, the Padova classification (Rugge *et al.*, 2000). It sets clear criteria to classify lesions as low grade or high grade, and includes a category of 'indefinite for dysplasia'. High-grade dysplasia is equivalent to carcinoma *in situ* with malignant nuclear characteristics but no clear stromal invasion.

Although multiple molecular alterations have been reported, no clear or constant model of progression has been identified. In the well-differentiated or 'intestinal' type of gastric carcinoma, K-*ras* and *p53* mutations are frequent. In the poorly differentiated or 'diffuse' type of gastric carcinoma, multifocal atrophy and metaplasia are not prominent. In such cases, individual neoplastic cells invade the stroma. Lack of cohesion between cells characterizes such tumours and has been linked to a defect in adhesion molecules, especially the calcium-dependent adhesion molecules (cadherins) (Becker *et al.*, 1994). They are either absent or malfunctioning in tumour cells, allowing the cells to migrate and invade freely. Molecular events are discussed in a separate chapter of this publication (Tahara, this volume).

Neoplastic and non-neoplastic outcomes

Gastroenterologists have reported historically that patients with peptic ulcer of the stomach are at increased risk of gastric carcinoma, whereas patients with peptic ulcer of the duodenum do not display such an increased risk. Two recent epidemiological studies have documented such differential risks. Hansson *et al.* (1996) linked hospital admission records and cancer registry data in Sweden. Patients with a past history of gastric ulcer had a significantly increased relative risk of developing gastric cancer (odds ratio, 1.8; confidence interval [CI], 1.6–2.0). Patients with duodenal ulcer had a decreased relative risk (odds ratio, 0.5; CI, 0.4–0.7) when compared with the general population. As discussed above, gastric ulcers are part of the MAG complex whereas duodenal ulcers are seen in patients with non-atrophic antral gastritis, both resulting from *H. pylori* infection. These results compare the outcome in ulcer patients with the general experience of Swedish cohorts, which at the time had high risks of gastric cancer. Another study recently published by Uemura *et al.* (2001) followed patients with *Helicobacter* infection in Japan for several years. In patients with MAG, *H. pylori* infection increased gastric cancer risk. In patients with duodenal ulcer and non-atrophic gastritis, *H. pylori* infection did not increase the gastric cancer risk.

It is therefore well documented that the same bacterial species (*H. pylori*) may induce a type of chronic inflammation (non-atrophic antral gastritis) that does not enter into a chain of events that leads to carcinogenesis. On the other hand, the same bacterial species induces a chronic inflammation (MAG) which is part of a precancerous process. Such a scenario represents a challenge and an opportunity to the scientific community. Scrutiny of the inflammatory response to the infection should identify forces that promote carcinogenesis as well as forces that inhibit it. The model of gastric carcinogenesis induced by *H. pylori* infection is a paradigm whose exploration may throw light into the causation as well as the prevention of human cancer.

Susceptibility to gastric cancer

It has long been recognized that gastric cancer may cluster in families and that some individuals develop the disease at a rather early age. The search for susceptibility markers has led to several possible candidates:

• Some HLA subtypes have been found more frequently in cancer patients (Magnusson *et al.*, 2001).
• Certain cytokines, linked to inflammatory response, are polymorphic. Interleukin (IL)-1β subtypes linked with decreased acid secretion in the gastric mucosa increase the risk of gastric cancer (El Omar, 2000). Other cytokines may have the same association.
• Molecular alterations of the E-cadherin gene are associated with susceptibility to diffuse adenocarcinoma (Tahara, this volume).
• Mucus secretion protects the epithelial cells from luminal toxins and irritants. MUC-1 is polymorphic. Subtypes with shorter components are markers of atrophy, suggesting that they afford less protection than larger phenotypes (Reis *et al.*, 1999).

It is possible that several traits may coincide in the same individual and may also coincide with infection by *H. pylori* strains with greater neoplastic potential (Hannig *et al.*, 2001). Such combinations of susceptibility genotypes in the host and in the causative agent may result in exponential increases in cancer risk.

Oxidative damage

Although the mechanisms by which *H. pylori* infection increases cancer risk are unknown, very suggestive evidence points to oxidative damage as a central player in gastric carcinogenesis. It has been well documented that *H. pylori* infection results in the expression of inducible nitric oxide synthase (iNOS) in inflammatory cells and in the epithelial cells (Figure 10) (Mannick *et al.*, 1996;

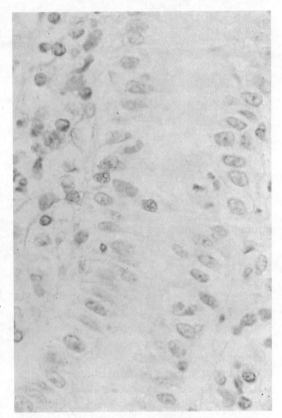

Figure 10. Gastric foveola stained for inducible nitric oxide synthase. Positively stained polymorphonuclear leukocytes are seen among epithelial cells and in the lumen.

Pignatelli *et al.*, 1998). Complex chemical reactions take place, which may result in the synthesis of several oxidative and mutagenic species such as peroxinitrate (ONOOH). They may interact with epithelial cells that are actively synthesizing DNA and replicating (Figure 11). In such circumstances, mutations may be induced and immortalized in the gastric epithelium (Correa & Miller, 1998).

Simultaneously with oxidative forces, antioxidant forces are expressed in the inflammatory cells after *H. pylori* infection. The most prominent antioxidant enzymes are: superoxide dismutase, catalase and glutathione peroxidase. Theoretically, these enzymes protect the DNA of replicating cells against mutagenic forces. Antioxidant

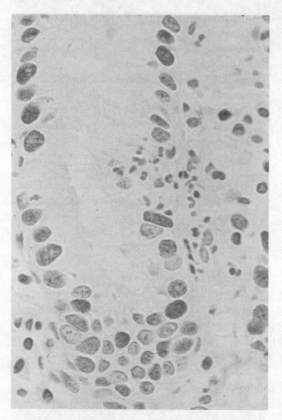

Figure 11. Gastric foveola stained for proliferating nuclear antigen indicating DNA synthesis. Positive cells are seen among epithelial cells migrating to the lumen.

micronutrients ingested with the diet find their way to the gastric mucosa. One of the most consistent findings in epidemiological studies of gastric cancer is the protective role played by fresh fruit and vegetables, rich in antioxidants such as ascorbic acid, carotenoids, tocopherols and folic acid. The mechanisms of protection at the tissue level are unknown but it is suspected that they protect nuclear DNA, mitochondria and lipid membranes against oxidative damage.

Epilogue

The complexity of gastric carcinogenesis induced by *H. pylori* infection is illustrated in Figure 12, which presents a diagrammatic outline of the events related to *H. pylori* infection in the gastric mucosa (adapted from Correa & Miller, 1998).

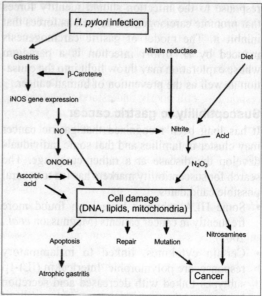

Figure 12. Diagrammatic representation of hypothetical events in the formation of oxidant species in the gastric microenvironment.

Factors related to the agent are only partially understood. The first marker of virulence identified with carcinogenic potential was the *Cag*A gene, as a marker of the pathogenicity island (Blaser *et al.*, 1995a; Covacci *et al.*, 1999). By itself, this marker is insufficient to explain carcinogenicity. Strains linked to gastric cancer are predominantly *Cag*A-positive, but so are those associated with duodenal ulcer, which is not implicated in carcinogenesis. The *Cag*A-positive strains have a type IV secretory apparatus shaped like a syringe which has been shown to inject CagA protein into the cytoplasm of the epithelial cells (Covacci *et al.*, 1999). This event is most probably a strong signal to initiate the inflammatory response. It stimulates the epithelial cell to secrete IL-8, with strong chemotactic attraction of neutrophils.

Genes associated with the vacuolating toxin VacA are polymorphic, especially in the signal (s) domain and the mid-portion (m) of the gene (Nogueira *et al.*, 2001). Strains with s_1m_1 genotype are more virulent and may have more carcinogenic potential than other strains such as s_2m_2. New research on the polymorphisms of

H. pylori genotypes may contribute to our understanding of the carcinogenic role of some strains.

Host factors related to susceptibility to carcinogenesis, i.e. HLA, cytokines and mucin markers, may play an important role in the process. The immunological modulation of the inflammatory response — still poorly understood — determines whether the outcome of the infection may or may not lead to neoplasia. The epithelial cell is the target of the inflammatory injury in neoplastic events. The mechanisms involved are not yet well understood, but some preliminary work points to cytoskeletal signalling pathways altered by *Helicobacter* infection.

External influences are also major determinants of the carcinogenic outcome of *H. pylori* infection. It has been reported that early infection in childhood increases cancer risk (Blaser *et al.*, 1995b). The circumstances of childhood infections are very poorly understood. The mode of transmission is mostly intrafamilial, especially from child to child, but the mode of transmission is unknown (Goodman & Correa, 2000). The immediate consequences of infection are also unknown. Some evidence points to iron-deficiency anaemia and decreased growth related to the infection. The histopathology of gastritis in children of high-risk populations is not well documented. It has been reported that children acquire and then lose the infection before developing persistent infection. It is speculated that this phenomenon reflects matching between bacterial genotypes and host genotypes.

The prevalence of infection in populations does not correlate with gastric cancer rates. Populations in Africa have a high prevalence of infection but a low incidence of gastric cancer (Holcombe, 1992). This so-called 'African enigma' is also found in people of Hindu extraction and people living in the coasts and valleys of Latin America.

The *Helicobacter*–gastric cancer model is a microcosmos in which carcinogenic and anticarcinogenic forces clash for decades before a neoplastic outcome becomes evident or is avoided.

Acknowledgements

Work supported by grant PO1-CA 28842 from the National Cancer Institute, and grant HEF (2000-05)-O3 from the Board of Regents of the State of Louisiana.

References

Becker, K.F., Atkinson, M.J., Reich, U., Becker, I., Nekarda, H., Siewert, J.R. & Hofler, H. (1994) E-Cadherin gene mutations provide clues to diffuse type of gastric carcinomas. *Cancer Res.*, **54**, 3845–3852

Blaser, M.J., Perez-Perez, G.I., Kleanthous, H., Cover, T.L., Peek, R.M., Chyou, P.H., Stemmerman, G.N. & Nomura, A. (1995a) Infection with *Helicobacter pylori* strains possessing cagA is associated with an increased risk of developing adenocarcinoma of the stomach. *Cancer Res.*, **55**, 2111–2115

Blaser, M.J., Chyou, P.H. & Nomura, A. (1995b) Age at establishment of *Helicobacter pylori* infection and gastric carcinoma, gastric ulcer and duodenal ulcer risk. *Cancer Res.*, **55**, 562–565

Brenes, F., Ruiz, B., Correa, P., Hunter, F., Rhamakrishnan, T., Fontham, E. & Shi, T.Y. (1993) *Helicobacter pylori* causes hyperproliferation of the gastric epithelium: pre- and post-eradication indices of proliferating cell nuclear antigen. *Am. J. Gastroenterol.*, **88**, 1870–1875

Correa, P. (1992) Human gastric carcinogenesis: a multistep and multifactorial process. *Cancer Res.*, **52**, 6735–6740

Correa, P. (1995) *Helicobacter pylori* and gastric carcinogenesis. *Am. J. Surg. Pathol.*, **19** (Suppl. 1), S37–S43

Correa, P. (1997) *Helicobacter pylori* and the cell cycle. *J. natl Cancer Inst.*, **89**, 836–837

Correa, P. & Miller, M.J.S. (1998) Carcinogenesis, apoptosis and cell proliferation. *Br. med. Bull.*, **54**, 151–162

Correa, P., Haenszel, W., Cuello, C., Tannenbaum, S. & Archer, M. (1975) A model for gastric cancer epidemiology. *Lancet*, **ii**, 58–60

Covacci, A., Telford, J.L., Del Giudice, G., Parsonnet, J. & Rappuoli, R. (1999) *Helicobacter pylori* virulence and genetic geography. *Science*, **284**, 1328–1333

Dixon, M.F., Genta, R.M., Yardley, J.H. & Correa, P. (1996) Classification and grading of gastritis. The updated Sydney System. International Workshop on the Histopathology of Gastritis, Houston. *Am. J. Surg. Pathol.*, **20**, 1161–1181

El Omar, E.M., Carrington, M., Chou, W.H., McColl, K.E., Bream, J.H., Young, H.A., Herrera, J., Lissowska, J., Yuan, C.C., Rothman, N., Lanyon, G., Martin, M., Fraumeni, J.R., Jr & Rabkin, C.S. (2000) Interleukin 1 polymorphisms associated with increased risk of gastric cancer. *Nature*, **404**, 398–402

Goodman, K.J. & Correa P. (2000) Transmission of *Helicobacter pylori* among siblings. *Lancet*, **355**, 358–362

Hannig, E.E., Butruk, E. & Ostrowski, J. (2001) RACK1 protein interacts with *Helicobacter pylori* VacA cytotoxin: the yeast two-hybrid approach. *Biochem. biophys. Res. Commun.*, **289**, 103–110

Hansson, L.E., Nyren, O., Hsing, A.W., Bergstrom, R., Josefsson, S., Chow, W.H., Fraumeni, J.F., Jr & Adami, H.O. (1996) The risk of stomach cancer in patients with gastric and duodenal ulcer disease. *New Engl. J. Med.*, **335**, 242–249

Holcombe, C. (1992) *Helicobacter pylori*: the African enigma. *Gut*, **33**, 429–431

IARC (1994) *IARC Monographs on the Evaluation of Carcinogenic Risks to Humans*, Vol. 61, *Schistosomes, Liver Flukes and* Helicobacter pylori, Lyon, IARC*Press*

Magnusson, P.K.E., Enroth, H., Eriksson, I., Held, M., Nyren, O., Engstrand, L., Hansson, L.E. & Gyllensten, U.B. (2001) Gastric cancer and human leukocyte antigen: distinct DQ and DR alleles are associated with development of gastric cancer and infection by *Helicobacter pylori*. *Cancer Res.*, **61**, 2684–2689

Mannick, E.E., Bravo L.E., Zarama, G, Realpe J.L., Zhang X.J., Ruiz B., Fontham, E.T., Mera, R., Miller M.J.S. & Correa, P. (1996) Inducible nitric oxide synthase, nitrotyrosine, and apoptosis in *Helicobacter pylori* gastritis: effect of antibiotics and antioxidants. *Cancer Res.*, **56**, 3238–3243

Moss, S.F., Sordillo, E.M., Abdalla, A.M., Makarov,V., Hanzely, Z., Perez-Perez, G.I., Blaser, M.J. & Holt, P.R. (2001) Increased gastric epithelial cell apoptosis with colonization with Cag A+ *Helicobacter pylori* strains. *Cancer Res.*, **61**, 1406–1411

Nogueira, C., Figueiredo, C., Carneiro, F., Gomes, A.J., Barreira, R., Figueira, P., Salgado, C., Belo, L., Peixoto, A., Bravo, J.C., Bravo, L.E., Realpe, J.L., Plaisier, A.P., Quint, W.G., Ruiz, B., Correa, P. &

van Doom, L.-J. (2001) *Helicobacter pylori* genotypes may determine gastric histopathology. *Am. J. Pathol.*, **158**, 647–654

Peek, R.M., Jr, Blaser, M.J., Mays, D.J., Forsyth, M.H., Cover, T.L., Song, S.Y., Krishna, U. & Pietenpol, J.A. (1999) *Helicobacter pylori* strain specific genotypes and modulations of gastric epithelial cell cycle. *Cancer Res.*, **59**, 6124–6131

Pignatelli, B., Bancel, B., Esteve, J., Malaveille, C., Calmels, S., Correa, P., Patricot, L.M., Laval, M., Lyandrat, N. & Ohshima, H. (1998) Inducible nitric oxide synthase, anti-oxidant enzymes and *Helicobacter pylori* infection in gastritis and gastric precancerous lesions in humans. *Eur. J. Cancer Prev.*, **7**, 439–447

Reis, C.A., David, L., Correa, P., Carneiro, F., Bolos, C., Garcia, E., Mandel, U., Clausen, H. & Sobrinho-Simoes, M. (1999) Intestinal metaplasia of human stomach displays distinct patterns of mucin (MUC1, MUC2, MUC5AC, and MUC6) expression. *Cancer Res.*, **49**, 1003–1007

Rugge, M., Correa, P., Dixon, M.F., Hattori, T., Leandro, G., Lewin, K., Riddel, R.H., Sipponen, P. & Watanabe, H. (2000) Gastric dysplasia: the Padova international classification. *Am. J. Surg. Pathol.*, **24**, 167–176

Uemura, N., Okamoto, S., Yamamoto, S., Matsumura, N., Yamaguchi, S., Yamakido, M., Taniyama K., Sasaki, N. & Schlemper, R.J. (2001) *Helicobacter pylori* infection and the development of gastric cancer. *New Engl. J. Med.*, **345**, 784–789

Vogelstein, B., Fearon, E.R., Hamilton, S.R., Kern, S.E., Preisinger, A.C., Leppert, M., Nakamura, Y., White, R., Smits, A.M. & Bos, J.L. (1988) Genetic alterations during colorectal-tumor development. *New Engl. J. Med.*, **319**, 525–532

Corresponding author:

Pelayo Correa
Department of Pathology Louisiana
State University Medical Center
1901 Perdido Street
New Orleans, LA 70012, USA
correa@lsuhsc.edu

Mechanisms of Carcinogenesis: Contributions of Molecular Epidemiology
Patricia Buffler, Jerry Rice, Robert Baan, Michael Bird and Paolo Boffetta, eds
IARC Scientific Publications No. 157
International Agency for Research on Cancer, Lyon, 2004

Epidemiology of Gastric Cancer

Martyn Plummer, Silvia Franceschi and Nubia Muñoz

Summary
The most recent estimates of global cancer incidence indicate that in 1990 stomach cancer was
the second most frequent cancer in the world
(after lung cancer), with about 800 000 new cases
diagnosed every year (Parkin *et al.*, 1999). Steady
declines in incidence rates of gastric cancer have
been observed worldwide in the last few decades.
The exact causes of the decline are not well
understood, but may include improvements in
diet and food storage and a decline in the prevalence of *Helicobacter pylori* infection. Dietary
modifications remain potentially one of the most
important tools for the prevention of gastric
cancer. Control of *H. pylori* infection, by indirect
means such as improving the general sanitary
conditions or by direct intervention such as eradication or immunization, is also likely to offer
great potential for prevention.

Introduction
According to the most recent available estimates,
gastric cancer is the second most common cancer
worldwide, following lung cancer (Parkin *et al.*,
1999). Survival from gastric cancer is poor. In the
USA, the 5-year survival rate is less than 20% and
has improved little in the last few decades (Kosary
et al., 1995). The poor survival from gastric cancer
is reflected in the high mortality : incidence ratio,
which is 70–90% in most countries.

In this review, the geographical distribution
and time trends of gastric cancer are examined.
With respect to the etiology of gastric cancer,
priority is given here to the findings concerning
the gastric bacterium *Helicobacter pylori*. The
possibilities for primary prevention of gastric
cancer are also discussed.

Two subclassifications of gastric carcinoma
have been proposed with possible implications for
etiology. The histological classification of Jarvi

and Laurén divides cancers into 'intestinal' and
'diffuse' types. These are discussed by Tahara
(this volume). Gastric cancers may also be classified by subsite within the stomach: the most
important distinction being between cardia (the
proximal part of the stomach) and non-cardia.
These two subclassifications will be mentioned
where appropriate.

Descriptive epidemiology
Geographical variation
Gastric cancer incidence shows a 15–20-fold
variation in risk between the highest and the
lowest-risk populations. Figure 1 shows a map of
the incidence of gastric cancer in men, standardized to the world population (Globocan, 2000;
Ferlay *et al.*, 2001). Incidence rates in women
follow a similar pattern, but are about 50% lower.
The high-risk areas are in Japan, China, eastern
Europe, Portugal and certain countries in Latin
America. Low-risk populations are seen among
whites in North America, India, the Philippines,
most countries in Africa, some western European
countries and Australia. Substantial variations in
the incidence of gastric cancer may also be found
within countries, a good example being Italy
where, for instance, male incidence rates range
from 36.3/100 000 in Florence to 13.2/100 000 in
Ragusa (Parkin *et al.*, 1997).

Time trends
Gastric cancer incidence and mortality rates have
been declining worldwide for several decades
(Coleman *et al.*, 1993). The precise reasons for
this decline are unknown, and it has consequently
been described as an 'unplanned triumph'
(Howson *et al.*, 1986). Figure 2 shows gastric
cancer mortality rates for a selection of countries
between 1960 and 1998, using data from the WHO
mortality database. The rates are plotted on a log

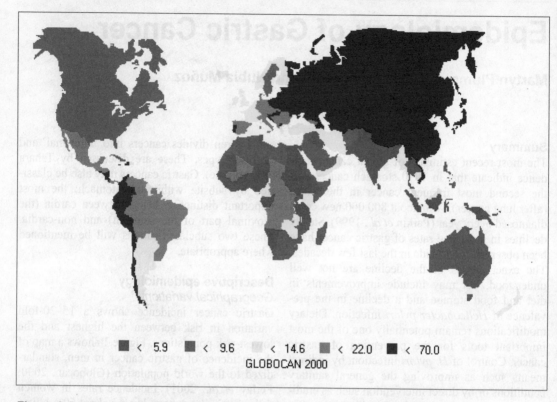

Figure 1. Incidence of stomach cancer in men. Age-standardized rate (world population). From Ferlay *et al.* (2001)

scale to show that the rate of decline is very similar (about 3%) for both high- and low-risk countries.

For gastric cardia cancer specifically, the incidence rates show a strong increase in some industrialized countries (Devesa *et al.*, 1998). This may be partly due to changes in diagnostic criteria (Ekström *et al.*, 1999) but, in the USA at least, it appears to be a genuine increase (Devesa & Fraumeni, 1999). The distinct time trend shown by cardia cancer might indicate that it has a different etiology. There has been a concomitant rise in the incidence of adenocarcinoma of the esophagus, which suggests that it shares some risk factors with carcinoma of the gastric cardia, namely obesity, gastric reflux and subsequent Barrett esophagus.

Migrant studies
Many studies have shown that migrants from high-risk to low-risk countries maintain the high gastric cancer risk of their country of origin. This has been

observed for migrants from Japan to Hawaii (Haenszel & Kurihara, 1968), from Iceland to Canada (Choi *et al.*, 1971), from various countries to Israel (Muñoz & Steinitz, 1971) and from Europe to Australia (McMichael *et al.*, 1980). Correa *et al.* (1970) observed the same pattern in migrants from different regions of Colombia to the capital, Cali. Together, these migrant studies strongly suggest that exposures early in life are important in determining gastric cancer risk.

Risk factors for gastric cancer
The focus of this review is on *H. pylori*, but in this section we briefly review other risk factors, referring to more detailed review articles when appropriate.

Diet
A panel of experts reviewed the available laboratory and epidemiological evidence on diet and

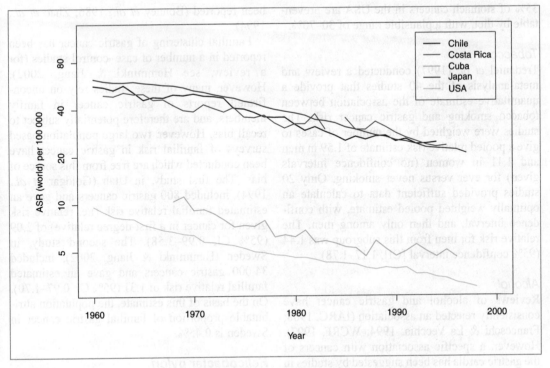

Figure 2. Mortality from gastric cancer, 1960–98. ASR, age-standardized rate

gastric cancer as part of a general review of nutrition and cancer (WCRF, 1997). The panel divided levels of evidence into 'convincing', 'probable', 'possible' and 'inadequate'. The hypotheses that they considered convincing or probable were as follows:

• There was convincing evidence that a diet high in vegetables and fruit decreases risk. The most likely anticarcinogenic compounds contained in vegetables and fruits are antioxidant vitamins (e.g. vitamin C, β-carotene and vitamin E).

• Evidence that vitamin C reduces risk was considered probable.

• Evidence that a diet high in salt intake increases risk was considered probable.

• There was convincing evidence that use of refrigeration to preserve food decreases risk. This effect may be mediated either through an increased intake of fresh fruit and vegetables or a decreased reliance on salted food.

• Other dietary effects that were classified as 'possible' were a protective effect of wholegrain cereals, allium compounds and green tea and an increased risk from consumption of starch and grilled or barbecued meat and fish. The panel concluded that there was insufficient evidence to evaluate the possible protective effects of fibre, selenium and garlic and the possible increased risk from cured meats and N-nitroso compounds.

The conclusions of the WCRF (1997) expert committee are not quantitative. They give only the strength of the evidence without reference to the size of the effect. Estimating the proportion of any cancer attributable to diet is extremely difficult. A summary of the causes of cancer in the USA by Doll and Peto (1981) estimated that 90% of stomach and large-bowel cancers may be preventable by dietary change, although they emphasized that this figure is a 'guesstimate'. In a follow-up exercise, Willett (1995) estimated that

35% of stomach cancers in the USA are preventable by diet, with a plausible range of 30–70%.

Tobacco

Trédaniel *et al.* (1997) conducted a review and meta-analysis of the 40 studies that provide a quantitative estimate of the association between tobacco smoking and gastric cancer risk. The studies were weighted by the number of cases to give a pooled relative risk estimate of 1.59 in men and 1.11 in women (no confidence intervals given) for ever versus never smoking. Only 20 studies provided sufficient data to calculate an optimally weighted pooled estimate, with confidence interval, and then only among men. The relative risk for men from this subgroup was 1.44 (95% confidence interval [CI], 1.17–1.78).

Alcohol

Reviews of alcohol and gastric cancer have consistently rejected an association (IARC, 1988; Franceschi & La Vecchia, 1994; WCRF, 1997). However, a specific association with cancers of the gastric cardia has been suggested by studies in the USA (Wu-Williams *et al.*, 1990), Italy (Palli *et al.*, 1992) and Spain (González *et al.*, 1994).

Socio-economic status

A strong association with socioeconomic status has been frequently observed, with individuals of lower status having higher risk. Socioeconomic status is, of course, not a causal factor, but is a surrogate for many other factors including sanitary conditions and nutrition.

Genetic susceptibility

The descriptive epidemiology of gastric cancer strongly indicates that the risk is dominated by environmental causes. There may, however, still be a role for genetic factors. Individuals with blood group A have been known for decades to have an approximately 20% excess risk of gastric cancer compared with those with other blood groups (Langman, 1988). Germline mutations in a gene encoding the cell adhesion protein E-cadherin (CDH1) have been found in familial diffuse gastric cancer (Guilford *et al.*, 1998). A genetic predisposition to precancerous lesions has also

been reported (Bonney *et al.*, 1986; Zhao *et al.*, 1994).

Familial clustering of gastric cancer has been reported in a number of case–control studies (for a review, see Hemminki & Jiang, 2002). However, many of these studies rely on unconfirmed reports of gastric cancer in family members, and are therefore potentially subject to recall bias. However, two large population-based surveys of familial risk in gastric cancer have been conducted which are free from this source of bias. The first study, in Utah (Goldgar *et al.*, 1994), included 800 gastric cancers and gave an estimated familial relative risk (i.e. relative risk given for cancer in a first-degree relative) of 2.09 (95% CI, 0.99–3.58). The second study, in Sweden (Hemminki & Jiang, 2002), included 34 000 gastric cancers and gave an estimated familial relative risk of 1.31 (95% CI, 0.97–1.70). On the basis of this estimate, the population attributable proportion of familial gastric cancer in Sweden is 0.45%.

Helicobacter pylori

H. pylori is a spiral gram-negative bacterium that colonizes the stomach. It is one of the most common infections in humans, with an estimated prevalence of 50% worldwide and 90% in developing countries. In high-prevalence populations, infection is rapidly acquired in childhood and persists throughout life. Prevalence of *H. pylori* infection is declining in many developed countries, probably because of a decline in the prevalence of infection in successive birth cohorts.

Substantial evidence indicates that *H. pylori* is the main cause of chronic gastritis and peptic ulcer. The final proof of causation for these diseases has been derived from experiments in humans showing that ingestion of *H. pylori* causes acute gastritis (Marshall *et al.*, 1985) and from controlled intervention trials showing that eradication of *H. pylori* has consistently led to resolution of the gastritis and of the peptic ulcer (Valle *et al.*, 1991).

In 1994, an expert working group convened by IARC classified *H. pylori* as carcinogenic to humans (IARC, 1994). This classification was made entirely on the basis of epidemiological evidence. At the time, the evidence from animal studies was considered inadequate. Since then, the Mongolian gerbil has been established as an animal model in which infection with *H. pylori* alone causes gastric cancer (for a review, see Fujioka *et al.*, 2000). Further epidemiological studies have also been conducted which clarify the relationship between *H. pylori* and gastric cancer in humans.

Epidemiological studies can be divided into three categories: ecological studies, retrospective studies and prospective studies. We consider each of these in turn.

Ecological studies

The limitations of ecological studies are well known. Nevertheless, large variations in gastric cancer risk between different populations have prompted a number of epidemiological studies using aggregate data. All but two of these studies have included 2–8 areas (Correa *et al.*, 1990; Sierra *et al.*, 1992; Fukao *et al.*, 1993; Palli *et al.*, 1993; Tsugane *et al.*, 1993; Lin *et al.*, 1995a; Chen *et al.*, 1997; Perez-Perez *et al.*, 1997) or ethnic groups (Fraser *et al.*, 1996; Fock *et al.*, 1997). With only a small number of groups for comparison, these studies are highly susceptible to problems of confounding. Not surprisingly, they have produced equivocal results. Five of the above studies found a significant association between *H. pylori* and gastric cancer and five did not.

Two large ecological studies have been conducted on *H. pylori* and gastric cancer. One study of 46 counties in rural China found a correlation of 0.4 between gastric cancer mortality and *H. pylori* prevalence. No significant correlation was observed between *H. pylori* and any other cancer (Forman *et al.*, 1990). A follow-up analysis showed that this association was not statistically significant ($p > 0.10$) when serum levels of selected micronutrients were controlled for (Kneller *et al.*, 1992). The EUROGAST study group examined 17 populations in 13 countries (EUROGAST Study Group, 1993). They found significant correlation between *H. pylori* seropositivity and both cancer incidence ($p = 0.0002$) and mortality ($p = 0.0002$), concluding that a

population with 100% prevalence of *H. pylori* would have a sixfold increase in gastric cancer risk compared with a population free of *H. pylori*.

The 'African enigma'

Discussion of the causal role of *H. pylori* has been dominated by the so-called 'African enigma' – the observation by Holcombe (1992) that some populations in Africa have high prevalence of *H. pylori* but low prevalence of diseases associated with *H. pylori* infection, including gastric cancer. Similar observations are often made about India. The term 'African enigma' is unfortunate because it suggests that the African continent is homogeneous. However, data from selected cancer registries in Africa show a fourfold variation in cancer risk. There is also a twofold variation in cancer risk in India (Parkin *et al.*, 1997).

The existence of populations with high *H. pylori* prevalence but low gastric cancer incidence does not rule out *H. pylori* as a causal factor. Gastric cancer is a multifactorial disease, and the presence or absence of other risk factors may influence the importance of *H. pylori*. One hypothesis that has recently been advanced is that progression of *Helicobacter*-induced gastritis and gastric atrophy may be mediated by concurrent parasitic infection (Fox *et al.*, 2000). This hypothesis, derived from an animal model, has generated considerable interest (Feldmeier & Krantz, 2000; Gordon, 2000; MacDonald, 2001). There is currently little evidence from human studies, although one early report (Mitchell *et al.*, 2000) supports the hypothesis.

Wabinga (2003) provides a comprehensive review of gastric cancer in Africa, concluding that the burden and heterogeneity of gastric cancer in Africa is difficult to assess because its diagnosis requires access to endoscopic facilities that are not always available. This observation suggests that one should be cautious before making generalizations about gastric cancer in Africa.

Retrospective studies

Retrospective studies of *H. pylori* and gastric cancer are summarized in Figure 3. There is considerable heterogeneity between studies, which makes the results difficult to interpret.

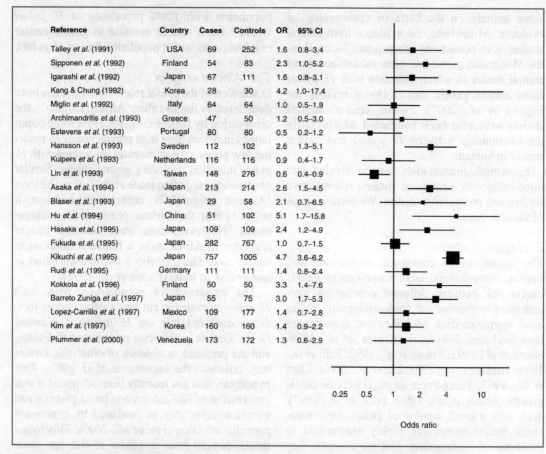

Reference	Country	Cases	Controls	OR	95% CI
Talley *et al.* (1991)	USA	69	252	1.6	0.8–3.4
Sipponen *et al.* (1992)	Finland	54	83	2.3	1.0–5.2
Igarashi *et al.* (1992)	Japan	67	111	1.6	0.8–3.1
Kang & Chung (1992)	Korea	28	30	4.2	1.0–17.4
Miglio *et al.* (1992)	Italy	64	64	1.0	0.5–1.9
Archimandritis *et al.* (1993)	Greece	47	50	1.2	0.5–3.0
Estevens *et al.* (1993)	Portugal	80	80	0.5	0.2–1.2
Hansson *et al.* (1993)	Sweden	112	102	2.6	1.3–5.1
Kuipers *et al.* (1993)	Netherlands	116	116	0.9	0.4–1.7
Lin *et al.* (1993)	Taiwan	148	276	0.6	0.4–0.9
Asaka *et al.* (1994)	Japan	213	214	2.6	1.5–4.5
Blaser *et al.* (1993)	Japan	29	58	2.1	0.7–6.5
Hu *et al.* (1994)	China	51	102	5.1	1.7–15.8
Hasaka *et al.* (1995)	Japan	109	109	2.4	1.2–4.9
Fukuda *et al.* (1995)	Japan	282	767	1.0	0.7–1.5
Kikuchi *et al.* (1995)	Japan	757	1005	4.7	3.6–6.2
Rudi *et al.* (1995)	Germany	111	111	1.4	0.8–2.4
Kokkola *et al.* (1996)	Finland	50	50	3.3	1.4–7.6
Barreto Zuniga *et al.* (1997)	Japan	55	75	3.0	1.7–5.3
Lopez-Carrillo *et al.* (1997)	Mexico	109	177	1.4	0.7–2.8
Kim *et al.* (1997)	Korea	160	160	1.4	0.9–2.2
Plummer *et al.* (2000)	Venezuela	173	172	1.3	0.6–2.9

Odds ratio

Figure 3. Case–control studies of gastric cancer. OR, odds ratio; CI, confidence interval

Various hypotheses have been put forward to explain the diverse results.

Huang *et al.* (1998) conducted a formal meta-analysis of 14 of these studies, along with five cohort studies (other studies listed here did not meet their inclusion criteria). Their summary odds ratio for gastric cancer in *H. pylori* infected subjects was 1.92 (95% CI, 1.32–2.78). They also examined sources of heterogeneity between studies, concluding that differences in the selection of controls, age of the subjects, and the site and stage of gastric cancer were responsible for the heterogeneity.

Differences in *H. pylori* genotype between different populations may also explain the differing results. *H. pylori* may be classified into two types based on the presence (type I) or absence (type II) of a 40-kbp pathogenicity island (Censini *et al.*, 1996). Since only type I strains have the gene for CagA (cytotoxin-associated antigen A), antibodies to CagA can be used as a marker of infection with type I strains. Among *H. pylori*-infected individuals, the presence of antibodies to *CagA*-positive strains has been associated with an increased risk of atrophic gastritis (Kuipers *et al.*, 1995) and gastric cancer (Blaser *et al.*, 1995; Ekström *et al.*, 2001).

Another possible source of heterogeneity is error in the assay used to diagnose *H. pylori* infection. On the basis of a comparative study in Thailand, Bodhidatta *et al.* (1994) suggested that the sensitivity of an ELISA may be improved by using antigens derived from local strains of *H. pylori* instead of strains from industrialized countries. However, this finding was not reproduced in a study in China, which showed equally high sensitivity for ELISAs based on a pool of Chinese strains and a pool of US strains (Groves *et al.*, 1997). A study in Venezuela compared four different ELISAs, including one based on local strains (Plummer *et al.*, 2000). This study found good agreement between the different assays when the results were expressed in terms of antibody titres (Spearman correlation coefficient, 0.7–0.8). The main reason for disagreement between assays was the choice of cut-off point for determining positivity.

This observation raises the more general issue of whether classifying subjects as 'positive' and 'negative' is the best approach in epidemiological studies. An alternative approach is to look at antibody levels. This approach has been successfully used to correlate Epstein–Barr virus with Hodgkin disease (IARC, 1997) and Burkitt lymphoma (Geser *et al.*, 1982) in populations with a high prevalence of the virus.

A major methodological problem with retrospective studies of *H. pylori* is that the disease itself may alter the measurement of exposure. In particular, extensive atrophy, which is a precursor of gastric cancer, may lead to a reduced burden of infection in the stomach and consequently lower antibody levels (for a review, see Plummer *et al.*, 2000). Measurements of *H. pylori* antibodies taken at the time of cancer incidence, or even a few years previously, may not therefore be a valid measure of the original exposure to *H. pylori*. Further progress using retrospective studies requires a marker of past infection to *H. pylori*. Ekström *et al.* (2001) suggest that one such marker may be antibodies to CagA. In a population-based case–control study, they found that anti-CagA antibodies detected by immunoblot were more strongly correlated with gastric cancer risk than antibodies to *H. pylori* detected by ELISA. They attribute this difference to the greater persistence of anti-CagA antibodies after disappearance of *H. pylori* (Sorberg *et al.*, 1997), rather than increased carcinogenicity of CagA-positive strains.

Prospective studies

Twelve cohort studies on *H. pylori* and gastric cancer have been published (Forman *et al.*, 1991; Nomura *et al.*, 1991; Parsonnet *et al.*, 1991; Lin *et al.*, 1993, 1995b; Aromaa *et al.*, 1996; Webb *et al.*, 1996; Simán *et al.*, 1997; Watanabe *et al.*, 1997; Hansen *et al.*, 1999; Yamagata *et al.*, 2000; Limburg *et al.*, 2001; Uemura *et al.*, 2001). All but two of these were analysed using a nested case–control design, and the results are summarized in Figure 4. In these studies, *H. pylori* antibody levels were measured in sera collected years before the cancer diagnosis. This reduces (and for long periods of follow-up eliminates) any effect of the carcinogenic process on *H. pylori* load in the gastric mucosa and, thus, serum antibody levels. All of the studies show an increased risk of gastric cancer for *H. pylori* infection, except for one Japanese study, where there was no association for women (Yamagata *et al.*, 2000).

A combined analysis of 10 of these studies and two additional unpublished studies has been undertaken using the original data (Helicobacter and Cancer Collaborative Group, 2001). The combined results give an odds ratio of 3.0 (95% CI, 2.3–3.8) for non-cardia cancers which was increased (odds ratio, 5.9; 95% CI, 3.4–10.3) when the blood sample for *H. pylori* serology was collected more than 10 years before diagnosis. *H. pylori* was not associated with an increased risk of cancer of the gastric cardia (odds ratio, 1.0; 95% CI, 0.7–1.4). Seven of the 12 studies in the meta-analysis included data on histological type. Among these, the association with *H. pylori* did not differ by histological type ($p = 0.5$).

This combined analysis represents the strongest epidemiological evidence for the association between *H. pylori* and gastric cancer. This evidence is imperfect, however, since only three of these studies controlled for potential confounders. Hansen *et al.* (1999) controlled for smoking and various indicators of socioeconomic status. Webb *et al.* (1996) controlled for education, smoking, alcohol consumption and some dietary components selected from a food frequency questionnaire (fresh fruit and vegetables, salted vegetables and cured meats). Aromaa *et al.* (1996) controlled for occupation, smoking and some serum micronutrient levels

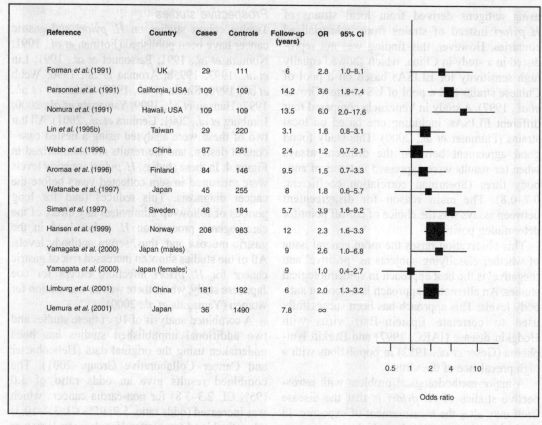

Reference	Country	Cases	Controls	Follow-up (years)	OR	95% CI
Forman et al. (1991)	UK	29	111	6	2.8	1.0–8.1
Parsonnet et al. (1991)	California, USA	109	109	14.2	3.6	1.8–7.4
Nomura et al. (1991)	Hawaii, USA	109	109	13.5	6.0	2.0–17.6
Lin et al. (1995b)	Taiwan	29	220	3.1	1.6	0.8–3.1
Webb et al. (1996)	China	87	261	2.4	1.2	0.7–2.1
Aromaa et al. (1996)	Finland	84	146	9.5	1.5	0.7–3.3
Watanabe et al. (1997)	Japan	45	255	8	1.8	0.6–5.7
Siman et al. (1997)	Sweden	46	184	5.7	3.9	1.6–9.2
Hansen et al. (1999)	Norway	208	983	12	2.3	1.6–3.3
Yamagata et al. (2000)	Japan (males)			9	2.6	1.0–6.8
Yamagata et al. (2000)	Japan (females)			9	1.0	0.4–2.7
Limburg et al. (2001)	China	181	192	6	2.0	1.3–3.2
Uemura et al. (2001)	Japan	36	1490	7.8	∞	

Figure 4. Prospective studies of gastric cancer. OR, odds ratio; CI, confidence interval

(α-tocopherol, β-carotene, retinol and selenium). In each case, the authors concluded that including confounding variables in the model did not alter the relative risk estimates. Nevertheless, it is unlikely that diet has been fully controlled for in these analyses. There are two methodological problems involved in controlling for diet as a confounder. The first is the extreme difficulty of measuring habitual diet accurately. The second is the definition of the exposure window. Aromaa et al. (1996) note that the subjects in their study would have had a traditional agricultural diet during their early years. This would be rather different from their diet at the time of blood collection. The main consequence of all these problems is that it is not possible, with current epidemiological data, to separate the relative contributions of diet and *H. pylori* to gastric cancer risk.

Prevention of gastric cancer

The two major changes that could be made at a population level to reduce gastric cancer incidence are improvement in diet and reduction in the prevalence of *H. pylori*. These changes are already taking place in many populations, and may explain the observed decline in gastric cancer incidence. Active intervention in a population requires proof that the intervention is effective, and this can only come from randomized trials.

Trials of vitamin supplementation

There have been no intervention trials on diet using cancer as an end-point. However, several trials have been conducted using supplementation with selected vitamins as an intervention. Vitamin supplementation can simulate improved diet in a population with low vitamin-intake levels, assuming that the protective micronutrients in a healthy diet have been identified correctly.

An intervention trial was conducted in the general adult population of Linxian, China, an area with a high incidence of cancer of the esophagus and the gastric cardia. Four different interventions were tested:

- retinol and zinc
- riboflavin and niacin
- vitamin C and molybdenum
- β-carotene, vitamin E and selenium.

During the 5.25-year follow-up period a significant reduction in gastric cancer mortality (relative risk, 0.79; 95% CI, 0.64–0.99) was observed in those receiving β-carotene, vitamin E and selenium. Reductions in total mortality and total cancer mortality were also observed in this group (Blot et al., 1993).

Gastric cancer is preceded by a sequence of changes to the gastric mucosa that may be identified histologically (Correa, this volume). Several trials have used changes in precancerous lesions as an end-point. In the Linxian trial, an endoscopic survey was conducted at the end of follow-up to compare the prevalence of gastric dysplasia and cancer between the different treatment groups. No significant differences were observed (Wang et al., 1994). The ATBC study was a trial of α-tocopherol and/or β-carotene in subjects at high risk of lung cancer. The main end-point of the ATBC study was lung cancer mortality, but an endoscopic survey was also conducted at the end of the 5–8-year follow-up period in a subsample. No difference in the prevalence of gastric dysplasia was found between the different treatment groups (Varis et al., 1998). A chemoprevention trial on precancerous lesions of the stomach has been conducted in Colombia (Correa et al., 2000). The trial compared treatment with ascorbic acid, β-carotene and anti-H. pylori treatment in a factorial design. Unlike the trials described above, the Colombian trial was specifically designed to look at precancerous lesions and included a gastroscopy at the beginning and at the end of the 6-year follow-up period. All seven groups receiving treatment showed higher regression of precancerous lesions (19–29% regression) than the control group (7% regression).

Other chemoprevention trials are underway in Venezuela (Muñoz et al., 1996), the Shandong province of China (Gail et al., 1998) and Europe (Biasco & Paganelli, 1999).

Trials of H. pylori eradication

Several treatment regimens have been used to eradicate H. pylori infection, but triple therapy including bismuth salts, amoxicillin and clarithromycin is currently the regimen of choice.

The only randomized trial to examine the effect of H. pylori eradication on precancerous lesions of the stomach is the chemoprevention trial in Colombia (Correa et al., 2000) described above. This showed a protective effect of H. pylori eradication that, like the antioxidant vitamin treatment, increased the rate of regression of precancerous lesions. However, a combination of H. pylori eradication and vitamin supplementation did not show an increased benefit over either intervention given separately. One possible interpretation of this finding is that the antioxidant treatment blocks the effect of H. pylori. However, this requires confirmation from other trials that are currently under way.

Issues with large-scale H. pylori eradication

Moving from the results of randomized trials to population intervention requires consideration of several issues. The first is effectiveness of anti-H. pylori treatment in eradicating H. pylori. Difficulties in eradicating H. pylori have been reported in Venezuela (Buiatti et al., 1994) and Costa Rica (Sierra et al., 1998), two countries with high risk of gastric cancer, although these studies used an H. pylori therapy that may be considered suboptimal. In the Colombian intervention trial, the prevalence of H. pylori infection was reduced from 96% to 26% over 6 years using two courses of anti-H. pylori treatment (Correa et al., 2000). A trial of H. pylori eradication in Iran showed an eradication rate of only 24% from a 1-week course of triple therapy. The rate was higher (36%) when treatment was given for 2 weeks and was higher still (63%) when an H_2-receptor antagonist was administered at the same time (Kaviani et al., 2001). These contrasting results highlight the need to find an effective treatment in the local population before widespread use of anti-*H. pylori* therapy can be considered.

H. pylori eradication using triple therapy may not be effective in the long term if subjects are rapidly reinfected. This possibility has led to an interest in vaccines against *H. pylori* which could offer lasting protection. Vaccines against *H. pylori* are currently under development and will soon be tested in humans. The current status of *H. pylori* vaccine development is reviewed by Alsahli *et al.* (2001).

A theoretical problem with *H. pylori* eradication is the possibility of harmful side-effects. It has been suggested that, on account of its pH-raising action, *H. pylori* is negatively associated with gastric reflux, Barrett esophagus and cancer of the gastric cardia and esophagus, with the implication that eradication of *H. pylori* might increase the risk of these diseases (Blaser, 1998; Chow *et al.*, 1998). This issue clearly has cost–benefit implications for eradication of *H. pylori* by any method.

Conclusions

Geographical distribution and time trends suggest that the risk of gastric cancer is strongly determined by environmental factors. Etiological studies point to infection with *H. pylori* and a poor diet as the main determinants of gastric cancer risk. Despite the long-term decline in incidence of gastric cancer in many populations, there is plenty of scope for active intervention to reduce the risk of gastric cancer, notably by eradication of *H. pylori*.

References

Archimandritis, A., Bitsikas, J., Tjivras, M., Anastasakou, E., Tsavaris, N., Kalogeras, D., Davaris, P. & Fertakis, A. (1993) Non-cardia gastric adenocarcinoma and *Helicobacter pylori* infection. *Ital. J. Gastroenterol.*, **25**, 368–371

Asaka, M., Kimura, T., Kato, M., Kudo, M., Miki, K., Ogoshi, K., Kato, T., Tasuta, M. & Graham, D.Y. (1994) Possible role of *Helicobacter pylori* infection in early gastric cancer development. *Cancer*, **73**, 2691–2694

Asaka, M., Kato, M., Kudo, M., Katagiri, M., Nishikawa, K., Yoshida, J., Takeda, H. & Miki K.

(1995) Relationship between *Helicobacter pylori* infection, atrophic gastritis and gastric carcinoma in a Japanese population. *Eur. J. Gastroenterol. Hepatol.*, **6** (Suppl. 1), S7–S10

Alsahli, M., Farrell, R.J. & Michetti, P. (2001) Vaccines: an ongoing promise? *Dig. Dis.*, **19**, 148–157

Aromaa, A., Kosunen, T.U., Knekt, P., Maatela, J., Teppo, L., Heinonen, O.P., Harkonen, M. & Hakama, M.K. (1996) Circulating anti-*Helicobacter pylori* immunoglobulin A antibodies and low serum pepsinogen I level are associated with increased risk of gastric cancer. *Am. J. Epidemiol.*, **144**, 142–149

Barreto-Zuniga, R., Maruyama, M., Kato, Y., Aizu, K., Ohta, H., Takekoshi, T. & Bernal, S.F. (1997) Significance of *Helicobacter pylori* infection as a risk factor in gastric cancer: serological and histological studies. *J. Gastroenterol.*, **32**, 289–294

Biasco, G. & Paganelli, G.M. (1999) European trials on dietary supplementation for cancer prevention. *Ann. N.Y. Acad. Sci.*, **889**, 152–156

Blaser, M.J. (1998) Helicobacter are indigenous to the human stomach: duodenal ulceration is due to changes in gastric microecology in the modern era. *Gut*, **43**, 721–727

Blaser, M.J., Kobayashi, K., Cover, T.L., Cao, P., Feurer, I.D. & Perez-Perez, G.I. (1993) *Helicobacter pylori* infection in Japanese patients with adenocarcinoma of the stomach. *Int. J. Cancer*, **55**, 799–802

Blaser, M.J., Perez-Perez, G.I., Kleanthous, H., Cover, T.L., Peek, R.M., Chyou, P.H., Stemmermann, G.N. & Nomura, A. (1995) Infection with *Helicobacter pylori* strains possessing CagA is associated with an increased risk of developing adenocarcinoma of the stomach. *Cancer Res.*, **55**, 2111–2115

Blot, W.J., Li, J.Y., Taylor, P.R., Guo, W., Dawsey, S.M., Wang, G.Q., Yang, C.S., Zheng, S.F., Gail, M., Li, G.Y., Yu, Y., Liu, B.Q., Tangrea, J., Sun, Y.H., Liu, F., Fraumeni, J.F., Jr, Zhang, Y.H. & Li, B. (1993) Nutrition intervention trials in Linxian, China: supplementation with specific vitamin/mineral combinations, cancer incidence, and disease-specific mortality in the general population. *J. natl Cancer Inst.*, **85**, 1483–1492

Bodhidatta, L., Hoge, C.W., Churnratanakul, S., Nirdnoy, W., Sampathanukul, P., Tungtaem, C.,

Raktham, S., Smith, C.D. & Echeverria, P. (1994) Diagnosis of *Helicobacter pylori* infection in a developing country; comparison of two ELISAs and a seroprevalence survey. *J. infect. Dis.*, **168**, 1549–1553

Bonney, G.E., Elston, R.C., Correa, P., Haenszel, W., Zavala, D.E., Zarama, G., Collazos, T. & Cuello, C. (1986) Genetic etiology of gastric carcinoma: I. Chronic atrophic gastritis. *Genet. Epidemiol.*, **3**, 213–224

Buiatti, E., Muñoz, N., Vivas, J., Cano, E., Peraza, S., Carillo, E., Castro, D., Sanchez, V., Andrade, O., Benz, M., de Sanjose, S. & Oliver, W. (1994) Difficulty in eradicating *Helicobacter pylori* in a population at high risk for stomach cancer in Venezuela. *Cancer Causes Control*, **5**, 249–254

Censini, S., Lange, C., Xiang, Z., Crabtree, J.E., Ghiara, P., Borodovsky, M., Rappuoli, R. & Covacci, A. (1996) Cag, a pathogenicity island of *Helicobacter pylori*, encodes type I- specific and disease-associated virulence factors. *Proc. natl Acad. Sci. USA*, **93**, 14648–14653

Chen, S.Y., Liu, T.Y, Chen, M.J., Lin, J.T., Sheu, J.C. & Chen, C.J. (1997) Seroprevalence of hepatitis B and C viruses and *Helicobacter pylori* in a small isolated population at high risk of gastric and liver cancer. *Int. J. Cancer*, **71**, 776–779

Choi, N.W., Entwistle, D.W., Michaluk, W. & Nelson, N. (1971) Gastric cancer in Icelanders in Manitoba. *Isr. J. med. Sci.*, **7**, 1500–1508

Chow, W.H., Blaser, M.J., Blot, W.J., Gammon, M.D., Vaughan, T.L., Risch, H.A., Perez-Perez, G.I., Schoenberg, J.B., Stanford, J.L., Rotterdam, H., West, A.B. & Fraumeni, J.F., Jr (1998) An inverse relation between CagA+ strains of *Helicobacter pylori* infection and risk of esophageal and gastric cardia adenocarcinoma. *Cancer Res.*, **58**, 588–590

Coleman, M.P., Estève, J., Damiecki, P., Arslan, A. & Renard, H., eds (1993) *Trends in Gastric Cancer Incidence and Mortality* (IARC Scientific Publications No. 121), Lyon, IARC*Press*

Correa, P., Cuello, C. & Duque, E. (1970) Carcinoma and intestinal metaplasia of the stomach in Colombian migrants. *J. natl Cancer Inst.*, **44**, 297–306

Correa, P., Fox, J., Fontham, E.T., Ruiz, B., Lin, Y., Zavala, D., Taylor, N., Mackinley, D., de Lima, E., Portilla, H. & Zarama, G. (1990) *Helicobacter pylori* and gastric carcinoma: serum antibody pre-valence in populations with contrasting cancer risks. *Cancer*, **66**, 2569–2574

Correa, P., Fontham, E.T., Bravo, J.C., Bravo, L.E., Ruiz, B., Zarama, G., Realpe, J.L., Malcolm, G.T., Li, D., Johnson, W.D. & Mera, R. (2000) Chemoprevention of gastric dysplasia: randomized trial of antioxidant supplements and anti-*Helicobacter pylori* therapy. *J. natl Cancer Inst.*, **92**, 1881–1888

Devesa, S.S. & Fraumeni, J.F., Jr (1999) The rising incidence of gastric cardia cancer. *J. natl Cancer Inst.*, **91**, 747–749

Devesa, S.S., Blot, W.J. & Fraumeni, J.F., Jr (1998) Changing patterns in the incidence of esophageal and gastric carcinoma in the United States. *Cancer*, **83**, 2049–2053

Doll, R. & Peto, R. (1981) The causes of cancer: quantitative estimates of avoidable risks of cancer in the United States today. *J. natl Cancer Inst.*, **66**, 1191–1308

Ekström, A.M., Signorello, L.B., Hansson, L.E., Berström, R., Lindgren, A. & Nyrén, O. (1999) Evaluating gastric cancer misclassification: a potential explanation for the rise in cardia cancer incidence. *J. natl Cancer Inst.*, **91**, 786–790

Ekström, A.M., Held, M., Hansson, L.-E., Engstrand, L. & Nyrén, O. (2001) *Helicobacter pylori* in gastric cancer established by CagA immunoblot as a marker of past infection. *Gastroenterology*, **121**, 784–791

Estevens, J., Fidalgo, P., Tendeiro, T., Chagas, C., Ferra, A., Nobre Leitao, C. & Costa Mira, F. (1993) Anti-*Helicobacter pylori* antibodies prevalence and gastric adenocarcinoma in Portugal: report of a case control study. *Eur. J. Cancer Prev.*, **2**, 377–380

EUROGAST Study Group (1993) An international association between *Helicobacter pylori* infection and gastric cancer. *Lancet*, **341**, 1359–1362

Feldmeier, H. & Krantz, I. (2000) The 'African enigma' – another explanation [Letter]. *Nature Med.*, **6**, 1297–1298

Ferlay, J., Bray, F., Pisani, P. & Parkin, D.M. (2001) *GLOBOCAN 2000: Cancer Incidence, Mortality and Prevalence Worldwide*, Version 1.0. IARC CancerBase No. 5, Lyon, IARC*Press*

Fock, K., Khor, C., Goh, K., Teoh, Y., Seow, A., Chia, K., Ho, B. & Ng, H. (1997) Seroprevalence of *Helicobacter pylori* infection and the incidence of gastric cancer in a multi-ethnic population, *Gut*, **41** (Suppl. 1), A50

Forman, D., Sitas, F., Newell, D.G., Stacey, A.R., Boreham, J., Peto, R., Campbell, T.C., Li, J. & Chen, J. (1990) Geographic association of *Helicobacter pylori* antibody prevalence and gastric cancer mortality in rural China. *Int. J. Cancer*, **46**, 608–611

Forman, D., Newell, D.G., Fullerton, F., Yarnell, J.W., Stacey, A.R., Wald, N. & Sitas, F. (1991) Association between infection with *Helicobacter pylori* and risk of gastric cancer: evidence from a prospective investigation. *Br. med. J.*, **302**, 1302–1305

Fox, J.G., Beck, P., Dangler, C.A., Whary, M.T., Wang, T.C., Shi, H.N. & Nagler-Anderson, C. (2000) Concurrent enteric helminth infection modulates inflammation and gastric immune responses and reduces helicobacter-induced gastric atrophy. *Nature Med.*, **6**, 536–542

Franceschi, S. & La Vecchia, C. (1994) Alcohol and the risk of cancers of the stomach and colon-rectum. *Dig. Dis.*, **12**, 276–289

Fraser, A.G., Scragg, R., Melcalf, P., McCullough, S. & Yeates, N.J. (1996) Prevalence of *Helicobacter pylori* infection in different ethnic groups in New Zealand children and adults. *Aust. N.Z. J. Med.*, **26**, 646–651

Fujioka, T., Honda, S. & Tokieda, M. (2000) *Helicobacter pylori* infection and gastric carcinoma in animal models. *J. Gastroenterol. Hepatol.*, **15** (Suppl.), D55–D59

Fukao, A., Komatsu, S., Tsubono, Y., Hisamichi, S., Ohori, H. & Kizawa, T. (1993) *Helicobacter pylori* infection and chronic atrophic gastritis among Japanese blood donors: a cross-sectional study. *Cancer Causes Control*, **4**, 307–312

Fukuda, H., Saito, D., Hayashi, S., Hisai, H., Ono, H., Yoshida, S., Oguro, Y., Noda, T., Sato, T., Katoh, M., Terada, M., & Sugimura, T. (1995) *Helicobacter pylori* infection, serum pepsinogen level and gastric cancer: a case–control study in Japan. *Jpn. J. Cancer Res.*, **86**, 64–71

Gail, M.H., You, W.C., Chang, Y.S., Zhang, L., Blot, W.J., Brown, L.M., Groves, F.D., Heinrich, J.P., Hu, J., Jin, M.L., Li, J.Y., Liu, W.D., Ma, J.L., Mark, S.D., Rabkin, C.S., Fraumeni, J.F., Jr & Xu, G.W. (1998) Factorial trial of three interventions to reduce the progression of precancerous gastric

lesions in Shandong, China: design issues and initial data. *Control. clin. Trials*, **19**, 352–369

Geser, A., de Thé, G., Lenoir, G., Day, N.E. & Williams, E.H. (1982) Final case reporting from the Ugandan prospective study of the relationship between EBV and Burkitt's lymphoma. *Int. J. Cancer*, **29**, 397–400

Goldgar, D.E., Easton, D.F., Cannon-Albright, L.A. & Skolnick, M.H. (1994) Systematic population-based assessment of cancer risk in first-degree relatives of cancer probands. *J. natl Cancer Inst.*, **86**, 1600–1608

González, C.A., Riboli, E., Badosa, J., Batiste, E., Cardona, T., Pita, S., Sanz, J.M., Torrent, M. & Agudo, A. (1994) Nutritional factors and gastric cancer in Spain. *Am. J. Epidemiol.*, **139**, 466–473

Gordon, D. (2000) Solving the African enigma: parasites may have their place. *Gastroenterology*, **119**, 611–612

Groves, F.D., Zhang, L., Li, J.Y., You, W.C., Chang, Y.S., Zhao, L., Liu, W.D., Rabkin, C.S., Perez-Perez, G.I., Blaser, M.J. & Gail, M.H. (1997) Comparison of two enzyme-linked immunosorbent assay tests for diagnosis of *Helicobacter pylori* infection in China. *Cancer Epidemiol. Biomarkers Prev.*, **6**, 551–552

Guilford, P., Hopkins, J., Harrawy, J., McLeod, M., McLeod, N., Harawira, P., Taite, H., Scoular, R., Miller, A. & Reeve, A. (1998) E-Cadherin germline mutations in familial gastric cancer. *Nature*, **392**, 402–405

Haenszel, W. & Kurihara, M. (1968) Studies of Japanese migrants. I. Mortality from cancer among Japanese in the United States. *J. natl Cancer Inst.*, **40**, 43–68

Hansen, S., Melby, K.K., Aase, S., Jellum, E. & Vollset, S.E. (1999) *Helicobacter pylori* infection and risk of cardia cancer and non-cardia gastric cancer. A nested case–control study. *Scand. J. Gastroenterol.*, **34**, 353–360

Hansson, E., Engstrand, L., Nyren, O., Evans, D.J., Jr, Lindgren, A., Bergstrom, R., Andersson, B., Athlin, L., Bendtsen, O. & Tracz, P. (1993) *Helicobacter pylori* infection: independent risk indicator of gastric adenocarcinoma. *Gastroenterology*, **105**, 1098–1103

Helicobacter and Cancer Collaborative Group (2001) Gastric cancer and *Helicobacter pylori*: a combined analysis of 12 case control studies nested within prospective cohorts. *Gut*, **49**, 347–353

Hemminki, K. & Jiang, Y. (2002) Familial and second gastric carcinomas: a nationwide epidemiologic study from Sweden. *Cancer*, **94**, 1157–1165

Holcombe, C (1992) *Helicobacter pylori*: the African enigma. *Gut*, **33**, 429–431

Howson, C.P., Hiyama, T. & Wynder, E.L. (1986) The decline in gastric cancer: epidemiology of an unplanned triumph. *Epidemiol. Rev.*, **8**, 1–27

Hu, P.J., Mitchell, H.M., Li, Y.Y., Zhou, M.H. & Hanzell, S.L. (1994) Association of *Helicobacter pylori* with gastric cancer and observations on the detection of this bacteria in gastric cancer cases. *Am. J. Gastroenterol.*, **89**, 1806–1810

Huang, J.-Q., Sridhar, S., Chen, Y. & Hunt, R.H. (1998) Meta-analysis of the relationship between *Helicobacter pylori* seropositivity and gastric cancer. *Gastroenterology*, **114**, 1169–1179

IARC (1988) *IARC Monographs on the Evaluation of Carcinogenic Risks to Humans*, Vol. 44, *Alcohol Drinking*, Lyon, IARCPress

IARC (1994) *IARC Monographs on the Evaluation of Carcinogenic Risks to Humans*, Vol. 61, *Schistosomes, Liver Flukes and* Helicobacter pylori, Lyon, IARCPress

IARC (1997) *IARC Monographs on the Evaluation of Carcinogenic Risks to Humans*, Vol. 70, *Epstein–Barr Virus and Kaposi's Sarcoma Herpesvirus/ Human Herpesvirus 8*, Lyon, IARCPress

Igarashi, H., Takahashi, S., Ishiyama, N., Nakamura, K., Masubuchi, N. & Sato, S. (1992) Is Helicobacter a causal agent in gastric cancer? *Irish J. med. Sci.*, **161** (Suppl. 10), 69

Kang, H. & Chung, I. (1992) *Helicobacter pylori* infection and gastric adenocarcinoma in Korea: prevalence and distribution of *Helicobacter pylori* in resected specimen of gastric cancer. *J. cath. med. Coll.*, **45**, 849–862

Kaviani, M.J., Malekzadeh, R., Vahedi, H., Sotoudeh, M., Kamalian, N., Amini, M. & Massarrat, S. (2001) Various durations of a standard regimen (amoxycillin, metronidazole, colloidal bismuth sub-citrate for 2 weeks or with additional ranitidine for 1 or 2 weeks) on eradication of *Helicobacter pylori* in Iranian peptic ulcer patients. A randomized controlled trial. *Eur. J. Gastroenterol. Hepatol.*, **13**, 915–919

Kikuchi, S., Wada, O., Kurosawa, M., Nakajima, T., Kobayashi, O., Yamazaki, T., Kikuichi, M., Mori, K., Oura, S., Watanabe, H., Nagawa, H., Otani, R., Inaba, Y., Okamoto, N., Anzai, H., Kubo, T., Konishi, T., Futagawa, S., Mozobuchi, N., Kobori, O., Kaise, R., Sato, T., Nishi, T., Sato, H., Ishibashi, T., Ichikawa, S., Hirata, T., Sato, N., Miki, K. & Myoga, A. (1995) Association between gastric cancer and *H. pylori* with reference to age. *Gut*, **45**, 319–323

Kim, H.Y., Cho, B.D., Chang, W.K., Kim, D.J, Kim, Y.B., Park, C.K., Shin, H.S. & Yoo, J.Y. (1997) *Helicobacter pylori* infection and the risk of gastric cancer among the Korean population. *J. Gastroenterol. Hepatol.*, **12**, 100–103

Kneller, R.W., Guo, W.D., Hsing, A.W., Chen, J.S, Blot, W.J., Li, J.Y., Forman, D. & Fraumeni, J.F., Jr (1992) Risk factors for stomach cancer in sixty-five Chinese counties. *Cancer Epidemiol. Biomarkers Prev.*, **1**, 113–118

Kokkola, A., Valle, J., Haapianen, R., Sipponen, P., Kivalaakso, E. & Puolakkainen, P. (1996) *Helicobacter pylori* infection in young patients with gastric carcinoma. *Scand. J. Gastroenterol.*, **31**, 643–647

Kosary, C.L., Ries, L.A. G, Miller, B.A., Hankey, B.F., Harras, A. & Edwards, B.K. (1995) *SEER Cancer Statistics Review, 1973–1992: Tables and Graphs.* (NIH Publ. No. 96–2789), Bethesda, MD, National Cancer Institute

Kuipers, E.J., Gracia-Casanova, M., Pena, A.S., Pals, G., van Kamp, G., Kok, A., Kurz-Pohlmann, E., Pels, N.F. & Meuwissen, S.G. (1993) *Helicobacter pylori* serology in patients with gastric carcinoma. *Scand. J. Gastroenterol.*, **28**, 433–437

Kuipers, E.J., Perez-Perez, G.I., Meuwissen, S.G. & Blaser, M.J. (1995) *Helicobacter pylori* and atrophic gastritis: importance of the cagA status. *J. natl Cancer Inst.*, **87**, 1777–1780

Langman, M. (1988) Genetic influences upon gastric cancer frequency. In: Reed, P. & Hill, M., eds, *Gastric Carcinogenesis*, Amsterdam, Excerpta Medica

Limburg, P., Qiao, Y., Mark, S., Wang, G, Perez-Perez, G., Blaser, M., Wu, Y., Zou, X., Dong, Z., Taylor, P. & Dawsey, S. (2001) *Helicobacter pylori* seropositivity and subsite-specific gastric cancer risks in Linxian, China. *J. natl Cancer Inst.*, **93**, 226–233

Lin, J.T., Wang, J.T., Wang, T.H., Wu, M.S., Lee, T.K. & Chen, C.J. (1993) *Helicobacter pylori* infection in a randomly selected population, healthy volunteers and patients with gastric ulcer and gastric adenocarcinoma. A seroprevalence study in Taiwan. *Scand. J. Gastroenterol.*, **28**, 1067–1072

Lin, J.T., Wang, L.Y, Wang, J.T, Wang, T.H. & Chen, C.J. (1995a) Ecological study of association between *Helicobacter pylori* infection and gastric cancer in Taiwan. *Dig. Dis. Sci.*, **40**, 385–388

Lin, J.T., Wang, L.Y, Wang, J.T., Wang, T.H., Yang, C.S. & Chen, C.J. (1995b) A nested case–control study on the association between *Helicobacter pylori* infection and gastric cancer risk in a cohort of 9775 men in Taiwan. *Anticancer Res.*, **15**, 603–606

Lopez-Carrillo, L., Fernandez-Ortega, C., Robles-Diaz, G., Rascon-Pacheco, R. & Ramirez-Iglesias, T. (1997) [*Helicobacter pylori* infection and gastric cancer in Mexico. A challenge for prevention and population control.] *Rev. Gastroenterol. Mex.*, **62**, 22–28 (in Spanish)

MacDonald, T.T (2001) The worm turns on *Helicobacter pylori*. *Gut*, **48**, 10–11

Marshall, B.J., Armstrong, J.A., McGechie, D.B. & Glancy, R.J. (1985) Attempt to fulfil Koch's postulates for pyloric campylobacter. *Med. J. Aust.*, **142**, 436–439

McMichael, A.J., McCall, M.G, Hartshorne, J.M. & Woodings, T.L. (1980) Patterns of gastro-intestinal cancer in European migrants to Australia: the role of dietary change. *Int. J. Cancer*, **25**, 431–437

Miglio, F., Miglio, M., Mazzeo, V., Holton, J., Mule, P. & Menegatti, M. (1992) Prevalence of *Helicobacter pylori* (HP) in patients with gastric carcinoma. *Irish J. med. Sci.*, **161** (Suppl. 10), 70

Mitchell, H.M., Ally, R., Wiseman, M., Ahmed, R. & Segal, I. (2000) The host immune response to *H. pylori* infection in Sowetans is significantly different from that in western subjects. *Gut*, **47**, A38

Muñoz, N. & Steinitz, R. (1971) Comparative histology of gastric cancer in migrant groups in Israel. *Isr. J. med. Sci.*, **7**, 1479–1487

Muñoz, N., Vivas, J., Buiatti, E. & Oliver, W. (1996) Chemoprevention trial on precancerous lesions of the stomach in Venezuela: summary of study design and baseline data. In: Stewart, B., McGregor, D. &

Kleihues, P., eds, *Principles of Chemoprevention* (IARC Scientific Publications No. 139), Lyon, IARC*Press*

Nomura, A., Stemmerman, G.N., Chyou, P.H., Kato, I., Perez-Perez, G.I. & Blaser, M.J. (1991) *Helicobacter pylori* infection and gastric carcinoma among Japanese Americans in Hawaii. *New Engl. J. Med.*, **325**, 1132–1136

Palli, D., Bianchi, S., Decarli, A., Cipriani, F., Avellini, C., Cocco, P., Falcini, F., Puntoni, R., Russo, A., Vindigni, C., Fraumeni, J.F., Jr, Blot, W.J. & Buiatti, E. (1992) A case control study of cancers of the gastric cardia in Italy. *Br. J. Cancer*, **65**, 263–266

Palli, D., Decarli, A., Cipriani, F., Sitas, F., Forman, D., Amadori, D., Avellini, C., Giacosa, A., Manca, P., Russo, A., Samloff, I.M., Fraumeni, J.F., Jr, Blot, W.J. & Buiatti, E. (1993) *Helicobacter pylori* antibodies in areas of Italy at varying gastric cancer risk. *Cancer Epidemiol. Biomarkers Prev.*, **2**, 37–40

Parkin, D.M., Whelan, S., Ferlay, J., Raymond, L. & Young, J., eds (1997) *Cancer Incidence in Five Continents* (IARC Scientific Publications No. 143), Lyon, IARC*Press*

Parkin, D.M., Pisani, P. & Ferlay, J. (1999) Estimates of the worldwide incidence of 25 major cancers in 1990. *Int. J. Cancer*, **80**, 827–841

Parsonnet, J., Friedman, G.D., Vandersteen, D.P., Chang, Y., Vogelman, J.H., Orentreich, N. & Sibley, R.K. (1991) *Helicobacter pylori* infection and the risk of gastric carcinoma. *New Engl. J. Med.*, **325**, 1127–1131

Perez-Perez, G.I., Bhat, N., Gaensbauer, J., Fraser, A., Taylor, D.N., Kuipers, E.J., Zhang, L., You, W.C. & Blaser, M.J. (1997) Country-specific constancy by age in CagA+ proportion of *Helicobacter pylori* infections. *Int. J. Cancer*, **72**, 453–456

Plummer, M., Vivas, J., Fauchere, J.L., Del Giudice, G., Pena, A.S., Ponzetto, A., Lopez, G., Miki, K., Oliver, W. & Muñoz, N. (2000) *Helicobacter pylori* and stomach cancer: a case–control study in Venezuela. *Cancer Epidemiol. Biomarkers Prev.*, **9**, 961–965

Rudi, J., Muller, M., von Herbay, A., Zuna, I., Raedsch, R., Stremmel, W. & Rath, U. (1995) Lack of association of *Helicobacter pylori* seroprevalence and gastric cancer in a population with low gastric cancer incidence. *Scand. J. Gastroenterol.*, **30**, 958–963

Sierra, R., Muñoz, N., Pena, A.S., Biemond, I., van Duijn, W., Lamers, C. B., Teuchmann, S., Hernandez, S. & Correa, P. (1992) Antibodies to *Helicobacter pylori* and pepsinogen levels in children from Costa Rica: comparison of two areas with different risks for stomach cancer. *Cancer Epidemiol. Biomarkers Prev.*, **1**, 449–454

Sierra, R., Salas, P., Mora-Zuniga, F., Sanabria, M., Chinnock, A., Pena, S., Quiros, E., Mora, W., Mena, F., Altman, R. & Muñoz, N. (1998) [Eradication of *Helicobacter pylori* in a population at high risk of gastric cancer.] *Acta med. costarricense*, **40**, 30–35 (in Spanish)

Simán, J., Forsgren, A., Berglund, A. & Floren, C.H. (1997) Association between *Helicobacter pylori* and gastric carcinoma in the city of Malmo, Sweden. A prospective study. *Scand. J. Gastroenterol.*, **32**, 1215–1221

Sipponen, P., Kosunen, T.U., Valle, J., Rihela, M. & Seppala, K. (1992) *Helicobacter pylori* infection and chronic gastritis in gastric cancer. *J. clin. Pathol.*, **45**, 319–323

Sorberg, M., Engstrand, L., Strom, M., Jonsson, K.A., Jorbeck, H. & Granstrom, M. (1997) The diagnostic value of enzyme immunoassay and immunoblot in monitoring eradication of *Helicobacter pylori*. *Scand. J. infect. Dis.*, **29**, 147–151

Talley, N.J., Zinsmeister, A.R., Weaver, A., DiMagno, E.P., Carpenter, H.A., Perez-Perez, G.I, & Blaser, M.J. (1991) Gastric adenocarcinoma and *Helicobacter pylori* infection. *J. natl Cancer Inst.*, **83**, 1734–1739

Trédaniel, J., Boffetta, P., Buiatti, E., Saracci, R. & Hirsch, A. (1997) Tobacco smoking and gastric cancer: review and meta-analysis. *Int. J. Cancer*, **72**, 565–573

Tsugane, S., Kabuto, M., Imai, H., Gey, F., Tei, Y., Hanaoka, T., Sugano, K. & Watanabe, S. (1993) *Helicobacter pylori*, dietary factors and atrophic gastritis in five Japanese populations with different gastric cancer mortality. *Cancer Causes Control*, **4**, 297–305

Uemura, N., Okamoto, S., Yamamoto, S., Matsumura, N., Yamaguchi, S., Yamakido, M., Taniyama, K., Sasaki, N. & Schlemper, R.J. (2001) *Helicobacter*

pylori infection and the development of gastric cancer. *New Engl. J. Med.*, **345**, 784–789

Valle, J., Seppälä, K., Sipponen, P. & Kosunen, T. (1991) Disappearance of gastritis after eradication of *Helicobacter pylori*. A morphometric study. *Scand. J. Gastroenterol.*, **26**, 1057–1065

Varis, K., Taylor, P.R., Sipponen, P., Samloff, I.M., Heinonen, O.P., Albanes, D., Harkonen, M., Huttunen, J.K., Laxen, F. & Virtamo, J. (1998) Gastric cancer and premalignant lesions in atrophic gastritis: a controlled trial on the effect of supplementation with alpha-tocopherol and beta-carotene. *Scand. J. Gastroenterol.*, **33**, 294–300

Wabinga, H. (2003) Stomach cancer. In: Parkin, D.M., Bah, E., Ferlay, J., Hamdi-Cherif, M., Sitas, F., Thomas, J., Wabinga, H. & Whelan, S., eds, *Cancer in Africa* (IARC Scientific Publications No. 153), Lyon, IARC*Press*, pp. 371–376

Wang, G.Q., Dawsey, S.M., Li, J.Y., Taylor, P.R., Li, B., Blot, W.J., Weinstein, W.M., Liu, F.S., Lewin, K.J., Wang, H., Wiggett, S., Gail, M.H. & Yang, C.S. (1994) Effects of vitamin/mineral supplementation on the prevalence of histological dysplasia and early cancer of the esophagus and stomach: results from the general population trial in Linxian, China. *Cancer Epidemiol. Biomarkers Prev.*, **3**, 161–166

Watanabe, Y., Kurata, J.H., Mizuno, S., Mukai, M., Inokuchi, H., Miki, K., Ozasa, K. & Kawai, K. (1997) *Helicobacter pylori* infection and gastric cancer. A nested case–control study in a rural area of Japan. *Dig. Dis. Sci.*, **42**, 1383–1387

WCRF (1997) *Food, Nutrition and the Prevention of Cancer: a Global Perspective*, Washington DC, World Cancer Research Fund/American Institute for Cancer Research

Webb, P.M., Yu, M.C., Forman, D., Henderson, B.E., Newell, D.G., Yuan, J.M., Gao, Y.T. & Ross, R.K. (1996) An apparent lack of association between *Helicobacter pylori* infection and risk of gastric cancer in China. *Int. J. Cancer*, **67**, 603–607

Willett, W.C. (1995) Diet, nutrition and avoidable cancer. *Environ. Health Perspect.*, **103** (Suppl. 8), 165–170

Wu-Williams, A.H., Yu, M.C. & Mack, T.M. (1990) Life-style, workplace and stomach cancer by subsite in young men of Los Angeles county. *Cancer Res.*, **50**, 2569–2576

Yamagata, H., Kiyohara, Y., Aoyagi, K., Kato, I., Iwamoto, H., Nakayama, K., Shimizu, H., Tanizaki, Y., Arima, H., Shinohara, N., Kondo, H., Matsumoto, T. & Fujishima, M. (2000) Impact of *Helicobacter pylori* infection on gastric cancer incidence in a general Japanese population: the Hisayama study. *Arch. intern. Med.*, **160**, 1962–1968

Zhao, L., Blot, W.J., Liu, W.D., Chang, Y.S., Zhang, J.S., Hu, Y.R., You, W.C., Xu, G.W. & Fraumeni, J.F., Jr (1994) Familial predisposition to precancerous gastric lesions in a high-risk area of China. *Cancer Epidemiol. Biomarkers Prev.*, **3**, 461–464

Corresponding author:

Silvia Franceschi
Unit of Field and Intervention Studies,
International Agency for Research on Cancer,
150 Cours Albert Thomas,
F-69372 Lyon cedex 08, France
franceschi@iarc.fr

Mechanisms of Carcinogenesis: Contributions of Molecular Epidemiology
Patricia Buffler, Jerry Rice, Robert Baan, Michael Bird and Paolo Boffetta, eds
IARC Scientific Publications No. 157
International Agency for Research on Cancer, Lyon, 2004

Genetic Pathways of Two Types of Gastric Cancer

Eiichi Tahara

Summary

Multiple genetic and epigenetic alterations in oncogenes, tumour-suppressor genes, cell-cycle regulators, cell adhesion molecules, DNA repair genes and genetic instability as well as telomerase activation are implicated in the multistep process of human stomach carcinogenesis. However, particular combinations of these alterations differ in the two histological types of gastric cancer, indicating that well-differentiated or intestinal-type and poorly differentiated or diffuse-type carcinomas have distinct carcinogenetic pathways. In the multistep process of well-differentiated-type carcinogenesis, the genetic pathway can be divided into three subpathways: an intestinal metaplasia→adenoma→carcinoma sequence, an intestinal metaplasia→carcinoma sequence and de novo. In the multistep process of well-differentiated-type or intestinal-type gastric carcinogenesis, infection with *Helicobacter pylori* may be a strong trigger for hyperplasia of hTERT-positive 'stem cells' in intestinal metaplasia. Genetic instability and hyperplasia of hTERT-positive stem cells precede replication error at the D1S191 locus, DNA hypermethylation at the D17S5 locus, *pS2* loss, *RARβ* loss, *CD44* abnormal transcripts and *p53* mutation, all of which accumulate in at least 30% of incomplete intestinal metaplasias. All of these epigenetic and genetic alterations are common events in intestinal-type gastric cancer. An adenoma→carcinoma sequence is found in about 20% of gastric adenomas with *APC* mutations. In addition to these events, *p53* mutation and loss of heterozygosity (LOH), reduced *p27* expression, *cyclin E* expression and the presence of c-*met* 6.0-kb transcripts allow malignant transformation from the above precancerous lesions to intestinal-type gastric cancer. *DCC* loss, *APC* mutations, 1q LOH, *p27* loss, reduced tumour growth factor (TGF)-β type I receptor expression, reduced *nm23* expression and c-*erb*B gene amplification are frequently associated with an advanced stage of intestinal-type gastric cancer. The de-novo pathway for carcinogenesis of well-differentiated gastric cancer involves LOH and abnormal expression of the *p73* gene that is responsible for the development of foveolar-type gastric cancers with pS2 expression.

On the other hand, LOH at chromosome 17p, mutation or LOH of *p53* and mutation or loss of E-cadherin are preferentially involved in the development of poorly differentiated gastric cancers. In addition to these changes, gene amplification of K-*sam*, and c-*met* and *p27* loss as well as reduced nm23 obviously confer progression, metastasis and diffusely productive fibrosis. Mixed gastric carcinomas composed of well-differentiated and poorly differentiated components exhibit some but not all of the molecular events described so far for each of the two types of gastric cancer.

Besides these genetic and epigenetic events, well-differentiated and poorly differentiated gastric cancers also organize different patterns of interplay between cancer cells and stromal cells through the growth factor/cytokine receptor system, which plays an important role in cell growth, apoptosis, morphogenesis, angiogenesis, progression and metastasis.

Meta-analysis of epidemiological studies and animal models show that both intestinal and diffuse types of gastric cancer are equally associated with *H. pylori* infection. However, *H. pylori* infection may play a role only in the initial steps of gastric carcinogenesis. Differences in *H. pylori* strain, patient age, exogenous or endogenous carcinogens and genetic factors such as DNA polymorphism and genetic instability may be implicated in two distinct major genetic pathways for gastric carcinogenesis.

Introduction

Striking advances in molecular dissection of pre-cancerous and cancerous lesions of the stomach indicate that genetic and epigenetic alterations in oncogenes, tumour-suppressor genes, DNA-repair genes, cell-cycle regulators, telomeres and telomerase, as well as genetic instability at micro-satellite foci are involved in the multistep process of human stomach carcinogenesis (Sano et al., 1991; Tahara, 1993; Tahara et al., 1996a).

There are several histological classifications of gastric cancer. Lauren (1965) divided gastric cancer into two types, intestinal and diffuse, and the Japan Research Society for Gastric Cancer (JRSGC, 1999) classified it into five common types. The JRSGC classification is similar to that of the World Health Organization (Hamilton & Aaltonen, 2000). In this chapter, we use a two-type classification: the intestinal or well-differen-tiated type (which includes the papillary and tubular adenocarcinomas of the JRSGC classi-fication), and the diffuse or poorly differentiated type (which includes the diffuse and signet-ring cell carcinomas of the JRSGC classification).

The genetic and epigenetic changes found in gastric carcinoma differ, depending upon the histological type of gastric cancer, indicating that different carcinogenetic pathways exist for intes-tinal and diffuse types of carcinomas (Table 1; Figures 1 and 2). In addition, cancer–stromal interaction through the growth factor/cytokine receptor system, which plays a pivotal role in morphogenesis, cancer progression and metas-tasis, is also much different between the two types of gastric carcinoma (Tahara et al., 1993, 1994).

This chapter provides a detailed overview of the molecular machinery that underlies stomach carcinogenesis.

Oncogenes

Several proto-oncogenes, including c-met, K-sam and c-erbB2, are frequently activated in gastric carcinomas. The amplification of the c-met gene encoding a receptor for hepatocyte growth factor/

scatter factor is found in 19% of intestinal and 39% of diffuse gastric cancers, frequently accom-panied by diffusely productive fibrosis of the scirrhous type (Kuniyasu et al., 1992). Most gastric carcinomas express two different c-met transcripts, one of 7.0 kb and the other of 6.0 kb. Expression of the 6.0-kb c-met transcript, which is expressed preferentially in cancer cells, correlates well with tumour staging, lymph node metastasis and depth of tumour invasion (Kuniyasu et al., 1993). Soman et al. (1991) reported that the tpr-met rearrangement is expressed in gastric carcino-mas and gastric precancerous lesions. However, we have not detected the tpr-met rearrangement in any gastric cancer or intestinal metaplasia.

The K-sam (KATO-III cell-derived stomach cancer amplified) gene has at least four trans-criptional variants. Type II encodes a receptor for keratinocyte growth factor (Katoh et al., 1992). Type II transcript is expressed only in carcinoma cells (not in cell lines from sarcomas). K-sam is preferentially amplified in 33% of advanced diffuse or scirrhous-type gastric carcinomas, but not in intestinal-type gastric carcinomas (Hattori et al., 1990). Moreover, K-sam is never seen in esophageal or colorectal carcinomas. Gastric cancers that overexpress K-sam protein are asso-ciated with a less favourable prognosis.

In contrast to K-sam, c-erbB2 is preferentially amplified in 20% of intestinal gastric cancers but not in diffuse-type gastric cancer (Yokota et al., 1988; Kameda et al., 1990). Overexpression of c-erbB2 associated with gene amplification is closely correlated with a poor prognosis and liver metas-tasis (Oda et al., 1990; Yonemura et al., 1991). The amplification of c-erbB1 and c-erbB3 is found in 3% (Kameda et al., 1990) and 0% (Katoh & Terada, 1993), respectively, of gastric cancers.

K-ras mutation is found in gastric intestinal metaplasias, adenomas and intestinal-type adeno-carcinomas (Sano et al., 1991; Lee et al., 1995; Isogaki et al., 1999), although its incidence is low (10–18%). However, K-ras mutation is not seen in diffuse-type gastric cancer. The hst-1 gene, iso-lated from a surgical specimen of human gastric cancer by the NIH/3T3 transformation assay, is rarely amplified in gastric cancer (2% of cases) (Yoshida et al., 1988).

**Table 1. Genetic and epigenetic alterations found
in two types of gastric cancer**

Genetic and epigenetic alterations	Incidence of cases with indicated alterations (%)	
	Well-differentiated[a]	Poorly differentiated[a]
Tumour suppressors		
p53 LOH, mutation	60	75
p73 LOH	53[b]	24
APC LOH, mutation	40–60	0
DCC LOH	50	0
LOH of chromosome 1q	44	0
LOH of chromosome 7q	53	33
LOH of chromosome 17q	0	40[c]
Loss of *pS2* expression	49	31
Loss of *RARβ*	64	0
Cell-cycle regulators		
Cyclin E amplification	33	7
Cyclin E overexpression	26	27
CDC25B overexpression	33	73
Loss of p16 expression	12	31
Loss of p27 expression	46	69
Oncogenes		
K-*ras* mutation	10	0
c-*met* amplification	19	39
K-*sam* amplification	0	33
c-*erbB2* amplification	20	0
Adhesion molecules		
E-cadherin mutation/loss	0	50
CD44 aberrant transcript	100	100
Microsatellite instability	20–40	20–70[c]
Histone deacetylation	61	82
Telomere/telomerase		
Telomere reduction	62	53
Telomerase activity	100	90
TERT expression	100	86

[a] According to the criteria of the JRSGC classification of gastric cancer
[b] Preferentially found in foveolar-type adenocarcinoma
[c] Preferentially found in patients younger than 35 years of age
LOH, loss of heterozygosity

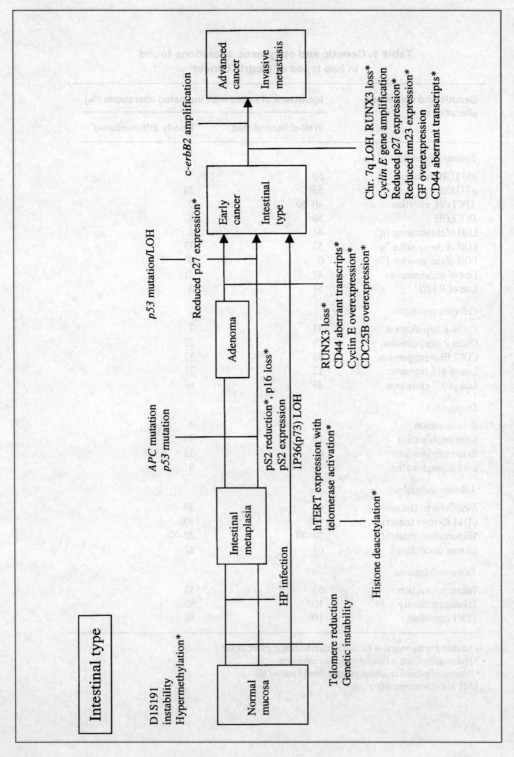

Figure 1. Multiple genetic and epigenetic alterations during human stomach carcinogenesis (intestinal type). * Epigenetic alterations. LOH, loss of heterozygosity; HP, *Helicobacter pylori*. From Tahara (2002)

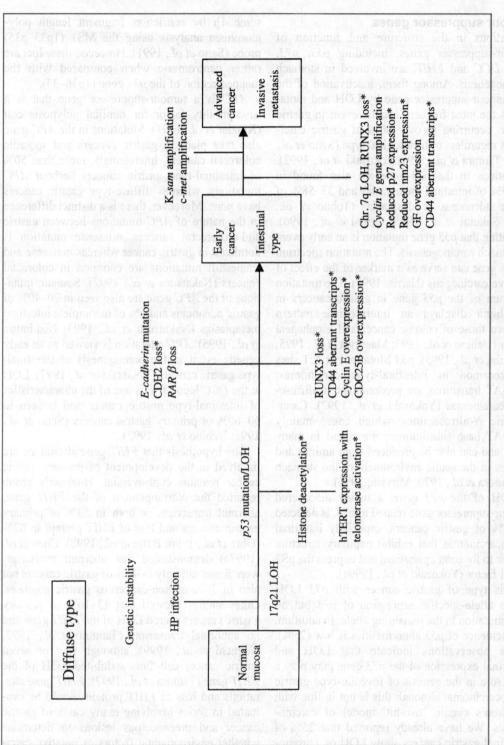

Figure 2. Multiple genetic and epigenetic alterations during human stomach carcinogenesis (diffuse type). * Epigenetic alterations. LOH, loss of heterozygosity; HP, *Helicobacter pylori*; GF, growth factor. From Tahara (2002)

Tumour suppressor genes

Alterations in the structure and function of tumour-suppressor genes, including *p53*, *p73*, *APC*, *DCC* and *FHIT*, are involved in stomach carcinogenesis. Among them, inactivation of the *p53* tumour-suppressor gene by LOH and mutation is the most frequent genetic event in gastric cancer, occurring in over 60% of gastric carcinomas regardless of histological type (Sano *et al.*, 1991; Tamura *et al.*, 1991; Yokozaki *et al.*, 1992). Alterations in the *p53* gene are also found in 13–37% of intestinal metaplasias and 33–58% of gastric adenomas or dysplasias (Tohdo *et al.*, 1993; Sakurai *et al.*, 1995; Ochiai *et al.*, 1996), indicating that *p53* gene mutation is an early event in stomach carcinogenesis. The mutation spectrum of this gene can serve as a marker of the effect of putative carcinogens (Harris, 1991). The mutation spectrum of the *p53* gene in gastric cancers in Hiroshima displays an intermediate pattern between those of colonic cancer and esophageal cancer (Uchino *et al.*, 1993; Maesawa *et al.*, 1995; Poremba *et al.*, 1995). *p53* Mutations at A:T sites are common in intestinal-type carcinomas; GC→AT transitions are predominant in diffuse-type carcinomas (Yokozaki *et al.*, 1992). Carcinogenic *N*-nitrosamines, which cause mainly GC→AT base substitutions, are found in many foods and can also be produced from amines and nitrates in the acidic environment of the stomach (Sugimura *et al.*, 1970; Mirvish, 1971).

LOH of the *p73* gene, a newly discovered tumour-suppressor gene related to *p53*, is detected in 38% of gastric cancers, especially intestinal adenocarcinomas that exhibit papillary structure similar to foveolar epithelium and express the pS2 trefoil factor (Yokozaki *et al.*, 1999a).

This type of gastric cancer with *p73* LOH shows allele-specific expression of *p73* but no gene mutation in the remaining allele. In addition, the incidence of *p53* abnormalities is low (25%). These observations indicate that LOH and abnormal expression of the *p73* gene may play a large role in the genesis of foveolar-type gastric adenocarcinoma, although this is not in line with Knudson's classic 'two-hit' model of carcinogenesis. We have already reported that 25% of intestinal gastric cancers show LOH on chromosome 1p by restriction fragment length polymorphism analysis using the MS1 (1p33–p35) probe (Sano *et al.*, 1991). However, these loci are rather centromeric when compared with the mapped region of the *p73* gene (1p36–33).

APC is a tumour-suppressor gene that is a susceptibility factor for familial polyposis coli (Kinzler *et al.*, 1991). Mutations in the *APC* gene also take place in gastric cancers and sporadic colorectal cancers. Interestingly, more than 50% of intestinal-type gastric cancers harbour *APC* mutations, whereas diffuse-type gastric cancers have none. Moreover, there is a distinct difference in the nature of *APC* mutations between gastric and colorectal cancers: missense mutation is dominant in gastric cancer whereas nonsense and frameshift mutations are common in colorectal cancers (Nakatsuru *et al.*, 1992). Somatic mutations of the *APC* gene are also seen in 20–40% of gastric adenomas and 6% of incomplete intestinal metaplasias (Nakatsuru *et al.*, 1993; Nishimura *et al.*, 1995). *APC* alteration is viewed as an early genetic event in the pathogenesis of intestinal-type gastric cancers (Yokozaki *et al.*, 1997). LOH at the *DCC* locus also is one of the characteristics of intestinal-type gastric cancer and is seen in 50–60% of primary gastric cancers (Sano *et al.*, 1991; Uchino *et al.*, 1992).

The hypothesis that *FHIT* gene alterations are involved in the development of primary gastric cancer remains controversial. Huebner's group reported the rearrangement of the *FHIT* gene, aberrant transcripts or both in 53% of primary gastric cancers and loss of FHIT protein in 67% (Ohta *et al.*, 1996; Baffa *et al.*, 1998). Chen *et al.* (1997a) demonstrated that aberrant transcripts were found not only in 46% of gastric cancers but also in 30% of non-cancerous gastric mucosas. Other studies showed that 13–16% of primary gastric cancers shared LOH of the *FHIT* gene and no abnormal transcripts (Tamura *et al.*, 1997; Noguchi *et al.*, 1999), although four of seven gastric cancer cell lines exhibited LOH of the *FHIT* gene (Tamura *et al.*, 1997). *FHIT* gene alterations and loss of FHIT protein should be evaluated in series involving many cases of gastric cancer and precancerous lesions to determine whether environmental factors or putative carcinogens are associated with differences between countries in frequency of FHIT abnormalities.

Several distinct chromosomal loci are deleted in gastric cancers. LOH at 1q and 7q are frequently associated with intestinal gastric cancer, whereas loss of 1p is relatively common in advanced diffuse gastric cancer (Sano *et al.*, 1991). Moreover, LOH at the *bcl*-2 gene locus is seen in many intestinal gastric cancers and colorectal cancers (Ayhan *et al.*, 1994). Our deletion mapping study on 7q shows that LOH at the D7S95 locus correlates well with peritoneal dissemination (Kuniyasu *et al.*, 1994a). Recently, investigators in a study on allelic loss in xenografted human gastric carcinomas reported a high degree of allelic loss on several chromosomal arms in 18 xenografted gastric adenocarcinomas: 3p (81%), 4p (64%), 5q (69%), 8p (57%), 13q (59%), 17p (80%) and 18q (61%) (Yustein *et al.*, 1999). From these assigned loci, candidates for the tumour-suppressor gene responsible for stomach carcinogenesis may be identified in the future.

pS2, a gastric-specific trefoil factor normally expressed in the gastric foveolar epithelial cells, may function as a gastric-specific tumour suppressor, since the inactivation of the *pS2* gene by gene targeting causes dysplasia, adenoma and adenocarcinoma of the glandular stomach in mice (Masiakowski *et al.*, 1982; Lefebvre *et al.*, 1996). Recently, we found that the reduction or loss of the *pS2* gene by DNA methylation at the promoter region occurs in intestinal metaplasias and gastric adenomas. Conversely, 32% of gastric cancers display strong expression of the *pS2* gene and 40% of gastric cancers, especially the intestinal type, show no expression (Fujimoto *et al.*, 2000). Reduced expression or loss of the *pS2* gene by promoter methylation may play a role in the early stages of carcinogenesis of intestinal stomach carcinoma.

Recent in-vivo and in-vitro studies suggest that the nuclear retinoic acid receptor β (RARβ) functions as a tumour suppressor and that loss of *RARβ* by CpG promoter hypermethylation is associated with tumorigenesis (Lotan *et al.*, 1995; Seewaldt *et al.*, 1995; Hayashi *et al.*, 2001a). More recently, we found that hypermethylation of

the *RARβ* gene promoter is preferentially observed in 64% of intestinal gastric cancers associated with reduced expression (Hayashi *et al.*, 2001b), but not in the diffuse type. Promoter hypermethylation is also detected in gastric intestinal metaplasia. Three gastric cancer cell lines (MKN-28, -45 and -74), all of which are derived from intestinal-type adenocarcinomas, exhibit a loss of *RARβ* expression by promoter methylation. *RARβ* expression is restored in these cell lines by 5-azacytidine or the histone deacetylase inhibitor trichostatin A. Overexpression of the RARβ in MKN-28 cells induces G_0–G_1 arrest, followed by down-regulation of the DNA methyltransferase 3α and DNA demethylase, and up-regulation of the acetylated histone H4. These results suggest that inactivation of RARβ as well as pS2 is implicated in gastric carcinogenesis of the intestinal type.

Cell-cycle regulators

Genetic and epigenetic abnormalities in cell-cycle regulators are involved in the development and progression of gastric cancer by causing unbridled proliferation. Most gastric cancers are associated with overexpression of positive regulators and reduction or loss of negative regulators, both of which co-operate to drive normal cells into malignancy.

The *cyclin E* gene is amplified in 15–20% of gastric carcinomas that are associated with its overexpression. The gene amplification or overexpression of cyclin E, or both cause aggressiveness and lymph node metastasis (Akama *et al.*, 1995). *Cyclin D1* gene amplification, on the other hand, is exceptional in gastric carcinomas but frequently occurs in esophageal carcinoma (Yoshida *et al.*, 1996).

CDC25 phosphatases dephosphorylate threonine and tyrosine residues at positions 14 and 15 in the cyclin-dependent kinases (CDKs) and then activate them (Honda *et al.*, 1993). Three types of CDC25 have been identified: CDC25A, -B and -C (Nagata *et al.*, 1991). CDC25A is expressed early in the G_1 phase of the cell cycle; CDC25B is expressed in both the G_1/S and G_2 phases (Jinno *et al.*, 1994) and CDC25C is predominantly expressed in the G_2 phase. CDC25B is overexpressed in more than 70% of gastric cancers regardless of histological type and is closely correlated with tumour invasion and nodal metastasis (Kudo *et al.*, 1997). On the other hand, only 2% of gastric adenomas overexpress CDC25B. However, no gene amplification of *CDC25B* has been found in any gastric cancer. In 38% of gastric cancers, CDC25A is overexpressed but CDC25C is at very low or undetectable levels. Thus, the overexpression of CDC25B in tumour cells may stimulate progression of gastric cancer.

With regard to negative-cell cycle regulators, the p53-inducible CDK inhibitor p21 is associated with the senescence of non-neoplastic gastric epithelial cells (Harper *et al.*, 1993). In neoplastic lesions, the expression of p21 is seen in 78% of gastric adenomas and 76% of gastric adenocarcinomas regardless of *p53* gene mutation, suggesting that a *p53*-independent pathway is substantially involved in the induction of *p21* in gastric tumours (Yasui *et al.*, 1996a). In fact, the growth inhibition of transforming growth factor (TGF)-β or retinoic acid is associated with *p53*-independent induction of *p21* in a gastric cancer cell line (Akagi *et al.*, 1996). Moreover, the strong expression of p21 in cancer cells is frequently observed in advanced cancers and nodal metastasis, whereas there is no inverse correlation between p21 expression and proliferative activity measured by Ki-67. These findings indicate overall that the proliferative activity of gastric cancer cells is not solely dependent on control of the cell cycle by p21. In addition, mutation of the *p21* gene is exceptional in gastric cancer (Akama *et al.*, 1996a) and a codon 31 polymorphism does not affect the expression levels of p21 (Akama *et al.*, 1996b).

p27, a member of the cip/kip family of CDK inhibitors, binds to a wide variety of cyclin/CDK complexes and inhibits kinase activity. We have found that growth suppression of interferon-β is associated with the induction of p27 in a gastric cancer cell, TMK-1 (Kuniyasu *et al.*, 1997a). More importantly, reduction in p27 expression is frequently seen in advanced gastric cancers, whereas p27 is well preserved in 90% of gastric adenomas and 85% of early cancers (Yasui *et al.*, 1997). Gastric adenomas with reduction or loss of

p27 are capable of developing into malignancies. Reduced expression of p27 significantly correlates with depth of tumour invasion and nodal metastasis. Moreover, metastatic tumour cells in lymph nodes express p27 at lower levels than do cells in primary tumours, suggesting that tumour cells with reduction or loss of p27 may selectively metastasize to lymph nodes or distant organs (Yasui *et al.*, 1999a). The expression of p27 in gastric cancer is inversely correlated with the expression of cyclin E (Igaki *et al.*, 1995). Loss of p27 function and gain of cyclin E evidently stimulate progression and metastasis of gastric carcinomas. Reduction in p27 expression occurs at post-translational levels, resulting from ubiquitin-mediated proteosomal degradation rather than genetic abnormalities (Yasui *et al.*, 1999a).

Deletion or mutations of the *p16* gene are uncommon in primary gastric carcinomas (Igaki *et al.*, 1995; Lee *et al.*, 1997; Gunther *et al.*, 1998), but homozygous deletion of this gene has been found in two of eight gastric cancer cell lines and lack of p16 protein expression in five of eight gastric cancer cell lines (Akama *et al.*, 1996b). Another mechanism of *p16* gene silencing is hypermethylation of the 5′CpG island (Merlo *et al.*, 1995). Reduced expression of p16 protein, probably by gene methylation, is found in about 20% of primary gastric cancers regardless of their histological type (Yasui *et al.*, 1996b). In particular, loss of p16 protein is often seen in advanced cancers with nodal metastasis. Loss of p16 and p27 proteins may be associated with the progression of gastric carcinoma. Chen *et al.* (1997b) reported that aberrant RNA transcripts of the *p16* gene is noted in 30–45% of primary gastric cancers.

Iida *et al.* (2000) reported that the *p14* (*ARF*) gene is more frequently inactivated by LOH or DNA methylation in diffuse-type gastric cancer than in those of the intestinal type, suggesting that alterations of *p14* (*ARF*) may be involved in diffuse-type gastric carcinogenesis.

Major alterations in the *Rb* gene are also infrequent in primary gastric cancers (Constancia *et al.*, 1994). All primary tumours and all gastric cancer cell lines express pRb (Akama *et al.*, 1996b).

An important downstream target of cyclin/ CDKs at the G1/S transition is a family of E2F transcription factors. Gene amplification of *E2F-1* is seen in 4% of gastric cancers and 25% of colorectal cancers. Overexpression of E2F is found in 40% of primary gastric carcinomas (Suzuki *et al.*, 1999). Moreover, E2F and cyclin E tend to be co-expressed in gastric cancer. In contrast, 70% of gastric cancers exhibit lower levels of E2F-3 expression than corresponding non-neoplastic mucosas. These results suggest that gene amplification and anomalous expression of the *E2F* gene may permit the development of gastric cancer.

Cell-adhesion molecules and metastasis-related genes

Cell-adhesion molecules may also work as tumour suppressors. Mutations in the *E-cadherin* gene have been reported to occur preferentially in 50% of diffuse gastric carcinomas (Becker *et al.*, 1994). *E-cadherin* gene mutation is found in the diffuse component of mixed gastric carcinomas composed of both intestinal and diffuse types (Machado *et al.*, 1999). The results of Handschuh *et al.* (1999) indicate that *E-cadherin* mutations affecting exons 8 or 9 induce the scattered morphology, decrease cellular adhesion and increase cellular motility of diffuse gastric cancers. The mutations are even detected in intramucosal carcinoma (Muta *et al.,* 1996). *E-cadherin* germ-line mutations in familial gastric cancer have been reported since 1998, but their frequency is extremely rare (Guilford *et al.*, 1998; Iida *et al.*, 1999; Keller *et al.*, 1999; Yoon *et al.*, 1999). Kawanishi *et al.* (1995) found that a diffuse gastric carcinoma cell line, HSC-39, contained a mutation of the *β-catenin* gene. Moreover, Caca *et al.* (1999) reported that *β-* and *γ-catenin* mutations but not E-cadherin inactivation brought about constitutive Tcf transcriptional activity in gastric and pancreatic cancer cells. In addition to genetic alterations in *E-cadherin* and *β-catenin*, crosstalk between β-catenin and receptor tyrosine kinases including c-*met*, epidermal growth factor (EGF) receptor and c-*erb*B2 takes place in gastric cancer cells *in vitro* and *in vivo*, leading to diffuse spreading or scattering of gastric cancer cells

(Ochiai *et al.*, 1994; Shibata *et al.*, 1996). These results indicate that genetic and epigenetic alterations in E-cadherin and catenins are involved in the development and progression of diffuse and scirrhous-type gastric cancers.

The *CD44* gene contains at least 20 exons, 12 of which can be alternatively spliced to make up a wide variety of molecular variants (Cooper *et al.*, 1992; Matsumura & Tarin, 1992). We have found that expression of abnormal CD44 transcripts, including exon 11, is frequently associated with primary gastric carcinomas and metastatic tumours (Yokozaki *et al.*, 1994). Moreover, the pattern of abnormal CD44 transcripts in the tumours differs between intestinal and diffuse gastric cancers. More importantly, all gastric cancer tissues and gastric cancer cell lines show overexpression of abnormal CD44 transcripts containing the intron 9 sequence (Higashikawa *et al.*, 1996), suggesting that the abnormal CD44 transcript containing the intron 9 sequence is presumably an effective biomarker for early detection of gastric cancers. Sixty per cent of gastric intestinal metaplasias express CD44 variants containing an intron 9 sequence; normal gastric mucosa does not express these variants (Yoshida *et al.*, 1995).

Osteopontin (OPN), also termed Eta-1 (early T-lymphocyte activation-1), which is a reported protein ligand of CD44, is overexpressed in 73% of gastric carcinomas (Weber *et al.*, 1996). The co-expression of OPN and CD44v9 in tumour cells correlates with the degree of invasion of lymphatic vessels or distant lymph node metastasis in diffuse gastric cancer (Ue *et al.*, 1998). In particular, clustering of the tumour cells in lymphatic vessels shows strong co-expression of OPN and Cd44v9. Therefore, mutual interactions between OPN and CD44v9 on the tumour cells may be used by CD44-bearing diffuse gastric carcinomas to promote lymphogenous metastasis.

A candidate suppressor gene related to metastasis, *nm*23, encodes nucleoside diphosphate kinase which may activate c-*myc* transcription factor. Although LOH of the *nm*23 gene in gastric cancer is rare, the reduced expression of *nm*23, presumably as a result of epigenetic mechanisms, is frequently associated with metastasis of gastric cancer (Nakayama *et al.*, 1993). In addition to *nm*23, galectin-3 (known as lactoside-binding lactin L-31), which belongs to a family of galactoside-binding proteins, is frequently overexpressed in primary tumours and liver metastases of gastric cancer of the intestinal type (Lotan *et al.*, 1994). This higher expression of galectin-3 in gastric cancers and metastases implicates this lectin in the metastatic phenotype.

Amplification of c-*met* or K-*sam* in gastric cancer evidently contributes to progression and peritoneal invasion of diffuse gastric carcinoma. In addition, peritoneal dissemination requires LOH of 7q. Our study on deletion mapping of 7q has already demonstrated that LOH at the D7S95 locus is frequently associated with peritoneal dissemination (Kuniyasu *et al.*, 1994a). The D7S95 locus may contain a candidate suppressor gene for the progression and metastasis of gastric cancer.

Genetic instability

Two types of genetic instability involved are microsatellite instability (MSI) and chromosomal instability. MSI is caused by altered DNA mismatch repair. MSI has been found in 15–39% of sporadic gastric carcinomas worldwide (Semba *et al.*, 1996; Yokozaki *et al.*, 1999b). Gastric carcinomas with a high frequency of MSI (MSI-H) can be divided into two subtypes, intestinal and diffuse carcinomas, each of which has specific clinicopathological characteristics. Intestinal-type gastric cancers with MSI-H are often seen in patients over 73 years of age and often occur in the *antrum pylori*. They are frequently associated with abundant lymphoid infiltration, a putative favourable prognosis, and multiple tumours (Wu *et al.*, 1998; Leung *et al.*, 1999). Hypermethylation of the *hMLH1* gene promoter occurs in over 70% of cases with this type of gastric cancer and is often associated with downregulation or loss of *hMLH1* (Fleisher *et al.*, 1999; Leung *et al.*, 1999). This evidence indicates that MSI-H in intestinal-type gastric cancer is mostly due to epigenetic inactivation of the *hMLH1* gene.

On the other hand, diffuse-type gastric cancers with MSI-H occur mostly in patients under 35 years of age, and are often accompanied by scirrhous-type carcinoma with diffusely produc-

tive fibrosis (Semba *et al.*, 1998). However, diffuse-type gastric cancers harbour no germline mutation of *hMLH*1 and *hMSH2* and no alteration at *BAT-RII*. This type of gastric cancer is frequently associated with LOH on chromosome 17q21, including the *BRCA1* gene. However, we have found no mutation of the *BRCA1* gene. This raises two possibilities: (1) chromosome 17q12–21, including the *BRCA1* locus, may contain a candidate tumour suppressor gene; (2) allelic loss of the *BRCA1* gene may be linked to frequent genetic instability in young patients with gastric cancer.

Microsatellite instability at the locus D1S191 (chromosome 1q) is found in 46% of intestinal gastric cancers but not in diffuse-type gastric carcinomas. Microsatellite alteration at the same locus is also seen in 26% of incomplete-type intestinal metaplasias adjacent to primary gastric cancers. Moreover, an identical pattern of microsatellite alteration at the locus D1S191 is detected in both intestinal-type adenocarcinoma and the adjacent intestinal metaplasia, suggesting the sequential development of intestinal adenocarcinoma from incomplete intestinal metaplasia (Hamamoto *et al.*, 1997). The results described above indicate that MSI at the D1S191 locus is one of the early events in the multistep process of stomach carcinogenesis.

Chromosomal instability leading to DNA aneuploidy is also an underlying factor in stomach carcinogenesis. Telomere length is necessary for maintaining chromosomal stability. Recent evidence indicates that in the absence of telomerase, telomere shortening can produce telomere dysfunction that causes both DNA breaks and chromosome gain or loss (Chin *et al.*, 1999; Hackett *et al.*, 2001). Therefore, telomere dysfunction may initiate chromosomal instability in tumorigenesis. Conversely, telomerase can inhibit chromosomal instability (Hackett *et al.*, 2001). Most intestinal carcinomas have remarkably shortened telomere length, associated with high levels of telomerase activity and significant expression of human telomerase reverse transcriptase (hTERT) (Tahara *et al.*, 1995; Yasui *et al.*, 1998). More importantly, over 50% of intestinal metaplasias, as well as adenomas, express low levels of telomerase activity equivalent to about one-tenth of the activity in gastric carcinomas (Yasui *et al.*, 1999b).

Immunohistochemistry shows that the hTERT protein is strongly expressed in the nuclei of the tumour cells of all carcinomas but weakly expressed in the nuclei of epithelial cells of intestinal metaplasia and gastric adenoma and in normal fundic mucosa (Yasui *et al.*, 1998). Thus, hTERT-positive epithelial cells in the above precancerous lesions and normal gastric mucosa may be viewed as epithelial 'stem cells'. Moreover, the prevalence of *H. pylori* infection in gastric mucosa correlates well with the grade of intestinal metaplasia and the levels of hTERT and of telomerase activity; the latter is frequently associated with hyperplasia of hTERT-positive epithelial cells (Kuniyasu *et al.*, 1997b; Yasui *et al.*, 1999b). These observations indicate that *H. pylori* infection may be a strong trigger for hyperplasia of hTERT-positive cells in intestinal metaplasia, followed by increased telomerase activity and telomere reduction. Hyperplasia of hTERT-positive cells caused by *H. pylori* may induce 'chronic mitogenesis' which can facilitate increased mutagenesis. In fact, DNA hypermethylation at the D17S5 locus, *pS2* loss, abnormal CD44 transcripts, CA repeat instability at the D1S19 locus, and *APC* and *p53* mutations, all of which are commonly seen in intestinal gastric cancer, occur in over 30% of incomplete intestinal metaplasias (Tahara, 1998).

These data all indicate that telomere reduction and hTERT overexpression due to stem-cell hyperplasia are very early events in the multistep development of intestinal-type gastric cancer, followed by the above-mentioned epigenetic and genetic alterations. The frequent development of intestinal-type gastric cancer in elderly patients with *H. pylori* infection suggests that this type of gastric cancer is a disease of a 'chronically afflicted genome' rather than a genetic disease.

Telomerase-negative gastric carcinomas are only of the diffuse type, not the intestinal type, although their incidence is 13–15% (Tahara *et al.*, 1995). Diffuse-type gastric cancers occasionally harbour extremely long telomere length and have genetic alterations that are different from those of

carcinomas of the intestinal type. Hence, a telomerase-independent or alternative mechanism may be involved in neoplastic transformation and immortalization of the cells of some diffuse-type gastric cancers.

Mutations in the *p53* gene are also implicated in chromosomal instability. Recently Kaplan and co-workers found that mutation in *APC* may be responsible for chromosomal instability in colon cancer (Kaplan *et al.*, 2001). APC protein directly binds to a kinetochore protein and is an avid in-vitro substrate of the mitotic check-point protein Bub1 (Pellman, 2001). It remains to examine whether gastric cancer cells carrying a truncated *APC* gene are defective in chromosome segregation. Mutations of the *hBub1* gene have been reported in colon cancers (Cahill *et al.*, 1998). However, there is no mutation in the *hBub1* gene in gastric carcinomas (Shigeishi *et al.*, 2001).

Growth factors and cytokines

Gastric cancer cells express a broad spectrum of growth factors, cytokines or both, including TGF-α, TGF-β1, EGF, amphiregulin (AR), cripto, heparin binding (HB)-EGF, platelet-derived growth factor (PDGF), insulin-like growth factor (IGF) II, basic fibroblast growth factor (bFGF), interleukin (IL)-1α, IL-6, IL-8 and OPN (Tahara, 1993; Tahara *et al.*, 1994, 1996b; Tahara, 1997). These growth factors and cytokines function as autocrine, paracrine and juxtacrine modulators of the growth of cancer cells, and they organize the complex interaction between cancer cells and stromal cells which plays a key role in morphogenesis, invasion, neovascularization and metastasis. Interestingly, the expression of these growth factors, cytokines or both by cancer cells differs in the two histological types of gastric carcinoma. The EGF family, including EGF, TGF-α and cripto, is commonly overexpressed in intestinal-type gastric carcinoma, whereas TGF-β, IGF-II and bFGF are predominantly overexpressed in the diffuse type (Tahara *et al.*, 1999). Co-expression of EGF/TGF-α, EGF receptor and cripto correlates well with the biological malignancy of gastric cancer, because these factors induce metalloproteinases (Yasui *et al.*, 1988; Yoshida *et al.*, 1990; Kuniyasu *et al.*, 1994b). Overexpression of cripto is frequently associated with intestinal metaplasia and gastric adenoma (Kuniyasu *et al.*, 1991).

AR, a member of the EGF family which is overexpressed in more than 60% of gastric carcinomas regardless of histological type (Kitadai *et al.*, 1993a), works as an autocrine growth factor and induces the expression of AR itself, TGF-α and EGF receptors by gastric cancer cells (Akagi *et al.*, 1995). Overexpression of the EGF family in gastric cancer usually does not accompany gene amplifications. The relative expression levels of positive transcription factor, Sp-1, and negative transcription factor, GC factor, may regulate gene expression of these growth factors and receptors (Kitadai *et al.*, 1993b).

IL-1α is a cytokine mainly produced by activated macrophages and mediates many of the local and systemic responses to infection and inflammation (Dinarello, 1992). It is also produced by gastric cancer cells. We have found that IL-1α evidently acts as an autocrine growth factor for gastric carcinoma cells and plays a pivotal role as a trigger for induction of EGF and EGF receptor expression (Ito *et al.*, 1993). The expression of IL-1α by tumour cells is induced by either IL-1α, EGF or TGF-α, while IL-1α up-regulates the expression of TGF-α and EGF receptor by tumour cells themselves, indicating that an intimate interplay between IL-1α and the EGF/receptor system stimulates the growth of gastric cancer.

In addition to IL-1α, IL-6 is also an autocrine growth stimulator for gastric cancer cells. The expression of IL-1α by tumour cells is induced by IL-6, while IL-1α increases the expression of IL-6 by tumour cells themselves (Ito *et al.*, 1997).

Stromal cells, especially fibroblasts stimulated by growth factors or cytokines such as IL-α, TGF-α and TGF-β, secrete HGF/SF (hepatocyte growth factor/scatter factor), which can function in a paracrine manner as a morphogen or motogen of tumour cells. For example, in the case of a clone maintaining expression of cell-adhesion molecules, HGF/SF promotes tubular formation of tumour cells, resulting in intestinal-type gastric cancer. Conversely, in the case of a clone with reduced expression of cell-adhesion molecules, HGF/SF can act as a motogen and induce scatte-

ring of tumour cells, resulting in diffuse gastric cancer (Tahara, 1993; Yokozaki *et al.*, 1997). Our recent findings suggest that interaction between c-*met* overexpressed in tumour cells and HGF/SF from stromal cells is related to the morphogenesis and progression of gastric cancer *in vivo*.

The negative growth factor TGF-β1 is commonly overexpressed in gastric carcinoma, particularly in diffuse-type carcinoma with diffusely productive fibrosis (Yoshida *et al.*, 1989). However, most human gastric cancer cells have escaped from TGF-β-induced growth inhibition at the receptor or post-receptor levels. TGF-β inhibited the growth of only one (TMK-1) of seven gastric carcinoma cell lines; this inhibition is associated with p53-independent induction of p21 which induces suppression of cyclin-dependent kinase activity, reduced phosphorylation of Rb and a decrease in cyclin A (Ito *et al.*, 1992a; Akagi *et al.*, 1996). Various mutations in the *TGF-β* receptor type II (RII) gene have been reported in gastric cancer. One type of mutation in the *TGF-βRII* gene is mutation in the polyA tract (i.e. deletion or insertion of 1–2 bases) that frequently occurs in the hereditary non-polyposis colon cancer syndrome (Markowitz *et al.*, 1995) and in gastric carcinoma with MSI-H (Yokozaki *et al.*, 1999b). Another type of mutation in the *TGF-βRII* gene involves abnormal amplification and truncation of the gene (Yang *et al.*, 1999). However, we have not seen genetic alterations of the *TGF-βRII* gene in any gastric carcinoma cell lines. Moreover, results of a study on expression of TGF-βRI in TGF-β-resistant gastric cancer cell lines that contain no discernible alteration in the *TGF-βRII* gene suggest that hypermethylation of a CpG island in the 5' region of the *TGF-βRI* gene is involved in another potentially important mechanism of escape from negative growth control by TGF-β (Kim *et al.*, 1999). We have already found that most gastric carcinomas show reduced levels of TGF-βRI and that this correlates well with the depth of tumour invasion (Ito *et al.*, 1992b).

A large number of angiogenic factors have been identified in human malignancy. Among them are vascular endothelial growth factor (VEGF), basic fibroblast growth factor (bFGF) and IL-8, which are derived from tumour cells and participate mainly in neovascularization within gastric carcinoma tissues. We have shown that all eight gastric cancer cell lines secrete VEGF into conditioned media (Yamamoto *et al.*, 1998). EGF or IL-1α up-regulates VEGF expression by tumour cells, whereas interferon-γ down-regulates it. Moreover, VEGF promotes angiogenesis and the progression of gastric carcinomas, especially carcinomas of the intestinal type (Takahashi *et al.*, 1996). On the other hand, bFGF produced by tumour cells is frequently associated with angiogenesis and extensive fibrosis in diffuse gastric carcinomas, particularly those of the scirrhous type (Tanimoto *et al.*, 1991).

IL-8, a member of the CXC chemokine family, induces haptotactic migration and proliferation of melanoma cells and angiogenesis. More importantly, gastric carcinoma cell lines express mRNA and protein for IL-8 and IL-8 receptors (IL-8RA and IL-8RB) (Kitadai *et al.*, 1998, 2000). More than 80% of gastric carcinomas co-express IL-8 and IL-8 receptors; this co-expression correlates directly with tumour vascularity and disease progression. IL-8 enhances the expression of EGF receptor, type IV collagenase (metalloproteinase (MMP)-9), VEGF and IL-8 mRNA itself by gastric cancer cells, whereas IL-8 decreases expression of E-cadherin mRNA. In addition, IL-8 also increases MMP-9 activity and the ability of gastric cancer cells to invade through Matrigel. Altogether, IL-8 may play an important role in the growth and progression of gastric carcinoma by autocrine and paracrine mechanisms.

Factors associated with increased incidence of gastric cancer

Three major factors, including environmental factors, host factors and genetic factors, cooperatively affect the genesis of gastric cancer (Table 2). Of these, environmental factors are the most important, as diet and cigarette smoking are primary offenders; in particular, the presence of carcinogens such as *N*-nitroso compounds and benzo[*a*]pyrene is directly linked to carcinogenesis. As already described, the mutation spectrum of the *p53* gene differs between intestinal-type and diffuse-type gastric cancers,

Table 2. Factors associated with increased incidence of gastric carcinoma

Environmental factors	Diet (nitrites derived from nitrates, smoked and salted food, pickled vegetables, lack of fresh fruit and vegetables) Cigarette smoking
Host factors	*H. pylori* infection (chronic gastric and intestinal metaplasia) Partial gastrectomy Barrett esophagus
Genetic factors	Hereditary diffuse gastric cancer Hereditary non-polyposis colon cancer DNA polymorphism Genetic instability

suggesting that different carcinogens may be implicated in the two types of gastric carcinogenesis (Yokozaki *et al.*, 1997). Palli *et al.* (2001) found that the risk of MSI-H gastric cancer was positively associated with high consumption of red meat and meat sauce, and negatively associated with consumption of white meat.

With regard to host factors, meta-analysis of the relationship between *H. pylori* infection and gastric cancer has indicated that *H. pylori* infection is associated with a twofold increased risk of gastric cancer (Huang *et al.*, 1998; Eslick *et al.*, 1999). Younger *H. pylori*-infected patients have a higher relative risk for gastric cancer than older patients. *H. pylori* infection is equally associated with intestinal-type and diffuse-type gastric cancers (Huang *et al.*, 1998). In fact, the findings in a Mongolian gerbil model of stomach carcinogenesis indicate that *H. pylori* infection promotes stomach carcinogenesis induced by chemical carcinogens, and that histological types of gastric carcinoma may depend on the concentration of chemical carcinogens rather than on *H. pylori* infection (Shimizu *et al.*, 1999). Eradication of the bacteria evidently decreases the incidence of gastric carcinomas in the Mongolian gerbil model (Shimizu *et al.*, 2000).

H. pylori infection produces reactive oxygen and nitrogen species that cause DNA damage, followed by chronic gastric and intestinal metaplasia (Correa *et al.*, 1997). Goto *et al.* (1999) reported that the expression of inducible nitric oxide synthase (iNOS) and nitrotyrosine in the gastric mucosa was significantly high in *H. pylori*-infected patients who developed gastric cancer at least 2 years after the initial biopsies. These findings suggest that high production of iNOS and nitrotyrosine in the gastric mucosa by *H. pylori* may contribute to gastric carcinogenesis.

Cyclooxygenase-2 (Cox-2) expression is also induced by *H. pylori* infection (Sung *et al.*, 2000). Successful eradication of *H. pylori* leads to down-regulation of Cox-2 in the epithelial and stromal cells. High expression of Cox-2 mRNA, protein and enzymatic activity is detected preferentially in the tumour cells of intestinal-type gastric cancer (Saukkonen *et al.*, 2001). Loss of Cox-2 promoter methylation may enhance Cox-2 expression and promote gastric carcinogenesis associated with *H. pylori* infection (Akhtar *et al.*, 2001).

It should not be forgotten that in Japan the annual incidence of gastric cancer is about 100 000, accounting for 0.16% of 60 million individuals with *H. pylori* infection. Moreover, analysis of chromosomal aberrations in gastric cancer shows that they do not differ between *H. pylori*-related and non-related gastric cancers (van Grieken *et al.*, 2000). Genetic factors play a critical role in susceptibility to stomach carcinogenesis (Table 3).

Prinz *et al.* (2001) reported that cagA+/vacAs1+ strains of *H. pylori* that are blood-group antigen-binding adhesion (BabA2)-positive are associated with activity or chronicity of gastritis. Adherence of *H. pylori* via BabA2 may play a key role for efficient delivery of VacA and CagA.

In addition to *H. pylori* strains, DNA polymorphism including HLA, MUC1 (Carvalho *et al.*, 1997), T-cell helper 1 and IL-1β has been reported to be associated with an increased risk of both atrophic gastritis induced by *H. pylori* and gastric cancer (El-Omar *et al.*, 2000). More excitingly, Magnusson *et al.* (2001) found that distinct HLA class II DQ and DR alleles are associated with the development of gastric cancer and infection with *H. pylori*. The DQA1*0102 is associated with protection from *H. pylori* infection, whereas the DRB*1601 is associated with cancer deve-

Table 3. Susceptibility to disease caused by *H. pylori*	
Strain of *H. pylori*	CagA+/VacAs1+strains that are BabA2-positive (Printz *et al.*, 2001)
Genetic factors	*HLA* polymorphism: *HLA*-DQA1 genetic typing
	MUC1 polymorphism
	T-cell helper 1 phenotype
	IL-1β polymorphism
	HLA DR and DQ alleles: DQA1*0102 is associated with protection from infection by *H. pylori*, whereas DRB*1601 is associated with cancer development, particularly *H. pylori*-negative diffuse type (Magnusson *et al.*, 2001).

lopment, particularly *H. pylori*-negative diffuse gastric cancer. These host genetic factors may determine why some individuals infected with *H. pylori* develop gastric cancer while others do not. However, these studies need confirmation by a large number of prospective investigations in each of the countries concerned.

Conclusion

Overall, the observations on the molecular events of gastric cancer may provide supporting evidence for our working hypothesis that there are two distinct major genetic pathways for stomach carcinogenesis (Figure 1). Genetic and epigenetic alterations found in two types of gastric cancer are summarized in Table 1. Among them, genetic instability including MIS and telomere reduction and immortality (activation of telomerase and expression of hTERT) are implicated in an initial step of stomach carcinogenesis. In the multistep process of intestinal-type gastric carcinogenesis, infection with *H. pylori* may be a strong trigger for hyperplasia of hTERT-positive stem cells in intestinal metaplasia. Genetic instability and hyperplasia of hTERT-positive stem cells may precede replication error at the D1S191 locus, DNA hypermethylation at the D17S5 locus, *pS2* loss, *RARβ* loss, CD44 abnormal transcripts and *p53* mutation, all of which accumulate in at least 30% of incomplete intestinal metaplasias. All of these epigenetic and genetic alterations are common events in intestinal-type gastric cancer. Incomplete intestinal metaplasia that contains an accumulation of the above multiple molecular events – that is, 'metaplastic dysplasia' – may be viewed as a bud of intestinal-type gastric cancer at genetic and epigenetic levels. An adenoma→carcinoma sequence is found in about 20% of gastric adenomas with *APC* mutations. In addition to these events, *p53* mutation and LOH, reduced p27 expression, cyclin E expression and presence of c-*met* 6.0-kb transcripts allow malignant transformation from the precancerous lesions to intestinal-type gastric cancer. *DCC* loss, *APC* mutations, 1q LOH, *p27* loss, reduced TGF-βRI expression, reduced nm23 expression and c-*erb*B gene amplification are implicated in the progression and metastasis of intestinal-type gastric cancer. Another pathway for carcinogenesis of intestinal-type gastric cancer involves LOH and abnormal expression of the *p73* gene that may be responsible for the development of foveolar-type gastric cancers with pS2 expression.

On the other hand, LOH at chromosome 17p, mutation or LOH of *p53* and mutation or loss of *E-cadherin* are preferentially involved in the development of diffuse gastric cancers. In addition to these changes, gene amplification of K-*sam* and c-*met* and *p27* loss as well as reduced nm23 obviously confer progression, metastasis and diffusely productive fibrosis.

Mixed gastric carcinomas composed of intestinal and diffuse components exhibit some but not all of the molecular events described for each of the two types of gastric cancer.

References

Akagi, M., Yokozaki, H., Kitadai, Y., Ito, R., Yasui, W., Haruma, K., Kajiyama, G. & Tahara, E. (1995) Expression of amphiregulin in human gastric cancer cell lines. *Cancer*, **75**, 1460–1466

Akagi, M., Yasui, W., Akama, Y., Yokozaki, H., Tahara, H., Haruma, K. Kajiyama, G. & Tahara, E. (1996) Inhibition of cell growth by transforming growth factor beta-1 is associated with p53-independent induction of p21 in gastric cells. *Jpn. J. Cancer Res.*, **87**, 377–384

Akama, Y., Yasui, W., Yokozaki, H., Kuniyasu, H., Kitahara, K., Ishikawa, T. & Tahara, E. (1995) Frequent amplification of the cyclin E gene in human gastric carcinomas. *Jpn. J. Cancer Res.*, **86**, 617–621

Akama, Y., Yasui, W., Kuniyasu, H., Yokozaki, H., Akagi, M., Tahara, H., Ishikawa, T. & Tahara, E. (1996a) Genetic status and expression of the cyclin-dependent kinase inhibitors in human gastric carcinoma cell lines. *Jpn. J. Cancer Res.*, **87**, 824–830

Akama, Y., Yasui, W., Kuniyasu, H., Yokozaki, H., Akagi, M., Tahara, H., Ishikawa, T. & Tahara, E. (1996b) No point mutations but a codon 31 polymorphism and decreased expression of the p21 SDI1/WAF1/CIP1/MDA6 gene in human gastric carcinomas. *Mol. Cell Differ.*, **4**, 187–198

Akhtar, M., Cheng, Y., Magno, R.M., Ashktorab, H., Smoot, D.T., Meltszer, S. J. & Wilson, K.T. (2001) Promoter methylation regulates *Helicobacter pylori*-stimulated cyclooxygenase-2 expression in gastric epithelial cells. *Cancer Res.*, **61**, 2399–2403

Ayhan, A., Yasui, W., Yokozaki, H., Seto, M., Ueda, R. & Tahara, E. (1994) Loss of heterozygosity at the bcl-2 gene locus and expression of bcl-2 in human gastric and colorectal carcinomas. *Jpn. J. Cancer Res.*, **85**, 584–591

Baffa, R., Veronese, M.L., Santoro, R., Mandes, B., Palazzo, J.P., Rugge, M., Santoro, E., Croce, C.M. & Huebner, K. (1998) Loss of FHIT expression in gastric carcinoma. *Cancer Res.*, **58**, 4708–4714

Becker, K.F., Atkinson, M.J., Reich, U., Becker, I., Nekarda, H., Siewert, J.R. & Hofler, H. (1994) E-cadherin gene mutations provide clues to diffuse type gastric carcinomas. *Cancer Res.*, **54**, 3845–3852

Caca, K., Kolligs, F.T., Ji, X., Hayes, M., Qian, J., Yahanda, A., Rimm, D.L., Costa, J. & Fearon, E.R. (1999) Beta- and gamma-catenin mutations, but not E-cadherin inactivation, underlie T-cell factor/lymphoid enhancer factor transcriptional deregulation in gastric and pancreatic cancer. *Cell Growth Differ.*, **10**, 369–376

Cahill, D.P., Lengauer, C., Yu, J., Riggins, G.J., Willson, J.K.V., Markowitz, S.D., Kinzler, K.W. & Vogelstein, B. (1998) Mutations of mitotic checkpoint genes in human cancers. *Nature*, **392**, 300–303

Carvalho, F., Seruca, R., David, L., Amorim, A., Seixas, M., Bennett, E., Clausen, H. & Sobrinho-

Simoes, M. (1997) MUC1 gene polymorphism and gastric cancer – an epidemiological study. *Glycoconj. J.*, **14**, 107–111

Chen, Y.J., Chen, P.H., Lee, M.D. & Chang, J.G. (1997a) Aberrant FHIT transcripts in cancerous and corresponding non-cancerous lesions of the digestive tract. *Int. J. Cancer*, **17**, 955–958

Chen, Y.J., Chang, J.G., Shih, L.S., Chen, P.H., Endo, M., Whang-Peng, J. & Chen, Y.M. (1997b) Frequent detection of aberrant RNA transcripts of the CDKN2 gene in human gastric adenocarcinoma. *Int. J. Cancer*, **71**, 350–354

Chin, L., Artandi, S., Shen Q., Tam, A., Lee, S.-L., Gottlieb, G.J., Greider, C.W. & DePinho, R.A. (1999) p53 Deficiency rescues the adverse effects of telomere loss and cooperates with telomere dysfunction to accelerate carcinogenesis. *Cell*, **97**, 527–538

Constancia, M., Seruca, R., Carneiro, F., Silva, F. & Castedo, S. (1994) Retinoblastoma gene structure and product expression in human gastric carcinomas. *Br. J. Cancer*, **70**, 1018–1024

Cooper, D.L., Dougherty, G., Harn, H.J., Jackson, S., Baptist, E.W., Byers, J., Datta, A., Phillips, G. & Isola, N.R. (1992) The complex CD44 transcriptional unit; alternative splicing of three internal exons generates the epithelial form of CD44. *Biochem. biophys. Res. Commun.*, **182**, 569–578

Correa, P., Miller, M. & Mannick, E.E. (1997) Oxidative damage during the gastric precancerous process. In: Tahara, E., ed., *Molecular Pathology of Gastroenterological Cancer: Application to Clinical Practice*, Tokyo, Springer-Verlag, pp. 23–29

Dinarello, C.A (1992) The biology of interleukin-1. *Chem. Immunol.*, **51**, 1-32

El-Omar, E.M., Carrington, M., Chow, W.H., McColl, K.E., Bream, J.H., Young, H.A., Herrera, J., Lissowska, J., Yuan, C.C., Rothman, N., Lanyon. G., Martin, M., Fraumeni, J.F., Jr & Rabkin, C.S. (2000) Interleukin-1 polymorphisms associated with increased risk of gastric cancer. *Nature*, **404**, 398–402

Eslick, G.D., Lim, L.L., Byles, J.E., Xia, H.H. & Talley, N.J. (1999) Association of *Helicobacter pylori* infection with gastric carcinoma: a meta-analysis. *Am. J. Gastroenterol.*, **94**, 2373–2379

Fleisher, A.S., Esteller, M., Wang, S., Tamura, G., Suzuki, H., Yin, J., Zou, T.-T., Abraham, J.M.,

Kong, D., Smolinski, K.N., Shi, Y-Q., Rhyu, M.-G., Powell, S.M., James, S.P., Wilson, K.T., Herman, J.G. & Meltzer, S.J. (1999) Hypermethylation of the hMLH1 gene promoter in human gastric cancers with microsatellite instability. *Cancer Res.*, **59**, 1090–1095

Fujimoto, J., Yasui, W., Tahara, H., Tahara, E., Kudo, Y., Yokozaki, H. & Tahara, E. (2000) DNA hypermethylation at the pS2 promoter region is associated with early stage of stomach carcinogenesis. *Cancer Lett.*, **149**, 125–134

Goto, T., Haruma, K., Kitadai, Y., Ito, M., Yoshimura, M., Sumii, K., Hayakawa, N. & Kajiyama, G. (1999) Enhanced expression of inducible nitric oxide synthase and nitrotyrosine in gastric mucosa of gastric cancer patients. *Clin. Cancer Res.*, **5**, 1411–1415

van Grieken, N.C.T., Weiss, M.M., Meijer, G.A., Hermsen, M.A.J.A., Scholte, G.H.A. Lindeman, J., Craanen, M.E., Bloemena, E., Meuwissen, S.G.M., Baak, J.P.A. & Kuipers, E.J. (2000) *Helicobacter pylori*-related and -non-related gastric cancers do not differ with respect to chromosomal aberrations. *J. Pathol.*, **192**, 301–306

Guilford, P., Hopkins, J., Harraway, J., McLeod, M., McLeod, N., Harawira, P., Taite, H., Scoular, R. & Miller, A. & Reeve, A.E. (1998) E-Cadherin germline mutations in familial gastric cancer. *Nature*, **392**, 402–405

Gunther, T., Schneider-Stock, R., Pross, M., Manger, T., Malgertheiner, P., Lippert, H. & Roessner, A. (1998) Alterations of the p16/MTS1-tumor suppressor gene in gastric cancer. *Pathol. Res. Pract.*, **194**, 809–813

Hackett, J.A., Feldser, D.M. & Greider, C.W. (2001) Telomere dysfunction increases mutation rate and genomic instability. *Cell*, **106**, 275–286

Hamamoto, T., Yokozaki, H., Semba, S., Yasui, W., Yunotani, S., Miyazaki, K. & Tahara, E. (1997) Altered microsatellites in incomplete-type intestinal metaplasia adjacent to primary gastric cancers. *J. clin. Pathol.*, **50**, 841–846

Hamilton, S.R. & Aaltonen, L.A., eds (2000) *Pathology and Genetics of Tumours of the Digestive System* (World Health Organization Classification of Tumours), Lyon, IARC*Press*, p. 38

Handschuh, G., Candidus, S., Luber, B., Reich, U., Schott, C., Oswald, S., Becke, H., Hutzler, P.,

Birchmeier, W., Hofler, H. & Becker, K.F. (1999) Tumour-associated E-cadherin mutations alter cellular morphology, decrease cellular adhesion and increase cellular motility. *Oncogene*, **18**, 4301–4312

Harper, J.W., Adami, G.R., Wei, N., Keyomarsi, K. & Elledge, S.J. (1993) The p21 Cdk-interacting protein Cip1 is a potent inhibitor of G1 cyclin-dependent kinases. *Cell*, **75**, 805–816

Harris, C.C (1991) Chemical and physical carcinogenesis: advances and perspectives for the 1990s. *Cancer Res.*, **51** (Suppl. 18), 5023s–5044s

Hattori, Y., Odagiri, H., Nakatani, H., Miyagawa, K., Naito, K., Sakamoto, H., Katoh, O., Yoshida,T., Sugimura, T. & Terada, M. (1990) K-*sam*, an amplified gene in stomach cancer, is a member of the heparin-binding growth factor receptor genes. *Proc. natl Acad. Sci. USA*, **87**, 5983–5987

Hayashi, K., Yokozaki, H., Naka K., Yasui, W., Lotan, R. & Tahara, E. (2001a) Overexpression of retinoic acid receptor induces growth arrest and apoptosis in oral cancer cell lines. *Jpn. J. Cancer Res.*, **92**, 42–50

Hayashi, K., Yokozaki, H., Goodison, S., Oue, N., Suzuki, T., Lotan, R., Yasui, W. & Tahara, E. (2001b) Inactivation of retinoic acid receptor β by promoter CpG hypermethylation in gastric cancer. *Differentiation*, **68**, 13–21

Higashikawa, K., Yokozaki, H., Ue, T., Taniyama, K., Ishikawa, T., Tarin, D. & Tahara, E. (1996) Evaluation of CD44 transcription variants in human digestive tract carcinomas and normal tissues. *Int. J. Cancer*, **66**, 11–17

Honda, R., Ohba, Y., Nagata, A., Okayama, H. & Yasuda, H. (1993) Dephosphorylation of human p34cdc2 kinase on both Thr-14 and Tyr-15 by human cdc25B phosphatase. *FEBS Lett.*, **318**, 331–334

Huang, J.Q., Sridhar, S., Chen, Y. & Hunt, R.H. (1998) Meta-analysis of the relationship between *Helicobacter pylori* seropositivity and gastric cancer. *Gastroenterology*, **114**, 1169–1179

Igaki, H., Sasaki, H., Tachimori, Y., Kato, H., Watanabe, H., Kitamura, T., Harada, Y., Sugimura, T. & Terada, M. (1995) Mutation frequency of the p16/CDKN2 gene in primary cancers in the upper digestive tract. *Cancer Res.*, **55**, 3421–3423

Iida, S., Akiyama, Y., Ichikawa, W., Yamashita, T., Nomizu, T., Nihei, Z., Sugihara, K. & Yuasa, Y.

(1999) Infrequent germ-line mutation of the E-cadherin gene in Japanese familial gastric cancer kindreds. *Clin. Cancer Res.*, **5**, 1445–1447

Iida, S., Akiyama, Y., Nakajima, T., Ichikawa, W., Nihei, Z., Sugihara, K. & Yuasa, Y. (2000) Alterations and hypermethylation of the p14(ARF) gene in gastric cancer. *Int. J. Cancer*, **87**, 654–658

Isogaki, J., Shinmura, K., Yin, W., Arai, T., Kodo, K., Kimura, T., Kino, I. & Sugimura, H. (1999) Microsatellite instability and K-ras mutations in gastric adenomas, with reference to associated gastric cancers. *Cancer Detect. Prev.*, **23**, 204–214

Ito, M., Yasui, W., Kyo, E., Yokozaki, H., Nakayama, H., Ito, H. & Tahara, E. (1992a) Growth inhibition of transforming growth factor-beta on human gastric carcinoma cells: receptor and postreceptor signaling. *Cancer Res.*, **52**, 295–300

Ito, M., Yasui, W., Nakayama, H., Yokozaki, H., Ito, H. & Tahara, E. (1992b) Reduced levels of transforming growth factor-beta type I receptor in human gastric carcinomas. *Jpn. J. Cancer Res.*, **83**, 86–92

Ito, R., Kitadai, Y., Kyo, E., Yokozaki, H., Yasui, W., Yamashita, U., Nikai, H. & Tahara, E. (1993) Interleukin 1α acts as autocrine growth stimulator for human gastric carcinoma cells. *Cancer Res.*, **53**, 4102–4106

Ito, R., Yasui, W., Kuniyasu, H., Yokozaki, H. & Tahara, E. (1997) Expression of interleukin-6 and its effect on the cell growth of gastric carcinoma cell lines. *Jpn. J. Cancer Res.*, **88**, 953–958

JRSGC (Japanese Research Society for Gastric Cancer) (1999) *Japanese Classification of Gastric Carcinoma*, 13th Ed., Tokyo, Kanehara

Jinno, S., Suto, K., Nagata, A., Igarashi, M., Kanaoka, Y., Nojima, H. & Okayama, H. (1994) Cdc25A is a novel phosphatase functioning early in the cell cycle. *EMBO J.*, **13**, 1549–1556

Kameda, T., Yasui, W., Yoshida, K., Tsujino, T., Nakayama, H., Ito, M., Ito, H. & Tahara, E. (1990) Expression of ERBB2 in human gastric carcinomas: relationship between p185 ERBB2 expression and the gene amplification. *Cancer Res.*, **50**, 8002–8009

Kaplan, K.B., Burds, A.A., Swedlow, J.R., Bekir, S.S., Sorger, P.K. & Näthke, I.S. (2001) A role for the adenomatous polyposis coli protein in chromosome segregation. *Nature Cell Biol.*, **3**, 429–432

Katoh, M. & Terada, M (1993) Oncogenes and tumor suppressor genes. In: Nishi, M., Ichikawa, H., Nakajima, T., Maruyama, K., Tahara, E., eds, *Gastric Cancer*, Tokyo, Springer-Verlag, pp. 196–208

Katoh, M., Hattori, Y., Sasaki, H., Tanaka, M., Sugano, K., Yazaki, Y., Sugimura, T. & Terada, M. (1992) K-*sam* Gene encodes secreted as well as transmembrane receptor tyrosine kinase. *Proc. natl Acad. Sci. USA*, **89**, 2960–2964

Kawanishi, J., Kato, J., Sasaki, K., Fujii, S., Watanabe, N. & Niitsu, Y. (1995) Loss of E-cadherin-dependent cell-cell adhesion due to mutation of the beta-catenin gene in a human cancer cell line, HSC-39. *Mol. cell. Biol.*, **15**, 1175–1181

Keller, G., Vogelsang, H., Becker, I., Hutter, J., Ott, K., Candidus, S., Grundei, T., Becker, K.F., Meuller, J., Siewert, J.R. & Hofler, H. (1999) Diffuse type gastric and lobular breast carcinoma in a familial gastric cancer patient with an E-cadherin germline mutation. *Am. J. Pathol.*, **155**, 337–342

Kim, S.-J., Yang, H.K., Im, Y.-H., Bang, Y.J. & Yang, H.K. (1999) Mechanisms of TGF-β receptor inactivation and development of resistance to TGF-β in human gastric cancer. In: *Proceedings of the Third International Gastric Cancer Congress, Seoul*, Bologna, Monduzzi Editore, pp. 81–90

Kinzler, K.W., Nilbert, M.C., Su, L.K., Vogelstein, B., Bryan, T.M., Levy, D.B., Smith, K.J., Preisinger, A.C., Hedge, P., McKechnie, D., Finniear, R., Markham, A., Groffen, J., Boguski, M.S., Altschul, S.F., Horii, A., Miyoshi, Y., Miki, Y., Nishisho, I. & Nakamura, Y. (1991) Identification of FAP locus genes from chromosome 5q21. *Science*, **253**, 661–665

Kitadai, Y., Yasui, W., Yokozaki, H., Kuniyasu, H., Ayhan, A., Haruma, K., Kajiyama, G., Johnson, G.R. & Tahara, E. (1993a) Expression of amphiregulin, a novel gene of the epidermal growth factor family, in human gastric carcinomas. *Jpn. J. Cancer Res.*, **84**, 879–884

Kitadai, Y., Yamazaki, H., Yasui, W., Kyo, E., Yokozaki, H., Kajiyama, G., Johnson, A.C., Pastan, I. & Tahara, E. (1993b) GC factor represses transcription of several growth factor/receptor genes and causes growth inhibition of human gastric carcinoma cell lines. *Cell Growth Differ.*, **4**, 291–296

Kitadai, Y., Haruma, K., Sumii, K., Yamamoto, S., Ue, T., Yokozaki, H., Yasui, W., Ohmoto, Y., Kajiyama, G., Fidler, I.J. & Tahara, E. (1998) Expression of interleukin-8 correlates with vascularity in human gastric carcinomas. *Am. J. Pathol.*, **152**, 93–100

Kitadai, Y., Haruma, K., Mukaida, N., Ohmoto, Y., Matsutani, N., Yasui, W., Yamamoto, S., Sumii, K., Kajiyama, G., Fidler, I.J. & Tahara, E. (2000) Regulation of disease-progression genes in human gastric carcinoma cells by interleukin-8. *Clin. Cancer Res.*, **6**, 2735–2740

Kudo, Y., Yasui, W., Ue, T., Yamamoto, S., Yokozaki, H., Nikai, H. & Tahara, E. (1997) Overexpression of cyclin-dependent kinase-activating CDC25B phosphatase in human gastric carcinomas. *Jpn. J. Cancer Res.*, **88**, 947–952

Kuniyasu, H., Yoshida, K., Yokozaki, H., Yasui, W., Ito, H., Toge, T., Ciardiello, F., Persico, M.G., Saeki, T., Salomon, D.S. & Tahara, E. (1991) Expression of cripto, a novel gene of the epidermal growth factor family, in human gastrointestinal carcinomas. *Jpn. J. Cancer Res.*, **82**, 969–973

Kuniyasu, H., Yasui, W., Kitadai, Y., Yokozaki, H., Ito, H. & Tahara, E. (1992) Frequent amplification of the c-*met* gene in scirrhous type stomach cancer. *Biochem. biophys. Res. Commun.*, **189**, 227–232

Kuniyasu, H., Yasui, W., Yokozaki, H., Kitadai, Y. & Tahara, E. (1993) Aberrant expression of c-met mRNA in human gastric carcinomas. *Int. J. Cancer*, **55**, 72–75

Kuniyasu, H., Yasui, W., Yokozaki, H., Akagi, M., Akama, Y., Kitahara, K., Fujii, K. & Tahara, E. (1994a) Frequent loss of heterozygosity of the long arm of chromosome 7 is closely associated with progression of human gastric carcinomas. *Int. J. Cancer*, **59**, 597–600

Kuniyasu, H., Yasui, W., Akama, Y., Akagi, H., Tohdo, H., Ji, Z.-Q., Kitadai, Y., Yokozaki, H. & Tahara, E. (1994b) Expression of cripto in human gastric carcinomas: an association with tumor stage and prognosis. *J. exp. clin. Cancer Res.*, **13**, 151–157

Kuniyasu, H., Yasui, W., Kitahara, K., Naka, K., Yokozaki, H., Akama, Y., Hamamoto, T., Tahara, H. & Tahara, E. (1997a) Growth inhibitory effect of interferon-β is associated with the induction of cyclin-dependent kinase inhibitor p27 Kip1 in a human gastric carcinoma cell line. *Cell Growth Differ.*, **8**, 47–52

Kuniyasu, H., Domen, T., Hamamoto, T., Yokozaki, H., Yasui, W., Tahara, H. & Tahara, E. (1997b) Expression of human telomerase RNA is an early event of stomach carcinogenesis. *Jpn. J. Cancer Res.*, **88**, 103–107

Lauren, P. (1965) The two histological main types of gastric carcinoma. Diffuse and so-called intestinal type carcinoma. An attempt at histochemical classification. *Acta pathol. microbiol. Scand.*, **64**, 31–49

Lee, K.H., Lee, J.S., Suh, C., Kim, S.W., Kim, S.B., Lee, J.H., Lee, M.S., Park, M.Y., Sun, H.S. & Kim, S.H. (1995) Clinicopathologic significance of the K-ras gene codon 12 point mutation in stomach cancer. An analysis of 140 cases. *Cancer*, **75**, 2794–2801

Lee, Y.Y., Kang, S.H., Seo, J.Y., Jung, C.W., Lee, K.U., Choe, K.J., Kim, B.K., Kim, N.K., Koeffler, H.P. & Bang, Y.J. (1997) Alterations of p16INK4A and p15INK4B genes in gastric carcinomas. *Cancer*, **80**, 1889–1896

Lefebvre, O., Chenard, M.P., Masson, R., Linares, J., Dierich, A., LeMeur, M., Wendling, C., Tomasetto, C., Chambon, P. & Rio, M.C. (1996) Gastric mucosa abnormalities and tumorigenesis in mice lacking the pS2 trefoil protein. *Science*, **274**, 259–262

Leung, S.Y., Yuen, S.T., Chung, L.P., Chu, K.M., Chan, A.S.Y. & Ho, J.C.I. (1999) hMLH1 promoter methylation and lack of hMLH1 expression in sporadic gastric carcinomas with high-frequency microsatellite instability. *Cancer Res.*, **59**, 159–164

Lotan, R., Ito, H., Yasui, W., Yokozaki, H., Lotan, D. & Tahara, E. (1994) Expression of a 31-kDa lactoside-binding lectin in normal human gastric mucosa and in primary and metastatic gastric carcinomas. *Int. J. Cancer*, **56**, 474–480

Lotan, R., Xu, C., Lippman, S.M., Ro, J.Y., Lee, J.S., Lee, J.J. & Hong, W.K. (1995) Suppression of retinoic acid receptor β in premalignant oral lesions and its upregulation by isotretinoin. *New Engl. J. Med.*, **332**, 1405–1410

Machado, J.C., Soares, P., Carneiro, F., Rocha, A., Beck, S., Blin, N., Berx, G. & Sobrinho-Simoes, M. (1999) E-Cadherin gene mutations provide a genetic basis for the phenotypic divergence of mixed gastric carcinomas. *Lab. Invest.*, **79**, 459–465

Maesawa, C., Tamura, G., Suzuki, Y., Ogasawara, S., Sakata, K., Kashiwaba, M. & Satodate, R. (1995) The sequential accumulation of genetic alterations characteristic of the colorectal adenoma–carcinoma sequence does not occur between gastric adenoma and adenocarcinoma. *J. Pathol.*, **176**, 249–258

Magnusson, P.K.E., Enroth, H., Eriksson, I., Held, M., Nyren, O., Engstrand, L., Hansson, L.E. & Gyllensten, U.B. (2001) Gastric cancer and human leukocyte antigen. *Cancer Res.*, **61**, 2684–2689

Markowitz, S., Wang, J., Myeroff, L., Parsons, R., Sun, L., Lutterbaugh, J., Fan, R.S., Zborowska, E., Kinzler, K.W., Vogelstein, B., Brattain, M. & Willson, J.K.V. (1995) Inactivation of the type II TGF-β receptor in colon cancer cells with microsatellite instability. *Science*, **268**, 1336–1338

Masiakowski, P., Breathnach, R., Bloch, J., Gannon, F., Krust, A. & Chambon, P. (1982) Cloning of cDNA sequences of hormone-regulated genes from MCF-7 human breast cancer cell lines. *Nucleic Acids Res.*, **10**, 7895–7903

Matsumura, Y. & Tarin, D. (1992) Significance of CD44 gene products for cancer diagnosis and disease evaluation. *Lancet*, **340**, 1053–1058

Merlo, A., Herman, J.G., Mao, L., Lee, D.J., Gabrielson, E., Burger, P.C., Baylin, S.B. & Sidransky, D. (1995) 5'CpG island methylation is associated with transcriptional silencing of the tumor suppressor p16/CDKN2/MTS1 in human cancers. *Nature Med.*, **1**, 686–692

Mirvish, S.S. (1971) Kinetics of nitrosamide formation from alkylureas, N-alkylurethanes, and alkylguanidines: possible implications for the etiology of human gastric cancer. *J. natl Cancer Inst.*, **46**, 1183–1193

Muta, H., Noguchi, M., Kanai, Y., Ochiai, A., Nawata, H. & Hirohashi, S. (1996) E-Cadherin gene mutations in signet ring cell carcinoma of the stomach. *Jpn. J. Cancer Res.*, **87**, 843–848

Nagata, A., Igarashi, M., Jinno, S., Suto, K. & Okayama, H. (1991) An additional homolog of the fission yeast cdc25+ gene occurs in humans and is highly expressed in some cancer cells. *New Biol.*, **3**, 959–968

Nakatsuru, S., Yanagisawa, A., Ichii, S., Tahara, E., Kato, Y., Nakamura, Y. & Horii, A. (1992) Somatic mutation of the APC gene in gastric cancer: frequent mutations in very well differentiated adenocarcinoma and signet-ring cell carcinoma. *Hum. mol. Genet.*, **1**, 559–563

Nakatsuru, S., Yanagisawa, A., Furukawa, Y., Ichii, S., Kato, Y., Nakamura, Y. & Horii, A. (1993) Somatic mutations of the APC gene in precancerous lesion of the stomach. *Hum. mol. Genet.*, **2**, 1463–1465

Nakayama, H., Yasui, W., Yokozaki, H. & Tahara, E (1993) Reduced expression of nm23 is associated with metastasis of human gastric carcinomas. *Jpn. J. Cancer Res.*, **84**, 184–190

Nishimura, K., Yokozaki, H., Haruma, K., Kajiyama, G. & Tahara, E. (1995) Alterations of the APC gene in carcinoma cell lines and precancerous lesions of the stomach. *Int. J. Oncol.*, **7**, 587–592

Noguchi, T., Muller, W., Wirtz, H.C., Willers, R. & Gabbert, H.E. (1999) FHIT gene in gastric cancer: association with tumor progression and prognosis. *J. Pathol.*, **188**, 378–381

Ochiai, A., Akimoto, S., Kanai, Y., Shibata, T., Oyama, T. & Hirohashi, S. (1994) c-erbB-2 Gene product associates with catenins in human cancer cells. *Biochem. biophys. Res. Commun.*, **205**, 73–78

Ochiai, A., Yamauchi, Y. & Hirohashi, S. (1996) p53 Mutations in the non-neoplastic mucosa of the human stomach showing intestinal metaplasia. *Int. J. Cancer*, **69**, 28–33

Oda, N., Tsujino, T., Tsuda. T., Yoshida, K., Nakamura, H., Yasui, W. & Tahara, E. (1990) DNA ploidy pattern and amplification of ERBB and ERBB2 genes in human gastric carcinomas. *Virchows Arch. B. Cell Pathol. mol. Pathol.*, **58**, 273–277

Ohta, M., Inoue, H., Cotticelli, M.G., Kastury, K., Baffa, R., Palazzo, J., Siprashvili, Z., Mori, M., McCue, P., Druck, T., Croce, C.M. & Huebner, K. (1996) The FHIT gene, spanning the chromosome 3p14.2 fragile site and renal carcinoma-associated t(3;8) breakpoint, is abnormal in digestive tract cancers. *Cell*, **84**, 587–597

Palli, D., Russo, A., Ottini, L., Masala, G., Saieva, C., Amorosi, A., Cama, A., D'Amico, C., Falchetti, M., Palmirotta, R., Decarli, A., Costantini, R.M. & Fraumeni, J.F., Jr (2001) Red meat, family history, and increased risk of gastric cancer with microsatellite instability. *Cancer Res.*, **61**, 5415–5419

Pellman, D. (2001) Cancer. A CINtillating new job for the APC tumor suppressor. *Science*, **291**, 2555–2556

Poremba, C., Yandell, D.W., Huang, Q., Little, J.B., Mellin, W., Schmid, K.W., Bocker, W. & Dockhorn-Dworniczak, B. (1995) Frequency and spectrum of p53 mutations in gastric – a molecular genetic and immunohistochemical study. *Virchows Arch.*, **426**, 447–455

Prinz, C., Schoniger, M., Rad, R., Becker, I., Keiditsch, E., Wagenpfeil, S., Classen, M., Rosch, T., Schepp, W. & Gerhard, M. (2001) Key importance of the *Helicobacter pylori* adherence factor blood group antigen binding adhesin during chronic gastric inflammation. *Cancer Res.*, **61**, 1903–1909

Sakurai, S., Sano, T. & Nakajima, T. (1995) Clinico-pathological and molecular biological studies of gastric adenomas with special reference to p53 abnormality. *Pathol. int.*, **45**, 51–57

Sano, T., Tsujino, T., Yoshida, K., Nakayama, H., Haruma, K., Ito, H., Nakamura, Y., Kajiyama, G. & Tahara, E. (1991) Frequent loss of heterozygosity on chromosomes 1q, 5q, and 17p in human gastric carcinomas. *Cancer Res.*, **51**, 2926–2931

Saukkonen, K., Nieminen, O., Van Rees, B., Vilkki, S., Harkonen, M., Juhola, M., Mecklin, J.-P., Sipponen, P. & Ristimaki, A. (2001) Expression of cyclooxygenase-2 in dysplasia of the stomach and in intestinal-type gastric adenocarcinoma. *Clin. Cancer Res.*, **7**, 1923–1931

Seewaldt, V.L., Johnson, B.S., Parker, M.B., Collins, S.J. & Swisshelm, K. (1995) Expression of retinoic acid receptor-β mediates retinoic acid-induced growth arrest and apoptosis in breast cancer cells. *Cell Growth Differ.*, **6**, 1077–1088

Semba, S., Yokozaki, H., Yamamoto, S., Yasui, W. & Tahara, E. (1996) Microsatellite instability in precancerous lesions and adenocarcinomas of the stomach. *Cancer* (Suppl. 8), 77, 1620–1627

Semba, S., Yokozaki, H., Yasui, W. & Tahara, E. (1998) Frequent microsatellite instability and loss of heterozygosity in the region including BRCA1 (17q21) in young patients with gastric cancer. *Int. J. Oncol.*, **12**, 1245–1251

Shibata, T., Ochiai, A., Kanai, Y., Akimoto, S., Gotoh, M., Yasui, N., Machinami, R. & Hirohashi, S. (1996) Dominant negative inhibition of the association between beta-catenin and c-erbB-2 by N-terminally deleted beta-catenin suppresses the invasion and metastasis of cancer cells. *Oncogene*, **13**, 883–889

Shigeishi, H., Yokozaki, H., Kuniyasu, H., Nakagawa, H., Ishikawa, T., Tahara, E. & Yasui, W. (2001) No mutations of the *Bub1* gene in human gastric carcinomas. *Oncol. Rep.*, **8**, 791- 794

Shimizu, N., Inada, K., Nakanishi, H., Tsukamoto, T., Ikehara, Y., Kaminishi, M., Kuramoto, S., Sugiyama, A., Katsuyama, T. & Tatematsu, M. (1999) *Helicobacter pylori* infection enhances glandular stomach carcinogenesis in Mongolian gerbils treated with a chemical carcinogen. *Carcinogenesis*, **20**, 669–676

Shimizu, N., Ikehara, Y., Inada, K., Nakanishi, H., Tsukamoto, T., Nozaki, K., Kaminishi, M., Kuramoto, S., Sugiyama, A., Katsuyama, T. & Tatematsu, M. (2000) Eradication diminishes enhancing effects of *Helicobacter pylori* infection on glandular stomach carcinogenesis in Mongolian gerbils. *Cancer Res.*, **60**, 1512–1514

Soman, N.R., Correa, P., Ruiz, B.A. & Wogan, G.N. (1991) The TPR-MET oncogenic rearrangement is present and expressed in human gastric carcinoma and precursor lesions. *Proc. natl Acad. Sci. USA*, **88**, 4892–4896

Sugimura, T., Fujimura S. & Baba, T. (1970) Tumor production in the glandular stomach and alimentary tract of the rat by N-methyl-N′-nitro-N-nitrosoguanidine. *Cancer Res.*, **30**, 455–465

Sung, J.J., Leung, W.K., Go, M.Y., To, K.F., Cheng, A.S., Ng, E.K. & Chan, F.K. (2000) Cyclooxygenase-2 expression in *Helicobacter pylori*-associated premalignant and malignant gastric lesions. *Am. J. Pathol.*, **157**, 729–735

Suzuki, T., Yasui, W., Yokozaki, H., Naka, K., Ishikawa, T. & Tahara, E. (1999) Expression of the E2F family in human gastrointestinal carcinomas. *Int. J. Cancer*, **81**, 535–538

Tahara, E. (1993) Molecular mechanism of stomach carcinogenesis. *J. Cancer Res. clin. Oncol.*, **119**, 265–272

Tahara, E. (1997) Cell growth regulation and cancer: stromal interaction. In: Sugimura, T. & Sasako, M., eds, *Gastric Cancer*, New York, Oxford University Press, pp. 100–108

Tahara, E. (1998) Molecular mechanism of human stomach carcinogenesis implicated in *Helicobacter pylori* infection. *Exp. Toxicol. Pathol.*, **50**, 375–378

Tahara, E. (2002) Histone acetylation and retinoic acid receptor beta DNA methylation as novel targets for gastric cancer therapy. *Drug News Perspect.*, **15**, 581–585

Tahara, E., Yokozaki, H. & Yasui, W. (1993) Growth factors in gastric cancer. In: Nishi, M., Ichikawa, H., Nakajima, T., Maruyama, K. & Tahara, E., eds, *Gastric Cancer*, Berlin, Springer-Verlag, pp. 209–217

Tahara, E., Kuniyasu, H., Yasui, W. & Yokozaki, H. (1994) Abnormal expression of growth factors and their receptors in stomach cancer. In: Nakamura, T. & Matsumoto, K., eds, *Gann Monograph on Cancer Research Growth Factors: Cell Growth, Morphogenesis and Transformation*, Tokyo, Japan Scientific Society Press, pp. 163–173

Tahara, H., Kuniyasu, H., Yokozaki, H., Yasui, W., Shey, J.W., Ide, T. & Tahara, E. (1995) Telomerase activity in preneoplastic and neoplastic gastric and colorectal lesions. *Clin. Cancer Res.*, **1**, 1245–1251

Tahara, E., Semba, S. & Tahara, H. (1996a) Molecular biological observations in gastric cancer. *Semin. Oncol.*, **23**, 307–315

Tahara, E., Yasui, W. & Yokozaki, H. (1996b) Abnormal growth factor networks in neoplasia. In: Pusztai, L., Lewis, C.E. & Yap, E., eds, *Cell Proliferation in Cancer*, Oxford, Oxford University Press, pp.131–153

Tahara, E., Yokozaki, H. & Yasui, W. (1999) Stomach–genetic and epigenetic alterations of preneoplastic and neoplastic lesions. In: Srivastava, S., Henson, D.E. & Gazdar, A., eds, *Molecular Pathology of Early Cancer*, Amsterdam, IOS Press, pp. 341–361

Takahashi, Y., Cleary, K.R., Mai, M., Kitadai, Y., Bucana, C.D. & Ellis, L.M. (1996) Significance of vessel count and vascular endothelial growth factor and its receptor (KDR) in intestinal-type gastric cancer. *Clin. Cancer Res.*, **2**, 1679–1684

Tamura, G., Kihana, T., Nomura, K., Terada, M., Sugimura, T. & Hirohashi, S. (1991) Detection of frequent p53 gene mutations in primary gastric cancer by cell sorting and polymerase chain reaction single-strand conformation polymorphism analysis. *Cancer Res.*, **51**, 2056–3058

Tamura, G., Sakata, K., Nishizuka, S., Maesawa, C., Suzuki, Y., Iwaya, T., Terashima, M., Saito, K. & Satodate, R. (1997) Analysis of the fragile histidine triad gene in primary gastric carcinomas and gastric carcinoma cell lines. *Genes Chromosomes Cancer*, **20**, 98–102

Tanimoto, H., Yoshida, K., Yokozaki, H., Yasui, W., Nakayama, H., Ito, H., Ohama, K. & Tahara, E. (1991) Expression of basic fibroblast growth factor in human gastric carcinomas. *Virchows Arch. B. Cell Pathol. mol. Pathol.*, **61**, 263–267

Tohdo, H., Yokozaki, H., Haruma, K., Kajiyama. G. & Tahara, E. (1993) p53 Gene mutations in gastric adenomas. *Virchows Arch. B. Cell Pathol. mol. Pathol.*, **63**, 191–195

Uchino, S., Tsuda, H., Noguchi, M., Yokota, J., Terada, M., Saito, T., Kobayashi, M., Sugimura, T. & Hirohashi, S. (1992) Frequent loss of heterozygosity at the DCC locus in gastric cancer. *Cancer Res.*, **52**, 3099–3102

Uchino, S., Noguchi, M., Ochiai, A., Saito, T., Kobayashi, M. & Hirohashi, S. (1993) p53 Mutation in gastric cancer: a genetic model for carcinogenesis is common to gastric and colorectal cancer. *Int. J. Cancer*, **54** 759–764

Ue, T., Yokozaki, H., Kitadai, Y., Yamamoto, S., Yasui, W., Ishikawa, T. & Tahara, E. (1998) Co-expression of osteopontin and CD44V9 in gastric cancer. *Int. J. Cancer*, **79**, 127–132

Weber, G.F., Ashkar, S., Glimcher, M.J. & Cantor, H. (1996) Receptor-ligand interaction between CD44 and osteopontin (Eta-1). *Science*, **271**, 509–512

Wu, M.S., Lee, C.W., Shun, C.T., Wang, H.P., Lee, W.J., Sheu J.C. & Lin, J.T. (1998) Clinicopathological significance of altered loci of replication error and microsatellite instability-associated mutations in gastric cancer. *Cancer Res.*, **58**, 1494–1497

Yamamoto, S., Yasui, W., Kitadai, Y., Yokozaki, H., Haruma, K., Kajiyama, G. & Tahra, E. (1998) Expression of vascular endothelial growth factor in human gastric carcinomas. *Pathol. int.*, **48**, 499–506

Yang, H.-K., Kang, S.H., Kim, Y.-S., Won, K., Bang, Y.-J. & Kim, S.-J. (1999) Truncation of the TGF-beta type II receptor gene results in insensitivity to TGF-beta in human gastric cancer cells. *Oncogene*, **18**, 2213–2219

Yasui, W., Hata, J., Yokozaki, H., Nakatani, H., Ochiai, A., Ito, H. & Tahara, E. (1988) Interaction between epidermal growth factor and its receptor in progression of human gastric carcinoma. *Int. J. Cancer*, **41**, 211–217

Yasui, W., Akama, Y., Kuniyasu, H., Yokozaki, H., Semba, S., Shimamoto, F. & Tahara, E. (1996a) Expression of cyclin-dependent kinase inhibitor p21WAF1/CIP1 in non-neoplastic mucosa and neoplasia of the stomach: relation with p53 status and proliferative activity. *J. Pathol.*, **180**, 122–128

Yasui, W., Yokozaki, H., Kuniyasu, H., Shimamoto, F. & Tahara, E. (1996b) Expression of CDK inhibitor p16CDKN2/MTS1/INK4A in human gastric carcinomas. In: Tahara, E., Sugimachi, K. & Oohara, T., eds, *Recent Advances in Gastroenterological Carcinogenesis I*, Bologna, Monduzzi Editore, pp. 765–769

Yasui, W., Kudo, Y., Semba, S., Yokozaki, H. & Tahara, E. (1997) Reduced expression of cyclin-dependent kinase inhibitor p27Kip1 is associated with advanced stage and invasiveness of gastric carcinomas. *Jpn. J. Cancer Res.*, **88**, 625–629

Yasui, W., Tahara, H., Tahara, E., Fujimoto, J., Nakayama, J., Ishikawa, F., Ide, T. & Tahara, E. (1998) Expression of telomerase catalytic component, telomerase reverse transcriptase, in human gastric carcinomas. *Jpn. J. Cancer Res.*, **89**, 1099–1103

Yasui, W., Naka, K., Suzuki, T., Fujimoto, J., Hayahi, K., Matsutani, N., Yokozaki, H. & Tahara, E. (1999a) Expression of p27Kip1, cyclin E, and E2F-1 in primary and metastatic tumors of gastric carcinoma. *Oncol. Rep.*, **6**, 983–987

Yasui, W., Tahara, E., Tahara, H., Fujimoto, J., Naka, K., Nakayama J., Ishikawa, F., Ide, T. & Tahara, E. (1999b) Immunohistochemical detection of human telomerase reverse transcriptase in normal mucosa and precancerous lesions of the stomach. *Jpn. J. Cancer Res.*, **90**, 589–595

Yokota, J., Yamamoto, T., Miyajima, N., Toyoshima, K., Nomura, N., Sakamoto, H., Yoshida, T., Terada, M. & Sugimura T. (1988) Genetic alterations of the c-erbB-2 oncogene occur frequently in tubular adenocarcinoma of the stomach and are often accompanied by amplification of the v-erbA homologue. *Oncogene*, **2**, 283–287

Yokozaki, H., Kuniyasu, H., Kitadai, Y., Nishimura, K., Todo, H., Ayhan, A., Yasui, W., Ito, H. & Tahara, E. (1992) p53 Point mutations in primary human gastric carcinomas. *J. Cancer. Res. clin. Oncol.*, **119**, 67–70

Yokozaki, H., Ito, R., Nakayama, H., Kuniyasu, H., Taniyama, K. & Tahara, E. (1994) Expression of CD44 abnormal transcripts in human gastric carcinomas. *Cancer Lett.*, **83**, 229–234

Yokozaki, H., Kuniyasu, H., Semba, S., Yasui, W. & Tahara, E. (1997) Molecular bases of human stomach carcinogenesis. In: Tahara, E., ed., *Mole-*

cular *Pathology of Gastroenterological Cancer: Application to Clinical Practice*, Tokyo, Springer-Verlag, pp. 55–70

Yokozaki, H., Shitara, Y., Fujimoto, J., Hiyama, T., Yasui, W. & Tahara, E. (1999a) Alterations of p73 preferentially occur in gastric adenocarcinomas with foveolar epithelial phenotype. *Int. J. Cancer*, **83**, 192–196

Yokozaki, H., Semba, S., Fujimoto, J. & Tahara, E. (1999b) Microsatellite instabilities in gastric cancer patients with multiple primary cancers. *Int. J. Oncol.*, **14**, 151–155

Yonemura, Y., Ninomiya, I., Ohoyama, S., Kimura, H., Yamaguchi, A., Fushida, S., Kosaka, T., Miwa, K., Miyazaki, I., Endou, Y., Tanaka, M. & Sasaki, T. (1991) Expression of c-erbB-2 oncoprotein in gastric carcinoma: immunoreactivity for c-erbB-2 protein is an independent indicator of poor short-term prognosis in patients with gastric carcinoma. *Cancer*, **67**, 2914–2918

Yoon, K.A., Ku, J.L., Yang, H.K., Kim, W.H., Park, S.Y. & Park, J.G. (1999) Germline mutations of E-cadherin gene in Korean familial gastric cancer patients. *J. hum. Genet.*, **44**, 177–180

Yoshida, M.C., Wada, M., Satoh, H., Yoshida, T., Sakamoto, H., Miyagawa, K., Yokota, J., Koda, T., Kakinuma, K., Sugimura, T. & Terada, M. (1988) Human *HST1 (HSTF1)* gene maps to chromosome band 11q13 and co-amplifies with the *INT2* gene in human cancer. *Proc. natl Acad. Sci. USA*, **85**, 4861–4864

Yoshida, K., Yokozaki, H., Niimoto, M., Ito, H., Ito, M. & Tahara, E. (1989) Expression of TGF-α and pro-collagen type I and type III in human gastric carcinomas. *Int. J. Cancer*, **44**, 394–398

Yoshida, K., Tsujino, T., Yasui, W., Kameda, T., Sano, T., Nakayama, H., Toge, T. & Tahara, E. (1990) Induction of growth factor-receptor and metalloproteinase genes by epidermal growth factor and/or transforming growth factor-β in human gastric carcinoma cell lines MKN-28. *Jpn. J. Cancer Res.*, **81**, 793–798

Yoshida, K., Bolodeoku, J., Sugino, T., Goodison, S., Matasumura, Y., Warren, B.F., Toge, T., Tahara, E. & Tarin, D. (1995) Abnormal retention of intron 9 in CD44 gene transcripts in human gastrointestinal tumors. *Cancer Res.*, **55**, 4273–4277

Yoshida, K., Yasui, W., Kagawa, Y. & Tahara, E. (1996) Multiple genetic alterations and abnormal growth factor network in human esophageal carcinomas. In: Tahara, E., ed., *Molecular Pathology of Gastroenterological Cancer: Application to Clinical Practice*, Tokyo, Springer-Verlag, pp. 31–41

Yustein, A.S., Harper, J.C., Petroni, G.R., Cummings, O.W., Moskaluk, C.A. & Powell, S.M. (1999) Allelotype of gastric adenocarcinoma. *Cancer Res.*, **59**, 1437–1441

Corresponding author:

Eiichi Tahara
Radiation Effects Research Foundation
Hiroshima-Nagasaki, 5-2 Hijiyama Park,
Minami-ku, Hiroshima 732-0815, Japan
etahara@cisnet.or.jp

Mechanisms of Carcinogenesis: Contributions of Molecular Epidemiology
Patricia Buffler, Jerry Rice, Robert Baan, Michael Bird and Paolo Boffetta, eds
IARC Scientific Publications No. 157
International Agency for Research on Cancer, Lyon, 2004

Biological Models for Leukaemia and Lymphoma

Mel F. Greaves

Summary

Blood-cell cancers (leukaemias, lymphomas and myeloma) are a very diverse group of neoplasms derived from a variety of stem cells at different hierarchical levels of haemopoietic and lymphoid cell development. This biological heterogeneity is likely to be associated with a variety of different etiological mechanisms. Correspondingly, a large number of inherited normal allelic variations might be expected to contribute to risk. Leukaemias alone have more than 200 different acquired (non-constitutive) molecular abnormalities but some are much more prevalent than others and are associated with biological subtypes with distinctive clinical or prognostic features. Balanced chromosome translocations are very common, together with simple gains or losses of chromosomes. Gene deletions and mutations are also relatively common, especially in more advanced disease. In several types of leukaemia and lymphoma, a transition from benign to malignant status can be tracked together with concurrent accrual of additional molecular abnormalities (e.g. chronic myeloid leukaemia evolving into blast crisis and follicular lymphoma becoming diffuse).

The covert preclinical natural history of paediatric leukaemia has been revealed by 'backtracking' using chromosomal translocation-generated fusion gene sequences as clone-specific stable, specific and sensitive markers. Studies in identical twins, in archived neonatal blood spots of patients and in normal newborn cord bloods all support the contention that chromosomal translocations often initiate leukaemia in utero. Twin concordance rates (and animal modelling) suggest that further secondary genetic changes and exposures postnatally are, however, critical and this is endorsed by the finding that leukaemic fusion genes are present in normal newborn infants at a
rate that far exceeds the cumulative risk of leukaemia. The natural history of leukaemic subtypes provides a useful framework for molecular epidemiological studies and significant advances have been made in this respect with infant and childhood acute lymphoblastic leukaemia.

Diversity of blood-cell cancers

Cancers of the blood-cell system – leukaemia, lymphoma, myeloma and their subsets – are extraordinarily diverse. (For a comprehensive description of the classification of leukaemias and lymphomas with allied molecular genetics, see Jaffe *et al.*, 2001). This heterogeneity probably reflects both the variety of 'target' cells available for transformation and also the variable phenotypic impact of different molecular genetic abnormalities (Greaves, 1996; Barr, 1998). Somewhat unusually, the blood-cell system has a hierarchical cell population structure that includes several developmentally distinct cell types with stem cell properties, each of which has been associated with different types of malignancy (Figure 1). Superimposed upon this developmental-linked pattern of transformation, it is clear (from clonogenic cell assays and immunophenotypic analysis) that stem cells at any one level can undergo mutation and divergent clonal evolution to produce a variety of different neoplasms. For example, many of the morphological and molecularly distinct subtypes of acute myeloid leukaemia derive from the same multipotential myeloid or lymphomyeloid stem cells (Bonnet & Dick, 1997) but with distinct molecular genetic lesions producing apparent clonal expansion and/or differentiation arrest at different developmental levels downstream of the initial target cell. Transgenic modelling with leukaemia genes indicates a similar 'cell context'-dependent impact of leu-

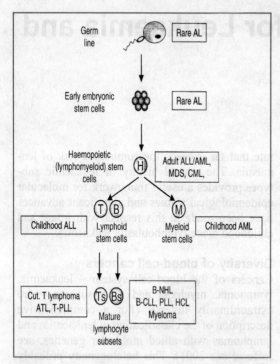

Figure 1. Developmental origins of blood cell cancers. AL, acute leukaemia; ALL, acute lymphoblastic leukaemia; AML, acute myeloblastic leukaemia; ATL, adult T-cell leukaemia (with human T-lymphotropic virus, HTLV-I); CLL, chronic lymphocytic leukaemia; CML, chronic myeloid leukaemia; Cut., cutaneous (T lymphoma); HCL, hairy-cell leukaemia; MDS, myelodysplastic syndrome (a pre-leukaemic condition); NHL, non-Hodgkin lymphoma; PLL, prolymphocytic leukaemia; Ts,Bs, subsets of mature T and B lymphocytes. Figure modified from Greaves (1996).

kaemia genes (Heisterkamp *et al.*, 1990; Corral *et al.*, 1996).

The extent of the cellular and molecular heterogeneity of blood-cell cancers poses a dilemma for molecular epidemiological studies. In the past, epidemiologists have often pooled (or 'lumped') subtypes of leukaemia/lymphoma together or used arbitrary age categories, and this may well have disguised important etiological associations. An example of this would be the causal link between human T-lymphotropic virus-I (HTLV-I) and mature T-cell leukaemia/lymphoma which was missed until immunophenotyping was intro-

duced. From our limited knowledge of causal mechanisms in blood-cell cancers, it is clear that several agents are linked with subtypes of disease (Table 1). Ionizing radiation has a broader spectrum of associations with disease subtype but this excludes chronic lymphocytic leukaemia and possibly some other subtypes of blood-cell cancer (Little *et al.*, 1999). It is therefore unclear in designing molecular epidemiological studies what prior assumptions concerning subtypes of disease should be made. In the largest study to date that has included cellular and molecular definitions of disease (the UK Childhood Cancer Study) (UK Childhood Cancer Study Investigators, 2000), a hierarchical classification of leukaemias was used (Figure 2) that provided the opportunity for subsequent analysis of different groupings. In this latter study, two hypotheses made prior predictions of subtype associations but most did not. This seems to be a biologically rational approach as well as a pragmatic one – provided, however, that adequate numbers of patients can be obtained for the smaller subgroups. In the extreme, all patients have a uniquely abnormal genotype and some non-random or consistent genetic changes are so rare that it will be difficult to analyse them separately for etiological associations.

Variety of genetic changes in blood cell cancers

Leukaemias and lymphomas have a similar, diverse spectrum of chromosomal and genetic abnormalities as most other cancers. Something like 5% of cases appear to involve inherited gene mutations, usually in association with a familial cancer syndrome with defective DNA damage repair, e.g. ataxia telangiectasia, and Li–Fraumeni and Bloom syndromes. Children with constitutive trisomy 21 and Down syndrome have a substantially increased risk (10–20-fold) of leukaemia, especially of the normally rare FABM7 megakaryoblastic subtype (Bhatia *et al.*, 1999). The molecular basis of this elevated risk is unknown, as are other molecular changes that may need to complement trisomy 21. A rare familial platelet disorder with predisposition to acute myeloid leukaemia (FPD/AML) has been linked to mutations (and haploinsufficiency) of the *AML1* gene, a

Table 1. Known 'causes' of leukaemia/lymphoma subtypes

Ionizing radiation
Atomic bomb in Japan[a]   ALL, CML, AML
Therapeutic irradiation   AML, CML

Genotoxic chemicals
Occupational – benzene   AML
Therapeutic – cancer drugs   AML[b]

Infectious microbes
Epstein–Barr virus (EBV)   Burkitt B-NHL[c]
Human T-lymphotrophic virus (HTLV-I)   Mature T cell leukaemia/lymphoma
Helicobacter pylori   Gastric (MALT) B-cell NHL

Inheritance of mutant genes (familial)
Li–Fraumeni syndrome (*p53*)[d]   ALL/AML
Bloom syndrome (*BLM*)   AML
Ataxia telangiectasia (*ATM*)   T-cell leukaemia

[a] Risk of ALL was highest in patients less than 15 years old at time of exposure. No cases of CLL were recorded. Relative risk of NHL was only slightly elevated (in males only) and no excess of adult T-cell leukaemia or myeloma was found (Preston *et al.*, 1994; Little *et al.*, 1999).
[b] Alkylating drugs associated with unbalanced translocations and deletions (5q⁻, 7q⁻); topoisomerase II-inhibiting drugs, epidophyllotoxins and anthracyclines associated with balanced translocations. Epidophyllotoxins, e.g. VP-16, linked to *11q23 MLL* gene fusions, especially in younger patients and with very short latencies (~18–24 months) (Andersen *et al.*, 1998; Felix, 1998).
[c] In the context of immunosuppression (from malaria, HIV or therapeutic immunosuppression) (Magrath, 1990).
[d] Genes involved given in parentheses.
ALL, acute lymphoblastic leukaemia; CML, chronic myeloid leukaemia; AML, acute myeloid leukaemia; NHL, non-Hodgkin lymphoma; MALT, mucosa-associated lymphoid tissue; HIV, human immunodeficiency virus

gene which is frequently involved in leukaemogenesis via acquired mutations or (more frequently) chromosomal translocation and gene fusion (see below) (Song *et al.*, 1999). Almost all other molecular abnormalities detected in leukaemic cells, of which over 200 have been described, are non-constitutional or acquired and are considered to arise in a single blood stem cell.

Leukaemias sharing the same haematological diagnosis – acute lymphoblastic leukaemia – have a striking variation in the major chromosome abnormalities in association with broad age groups at diagnosis (Figure 3). These predominant genetic changes have independent prognostic significance in the context of particular therapeutic regimens (Ferrando & Look, 2000) and help rationalize the differences in clinical outcome for infants, children and adults with acute lymphoblastic leukaemia. It is likely that these age-linked biological subtypes derive from different lymphomyeloid stem cells and **they may well have distinct etiologies**.

The most striking molecular abnormalities of blood-cell cancers, shared with sarcomas, but curiously only rarely detected in carcinomas (Kroll *et al.*, 2000), are the balanced (two-way or reciprocal) chromosomal translocations (Rabbitts, 1994; Look, 1997; Mrozek & Bloomfield, 1998; Rowley, 1998). These are stable markers expressed homogeneously by the leukaemic clone and contrast with the multiple unbalanced chromosomal breaks that are common in epithelial cancers and that are associated with a chromosomal instability phenotype (Lengauer, 2001).

The consequence of these gross genetic exchanges or recombinations in leukaemia is the

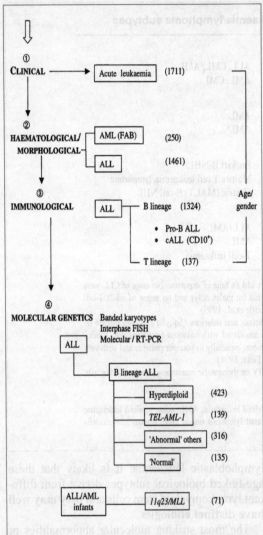

Figure 2. A hierarchical classification of acute leukaemia for a molecular epidemiological study (the United Kingdom Children's Cancer Study, UKCCS, a case–control study of the possible cause of childhood leukaemia, lymphoma and other cancers). Numbers in parentheses indicate the number of cases entered. The AML cases were also classified by molecular cytogenetics but the number of cases with particular common abnormalities, e.g. t(8;21) *AML1-ETO*, were too low for subgroup analysis. AML, acute myeloid leukaemia; ALL, acute lymphoblastic leukaemia; FISH, fluorescence in-situ hybridization; RT-PCR, reverse transcription-polymerase chain reaction.

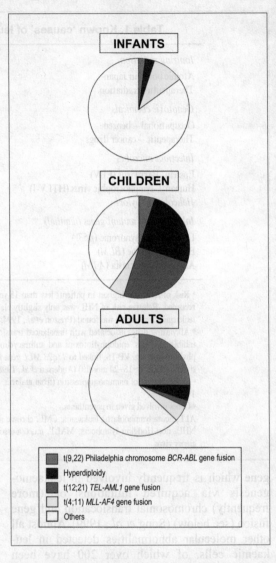

Figure 3. Molecular genetic heterogeneity of acute lymphoblastic leukaemia. Major molecular cytogenetic subgroups only shown. Infants, < 1 year of age. Children, 1–15 years. Adults, > 15 years. Redrawn from Greaves (1999).

generation of abnormal transcriptional units with either dysregulated (constitutive) activation of one partner gene or chimeric gene function (Figure 4). Several individual genes are very frequently involved in these illegitimate recombinants and may associate with multiple different or alterna-

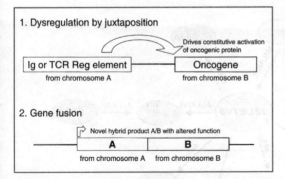

Figure 4. Two types of novel transcriptional units generated by chromosomal translocation in leukaemia/lymphoma. Ig, immunoglobulin; TCR, T-cell receptor; Reg, regulatory (element).

tive partners. For example, *MLL* (in infant acute leukaemia and 'secondary' therapy-associated acute myeloid leukaemia) has 50 or more alternative partner genes, more than 20 of which have been identified by cloning. *BL6* has multiple different partners in diffuse non-Hodgkin lymphoma (Dalla-Favera *et al.*, 1999). The retinoic acid receptor α gene has five alternative partner genes in acute promyelocytic leukaemia (Zelent *et al.*, 2001). *TEL* and *AML1* not only combine together to form the most common fusion gene in paediatric cancer (in paediatric acute lymphoblastic leukaemia) but have many alternative partners in acute lymphoblastic leukaemia or acute myeloid leukaemia (Greaves, 1999) (Figure 5). The product of the diverse fusions of *TEL* and *AML1* in both acute lymphoblastic leukaemia and acute myeloid leukaemia is usually either an activated kinase or a novel transcriptional regulatory protein (Figure 5).

The predominance of particular genes in blood-cell malignancy can be ascribed to the critical role that these same genes play in normal regulation of haemopoiesis or lymphoid-cell development (Tenen *et al.*, 1997; Enver & Greaves, 1998; Dalla-Favera *et al.*, 1999). *MLL* is a 'master' regulator of homeotic gene expression (plus downstream genes) and chromatin stability (Yu *et al.*, 1998). *MLL*, *TEL* and *AML1* are all essential for haemopoiesis as judged by knock-out experiments (Okuda *et al.*, 1996) and *BCL6* regulates germinal centre B-cell development

(Dalla-Favera *et al.*, 1999). *AML1* gene encodes a component of the CBF transcriptional complex (CBFA2 protein) that has several important myeloid genes as its target (Tenen *et al.*, 1997). Genes encoding other protein components of the same complex can be found in mutant varieties in acute leukaemia (Figure 6).

Several of these chimeric gene products, in acute myeloid leukaemia, acute promyelocytic leukaemia and acute lymphoblastic leukaemia, appear to be dominant negative regulators of target gene transcription resulting in differentiation arrest (Lutterbach & Hiebert, 2000). They appear to operate by recruitment of co-repressor proteins including N-COR, Sin3A and histone deacetylases (HDAC) that re-conform chromatin structure. Interestingly, these changes may be reversible by HDAC inhibitors endorsing the idea that an understanding of molecular pathogenesis could lead to novel and selective approaches to therapy (Redner *et al.*, 1999). An encouraging precedent for this has been provided with the selective kinase inhibitor ST1571 (Gleevec) in chronic myeloid leukaemia (Druker *et al.*, 2001).

Mechanisms of chromosomal translocation

Chromosomal translocations and deletions in leukaemia and lymphoma (and myeloma) appear to involve misdirection of the normal processors of DNA double-strand breakage repair or rearrangement (Ferguson & Alt, 2001; Rothkamm *et al.*, 2001).

Chromosomal rearrangements involving the lymphoid *Ig* and *TCR* genes may in some cases involve usage of the lymphoid RAG recombinases and Ig/TCR signal sequences (reviewed in Rabbitts, 1994; Küppers & Dalla-Favera, 2001). The recombinase may operate via signal sequences provided by both *TCR* **and** the partner gene or only impact direct on the *TCR* or *IGH* genes (see Table 2 and Marculescu *et al.*, 2002). In a broader sense, the mechanism of chromosomal recombination in leukaemia was, at one stage, thought to involve homologous recombination, via for example Alu repeats. This may be correct for some genetic changes – *MLL* gene self-fusion, for example (So *et al.*, 1997).

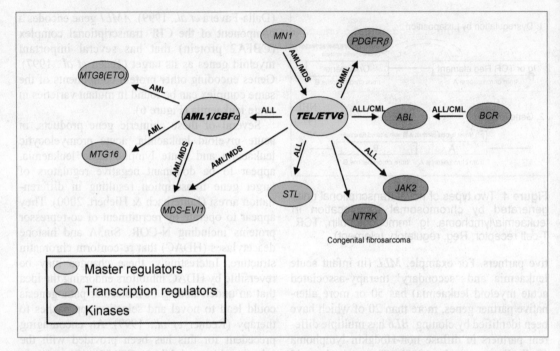

Figure 5. Chimeric fusion genes involving *TEL* and *AML1* and their functional impact. This diagram illustrates some, but not all, of the known genes involved in fusion with *TEL* and *AML1* (Greaves, 1999). AML, acute lymphoblastic leukaemia; MDS, myelodysplastic syndrome; CML, chronic myeloid leukaemia; CMML, chronic myelomonocytic leukaemia

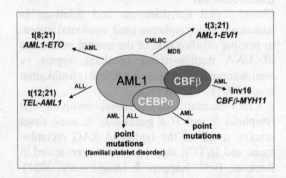

Figure 6. CBF transitional complex aberrations in leukaemias.

However, now that many leukaemia fusion genes have been sequenced at the genomic level, it seems that sequences that might facilitate homologous recombination are usually absent. This, plus the presence of small homologies (1–5 bp) and deletions at the break-points, has

suggested that, following double-stranded breaks (simultaneously in two chromosomes or more), the translocations arise predominantly by error-prone repair via non-homologous end-joining (see Table 2 and references therein). This is the common type of DNA-repair process in mammalian cells but raises the question of what causes the double-stranded DNA breaks in the first place. Breakage and illegitimate recombination of the *MLL* gene in infant acute leukaemia and chemotherapy-associated or 'secondary' acute myeloid leukaemia may be initiated by chemicals that bind to topoisomerase II sites (Ross *et al.*, 1994; Felix, 1998; Strissel *et al.*, 1998).

Natural history of leukaemia/lymphoma

Although blood-cell cancers do not have the histopathological correlates of transition from tumour to carcinoma seen with most adult cancers, there are many clear-cut examples of disease evolution or progression, most of which have adverse

Table 2. Recombination mechanisms in fusion genes, derived from chromosomal translocations

Disease	Fusion gene	Mechanism	Reference
ALL/AML	MLL–AF4	NHEJ	Gillert et al. (1999)
	MLL–other partners	(+/- topo II sites?)	Felix (1998); Lovett et al. (2001)
ALL	TEL–AML1	NHEJ	Wiemels & Greaves (1999)
AML	AML1–ETO	NHEJ	Xiao et al. (2001)
APML	PML–RARA	NHEJ	Yoshida et al. (1995)
B/T cell tumours	IGH/TCR-X[a]	V(D)J RAG 1/2 recombinases[b]	Haluska et al. (1990); Vaandrager et al. (2000); Küppers & Dalla-Favera (2001); Marculescu et al. (2002)
T-ALL	TAL-1 del SIL-TAL-1 rearrangement	V(D)J RAG 1/2 recombinases[c]	Breit et al. (1993)
Ewing sarcoma	EWS-FLI1	NHEJ	Zucman-Rossi et al. (1998)

[a] -X; various alternative partner genes for *IGH* and *TCR*. Recent data indicates that in some rearrangements, cryptic V(D)J recombinase signals on the partner gene are involved: T-cell receptor gene recombining with *TAL-1*, *TAL-2* and *LM02* as seen in translocation t(1;14), t(7;9) and t(11;14). In the translocations involving *IGH* with *BCL-1* and *BCL-2*, the evidence indicates that V(D)J recombinases are active on the *IGG* gene; their direct involvement in partner gene breakage is contentious (see Vaandrager et al., 2000; Marculescu et al., 2002).
[b] V(D)J, RAG-dependent recombination requires components of the NHEJ region complex (e.g. DNA-PK).
ALL, acute lymphoblastic leukaemia; AML, acute myeloid leukaemia; NHEJ, non-homologous end-joining; APML, acute promyelocytic leukaemia

clinical correlates and are associated with the acquisition of additional molecular genetic abnormalities. Some of the best-studied include chronic myeloid leukaemia evolving to blast crisis (Deininger et al., 2000) and follicular lymphoma transforming to diffuse lymphoma (Mrozek & Bloomfield, 1998; Horsman et al., 2001). Mucosa-associated lymphoid tissue, or gastric lymphoma, is a particularly informative example also (Figure 7) as its natural history can be linked with a pathogenic mechanism – chronic *Helicobacter pylori* infection and T-cell-driven proliferation of B cells (Du & Isaacson, 1998). Some 70–80% of gastric lymphomas regress after eradication of *H. pylori* with antibiotics (Wotherspoon et al., 1993).

A key issue for molecular epidemiological studies in this context is the time-frame involved. How long is the latency between initiation of disease and clinical diagnosis? What time period is usually required for transition from benign to malignant or metastatic disease and how many distinct molecular genetic abnormalities are

usually observed (and in what order, if any)? We know from leukaemias that occur after known single or chronic exposures (e.g. atomic bomb exposures in Japan, therapeutic exposure to irradiation or chemotherapy) that latency for chronic myeloid leukaemia and acute leukaemia can be extremely variable, from 12 months (induced by topoisomerase II inhibiting therapeutic drugs; Felix, 1998) to 25 years, although the risk may be maximum after 2–5 years. This is brief compared with the latency of disseminated adult carcinoma, e.g. breast cancer after radiation.

Given the young age of paediatric patients with leukaemia (average ~3 years), then these de-novo cases also must have a brief preclinical history. One plausible explanation for this apparent distinction between leukaemias and carcinomas is that leukaemias originate from mobile, active stem cells and require fewer independent genetic abnormalities before they become diffuse in the bone marrow and provoke diagnostic symptoms. In other words, they may be caught earlier in their evolutionary trajectory (Knudson, 1992; Greaves,

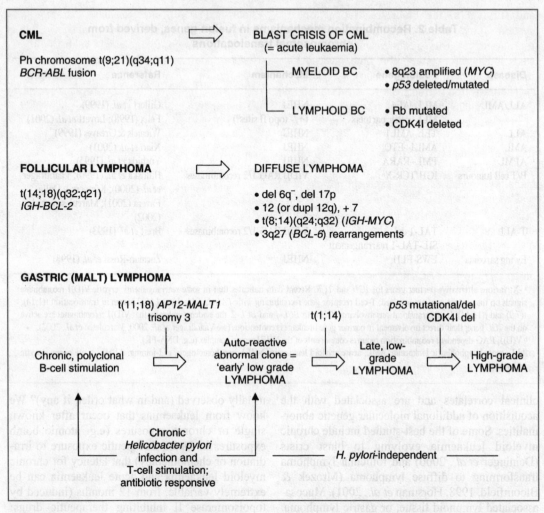

CML

Ph chromosome t(9;21)(q34;q11)
BCR-ABL fusion

⟹ **BLAST CRISIS OF CML**
(= acute leukaemia)

MYELOID BC
- 8q23 amplified (*MYC*)
- *p53* deleted/mutated

LYMPHOID BC
- Rb mutated
- CDK4I deleted

FOLLICULAR LYMPHOMA ⟹ DIFFUSE LYMPHOMA

t(14;18)(q32;q21)
IGH-BCL-2

- del 6q⁻, del 17p
- 12 (or dupl 12q), + 7
- t(8;14)(q24;q32) (*IGH-MYC*)
- 3q27 (*BCL-6*) rearrangements

GASTRIC (MALT) LYMPHOMA

t(11;18) *AP12-MALT1*
trisomy 3

t(1;14)

p53 mutational/del
CDK4I del

Chronic, polyclonal
B-cell stimulation

⟹ Auto-reactive
abnormal clone =
'early' low grade
LYMPHOMA

⟹ Late, low-
grade
LYMPHOMA

⟹ High-grade
LYMPHOMA

Chronic
Helicobacter pylori
infection and
T-cell stimulation;
antibiotic responsive

H. pylori-independent

Figure 7. Molecular pathogenesis and progression of leukaemia/lymphoma. CML, chronic myeloid leukaemia; MALT, mucosa-associated lymphoid tissue. Redrawn from Du and Isaacson (1998). Note that there is considerable heterogeneity in the molecular genetics of gastric lymphomas. Cases with t(11;18) *AP12-MLT1* fusion are less likely to respond to antibiotic therapy than those without this marker (e.g. with trisomy 3 only) (Liu *et al.*, 2001).

1999). This may also help to explain why they are curable in many (but not all) cases by combination chemotherapy, i.e. they have not yet evolved to the stage of widespread genetic instability or multiple genotypic lesions that corrupt apoptotic pathways and endow drug resistance. A similar argument might apply to other paediatric cancers originating in mobile, active stem cells early in development (e.g. Wilms tumour) and to

examples of 'young' adult cancers that are chemo-sensitive even when disseminated – choriocarcinoma and testicular cancer (Greaves, 2000). This needs not contradict the multistep paradigm that has emerged for carcinomas (Hanahan & Weinberg, 2000). In the latter cases, the emerging clone has to negotiate more hurdles or bottlenecks in order to disseminate, including the architectural constraints of epithelial tissue, anoxic conditions and survival in the bloodstream or lymphatic system. This more demanding evolutionary journey necessarily requires more mutational steps and therefore either more time, more genetic instability or both (Greaves, 2000).

The transition period from relatively benign to more malignant status in blood-cell cancers can clearly be extremely variable, resulting from either a stochastic process (of mutation accrual) or the requirement of some relevant, infrequent exposure. Intervals of 5–10 years, and occasionally 25 years or more, from chronic myeloid leukaemia to chronic myeloid leukaemia blast crisis or from low-grade follicular lymphoma to diffuse lymphoma are common. In contrast, it is also likely that, in many patients, this clonal, evolutionary transition or progression occurs in an entirely covert or clinically silent fashion with patients presenting with advanced disease, e.g. diffuse lymphoma with t(14;18) plus other changes or Philadelphia-positive (Ph$^+$) *BCR-ABL*-positive chronic myeloid leukaemia in blast crisis masquerading as primary acute lymphoblastic leukaemia (but reverting to chronic myeloid leukaemia in 'remission'). These transitions and variable presentations, as exemplified by chronic myeloid leukaemia with the Ph chromosome, can be best understood in terms of the stem-cell origins of disease (Figure 1) coupled with very variable dynamics. In this context, there is a parallel with some non-haemopoietic cancers, e.g. astrocytoma evolving into glioblastoma or presenting as a primary glioblastoma, i.e. a glial stem cell is the 'target' with or without further differentiation (Greaves, 1982). Pathologists may view these transitions and presentations quite differently (as distinctly separate cancers or as de-differentiation).

How many genetic 'steps' are required?

Leukaemic cell genotypes may appear simple or very complex and much may depend on the incisiveness of the tools used. Banded karyotypes, fluorescence in-situ hybridization (FISH) methods (M-FISH and SKY), expression microarrays and whole-genome mutation screening will paint different portraits. What is clear is that leukaemias that have progressed to relapse or that have been established as cell lines can have extraordinarily diverse molecular genetic abnormalities visible at the whole chromosome level (Veldman *et al.*, 1997) in addition to submicroscopic point mutations (e.g. in *Rb*, *p53*, *RAS*) or deletions (e.g. in *p53*, CDK4I). Some of this diversity may relate to the acquisition of genetic instability, a rare phenotype at diagnosis of leukaemia, and much of it is associated with progression of disease and intensive subclone selection (including that derived for therapeutic selective pressure). CDK4I deletions (Carter *et al.*, 2001) and *p53* mutations (Imamura *et al.*, 1994), for example, are found much more frequently in leukaemic cell populations from more advanced disease, relapses or cell lines, suggesting that they most often contribute to progression as relatively late selective events. However, what **can** happen in leukaemia is not the same as what is normally **required** to happen for a clinical diagnosis, and from the perspective of etiology and molecular epidemiology, minimal models may be more appropriate. These should incorporate an appropriate time frame of pre-clinical natural history with initiation (the first genetic hit) and promotion (a second hit) as the simplest scenario. Progress has been made in this respect with paediatric leukaemia.

Backtracking paediatric leukaemia and chromosomal translocations to fetal development

It is now clear that a substantial fraction of paediatric acute lymphoblastic and acute myeloid leukaemias are initiated prenatally during fetal development by chromosomal translocations. The evidence comes from three sources – a comparison of leukaemic cell gene fusion sequences in identical twins with acute lymphoblastic leukaemia, retrospective scrutiny of archived neonatal blood spots (Guthrie cards) of patients for fusion gene sequences and a screen of normal newborn cord bloods for chromosomal translocation-derived gene fusion mRNA.

Twins with leukaemia

Concordance of leukaemia in twins has been recognized since 1935 but most reports before 1993 were of single pairs with limited data on zygosity status and molecular cytogenetics. Since 1985, the Leukaemia Research Fund Centre at the Institute of Cancer Research has been accumulating such cases on a worldwide basis. Twenty pairs with paediatric acute lymphoblastic leukaemia have been identified, including two sets of triplets. Nine of these pairs have been evaluated extensively for clonal relationship using available molecular genetic markers:

- Three sets of monozygotic twin infants (aged 2–10 months) with acute lymphoblastic leukaemia had identical *MLL* gene fusions (Ford *et al.*, 1993). Two further such pairs have subsequently been reported (Gill Super *et al.*, 1994; Megonigal *et al.*, 1998).
- Three sets of monozygotic twin children (aged 2–14 years) had identical *TEL-AML1* genomic fusion sequences (Figure 8) (Ford *et al.*, 1998; Wiemels *et al.*, 1999a,b).
- In a set of triplets, the two monozygotic twins had acute lymphoblastic leukaemia with an identical *TEL-AML1* fusion gene but the third, dizygotic triplet was non-leukaemic and had no detectable fusion gene sequences (Maia *et al.*, 2001).

- One set of T-acute lymphoblastic leukaemia/ T-non-Hodgkin lymphoma twins shared an identical TCRβ gamma sequence including a 11-bp 'random' N region (Ford *et al.*, 1997).
- One set of twins with hyperdiploid acute lymphoblastic leukaemia shared the same karyotype plus a shared, clonotypic TCRδ sequence (Maia & Greaves, unpublished observations).

All of these molecular markers – *MLL* fusions, *TEL-AML1* and *IgH/TCR* breaks and rearrangements – are highly diverse (and random within circumscribed regions of DNA) and therefore both clone-specific and patient-specific (see Figure 8 for *TEL-AML1*) (Wiemels & Greaves, 1999). Now, since twins do not co-inherit these shared clonal markers, they must share the **same** leukaemic clone originating in one cell in one of the twins. This is plausible, as 60% of monozygotic twins share a single (monochorionic) placenta within which there are vascular anastomoses facilitating cell passage (Strong & Corney, 1967). Blood-cell chimerism in twins has been well recognized for many decades in cattle, and in humans, shared placental vasculature and blood cell transit is responsible for the twin–twin trans-

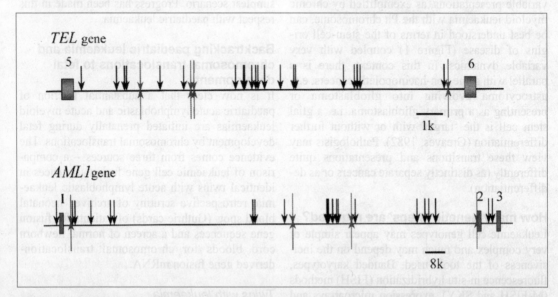

TEL gene

1k

AML1 gene

8k

Figure 8. Break-point positions in *TEL* and *AML1* in acute lymphoblastic leukaemia. Individual, unrelated patients compared with identical twins. Black arrows, individual patients; blue arrows above and below the lines, pairs of identical twins (4 shown). 1K, 4K, size scale of DNA in kilobases. Number red and green boxes, *TEL* and *AML1* exons.

fusion syndrome (Cincotta & Fisk, 1997). In these twin pairs therefore, acute lymphoblastic leukaemia was initiated prenatally. Latency is very short in the case of infant acute lymphoblastic leukaemia with *MLL* gene fusions but for common acute lymphoblastic leukaemia, it is clearly very variable and occasionally protracted (up to 14 years; Wiemels *et al.*, 1999b).

Guthrie card analysis

Confirmation of this interpretation of the twin data and more direct evidence comes from a polymerase chain reaction (PCR)-based analysis of neonatal blood spots or Guthrie cards. For analysis of both twins and Guthrie card DNA, the unique leukaemia fusion gene genomic fusion sequence must first be identified using long-distance PCR methods (Wiemels & Greaves, 1999). Primers can then be designed for conventional nested PCR that will detect fusion genes with low copy number (1–10).

Guthrie cards have so far been tested for *MLL-AF4* (in infant acute lymphoblastic leukaemia) (Gale *et al.*, 1997), *TEL-AML1* (in childhood common acute lymphoblastic leukaemia) (Wiemels *et al.*, 1999a; Maia *et al.*, 2001), *AML1-ETO* (in childhood acute myeloid leukaemia; Wiemels *et al.*, 2002) and for *IGH* sequences (in childhood acute lymphoblastic leukaemia; Fasching *et al.*, 2000; Yagi *et al.*, 2000). These studies are still ongoing, but it is clear that many cases of paediatric acute lymphoblastic leukaemia have a fetal origin with chromosomal translocations as the likely initiating event. Some Guthrie cards do give negative results but these are difficult to interpret (i.e. genuinely postnatal origin or a fetal origin but few cells to detect in the blood spot). It is unclear, therefore, exactly what proportion of paediatric leukaemias are prenatal in origin. A secure conclusion at present would be that all infant acute lymphoblastic leukaemias are prenatal, the majority of childhood acute lymphoblastic leukaemias (with *TEL-AML1*) are prenatal and a substantial fraction (~50%) of childhood acute myeloid leukaemias (with *AML1-ETO*) are prenatal. There is no reason to exclude the possibility that some paediatric acute lymphoblastic/acute myeloid leukaemias do arise postnatally.

A key issue that follows from these observations is whether the chromosomal translocation event *in utero* is sufficient for leukaemia or whether some additional postnatal or secondary changes are also necessary. Conventional wisdom in this field and transgenic animal modelling (Yuan *et al.*, 2001) would support the latter. The concordance **rates** for leukaemia in twins are informative in this regard. The rate for infants is not known with accuracy but appears to be exceptionally high, perhaps close to 100% for those twins with a single placenta (Greaves, 1999). This implies that a functional *MLL* fusion gene in the appropriate stem-cell type will inevitably generate a clinically overt leukaemic population within a very short period (i.e. months rather than years). It is unclear whether MLL fusion proteins achieve this potent transformation status via the simultaneous corruption of multiple signal pathways or by promoting the likelihood of rapid acquisition of other genetic changes, i.e. some form of genetic instability (Ayton & Cleary, 2001). This conclusion is of some etiological relevance as it implies that any relevant exposures are likely to be confined to the period of pregnancy, i.e. exposure of mother and transplacental exposure of the fetus. Some candidate chemical exposures have recently been identified (Alexander *et al.*, 2001) along with inherited susceptibility alleles (Wiemels *et al.*, 1999c, 2001).

For older children, the story is different. Concordance rates are much lower at somewhere between 5% and 15% (Buckley *et al.*, 1996; Hemminki & Jiang, 2002). This still represents a ~100-fold extra risk of leukaemia for the twin of a patient with the disease but clearly this implies that one or more postnatal secondary genetic changes (and associated exposure) are necessary **for which twins are usually discordant**. Several molecular genetic, chromosomal changes have been identified, at diagnosis, in association with *TEL-AML*. These include 9p⁻, 6q⁻ but, at high frequency, 12p⁻ in which the critical deleted region is the non-rearranged *TEL* allele (Bernard *et al.*, 1996). Evidence for the secondary nature of *TEL* deletions in acute lymphoblastic leukaemia comes from FISH analysis which reveals that *TEL* deletions are usually subclonal to *TEL-AML1*.

TEL deletion boundaries are variable and clonotypic. In a pair of twins sharing an identical *TEL-AML1* fusion sequence, *TEL* deletions (mapped by microsatellite loss of heterozygosity (LOH) were shown to be subclonal (by FISH) and had molecularly distinct boundaries (Maia *et al.*, 2001). *TEL* deletions most probably arise therefore as secondary, postnatal events. This might occur proximal to diagnosis as a 'precipitating' event but this is conjecture.

Chromosomal translocations in normal cord blood: frequent initiation of leukaemia, uncommon fruition

These data suggest the simple (or minimal) two-step model illustrated in Figure 9 for childhood acute leukaemias (the infant cases being different). If this is correct, then an important prediction follows. This is that for every child with acute lymphoblastic or acute myeloid leukaemia, there should be many more healthy normal children who are born with a functional leukaemia fusion gene and covert pre-leukaemic clone. We have tested this prediction by screening a large series of unselected newborn cord bloods by RT-PCR, RQ-PCR (Taqman) and FISH for *TEL-AML1* and *AML1-ETO* fusion genes (Mori *et al.*, 2002). The results are summarized in Table 3. The cumulative risk of any child developing acute lymphoblastic leukaemia by the age of 15 years is ~1 in 2000. For acute myeloid leukaemia this figure is ~1 in 10 000; for acute lymphoblastic leukaemia with *TEL-AML1* it is ~1 in 12 500; for acute myeloid leukaemia with *AML1-ETO* it is ~1 in 80 000.

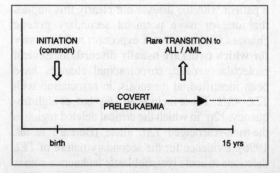

Figure 9. Natural history of paediatric acute leukaemias.

What the data provocatively suggest is that bonafide chromosomal translocations, fusion genes and presumptive pre-leukaemic clones are generated during normal fetal development at a rate that is some 100 times that of the corresponding overt leukaemia. This then implies that the postnatal exposure or secondary genetic event is a crucial bottleneck in the emergence of leukaemia in children. This finding may not be peculiar to leukaemia. Although no other paediatric cancer has been 'back-tracked' using molecular genetic markers, there is longstanding histopathological evidence from autopsy reports that something very similar may well occur with neuroblastoma and Wilms tumour. In both of these cases, and in around 1% of newborns (dying of non-malignant causes), there was evidence for covert adrenocortical and kidney tumours and, as in acute lymphoblastic leukaemia, this represents around 100 times the overt cancer rate. There is a parallel perhaps also with adult disease where breast, prostate and thyroid carcinomas exist subclinically (as judged by autopsy or screening) at rates that considerably exceeds their clinical incidence.

Implications for etiology

These patterns of natural history of paediatric leukaemias have several implications for molecular epidemiology. First, critical time windows for rate-limiting events can be described. Second, inherited alleles and exposures related to risk could be different for initiating and later promoting events. Third, whatever environmental and genetic risk factors are relevant to initiating events, they may be very much more common than the disease itself. Fourth, biologically defined subtypes of disease, e.g. acute lymphoblastic leukaemia positive for the *MLL* fusion gene, must be considered separately. Although this latter requirement may impose limitations on numbers of patients that can be accrued (and therefore statistical robustness), it has the advantage that if associations uncovered are **selective** for a disease subtype, then they are likely to be more credible – e.g. in Wiemels *et al.* (1999c); Alexander *et al.* (2001). The definition of all appropriate biological subgroups for molecular epidemiological studies is beyond the scope of this review (see UK Child-

Table 3. Cord blood screening for leukaemia fusion genes (data from Mori *et al.*, 2002)

	No. screened	No. positive		No. in frame	~Frequency of cells[a]
		By RT- PCR	Confirmed by Taqman	(by sequencing)	
TEL-AML1	567	6 (1%)	6	6	10⁻⁴–10⁻³
AML1-ETO	496	1 (~0.2%)	1	1	10⁻⁴

[a] Calculated range of frequencies of cells in individual cord bloods expressing *TEL-AML1* mRNA. This is based on Taqman quantitation but assumes that levels of mRNA for *TEL-AML1* in 'normal' and overtly leukaemic cells are similar. Fusion gene-positive cells were identified by immunomagnetic cell enrichment followed by combined antibody (cell type)/FISH three-colour staining. In cord bloods with *TEL-AML1*-positive PCR, the fusion gene-positive cells were all of lymphoid lineage (precursor and mature) phenotype. In the one case of *AML1-ETO* fusion gene-positive PCR, the positive cells were myeloid.

hood Cancer Study Investigators, 2000) but should include the following: *MLL* fusion gene-positive infant acute lymphoblastic/acute myeloid leukaemias, common B-cell precursor acute lymphoblastic leukaemia (with *TEL-AML1* or hyperdiploidy), acute myeloid leukaemia with balanced translocation versus monosomy or 5q, 7q deletions, and molecular subtypes of lymphomas. The grouping should recognize that one pathological or haematological subtype can transform into another, e.g. chronic myeloid leukaemia to Philadelphia-positive acute leukaemia, follicular lymphoma to diffuse. Note that, paradoxically, some groups that are often regarded as separate diseases might well be biologically and etiologically a single entity and should therefore be pooled, e.g. paediatric thymic acute lymphoblastic leukaemia and T-non-Hodgkin lymphoma, mature B-acute lymphoblastic leukaemia (FABL3) and Burkitt-like lymphoma. In the former cases of T-cell malignancy, the immunophenotypes and molecular aberrations may be identical and cases with blood-borne disease, diagnosed as T-acute lymphoblastic leukaemia, almost invariably have lymphomatous masses. Evidence supporting this comes from twin data referred to above: T-non-Hodgkin lymphoma and T-acute lymphoblastic leukaemia in a pair of monozygotic twins but deriving from the same single fetal clone (Ford *et al.*, 1997).

For paediatric acute lymphoblastic leukaemia, it remains uncertain what exposures are relevant

to etiology, and evaluation of disease susceptibility alleles is only just beginning. Models or hypotheses proposed several years ago to which new epidemiological and genetic data can now be added have, however, provided plausible mechanisms. For acute leukaemia in infants, the model (Figure 10) is transplacental (or *in utero*) exposure to chemicals that inhibits topoisomerase II (Ross *et al.*, 1994; Greaves, 1999) or other chemicals. In a recent international case–control study, Alexander *et al.* (2001) identified Baygon mosquitocidal and the drug dipyron as possible transplacental agents associated specifically with leukaemia positive for the *MLL* gene. Risk of infant leukaemia with *MLL* fusion genes is modified by

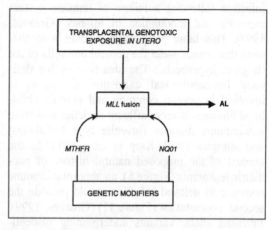

Figure 10. A causal mechanism for infant acute leukaemias.

a number of polymorphic genes including *MTHFR* and *NQO1* (Wiemels *et al.*, 1999c, 2001). This, in turn, implicates both folate metabolism and chemicals detoxified by NAD(P)H: quinone oxidoreductase, including benzene metabolites and quinone-containing substances such as flavonoids (topo II inhibitors). The *NQO1* link might, however, be via an impact on oxidative stress.

For infant leukaemia, there is an urgent need for new multinational molecular epidemiological studies, perhaps, linked to new clinical trials for the disease (e.g. Interfanta 99). These studies need to give careful consideration to the choice of controls but should focus specifically on infant cases with *MLL* gene fusions (acute lymphoblastic and acute myeloid leukaemia) and combine assessment of pregnant mothers' chemical exposures with extensive genotyping of both mother, father and child. The preliminary data on *NQO1* and *MTHFR* alleles require replicating and there are other genes/alleles that should be assessed, e.g. other genes in the folate metabolism pathway (M. Smith, personal communication), cytochrome P450s and glutathione *S*-transferases.

For childhood acute lymphoblastic leukaemias, one current model receiving considerable attention postulates an abnormal response to a common infection (Little *et al.*, 1999). This is postulated to arise as a consequence of either population mobility and mixing (Kinlen, 1995, 1998) or delayed infection following a failure of immune system exposure and modulation in infancy (Greaves, 1997). This latter perspective invokes a mechanism that comes under the general umbrella of the 'hygiene hypothesis'. The idea here is that deficient immunological exposure of infants is involved in several common and chronic childhood illnesses of more affluent societies including autoimmune diseases (juvenile type I diabetes) and allergies (Wills-Karp *et al.*, 2001). In the context of the proposed natural history of paediatric leukaemia (Figure 8), an abnormal immune response to delayed infection would provide the second, postnatal hit (Figure 11) (Greaves, 1999). Inherited allelic variants underpinning susceptibility to the sequential pre- and postnatal events might well be different. Alleles of type II HLA and

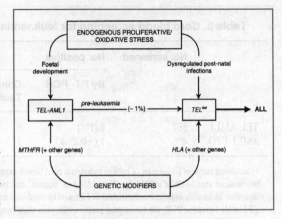

Figure 11. A causal mechanism for childhood acute lymphoblastic leukaemia.

of other genes regulating the immune response (Jepson, 1996) are predicted to modify the risk of the postnatal promotional event in childhood acute lymphoblastic leukaemia. Preliminary data implicates the HLA-DPβ1 0201 allele in increased risk for acute lymphoblastic leukaemia (Taylor *et al.*, 1995; Dearden *et al.*, 1996). Note that Hodgkin lymphoma in young adults is suggested to have a similar etiology to childhood acute lymphoblastic leukaemia, i.e. it is precipitated by an abnormal (delayed) immune response to common infection(s) in genetically susceptible individuals (Gutensohn & Cole, 1981). The concordance rate of Hodgkin lymphoma in young adult twins is also around 5% (Mack *et al.*, 1995); it is unclear if this is all explained by co-inheritance of susceptibility alleles or prenatal sharing of cells and chimerism.

Large case–control studies (e.g. see UK Childhood Cancer Study Investigators, 2000) are in progress in Europe and the USA to evaluate the infection hypothesis and at least two of these are incorporating biological subset analysis of leukaemia and aspects of genotyping or gene–environment interaction (the UK study and the California study; P. Buffler, personal communication). The delayed infection hypothesis makes some testable predictions concerning direct or proxy measures of infection in the two critical time windows. Children with acute lymphoblastic leukaemia are predicted to have evidence of fewer infections in infancy and fewer social contacts (i.e. proxy for infections) as reflected in number of siblings or attendance at playgroups of different sizes. The first-born should be more at risk than those with older siblings. Some types of vaccinations given in infancy might be expected to be protective. Some evidence for all of these associations is in fact already available (Table 4) but needs replicating in large, well-designed studies with appropriate control selection. Finally, reports of striking clusters of childhood acute lymphoblastic leukaemia (as in the recent case of Fallon, Nevada) should be considered not just in the emotionally charged context of local sources of genotoxic pollutants but in terms of recent population mixing as a setting for infection (Kinlen, 1995).

The infectious etiology hypotheses raise the obvious question of molecular screening for candidate agents but this may be less than rewarding if the exposure involves not a trans-forming virus (as in cat and chicken leukaemia) but an abnormal immune response to one, or perhaps several, infections and which could be bacterial. Nevertheless, molecular PCR-based screening for candidate viruses or viral families has been carried out. So far, the results have been negative for polyoma and herpes family members (MacKenzie *et al.*, 1999, 2001).

It will be critical to combine exposure data of biological subtypes of acute lymphoblastic leukaemia with genetic susceptibility data (e.g. allelic variation in immune response genes, *NQO1*); the combination of the two provides a platform for evaluating gene–environment interaction and might be expected to produce more convincing odds ratios. There are encouraging precedents from other infectious diseases where allelic variations have been linked to susceptibility (Cooke & Hill, 2001). In view of the finding of an association of *MTHFR* alleles and risk of paediatric

---

Table 4. Epidemiological evidence supporting an infectious aetiology of childhood acute lymphoblastic leukaemia

		Risk[a]	References
A.	The 'delayed infection' hypothesis		Greaves (1988, 1997)
	1. ↑ Common infections in infancy	↓	van Steensel-Moll *et al.* (1986); McKinney *et al.* (1999); Chan *et al.* (2002)
	2. ↑ Infections 3–12 months before diagnosis	↑	Chan *et al.* (2002)
	3. ↑ Social contacts in infancy:		Petridou *et al.* (1993, 1997); Infante-
	Attendance at playgroups	↓	Rivard *et al.* (2000); Ma *et al.* (2002);
	Older siblings	↓	Dockerty *et al.* (2001); Greaves (2001)
	4. Vaccinations in pregnancy	↓	Auvinen *et al.* (2000); Groves *et al.* (2001)
	Haemophilus influenzae		
	5. Seasonal variation (of onset)	↑↓	Badrinath *et al.* (1997); Westerbeek *et al.* (1998); Ross *et al.* (1999); Sørensen *et al.* (2001)
B.	The 'population mixing' hypothesis		Kinlen (1989, 1995, 1998)
	↑ Recent population mobility and mixing[b]	↑	Kinlen (1995); Alexander *et al.* (1997); Dickinson & Parker (1999); Kinlen & Balkwill (2001)

[a] Only supportive studies listed. Some other studies have produced contrary data but, in part, this may be due to differences in study design.

[b] Other clear-cut examples of space–time clustering of childhood acute lymphoblastic leukaemia also accord with an infectious etiology of acute lymphoblastic leukaemia (e.g. Heath & Hasterlik, 1963; Alexander, 1992; Alexander *et al.*, 1996, 1998) but are potentially open to other, 'non-infectious' interpretations.

leukaemia (as well as adult acute lymphoblastic leukaemia and lymphoma; see Smith *et al.*, this volume), dietary aspects of folate intake should be studied. In this respect, the recent finding that folate supplementation by pregnant women may decrease risk of acute lymphoblastic leukaemia in offspring is of particular interest (Thompson *et al.*, 2001) and should be replicated in the context of a molecular epidemiological study with *MTHFR* allele assessment. Indeed, folate metabolism may play a more critical role in leukaemogenesis (and other cancers) than previously suspected. It is well established that lowered folate levels can, via enhanced uracil incorporation and its excision repair in DNA, increase DNA breaks (Blount *et al.*, 1997). The interaction between folate intake during pregnancy and genotype may well have a decisive influence on the risk of chromosomal translocations and pre-leukaemic clones arising in the fetus.

There is an urgent need to develop equivalent natural history and etiological models and molecular epidemiological testing for adult leukaemia and lymphoma. A long-standing idea (see Magrath, 1990) is that malignancies of mature lymphoid cells (non-Hodgkin lymphoma, chronic lymphocytic leukaemia, prolymphocytic leukaemia) are initially driven by antigens (infectious or otherwise, including autoantigens), and that, as in gastric lymphoma with *H. pylori* (Wotherspoon *et al.*, 1993), the clone becomes more malignant when immunological networking control breaks down and antigen independence emerges. A similar scenario, perhaps, to that of estrogenic and androgenic drive of breast and prostate cancers? Lymphomas associated with chronic hepatitis C infection, cryoglobulinaemia and rheumatoid factor (Ig) production appear to provide another plausible example of lymphoma initiation via chronic antigenic stimulation (De Re *et al.*, 2000).

Many of these non-Hodgkin lymphoma cancers originate in B-cell subsets within the germinal centre – a hotbed of hypermutation, cell selection and apoptosis. This area deserves much more study. Adult non-Hodgkin lymphoma is a common cancer and is increasing significantly in incidence (for unknown reasons) in Europe and North America. Although often presenting in a benign, localized form it usually emerges, phoenix-like, after a silence of some years, as a lethal cancer.

Acknowledgements

The author's research is supported by the Leukaemia Research Fund, the Kay Kendall Leukaemia Fund and the Institute of Cancer Research.

References

Alexander, F.E. (1992) Space–time clustering of childhood acute lymphoblastic leukaemia: indirect evidence for a transmissible agent. *Br. J. Cancer*, **65**, 589–592

Alexander, F.E., Wray, N., Boyle, P., Bring, J., Coebergh, J.W., Draper, G., Levi, F., McKinney, P.A., Michaelis, J., Peris-Bonet, R., Petridou, E., Pukkala, E., Storm, H., Terracini, B. & Vatten, L. (1996) Clustering of childhood leukaemia: a European study in progress. *J. Epidemiol. Biostatist.*, **1**, 13–24

Alexander, F.E., Chan, L.C., Lam, T.H., Yuen, P., Leung, N.K., Ha, S.Y., Yuen, H.L., Li, C.K., Li, C.K., Lau, Y.L. & Greaves, M.F. (1997) Clustering of childhood leukaemia in Hong Kong: association with the childhood peak and common acute lymphoblastic leukaemia and with population mixing. *Br. J. Cancer*, **75**, 457–463

Alexander, F.E., Boyle, P., Carli, P.M., Coebergh, J.W., Draper, G.J., Ekbom, A., Levi, F., McKinney, P.A., McWhirter, W., Magnani, C., Michaelis, J., Olsen, J.H., Peris-Bonet, R., Petridou, E., Pukkala, E. & Vatten, L. (1998) Spatial temporal patterns in childhood leukaemia: further evidence for an infectious origin. EUROCLUS project. *Br. J. Cancer*, **77**, 812–817

Alexander, F.E., Patheal, S.L., Biondi, A., Brandalise, S., Cabrera, M.-E., Chan, L.C., Chen, Z., Cimino, G., Cordoba, J.-C., Gu, L.-J., Hussein, H., Ishii, E., Kamel, A.M., Labra, S., Magalhães, I.Q., Mizutani, S., Petridou, E., Pombo de Oliveira, M., Yuen, P., Wiemels, J.L. & Greaves, M.F. (2001) Transplacental chemical exposure and risk of infant leukemia with *MLL* gene fusion. *Cancer Res.*, **61**, 2542–2546

Andersen, M.K., Johansson, B., Larsen, S.O. & Pedersen-Bjergaard, J. (1998) Chromosomal abnormalities in secondary MDS and AML. Relationship to drugs and radiation with specific emphasis on the balanced rearrangements. *Haematologica*, **83**, 483–488

Auvinen, A., Hakulinen, T. & Groves, F. (2000) *Haemophilus influenzae* type B vaccination and risk of childhood leukaemia in a vaccine trial in Finland. *Br. J. Cancer*, **83**, 956–958

Ayton, P.M. & Cleary, M.L. (2001) Molecular mechanisms of leukemogenesis mediated by MLL fusion proteins. *Oncogene*, **20**, 5695–5707

Badrinath, P., Day, N.E. & Stockton, D. (1997) Seasonality in the diagnosis of acute lymphocytic leukaemia. *Br. J. Cancer*, **75**, 1711–1713

Barr, F.G. (1998) Translocations, cancer and the puzzle of specificity. *Nature Genet.*, **19**, 121–124

Bernard, O.A., Romana, S.P., Poirel, H. & Berger, R. (1996) Molecular cytogenetics of t(12;21)(p13; q22). *Leuk. Lymphoma*, **23**, 459–465

Bhatia, S., Ross, J.A., Greaves, M.F. & Robison, L.L. (1999) Epidemiology and etiology. In: Pui, C.-H., ed., *Childhood Leukemias*, Cambridge, Cambridge University Press, pp. 38–49

Blount, B.C., Mack, M.M., Wehr, C.M., MacGregor, J.T., Hiatt, R.A., Wang, G., Wickramasinghe, S.N., Everson, R.B. & Ames, B.N. (1997) Folate deficiency causes uracil misincorporation into human DNA and chromosome breakage: implications for cancer and neuronal damage. *Proc. natl Acad. Sci. USA*, **94**, 3290–3295

Bonnet, D. & Dick, J.E. (1997) Human acute myeloid leukemia is organized as a hierarchy that originates from a primitive hematopoietic cell. *Nature Med.*, **3**, 730–737

Breit, T.M., Mol, E.J., Wolvers-Tettero, I.L., Ludwig, W.-D., van Wering, E.R. & van Dongen, J.J.M. (1993) Site-specific deletions involving the *tal*-1 and *sil* genes are restricted to cells of the T cell receptor α/β lineage: T cell receptor δ gene deletion mechanism affects multiple genes. *J. exp. Med.*, **177**, 965–977

Buckley, J.D., Buckley, C.M., Breslow, N.E., Draper, G.J., Roberson, P.K. & Mack, T.M. (1996) Concordance for childhood cancer in twins. *Med. pediatr. Oncol.*, **26**, 223–229

Carter, T.L., Reaman, G.H. & Kees, U.R. (2001) *INK4A/ARF* deletions are acquired at relapse in childhood acute lymphoblastic leukaemia: a paired

study on 25 patients using real-time polymerase chain reaction. *Br. J. Haematol.*, **113**, 323–328

Chan, L.C., Lam, T.H., Li, C.K., Lau, Y.L., Li, C.K., Yuen, H.L., Lee, C.W., Ha, S.Y., Yuen, P., Leung, N.K., Patheal, S.L., Greaves, M.F. & Alexander, F.E. (2002) Is the timing of exposure to infection a major determinant of acute lymphoblastic leukaemia in Hong Kong? *Pediatr. perinat. Epidemiol.*, **16**, 154–165

Cincotta, R.B. & Fisk, N.M. (1997) Current thoughts on twin-twin transfusion syndrome. *Clin. Obstet. Gynecol.*, **40**, 290–302

Cooke, G.S. & Hill, A.V.S. (2001) Genetics of susceptibility to human infectious disease. *Nature Rev. Genet.*, **2**, 967–977

Corral, J., Lavenir, I., Impey, H., Warren, A.J., Forster, A., Larson, T.A., Bell, S., McKenzie, A.N.J., King, G. & Rabbitts, T.H. (1996) An *Mll-AF9* fusion gene made by homologous recombination causes acute leukemia in chimeric mice: a method to create fusion oncogenes. *Cell*, **85**, 853–861

Dalla-Favera, R., Migliazza, A., Chang, C.C., Niu, H., Pasqualucci, L., Butler, M., Shen, Q. & Cattoretti, G. (1999) Molecular pathogenesis of B cell malignancy: the role of BCL-6. *Curr. Top. Microbiol. Immunol.*, **246**, 257–263

De Re, V., De Vita, S., Marzotto, A., Rupolo, M., Gloghini, A., Pivetta, B., Gasparotto, D., Carbone, A. & Boiocchi, M. (2000) Sequence analysis of the immunoglobulin antigen receptor of hepatitis C virus-associated non-Hodgkin lymphomas suggests that the malignant cells are derived from the rheumatoid factor-producing cells that occur mainly in type II cryoglobulinemia. *Blood*, **96**, 3578–3584

Dearden, S.P., Taylor, G.M., Gokhale, D.A., Robinson, M.D., Thompson, W., Ollier, W., Binchy, A., Birch, J.M., Stevens, R.F., Carr, T. & Bardsley, W.G. (1996) Molecular analysis of *HLA-DQB1* alleles in childhood common acute lymphoblastic leukaemia. *Br. J. Cancer*, **73**, 603–609

Deininger, M.W.N., Goldman, J.M. & Melo, J.V. (2000) The molecular biology of chronic myeloid leukaemia. *Blood*, **96**, 3343–3356

Dickinson, H.O. & Parker, L. (1999) Quantifying the effect of population mixing on childhood leukaemia risk: the Seascale cluster. *Br. J. Cancer*, **81**, 144–151

Dockerty, J.D., Draper, G., Vincent, T., Rowan, S.D. & Bunch, K.J. (2001) Case–control study of parental age, parity and socioeconomic level in relation to childhood cancers. *Int. J. Epidemiol.*, **30**, 1428–1437

Druker, B.J., Talpaz, M., Resta, D.J., Peng, B., Buchdunger, E., Ford, J.M., Lydon, N.B., Kantarjian, H., Capdeville, R., Ohno-Jones, S. & Sawyers, C.L. (2001) Efficacy and safety of a specific inhibitor of the BCR-ABL tyrosine kinase in chronic myeloid leukaemia. *New Engl. J. Med.*, **344**, 1031–1037

Du, M.-Q. & Isaacson, P.G. (1998) Recent advances in our understanding of the biology and pathogenesis of gastric mucosa-associated lymphoid tissue (MALT) lymphoma. *FORUM Trends exp. clin. Med.*, **8**, 162–173

Enver, T. & Greaves, M.F. (1998) Loops, lineage, and leukaemia. *Cell*, **94**, 9–12

Fasching, K., Panzer, S., Haas, O.A., Marschalek, R., Gadner, H. & Panzer-Grümayer, E.R. (2000) Presence of clone-specific antigen receptor gene rearrangements at birth indicates an in utero origin of diverse types of early childhood acute lymphoblastic leukaemia. *Blood*, **95**, 2722–2724

Felix, C.A. (1998) Secondary leukemias induced by topoisomerase-targeted drugs. *Biochim. biophys. Acta*, **1400**, 233–255

Ferguson, D.O. & Alt, F.W. (2001) DNA double strand break repair and chromosomal translocation: lessons from animal models. *Oncogene*, **20**, 5572–5579

Ferrando, A.A. & Look, A.T. (2000) Clinical implications of recurring chromosomal and associated molecular abnormalities in acute lymphoblastic leukaemia. *Semin. Hematol.*, **37**, 381–395

Ford, A.M., Ridge, S.A., Cabrera, M.E., Mahmoud, H., Steel, C.M., Chan, L.C. & Greaves, M.F. (1993) *In utero* rearrangements in the trithorax-related oncogene in infant leukaemias. *Nature*, **363**, 358–360

Ford, A.M., Pombo-de-Oliveira, M.S., McCarthy, K.P., MacLean, J.M., Carrico, K.C., Vincent, R.F. & Greaves, M. (1997) Monoclonal origin of concordant T-cell malignancy in identical twins. *Blood*, **89**, 281–285

Ford, A.M., Bennett, C.A., Price, C.M., Bruin, M.C.A., Van Wering, E.R. & Greaves, M.F. (1998) Fetal origins of the *TEL-AML1* fusion gene in identical twins with leukaemia. *Proc. natl Acad. Sci. USA*, **95**, 4584–4588

Gale, K.B., Ford, A.M., Repp, R., Borkhardt, A., Keller, C., Eden, O.B. & Greaves, M.F. (1997) Backtracking leukaemia to birth: identification of clonotypic gene fusion sequences in neonatal blood spots. *Proc. natl Acad. Sci. USA*, **94**, 13950–13954

Gill Super, H.J., Rothberg, P.G., Kobayashi, H., Freeman, A.I., Diaz, M.O. & Rowley, J.D. (1994) Clonal, nonconstitutional rearrangements of the *MLL* gene in infant twins with acute lymphoblastic leukemia: in utero chromosome rearrangement of 11q23. *Blood*, **83**, 641–644

Gillert, E., Leis, T., Repp, R., Reichel, M., Hosch, A., Breitenlohner, I., Angermuller, S., Borkhardt, A., Harbott, J., Lampert, F., Griesinger, F., Greil, J., Fey, G.H. & Marschalek, R. (1999) A DNA damage repair mechanism is involved in the origin of chromosomal translocations t(4;11) in primary leukemic cells. *Oncogene*, **18**, 4663–4671

Greaves, M.F. (1982) 'Target' cells differentiation and clonal evolution in chronic granulocytic leukaemia: a 'model' for understanding the biology of malignancy. In: Shaw, M.T., ed., *Chronic Granulocytic Leukaemia*, New York, Praeger, pp. 15–47

Greaves, M.F. (1988) Speculations on the cause of childhood acute lymphoblastic leukaemia. *Leukemia*, **2**, 120–125

Greaves, M.F. (1996) The new biology of leukemia. In: Henderson, E.S., Lister, T.A. & Greaves, M.F., eds, *Leukemia*, Philadelphia, W.B. Saunders, pp. 34–45

Greaves, M.F. (1997) Aetiology of acute leukaemia. *Lancet*, **349**, 344–349

Greaves, M.F. (1999) Molecular genetics, natural history and the demise of childhood leukaemia. *Eur. J. Cancer*, **35**, 1941–1953

Greaves, M.F. (2000) *Cancer. The Evolutionary Legacy*, Oxford, Oxford University Press

Greaves, M.F. (2001) Commentary: birth order and risk of childhood acute lymphoblastic leukaemia (ALL). *Int. J. Epidemiol.*, **30**, 1438–1439

Groves, F.D., Sinha, D., Kayhty, H., Goedert, J.J. & Levine, P.H. (2001) *Haemophilus influenzae* type b serology in childhood leukaemia: a case–control study. *Br. J. Cancer*, **85**, 337–340

Gutensohn, N. & Cole, P. (1981) Childhood social environment and Hodgkin's disease. *New Engl. J. Med.*, **304**, 135–140

Haluska, F.G., Finger, L.R., Kagan, J. & Croce, C.M. (1990) Molecular genetics of chromosomal translocations in B- and T-lymphoid malignancies. In: Cossman, J., ed., *Molecular Genetics in Cancer Diagnosis*, New York, Elsevier, pp. 143–162

Hanahan, D. & Weinberg, R.A. (2000) The hallmarks of cancer. *Cell*, **100**, 57–70

Heath, C.W., Jr & Hasterlik, R.J. (1963) Leukemia among children in a suburban community. *Am. J. Med.*, **34**, 796–812

Heisterkamp, N., Jenster, G., ten Hoeve, J., Zovich, D., Pattengale, P.K. & Groffen, J. (1990) Acute leukaemia in *bcr/abl* transgenic mice. *Nature*, **344**, 251–253

Hemminki, K. & Jiang, Y. (2002) Risks among siblings and twins for childhood acute lymphoid leukaemia: results from the Swedish Family-Cancer Database. *Leukemia*, **16**, 297–298

Horsman, D.E., Connors, J.M., Pantzar, T. & Gascoyne, R.D. (2001) Analysis of secondary chromosomal alterations in 165 cases of follicular lymphoma with t(14;18). *Genes Chromosomes Cancer*, **30**, 375–382

Imamura, J., Miyoshi, I. & Koeffler, H.P. (1994) p53 in hematologic malignancies. *Blood*, **84**, 2412–2421

Infante-Rivard, C., Fortier, I. & Olson, E. (2000) Markers of infection, breast-feeding and childhood acute lymphoblastic leukaemia. *Br. J. Cancer*, **83**, 1559–1564

Jaffe, E.S., Harris, N.L., Stein, H. & Vardiman, J.W. (2001) *Pathology and Genetics of Tumours of Haematopoietic and Lymphoid Tissues (WHO Classification of Tumours)*, Lyon, IARCPress

Jepson, A.P. (1996) Infection . . . by the new genetics. *J. Infect.*, **33**, 1–5

Kinlen, L.J. (1989) Infective cause of childhood leukaemia. *Lancet*, **i**, 378–379

Kinlen, L.J. (1995) Epidemiological evidence for an infective basis in childhood leukaemia. *Br. J. Cancer*, **71**, 1–5

Kinlen, L.J. (1998) Infection and childhood leukaemia. *Cancer Causes Control*, **9**, 237–239

Kinlen, L.J. & Balkwill, A. (2001) Infective cause of childhood leukaemia and wartime population mixing in Orkney and Shetland, UK. *Lancet*, **357**, 858

Knudson, A.G. (1992) Stem cell regulation, tissue ontogeny, and oncogenic events. *Semin. Cancer Biol.*, **3**, 99–106

Kroll, T.G., Sarraf, P., Pecciarini, L., Chen, C.-J., Mueller, E., Spiegelman, B.M. & Fletcher, J.A. (2000) *PAX8-PPARγ1* fusion oncogene in human thyroid carcinoma. *Science*, **289**, 1357–1360

Küppers, R. & Dalla-Favera, R. (2001) Mechanisms of chromosomal translocations in B cell lymphomas. *Oncogene*, **20**, 5580–5594

Lengauer, C. (2001) How do tumors make ends meet? *Proc. natl Acad. Sci. USA*, **98**, 12331–12333

Little, M.P., Weiss, H.A., Boice, J.D., Darby, S.C., Day, N.E. & Muirhead, C.R. (1999) Risks of leukemia in Japanese atomic bomb survivors, in women treated for cervical cancer, and in patients treated for ankylosing spondylitis. *Radiat. Res.*, **152**, 280–292

Liu, H., Ruskon-Fourmestraux, A., Lavergne-Slove, A., Ye, H., Molina, T., Bouhnik, Y., Hamoudi, R.A., Diss, T.C., Dogan, A., Megraud, F., Rambaud, J.C., Du, M.-Q. & Isaacson, P.G. (2001) Resistance of t(11;18) positive gastric mucosa-associated lymphoid tissue lymphoma to *Helicobacter pylori* eradication therapy. *Lancet*, **357**, 39–40

Look, A.T. (1997) Oncogenic transcription factors in the human acute leukemias. *Science*, **278**, 1059–1064

Lovett, B.D., Lo Nigro, L., Rappaport, E.F., Blair, I.A., Osheroff, N., Zheng, N., Megonigal, M.D., Williams, W.R., Nowell, P.C. & Felix, C.A. (2001) Near-precise interchromosomal recombination and functional DNA topoisomerase II cleavage sites at *MLL* and *AF-4* genomic breakpoints in treatment-related acute lymphoblastic leukemia with t(4;11) translocation. *Proc. natl Acad. Sci. USA*, **98**, 9802–9807

Lutterbach, B. & Hiebert, S.W. (2000) Role of the transcription factor AML-1 in acute leukemia and hematopoietic differentiation. *Gene*, **245**, 223–235

Ma, X., Buffler, P.A., Selvin, S., Matthay, K.K., Wiencke, J.K., Wiemels, J.L. & Reynolds, P. (2002) Daycare/preschool attendance and the risk of childhood acute lymphoblastic leukaemia. *Br. J. Cancer*, **86**, 1419–1424

Mack, T.M., Cozen, W., Shibata, D.K., Weiss, L.M., Nathwani, B.N., Hernandez, A.M., Taylor, C.R., Hamilton, A.S., Deapen, D.M. & Rappaport, E.B. (1995) Concordance for Hodgkin's disease in identical twins suggesting genetic susceptibility to the young-adult form of the disease. *New Engl. J. Med.*, **332**, 413–418

MacKenzie, J., Perry, J., Ford, A.M., Jarrett, R.F. & Greaves, M. (1999) JC and BK virus sequences are not detectable in leukaemic samples from children with common acute lymphoblastic leukaemia. *Br. J. Cancer*, **81**, 898–899

MacKenzie, J., Gallagher, A., Clayton, R.A., Perry, J., Eden, O.B., Ford, A.M., Greaves, M.F. & Jarrett, R.F. (2001) Screening for herpesvirus genomes in common acute lymphoblastic leukaemia. *Leukemia*, **15**, 415–421

Magrath, I.T., ed. (1990) *The Non-Hodgkin's Lymphomas*, London, Edward Arnold

Maia, A.T., Ford, A.M., Jalali, G.R., Harrison, C.J., Taylor, G.M., Eden, O.B. & Greaves, M.F. (2001) Molecular tracking of leukemogenesis in a triplet pregnancy. *Blood*, **98**, 478–482

Marculescu, R., Le, T., Simon, P., Jaeger, U. & Nadel, B. (2002) V(D)J-mediated translocations in lymphoid neoplasms: a functional assessment of genomic instability by cryptic sites. *J. exp. Med.*, **195**, 85–98

McKinney, P.A., Juszczak, E., Findlay, E., Smith, K. & Thomson, C.S. (1999) Pre- and perinatal risk factors for childhood leukaemia and other malignancies: a Scottish case control study. *Br. J. Cancer*, **80**, 1844–1851

Megonigal, M.D., Rappaport, E.F., Jones, D.H., Williams, T.M., Lovett, B.D., Kelly, K.M., Lerou, P.H., Moulton, T., Budarf, M.L. & Felix, C.A. (1998) t(11;22)(q23;q11.2) in acute myeloid leukemia of infant twins fuses *MLL* with hCDC*rel*, a cell division cycle gene in the genomic region of deletion in DiGeorge and velocardiofacial syndromes. *Proc. natl Acad. Sci. USA*, **95**, 6413–6418

Mori, H., Colman, S.M., Xiao, Z., Ford, A.M., Healy, L.E., Donaldson, C., Hows, J.M., Navarrete, C. & Greaves, M. (2002) Chromosome translocations and covert leukemic clones are generated during normal fetal development. *Proc. natl Acad. Sci. USA*, **99**, 8242–8247

Mrozek, K. & Bloomfield, C.D. (1998) Major cytogenetic findings in non-Hodgkin's lymphoma. In: Canellos, G.P., Lister, T.A. & Sklar, J.L., eds, *The Lymphomas*, Philadelphia, W.B. Saunders, pp. 107–128

Okuda, T., van Deursen, J., Hiebert, S.W., Grosveld, G. & Downing, J.R. (1996) AML1, the target of multiple chromosomal translocations in human leu-

kemia, is essential for normal fetal liver hematopoiesis. *Cell*, **84**, 321–330

Petridou, E., Kassimos, D., Kalmanti, M., Kosmidis, H., Haidas, S., Flytzani, V., Tong, D. & Trichopoulos, D. (1993) Age of exposure to infections and risk of childhood leukaemia. *Br. med. J.*, **307**, 774

Petridou, E., Trichopoulos, D., Kalapothaki, V., Pourtsidis, A., Kogevinas, M., Kalmanti, M., Koliouskas, D., Kosmidis, H., Panagiotou, J.P., Piperopoulou, F. & Tzortzatou, F. (1997) The risk profile of childhood leukaemia in Greece: a nationwide case–control study. *Br. J. Cancer*, **76**, 1241–1247

Preston, D.L., Kusumi, S., Tomonaga, M., Izumi, S., Ron, E., Kuramoto, A., Kamada, N., Dohy, H., Matsui, T., Nonaka, H., Thompson, D.E., Soda, M. & Mabuchi, K. (1994) Cancer incidence in atomic bomb survivors. 3. Leukemia, lymphoma and multiple myeloma, 1950–1987. *Radiat. Res.*, **137** (Suppl.), S68–S97

Rabbitts, T.H. (1994) Chromosomal translocations in human cancer. *Nature*, **372**, 143–149

Redner, R.L., Wang, J. & Liu, J. (1999) Chromatin remodeling and leukemia: new therapeutic paradigms. *Blood*, **94**, 417–428

Ross, J.A., Potter, J.D. & Robison, L.L. (1994) Infant leukemia, topoisomerase II inhibitors, and the MLL gene. *J. natl Cancer Inst.*, **86**, 1678–1680

Ross, J.A., Severson, R.K., Swensen, A.R., Pollock, B.H., Gurney, J.G. & Robison, L.L. (1999) Seasonal variations in the diagnosis of childhood cancer in the United States. *Br. J. Cancer*, **81**, 549–553

Rothkamm, K., Kühne, M., Jeggo, P.A. & Löbrich, M. (2001) Radiation-induced genomic rearrangements formed by nonhomologous end-joining of DNA double-strand breaks. *Cancer Res.*, **61**, 3886–3893

Rowley, J.D. (1998) The critical role of chromosome translocations in human leukemias. *Annu. Rev. Genet.*, **32**, 495–519

So, C.W., Ma, Z.G., Price, C.M., Dong, S., Chen, S.J., Gu, L.J., So, C.K., Wiedemann, L.M. & Chan, L.C. (1997) *MLL* self fusion mediated by Alu repeat homologous recombination and prognosis of AML-M4/M5 subtypes. *Cancer Res.*, **57**, 117–122

Song, W.-J., Sullivan, M.G., Legare, R.D., Hutchings, S., Tan, X., Kufrin, D., Ratajczak, J., Resende, I.C., Haworth, C., Hock, R., Loh, M., Felix, C., Roy,

D.-C., Busque, L., Kumit, D., Willman, C., Gewirtz, A.M., Speck, N.A., Bushweller, J.H., Li, F.P., Gardiner, K., Poncz, M., Maris, J.M. & Gilliland, D.G. (1999) Haploinsufficiency of *CBFA2* causes familial thrombocytopenia with propensity to develop acute myelogenous leukaemia. *Nature Genet.*, **23**, 166–175

Sørensen, H.T., Pedersen, L., Olsen, J.H. & Rothman, K.J. (2001) Seasonal variation in month of birth and diagnosis of early childhood acute lymphoblastic leukaemia. *J. Am. med. Assoc.*, **285**, 168–169

van Steensel-Moll, H.A., Valkenburg, H.A. & van Zanen, G.E. (1986) Childhood leukemia and infectious diseases in the first year of life: a register-based case–control study. *Am. J. Epidemiol.*, **124**, 590–594

Strissel, P.L., Strick, R., Rowley, J.D. & Zeleznik-Le, N.J. (1998) An in vivo topoisomerase II cleavage site and a DNase I hypersensitive site colocalize near exon 9 in the *MLL* breakpoint cluster region. *Blood*, **92**, 3793–3803

Strong, S.J. & Corney, G. (1967) *The Placenta in Twin Pregnancy*, Oxford, Pergamon Press

Taylor, G.M., Robinson, M.D., Binchy, A., Birch, J.M., Stevens, R.F., Jones, P.M., Carr, T., Dearden, S. & Gokhale, D.A. (1995) Preliminary evidence of an association between HLA-DPB1*0201 and childhood common acute lymphoblastic leukaemia supports an infectious aetiology. *Leukemia*, **9**, 440–443

Tenen, D.G., Hromas, R., Licht, J.D. & Zhang, D.E. (1997) Transcription factors, normal myeloid development, and leukaemia. *Blood*, **90**, 489–519

Thompson, J.R., Gerald, P.F., Willoughby, M.L.N. & Armstrong, B.K. (2001) Maternal folate supplementation in pregnancy and protection against acute lymphoblastic leukaemia in childhood: a case–control study. *Lancet*, **358**, 1935–1940

UK Childhood Cancer Study Investigators (2000) The United Kingdom Childhood Cancer Study: objectives, materials and methods. *Br. J. Cancer*, **82**, 1073–1102

Vaandrager, J.-W., Schuuring, E., Philippo, K. & Kluin, P.M. (2000) V(D)J recombinase-mediated transposition of the *BCL2* gene to the *IGH* locus in follicular lymphoma. *Blood*, **96**, 1947–1952

Veldman, T., Vignon, C., Schröck, E., Rowley, J.D. & Ried, T. (1997) Hidden chromosome abnormalities in haematological malignancies detected by multi-colour spectral karyotyping. *Nature Genet.*, **15**, 406–410

Westerbeek, R.M., Blair, V., Eden, O.B., Kelsey, A.M., Stevens, R.F., Will, A.M., Taylor, G.M. & Birch, J.M. (1998) Seasonal variations in the onset of childhood leukaemia and lymphoma. *Br. J. Cancer*, **78**, 119–124

Wiemels, J.L. & Greaves, M.F. (1999) Structure and possible mechanisms of *TEL-AML1* gene fusions in childhood acute lymphoblastic leukaemia. *Cancer Res.*, **59**, 4075–4082

Wiemels, J.L., Cazzaniga, G., Daniotti, M., Eden, O.B., Addison, G.M., Masera, G., Saha, V., Biondi, A. & Greaves, M.F. (1999a) Prenatal origin of acute lymphoblastic leukaemia in children. *Lancet*, **354**, 1499–1503

Wiemels, J.L., Ford, A.M., Van Wering, E.R., Postma, A. & Greaves, M.F. (1999b) Protracted and variable latency of acute lymphoblastic leukemia after *TEL-AML1* gene fusion in utero. *Blood*, **94**, 1057–1062

Wiemels, J.L., Pagnamenta, A., Taylor, G.M., Eden, O.B., Alexander, F.E. & Greaves, M.F. (1999c) A lack of a functional NAD(P)H:quinone oxido-reductase allele is selectively associated with pediatric leukemias that have *MLL* fusions. *Cancer Res.*, **59**, 4095–4099

Wiemels, J.L., Smith, R.N., Taylor, G.M., Eden, O.B., Alexander, F.E. & Greaves, M.F. (2001) Methylenetetrahydrofolate reductase (MTHFR) polymorphisms and risk of molecularly defined subtypes of childhood acute leukaemia. *Proc. natl Acad. Sci. USA*, **98**, 4004–4009

Wiemels, J.L., Xiao, Z., Buffler, P.A., Maia, A.T., Ma, X., Dicks, B.M., Smith, M.T., Zhang, L., Feusner, J., Wiencke, J., Pritchard-Jones, K., Kempski, H. & Greaves, M. (2002) In-utero origin of t(8;21) *AML1-ETO* translocations in childhood acute myeloid leukaemia. *Blood*, **99**, 3801–3805

Wills-Karp, M., Santeliz, J. & Karp, C.L. (2001) The germless theory of allergic disease: revisiting the hygiene hypothesis. *Nature Rev. Immunol.*, **1**, 69–75

Wotherspoon, A.C., Doglioni, C., Diss, T.C., Pan, L., Moschini, A., de Boni, M. & Isaacson, P.G. (1993) Regression of primary low-grade B-cell gastric lymphoma of mucosa-associated lymphoid tissue type after eradication of *Helicobacter pylori*. *Lancet*, **342**, 575–577

Xiao, Z., Greaves, M.F., Buffler, P., Smith, M.T., Segal, M.R., Dicks, B.M., Wiencke, J.K. & Wiemels, J.L. (2001) Molecular characterization of genomic *AML1-ETO* fusions in childhood leukaemia. *Leukemia*, **15**, 1906–1913

Yagi, T., Hibi, S., Tabata, Y., Kuriyama, K., Teramura, T., Hashida, T., Shimizu, Y., Takimoto, T., Todo, S., Sawada, T. & Imashuku, S. (2000) Detection of clonotypic IGH and TCR rearrangements in the neonatal blood spots of infants and children with B-cell precursor acute lymphoblastic leukaemia. *Blood*, **96**, 264–268

Yoshida, H., Naoe, T., Fukutani, H., Kiyoi, H., Kubo, K. & Ohno, R. (1995) Analysis of the joining sequences of the t(15;17) translocation in human acute promyelocytic leukemia: sequence non-specific recombination between the *PML* and *RARA* genes within identical short stretches. *Genes Chromosomes Cancer*, **12**, 37–44

Yu, B.D., Hanson, R.D., Hess, J.L., Horning, S.E. & Korsmeyer, S.J. (1998) MLL, a mammalian *trithorax*-group gene, functions as a transcriptional maintenance factor in morphogenesis. *Proc. natl Acad. Sci. USA*, **95**, 10632–10636

Yuan, Y., Zhou, L., Miyamoto, T., Iwasaki, H., Harakawa, N., Hetherington, C.J., Burel, S.A., Lagasse, E., Weissman, I.L., Akashi, K. & Zhang, D.-E. (2001) AML1-ETO expression is directly involved in the development of acute myeloid leukemia in the presence of additional mutations. *Proc. natl Acad. Sci. USA*, **98**, 10398–10403

Zelent, A., Guidez, F., Melnick, A., Waxman, S. & Licht, J.D. (2001) Translocations of the *RARα* gene in acute promyelocytic leukaemia. *Oncogene*, **20**, 7186–7203

Zucman-Rossi, J., Legoix, P., Victor, J.-M., Lopez, B. & Thomas, G. (1998) Chromosome translocation based on illegitimate recombination in human tumors. *Proc. natl Acad. Sci. USA*, **95**, 11786–11791

Corresponding author:

Mel F. Greaves
Leukaemia Research Fund Centre,
Institute of Cancer Research,
Chester Beatty Laboratories,
237 Fulham Road,
London SW3 6JB, UK
m.greaves@icr.ac.uk

Mechanisms of Carcinogenesis: Contributions of Molecular Epidemiology
Patricia Buffler, Jerry Rice, Robert Baan, Michael Bird and Paolo Boffetta, eds
IARC Scientific Publications No. 157
International Agency for Research on Cancer, Lyon, 2004

Causal Models of Leukaemia and Lymphoma

Martyn T. Smith, Christine F. Skibola, James M. Allan and Gareth J. Morgan

Summary

In this chapter, we apply the molecular epidemiological paradigm of biomarkers of exposure, early effect and susceptibility to causal models of leukaemia and lymphoma. The aim is to enhance the development of biomarkers for use in studying the causes of these haematopoeitic cancers in the general population. Two causal models of acute myeloid leukaemia are discussed in detail: chemotherapy-induced and benzene-induced acute myeloid leukaemia. Specific chromosomal changes found in acute myeloid leukaemia may serve as useful biomarkers of early effect in these models, and genetic variants in glutathione S-transferases, NQO1 and DNA-repair enzymes may serve as useful biomarkers of susceptibility. Several causal models of lymphoma exist in which biomarkers could be developed and validated. These include human immunodeficiency virus (HIV) immunosuppression, families with inherited disorders and workers exposed to petroleum products, pesticides or organochlorines. Biomarkers of early effect could include markers of DNA double-strand breaks and aberrant V(D)J recombination, and susceptibility may be related to polymorphisms in genes controlling DNA repair and immunological status. We predict that biomarkers of susceptibility will continue to be studied in the case–control format, perhaps in large pooled studies, but that for biomarkers of early effect, there will be a move away from the study of diseased populations to the study of individuals 'at risk' in the causal models described above.

Introduction

Leukaemias and related disorders originate in pluripotential precursor cells located in the bone marrow that normally give rise to all blood cells.

Disruptions of the normal hierarchy of maturation result in haematological disorders characterized by either excesses or deficiencies of the mature effector cells (Lee et al., 1999). The disorders of myeloid origin include acute myeloid leukaemia, myelodysplastic syndromes and myeloproliferative disorders such as chronic myeloid leukaemia. The disorders of lymphoid origin include acute lymphocytic leukaemia and may affect B or T cells and their precursors. Lymphomas also have a lymphoid origin but arise outside the bone marrow, possibly in the germinal centres. They are highly diverse in their pathological features and are classified by the Revised European American Lymphoma (REAL) system. In the present chapter, we consider causal models of the myeloid disorders, acute myeloid leukaemia/myelodysplastic syndrome and the lymphoid disorders acute lymphoblastic leukaemia and non-Hodgkin lymphoma. For discussion purposes, these causal models will be placed in the familiar molecular epidemiological paradigm of biomarkers of exposure, early effect and susceptibility.

Biology of acute myeloid leukaemia and related disorders

The inter-relationship of myeloid disorders becomes clearer when the stem-cell origin of these conditions is considered. Acute myeloid leukaemia is characterized by maturation block and an increased rate of proliferation. Myelodysplastic syndrome, in contrast, is the clinical consequence of disordered maturation (Lee et al., 1999). Myelodysplastic syndrome is a preleukaemic condition and may transform to acute myeloid leukaemia. From the epidemiological perspective, it is important to recognize the variable antecedent history of acute myeloid leukaemia. Although morphologically similar in appearance, acute myeloid leukaemia may arise *de novo* or follow a myelodysplastic or myeloproliferative state. The antecedent history of acute myeloid leukaemia is taken into account in the WHO classification in the designation of secondary acute myeloid leukaemia, which arises after an earlier myelodysplastic syndrome phase, and of therapy-related acute myeloid leukaemia, which arises after treatment with leukaemogenic agents. Therapy-related myelodysplastic syndrome and therapy-related acute myeloid leukaemia are part of the same disease spectrum, although the specific cytogenetic and molecular characteristics of chemotherapy-related acute myeloid leukaemia may differ according to the form of chemotherapy used (van Leeuwen, 1996).

Cytogenetic studies of acute myeloid leukaemia and myelodysplastic syndrome have shown that most people with these diseases have acquired chromosomal aberrations, including the most commonly recurrent balanced rearrangements t(15;17), t(8;21) and inv(16); partial deletions or loss of whole chromosomes 5q or 7q; and numerical changes, such as trisomy 21 and trisomy 8. These chromosomal aberrations may be meaningful if related to specific exposures rather than evidence of genomic instability (Rowley, 1998).

The abnormality t(15;17), seen almost exclusively in acute promyelocytic leukaemia (FAB subtype M3) (Grignani *et al.*, 2000), results from fusion of the *PML* gene from chromosome 15 to the *RAR*-α gene from chromosome 17 to generate the *PML/RAR*-α fusion, and occurs in about 90% of cases (Sainty *et al.*, 2000). The abnormality t(8;21), most often associated with acute myeloid leukaemia M2, occurs when the *ETO* gene from chromosome 8 is fused to the *AML1* gene from chromosome 21 (Hagemeijer *et al.*, 1998). The inv(16) abnormality, often linked with trisomy 22 in myelomonocytic leukaemia or M4 (Wong & Kwong, 1999), results from an inversion of the telomeric sequences of chromosome 16 that generates a fusion gene of *MYH11* and *CBFb*. The molecular mechanisms responsible for translocations may give important clues about environmental exposures, for example the binding sites for topoisomerase II inhibitors at the 11q23 break-

points (Broeker *et al.*, 1996) and the microclustering of breakpoints observed in the *AML1* gene in t(12;21) and t(8;21) (Wiemels *et al.*, 2000).

Interstitial deletions of the long arms or even loss of a whole copy of chromosomes 5 and 7 in acute myeloid leukaemia and myelodysplastic syndrome are also common, especially in therapy-related acute myeloid leukaemia from alkylating agents and in de-novo acute myeloid leukaemia in elderly people. Monosomy of chromosome 7 can also be a congenital condition and is associated with a high risk of childhood myelodysplastic syndrome. Trisomy of chromosome 8 has been linked with myelodysplastic syndrome, and appears to predispose affected people with this disease to a higher risk of acute leukaemic transformation (Solé *et al.*, 2000). Similar cytogenetic abnormalities characterize de-novo acute myeloid leukaemia occurring in elderly people and secondary myelodysplastic syndrome and acute myeloid leukaemia (Rossi *et al.*, 2000), perhaps suggesting overlapping pathogenic or etiological factors. Other molecular abnormalities seen in acute myeloid leukaemia and myelodysplastic syndrome include *RAS* and *p53* mutations, microsatellite instability and endoduplications of the Flt 3 receptor (Willman, 1999).

Causes and causal models of acute myeloid leukaemia and myelodysplastic syndromes

The established risk factors for acute myeloid leukaemia and myelodysplastic syndrome include ionizing radiation associated with people exposed to atomic bomb blasts, X-rays at work and radiotherapy (Little, 1993); alkylating agents and topoisomerase II inhibitor chemotherapeutic drugs (van Leeuwen, 1996; Felix, 1998); occupational exposure to benzene (Aksoy, 1985; Hayes *et al.*, 1997); smoking (Garfinkel & Boffetta, 1990; Kane *et al.*, 1999); and genetic components such as Down syndrome, Fanconi anaemia and familial monosomy 7 (Alter, 1996; Hasle *et al.*, 2000; Kwong *et al.*, 2000). Studies of people exposed to radiation, chemotherapy and benzene could form good causal models for acute myeloid leukaemia and myelodysplastic syndrome allowing novel biomarkers to be developed, as could familial studies of people with genetic predisposition. Here, because of limited space, we focus on two potential causal models: people treated with chemotherapy drugs and workers occupationally exposed to benzene. We consider them under the typical molecular epidemiological paradigm of biomarkers of exposure, effect and susceptibility.

Cancer chemotherapy as a causal model for acute myeloid leukaemia

Numerous chemotherapeutic alkylating agents and topoisomerase II inhibitors have been linked with increased risks of acute myeloid leukaemia and myelodysplastic syndrome (Table 1) (van Leeuwen, 1996). Therapy-related myelodysplastic syndrome and acute myeloid leukaemia have been reported subsequent to treatment with alkylating agents for many different cancers. Typically they occur at 5–7 years after treatment and risk is related to cumulative dose of the alkylating drug. These conditions are frequently characterized by a preleukaemic phase, trilineage dysplasia and cytogenetic abnormalities involving partial deletions of chromosomes 5 and 7 (Table 1). Certain agents, such as melphalan, pose a higher risk than others, such as cyclophosphamide (Curtis et al., 1992; Krishnan et al., 2000). Therapy-related acute myeloid leukaemia induced by an alkylating agent therefore provides a poten-

tially interesting causal model for secondary acute myeloid leukaemia and for cases carrying the $5q^-/7q^-$ deletion which typically occur in elderly people. These entities have a number of features in common, including interstitial deletions, TP53 mutation, mismatch-repair defects and a poor outcome with treatment.

Various biomarkers of exposure, early effect and susceptibility have been and could be further applied in people treated with alkylating agents (Table 2). DNA and protein adducts could be used as biomarkers of exposure and dose to specific target sites. Cytogenetic changes relevant to induction of acute myeloid leukaemia, such as the loss of chromosomes 5 and 7 and interstitial deletions on the q arms of these chromosomes, could be measured as biomarkers of early effect (Table 2). The clonal lymphocyte HPRT mutation assay could also be used to study the potential role of clonal selection in haematopoietic tumour development. Polymorphisms in metabolism and DNA-repair genes could serve as biomarkers of susceptibility. For example, the metabolism of alkylating chemotherapeutic drugs is well understood and glutathione S-transferase P1 (GST-P1) seems to be particularly important in this respect. Known substrates of GST-P1 include melphalan, cyclophosphamide, platinum and busulphan, all of which have been implicated in the etiology of therapy-related acute myeloid leukaemia (Table 1). The genetic variant of GST-P1 that carries an isoleucine to valine amino acid change at position 105 is associated with impaired activity of this enzyme and an increased risk of therapy-related acute myeloid leukaemia. This increased risk is particularly high when there has been exposure to a known substrate of GST-P1 (odds ratio, 4.34; 95% confidence interval [CI], 1.43–13.20) (Allan et al., 2001).

A second group of therapy-related acute myeloid leukaemia is linked with drugs called topoisomerase II inhibitors, including the epipodophyllotoxin etoposide. Therapy-related acute myeloid leukaemia associated with treatment with these agents is often not preceded by a preleukaemic phase and develops after a shorter latency period (typically 2 years), but is apparently not related to cumulative dose (Smith et al., 1999) (Table 1).

Table 1. Therapy-related acute myeloid leukaemia/myelodysplastic syndrome

Karyotype	Age	Latency (years)	Chemotherapy
			Alkylating agents
−5/del(5q)	Older	5–7	Melphalan
−7/del(7q)			Chlorambucil
			Cyclophosphamide
			Procarbazine
			Topo II inhibitors
t(11q23)	Younger	1–5	Etoposide
t(21q22)			Actinomycin D
t(3q26)			Doxorubicin
			Mitoxantrone

Table 2. Biomarkers in the study of therapy-related and benzene-induced acute myeloid leukaemia

Biomarker	Therapy-related acute myeloid leukaemia		Benzene
	Alkylating agent	Topo II	
Exposure	O^6-methylguanine	Enzyme inhibition	Protein adducts of 1,4 BQ, BO
	Protein adducts	Protein adducts	
	Urine adducts	Urine adducts	5-PMA, ttMA
Early effect	−5, −7, 5q–/7q–	t(11q23)	−5, −7, 5q–/7q–
	TP53 mutation	MLL breakage	t(8;21)
Susceptibility	GSTP1	CYP3A4	CYP2E1 phenotype
	NQO1	DNA repair	NQO1
	DNA repair		
	GSTT1		
	GSTA1		

The pattern of cytogenetic abnormalities is also different with balanced translocations involving the *MLL* gene at 11q23 being the most characteristic abnormality; less often, other balanced translocations such as t(8;21) are seen (Andersen *et al.*, 1998; Felix, 1998) (Table 1). Translocations or breaks in the *MLL* gene at 11q23 may therefore serve as useful biomarkers of early effect for topoisomerase II inhibitors (Table 2). Indeed, Megonigal *et al.* (2000) showed that a *MLL* translocation t(11;17) was detectable after only 6 weeks of therapy in a neuroblastoma patient treated with topoisomerase II inhibitors and acted as a biomarker of early effect for the subsequent development of therapy-related acute myeloid leukaemia in this patient. Genetic variants that affect the metabolism of topoisomerase II inhibitors would also be ideal candidates for biomarkers of susceptibility (Table 2). A variant in *CYP3A4* has been investigated in this respect and has been suggested to be of particular importance (Felix *et al.*, 1998; Felix, 2001).

Benzene as a causal model for an environmentally encountered xenobiotic

Although cytotoxic chemotherapy provides one broad group of agents capable of causing acute myeloid leukaemia, it does not encompass all of the potential environmental exposures that may

be important in the aetiology of this leukaemia. Benzene, which is perhaps the best known chemical leukaemogen (Aksoy, 1985), has been the subject of numerous mechanistic and epidemiological studies over the years. An approximate 2–10-fold increase in leukaemia (mostly acute myeloid leukaemia) has been reported in cohort and case–control studies of benzene-exposed painters, printers and workers employed in petroleum refining and in chemical, rubber, Pliofilm and shoe manufacturing (Rinsky *et al.*, 1987; Hayes *et al.*, 1997). Although benzene has been most strongly associated with acute myeloid leukaemia and aplastic anaemia, there is evidence to suggest that other subtypes of leukaemia, myelodysplastic syndrome, non-Hodgkin lymphoma and possibly other haematopoietic and lymphoproliferative malignancies and related disorders are linked with exposure to this chemical (Hayes *et al.*, 1997; Savitz & Andrews, 1997; Hayes *et al.*, 2001).

The cytogenetic features of benzene-induced leukaemias are less well established than those of therapy-related acute myeloid leukaemia, but a recent thorough review of the literature (Zhang *et al.*, 2002) showed that they are more likely to contain clonal chromosomal aberrations than those arising de-novo in the general population. These are not solely losses of chromosomes 5 and 7 and interstitial deletions on the q arms of these chromosomes, but also include translocations especially involving t(21q22). A preleukaemic phase often precedes acute myeloid leukaemia from exposure to benzene and the latency is usually 7–10 years, but can also be much shorter (Irons & Stillman, 1996; Zhang *et al.*, 2002). Thus, acute myeloid leukaemia induced by benzene has many features in common with therapy-related acute myeloid leukaemia produced by alkylating agents but is not identical.

Workers exposed to benzene have been shown to have higher levels of acute myeloid leukaemia-specific aberrations, including –5, –7, del(5q31), del(7q) and t(8;21), in metaphase spreads prepared from their peripheral blood lymphocytes (Smith *et al.*, 1998; Zhang *et al.*, 1998a). In these studies, chromosomes 8 and 21 were painted in lymphocyte metaphases of 44 workers exposed to benzene and 44 matched controls. Exposure to benzene was associated with significant increases in hyperdiploidy of chromosome 8, and translocations between chromosomes 8 and 21 were increased up to 15-fold in highly exposed workers. In one highly exposed individual, these translocations were also detectable by reverse-transcriptase polymerase chain reaction (RT-PCR) (Smith & Zhang, 1998; Smith *et al.*, 1998). Analysis by fluorescence in-situ hybridization (FISH) of chromosomes 5 and 7 in these same workers also showed that exposure to benzene was associated with increases in the rates of monosomies 5 and 7 and the long arm deletion of chromosomes 5 and 7 in a dose-dependent fashion (Zhang *et al.*, 1998a). These same changes have also been shown to be induced by benzene metabolites *in vitro* (Zhang *et al.*, 1998b). These data indicate a potential role for t(8;21) and changes in chromosomes 5 and 7 in benzene-induced leukaemogenesis, and demonstrate that detection of leukaemia-specific chromosomal aberrations may be a useful biomarker of early effect for increased risk of leukaemia from exposure to benzene (Table 2).

It has been clearly demonstrated that benzene must be metabolized in order for it to induce its haematotoxic and leukaemogenic effects (Valentine *et al.*, 1996; Snyder, 2000). Initial metabolism of benzene takes place in the liver (Ross, 1996) where cytochrome P450, in particular CYP2E1 (Valentine *et al.*, 1996), converts it to a number of reactive intermediates (Figure 1). The initial metabolite of benzene is benzene oxide. This spontaneously rearranges mainly to phenol, but it may also be conjugated with glutathione by GST to form pre-phenyl mercapturic acid or be metabolized by epoxide hydrolase to benzene dihydrodiol (Ross, 1996; Snyder, 2000) (Figure 1). Benzene dihydrodiol can then undergo dehydrogenation to form catechol, which can be conjugated with sulfate or glucuronic acid and excreted in the urine (Figure 1). Benzene oxide can also form an oxepin which ring-opens to *trans,trans*-muconaldehyde, a highly reactive compound that may have toxic effects. The primary metabolite, however, is phenol which can be further metabolized by CYP2E1 to hydroquinone, which can in turn be further hydroxylated to 1,2,4-benzenetriol (Figure 1). The three polyphenols – hydroquinone, catechol and benzenetriol – accumulate in bone marrow and are readily oxidized to highly toxic benzoquinones by peroxidase enzymes such as bone marrow myeloperoxidase (MPO), a process enhanced by the presence of phenol (Smith, 1996). The main protection against the toxic effects of these benzoquinones is NAD(P)H:quinone oxidoreductase 1 (NQO1), originally called DT-diaphorase (Ross, 1996; Smith, 1999) (Figure 1). Thus, people who have low NQO1 activity but high CYP2E1 activity would potentially be more susceptible to the toxic effects of benzene than those with low CYP2E1 and high NQO1 activities. In a case–control study of benzene-poisoned workers in China, Rothman *et al.* (1997) showed that this was indeed true, with people lacking NQO1 activity being about 2.5-fold more susceptible to benzene-induced leukopenia, and that high versus low CYP2E1 activity conferred an additional 2.5-fold increased susceptibility. People with the combination of high CYP2E1 activity and null NQO1 activity were at highest risk from benzene poisoning (odds ratio, 7.6) (Rothman *et al.*, 1997). Thus, CYP2E1 and NQO1 activities are potential biomarkers of susceptibility to benzene-induced acute myeloid leukaemia and related disorders.

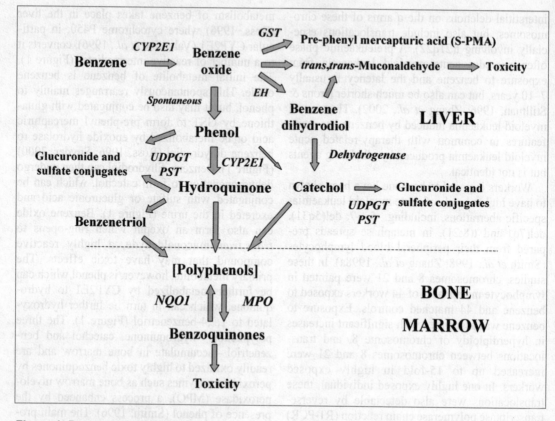

Figure 1. Benzene metabolism

Low NAD(P)H:quinone oxidoreductase activity is associated with acute leukaemia

NQO1 activity is closely correlated with genotypic differences affecting the coding region of the *NQO1* gene. A single nucleotide polymorphism (C→T) at position 609 in the *NQO1* gene was first identified in a human colon cancer cell line with very low NQO1 activity (Traver *et al.*, 1992). This mutation produces a proline→serine substitution that inactivates the enzyme. People who are homozygous for the variant allele completely lack NQO1 activity, and heterozygotes have low intermediate activity compared with the wild-type (Siegel *et al.*, 1999). There have now been a number of studies examining NQO1 genotype as a potential risk factor for leukaemia (Table 3).

The Smith laboratory in Berkeley, with Richard Larson's group in Chicago, examined the evidence that the *NQO1 C609T* variant allele was over-

represented in therapy-related myelodysplastic syndrome and acute myeloid leukaemia, especially in people with specific chromosomal aberrations, in a series of 104 cases (Larson *et al.*, 1999) (Table 3). These studies encouraged us to examine the effects of the *NQO1* polymorphism in de-novo acute leukaemias in the general population (Smith *et al.*, 2001). DNA samples from a population-based case–control study in England of 493 adult de-novo acute leukaemia patients and their 838 unaffected controls matched for age, sex and geographical location were genotyped for *NQO1 C609T*. The frequency of cases with low or null NQO1 activity (heterozygote + homozygous mutant) was significantly higher among total acute leukaemia cases compared with their matched controls (Table 3). Cases of both acute lymphoblastic and myeloid leukaemia exhibited a higher ratio of genotypes that conferred low or null

Table 3. NQO1 and leukaemia risk

Leukaemia type	Odds ratio	References
Therapy-related acute myeloid leukaemia	1.4	Larson et al. (1999)
	2.62	Naoe et al. (2000)
Benzene-induced	2.5	Rothman et al. (1997)
De-novo acute myeloid leukaemia	1.47	Smith et al. (2001)
with translocations	2.39	Smith et al. (2001)
with Inv(16)	8.13	Smith et al. (2001)
Infant leukaemia		
with 11q23	2.5	Wiemels et al. (1999)
	2.26	Smith et al. (unpublished)
with t(4;11)	8.12	Wiemels et al. (1999)
	10.82	Smith et al. (unpublished)

NQO1 activity than did controls (Smith et al., 2001). Among de-novo cases of acute myeloid leukaemia, genotypes conferring low or null NQO1 activity were significantly associated with cases harbouring translocations and inversions, especially those having inversion(16) (Table 3). In addition, a small British study has suggested that *NQO1 C609T* is associated with an increased risk of infant leukaemias with *MLL* translocations, especially infant acute lymphoblastic leukaemia with t(4;11) (Wiemels et al., 1999) (Table 3). Low or null NQO1 activity therefore seems to be a bio-marker of susceptibility to leukaemia.

By inference, the above data indicate that environmental agents that are normally detoxified by NQO1 are risk factors for producing acute lymphoblastic and myeloid leukaemia in the general population. This suggests that exposure to benzene from gasoline, cigarette smoking, and air pollution may be a risk factor for some forms of leukaemia. However, although benzene may contribute to some de-novo leukaemias, it is likely that for most people environmental exposures to benzene are too low to be a significant risk factor. In our studies of benzene-exposed individuals and matched controls, we noticed a large background of protein adducts of benzene's quinone metabolite 1,4-benzoquinone in the controls (Waidyanatha et al., 1998; Yeowell-O'Connell et al., 2001). This high background was first observed by McDonald et al.

(1993, 1994) in rats. With McDonald, the Smith laboratory investigated the source of this high background and concluded that the most important source of phenol and hydroquinone, which are precursors of 1,4-benzoquinone, is the diet and the intestinal breakdown of tyrosine derived from protein (McDonald et al., 2001). These dietary sources outweigh environmental exposure to benzene and it is possible that phenols derived mainly from diet are risk factors for acute leukaemia (McDonald et al., 2001). This hypothesis is undergoing further testing in collaboration with Stephen Rappaport's laboratory, which developed the 1,4-benzoquinone protein adduct assays as biomarkers of exposure to benzene (Waidyanatha et al., 1998). This demonstrates how using causal models may lead to interesting avenues for further research into general disease causation.

Models appropriate for the study of leukaemias with balanced translocations

As discussed earlier, various specific chromosomal translocations and inversions including inv(16), t(8;21), t(9;22) and t(15;17) are associated with particular types of myeloid leukaemia. Further, translocation t(12;21) is common (~25%) in childhood acute lymphoblastic leukaemia and, in non-Hodgkin lymphoma, the translocation t(14;18) is found in follicular lymphoma. These chromosomal rearrangements may therefore serve as potential biomarkers of early effect for leukaemias and follicular non-Hodgkin lymphoma. Indeed, certain chromosomal rearrangements, including t(9;22) and t(14;18), have been detected by the PCR in smoking and nonsmoking members of the general population (Liu et al., 1994; Bell et al., 1995; Biernaux et al., 1995; Fuscoe et al., 1996). Both translocations were found to increase with age, and the t(14;18) translocation was increased in cigarette smokers (Bell et al., 1995). Studies from our laboratory showing detectable t(8;21) by RT-PCR in an otherwise healthy benzene-exposed worker (Smith et al., 1998) also show the potential of RT-PCR for monitoring specific aberrations in populations exposed to suspected or established leukaemogens. Because many of these transloca-tions have multiple breakpoints or translocation partners, multiplex assays have also been deve-loped to detect multiple or unknown rearrange-ments. Despite recent improvements in sensitivity and applicability, conventional PCR methods remain semi-quantitative. However, with the recent advent of real-time PCR, quantitation is no longer an obstacle and a whole new avenue of biological monitoring for early detection of leukaemia and lymphoma becomes available. With this in mind, our laboratories have further developed and refined real-time RT-PCR methods so that they permit the quantification of t(8;21), t(15;17), inv(16), t(11q23), t(14;18), t(12;21) and t(1;19) fusion gene expression at very low levels (1 transcript per 100 000 cells) (Doelken et al., 1998; Luthra et al., 1998; Marcucci et al., 1998). This has enabled us to begin to examine the levels of these translocations in adult and cord blood of individuals in the general population, in workers exposed to benzene and in people given chemotherapeutic drugs. We have found that a significant number of normal indivi-duals express measurable levels of the specific translocations and that mitogen-stimulated blood culture enhances the expression of several trans-locations. This raises questions as to how predic-tive these measurements will be and in what models they should be tested.

Leukaemias harbouring translocations have a different age distribution from those that do not, and occur with almost constant frequency through-out life (Moorman et al., 2001), suggesting that studies aimed at understanding their etiology should be different from those aimed at understan-ding secondary leukaemias. In many respects, adult leukaemias with translocations are analogous to the paediatric leukaemias where there is a variable but relatively short latency between the development of the translocation and the onset of clinical disease. There are a number of potential variables that will affect the likelihood of developing leukae-mia as a result of a balanced translocation. These factors include the rate of acquisition of trans-locations, the rate of extinction of clones carrying the abnormality and the likelihood of a clone being immortalized. The other important variable is the cell in which the translocation occurs, because it is likely that it can potentially give rise to leukaemia only if it occurs in an appropriate target. The environment can interact with any of these factors, increasing the likelihood of developing leukaemia. There are very few data on any of these issues, making this a very fertile area for research.

The biology and classification of adult acute lymphoblastic leukaemia

Acute lymphoblastic leukaemia is morphologically more homogeneous than acute myeloid leukaemia but it is also a heterogeneous disease and there are marked differences between adult and paediatric disease. Lymphoblastic leukaemia is recognized clinically as a malignant proliferation of lymphoid blast cells. In most cases, paediatric acute lympho-blastic leukaemia results from the transformation of a lymphoid-committed precursor cell that carries the machinery to undergo apoptosis. In adult disease, the target cell is thought to be a stem cell that differentiates along the lymphoid lineage and is inherently resistant to apoptosis. Paediatric acute lymphoblastic leukaemia is distinct from adult disease in its epidemiology, having a peak at age 5, whereas the incidence of adult disease increases with increasing age.

Cytogenetics of acute lymphoblastic leukaemia

The molecular subgroups are also different with t(12;21) predominating in paediatric disease, whereas in adult disease the percentage of cases carrying the t(9;22) increases with age and comprises up to 20–30% of total genetic abnormalities in older age groups. The biology of t(9;22) is well known, the p190 variant being associated with de-novo cases and the p210 variants with transformed chronic myeloid leukaemia. The t(4;11) translocation is associated with cases which express myelomonocytic antigens and is seen in up to 70% of infant acute lymphoblastic leukaemia. Although rarely seen in the total group of acute lymphoblastic leukaemia, t(1;19) is the most common abnormality in pre-B acute lymphoblastic leukaemia. The ability to maintain chromosomal number is lost in a significant proportion of paediatric and adult cases, and results in hyperdiploidy. Although acute lymphoblastic leukaemia is a disease of cells in the process of rearranging their immunoglobulin genes, it is of some interest that chromosomal translocations involving the immunoglobulin genes are only rarely seen in B lineage disease. This is in marked contrast to T-cell acute lymphoblastic leukaemia where rearrangements of the T-cell receptor genes are frequently involved in aberrant chromosomal translocations.

Implications for etiological studies

Acute lymphoblastic leukaemia is a very rare disease in adults, which makes analysis of its epidemiology difficult. It is important to consider adult and paediatric acute lymphoblastic leukaemia as different entities, as well as to distinguish T from B lineage disease. Differentiating disease with and without a t(9;22) may also be important. Other major cytogenetic groups include the group with hyperdiploidy, but no other major cytogenetic groups are suitable for analysis.

The folate pathway and leukaemia

Folate metabolism is important in the maintenance of the integrity of DNA and is, therefore, a candidate for mediating leukaemia risk. Depleted folic acid levels increase plasma homocysteine levels and lead to disruptions in DNA methylation. They also result in elevated uracil incorporation into DNA (Blount et al., 1997; Pogribny et al., 1997) and diminished DNA-repair capacity (Choi et al., 1998), resulting in DNA strand breaks (Kim et al., 1997) and chromosomal damage (Fenech, 2001).

The 5,10-methylenetetrahydrofolate reductase (MTHFR) enzyme, critical in the regulation of folate and methionine metabolism, catalyses the reduction of 5,10-methylenetetrahydrofolate (required for purine and pyrimidine synthesis) to 5-methyltetrahydrofolate. There are two common polymorphisms (C677T and A1298C) in the MTHFR gene that result in reduced enzyme activity (Frosst et al., 1995) and enhance the flux of folate towards DNA synthesis and repair processes. We have tested whether carriers of variant alleles for MTHFR C677T and A1298C were protected from adult acute leukaemia in a case–control study based in England of 308 acute leukaemia cases and 491 controls (Skibola et al., 1999). We found a significant association for carriers of the variant alleles of MTHFR C677T and MTHFR A1298C and a reduced risk of acute lymphoblastic leukaemia. Specifically, we observed a 4–14-fold reduced risk of acute lymphoblastic leukaemia in individuals with the MTHFR 677TT, MTHFR 1298AC and 1298CC genotypes. This protective effect was not evident in acute myeloid leukaemia. Similar findings in molecularly defined subgroups of childhood leukaemias have been reported by Wiemels et al. (2001) where the variant MTHFR C677T and MTHFR A1298C alleles were associated with a reduced risk of MLL-positive and hyperdiploid leukaemias, respectively. These protective effects may be real or may be the result of chance, bias, confounding or linkage disequilibrium. Further studies are needed to confirm these observations. However, if they are real, they are likely due to increased levels of the methyl group donor 5,10-methylenetetrahydrofolate being available for DNA synthesis, thereby reducing levels of incorporation of the abnormal base uracil instead of thymidine into DNA. Uracil misincorporation has been shown to cause DNA double-strand breaks (Blount et al., 1997) presumably through the deficient methylation of dUMP to dTMP. Failure to repair DNA double-strand breaks could result in the formation of chromosomal translocations and deletions common in leukaemia.

To examine further the role of the folate pathway in leukaemia susceptibility and to test further the significance of the DNA synthesis pathway in risk for acute lymphoblastic leukaemia, we are currently examining another group of genes involved in folate metabolism and uptake that could affect the homeostasis of the one-carbon pool and may be significant in acute lymphoblastic leukaemia. In this group are genes involved in homocysteine remethylation and transulfuration pathways, the DNA synthesis pathway, as well as folate receptor and transport genes. Our preliminary results look very promising. Folate metabolism is also likely to be similarly important in lymphoma susceptibility, since this malignancy is also of lymphoid tissue origin. We further plan to investigate these candidate genes to determine their potential effect in lymphoma risk in two large case–control studies, one based in the United Kingdom involving 400 cases of germinal centre lymphomas (follicular and diffuse large B-cell) and 400 controls, and another based in the San Francisco Bay area consisting of more than 1000 cases and 1000 controls.

Biology of lymphoma

In seeking to explain the etiology of lymphoma, it is important to develop plausible pathogenic and causal models which integrate recent developments in understanding of lymphocyte biology with environmental exposures that may affect these processes. Important aspects to consider in this respect are that lymphoproliferative disorders are diverse and each entity may have its own specific etiological factor; DNA instability is generated during the development of lymphocytes and different components are active at different stages of lymphoid development; and the lymphoid system has developed specifically to deal with environmentally encountered infectious agents and is directly shaped by the infections it has encountered. In this manner, common exposures may affect the risk of developing lymphoid tumours by modulating the immune response or deleting highly reactive clones. Further, chronic inflammation and immunosuppression are associated with an increased risk of lymphoma.

Lymphoproliferative disorders are diverse

It has been recognized for about 100 years that lymphoproliferative disorders are diverse in their cellular composition and clinical outcomes. The publication of the REAL classification and the WHO classification in 1994 and 2001 were landmarks in this regard (Harris *et al.*, 1999) and showed that, when a very wide range of clinical and biological factors are considered, only a relatively small number of entities emerge. These entities are defined in terms of cellular morphology, cytogenetics, immunophenotype and clinical behaviour. Despite the complexity of current classifications, a limited number of entities are responsible for the bulk of the lymphomas. Most cases are made up of follicular lymphoma, diffuse large B-cell lymphoma, Hodgkin disease and chronic lymphoblastic leukaemia. Even these are not homogeneous entities. Diffuse large B-cell lymphoma is a biologically and clinically heterogenous form of lymphoma that has recently been shown, through the application of cDNA expression micro-array analysis, to consist of two distinct groups, the first corresponding to a germinal centre stage of differentiation and the second corresponding to an activated lymphocyte. The definition of chronic lymphoblastic leukaemia is very clear, but again recent data suggest that this may include two quite different entities based on the extent of hypermutation. The relevance of these groups for the study of the etiology of lymphoma has yet to be tested, but it serves to illustrate the way that classifications will continue to evolve in the future.

Mechanisms of lymphoid-specific DNA instability and the generation of chromosomal translocations

Chromosomal translocations affecting immunoglobulin (Ig) genes are characteristic features of lymphoma and thus their origin may give insight into the causes of lymphoma. Lymphocytes are unique in being the only cell types in which a specific mechanism has evolved that can rearrange and mutate genomic DNA (Harris *et al.*, 1999). Both T and B lymphocytes undergo genetic recombination and mutation as part of their normal life cycle. Diversity of antigenic specificity is generated in T and B cells through a number of distinct steps, including recombination of Ig and T-cell receptor genes, that occurs in lymphocyte precursor cells within the bone marrow (Ramsden *et al.*, 1997; Melek *et al.*, 1998). Lymphocytes that are autoreactive or have generated aberrant receptors are deleted by apoptosis and the rest leave the bone marrow and enter the peripheral lymphoid tissues as mature immunocompetent cells. Antigen encountered from the environment leads to clonal expansion of reactive B cells and the formation of germinal centres. Mutation of the Ig genes takes place within these structures and, when combined with antigen-driven selection, leads to the emergence of subclones of B cells with higher antigenic affinity than their predecessors (Goossens *et al.*, 1998). The mechanism of this process is the subject of intense investigation, but current hypotheses suggest that double-stranded breaks combined with error-prone DNA repair are a key (Kelsoe, 1998; Kim & Storb, 1998; Kong *et al.*, 1998; Storb *et al.*, 2001). Thus, double-strand breaks generated by derangement of physiological processes or by environmentally encountered DNA-damaging agents may be central features in the causation of lymphoma-specific translocations.

In mammalian cells, double-strand breaks trigger several damage-response mechanisms including cell-cycle checkpoint arrest and apoptosis. In addition to these responses, DNA-repair processes act on the breaks catalysing the rearrangement, and both non-homologous end joining and homologous recombination function in this pathway (Takata *et al.*, 1998). The result is

typically a chromosomal translocation involving 14q32, the site of the Ig heavy-chain gene locus. The t(14;18) translocation characteristic of follicular lymphoma is the most common of these Ig translocations of lymphoma and has been well characterized at the molecular level. The current hypothesis is that aberrant recombinase-mediated V(D)J recombination at the Ig locus, possibly occurring during reception editing, combined with double-strand breaks in the target gene are important mechanisms. It has also been suggested that these double-strand breaks may be targeted by the somatic hypermutation mechanism. Examples of this targeting have recently been described for *BCL6*, *PAX 5* and *Rho TTF* (Pasqualucci *et al.*, 1998, 2001), where the sites of mutation seen in germinal centre-cell tumours correspond to the site of translocation. A further process involved in B-cell tumours is aberrant switch recombination. Another important disease-associated translocation is the t(11;14) associated with mantle-cell lymphoma and deregulation of cyclin D1. Both t(14;18) and t(11;14) may therefore be good biomarkers of early effect for lymphoma (Table 4). As described above, double-strand breaks are important transitional events in the generation of translocations, and the induction of double-strand breaks, aberrant recombination and specific lymphoma-related translocations in peripheral blood lymphocytes may be good biomarkers of exposure and early effect for potential causes of lymphoma (Table 4).

Table 4. Possible biomarkers in the study of causal models of lymphoma

Exposure	Early effect	Susceptibility
Viral DNA (HIV, EBV)	DNA double-strand breaks (Comet)	HLA allelles
Antibodies to bacteria associated with contact and hygiene	Aberrant V(D)J recombination, e.g. inv(7), del(1p), t(14q32)	Polymorphisms in genes controlling susceptibility to infection
Organophosphate or benzene metabolites in urine	CLL cells Cytokine levels	Cytokine/chemokine polymorphisms
PCBs in serum	CD4 TH1/TH2 ratio	DNA-repair genes

HIV, human immunodeficiency virus; EBV, Epstein-Barr virus; HLA, human leukocyte antigen; CLL, chronic lymphoblastic leukaemia; PCB, polychlorinated biphenyl

Ataxia telangiectasia and Nijmegen breakage syndrome as causal models of lymphoma

If the production of double-strand breaks, non-homologous end-joining and homologous recombination are important in the etiology of lymphoma, humans with inherited mutations in genes of these pathways would be predicted to be at increased risk of lymphoma (Taccioli et al., 1993; Zhu et al., 1996). This is indeed the case. For example, there are a number of inherited disorders which predispose to the development of lymphoma including ataxia telangiectasia (ATM; Xu et al., 1998), Nijmegen breakage syndrome (Nbs1) and a variant form of ataxia telangiectasia called ataxia telangiectasia-like disorder (Mre11) (Digweed et al., 1999; Liao & Van Dyke, 1999; Stewart et al., 1999). All have higher rates of aberrant recombination in lymphocytes than control individuals. Thus people with ataxia telangiectasia and Nijmegen breakage syndrome may serve as good causal models for the development of lymphoma (Table 5), but the diseases are rare and the families involved are perhaps over-utilized as research subjects. More subtle abnormalities of these pathways mediated by inherited single-nucleotide polymorphisms are, however, good candidates for mediating the observed inter-individual risk for lymphoid tumours.

Table 5. Potential causal models of lymphoma

HIV immunosuppression

EBV and endemic Burkitt lymphoma

Families with ataxia telangiectasia

Patients with autoimmune disorders such as rheumatoid arthritis, Hashimoto's thyroiditis, etc.

Refinery workers – mildly immunosuppressed from benzene

Pesticide applicators

People with high serum PCB and/or dioxin levels

HIV, human immunodeficiency virus; EBV, Epstein-Barr virus; PCB, polychlorinated biphenyl

Infection and autoimmunity in the pathogenesis of lymphoma

The induction of chromosomal translocations and aberrant recombination are seen in normal as well as diseased individuals and cannot, on their own, explain lymphoma induction. It should be remembered that lymphomas are cancers of the immune system and that the immune system is highly responsive to the external environment. Exposure to external infective agents or the development of autoimmune states can lead to massive clonal expansion, in some cases extending over months or years. Antigenic stimulation and inflammation can therefore act as a powerful tumour promoter increasing the target population for malignant change as well as potentiating the lymphoid-specific mechanisms thought to be important in the pathogenesis of lymphoma. A good example of this process is gastric (mucosa-associated lymphoid tissue) lymphoma where the development of extra-nodal lymphoid tissue due to chronic infection with Helicobacter pylori is an essential prerequisite for the development of lymphoma (Isaacson et al., 1986). Risks of non-Hodgkin lymphoma, ranging from two- to 44-fold, have also been observed in people with various autoimmune or connective tissue disorders. The firmest associations are with the organ-specific autoimmune diseases Hashimoto thyroiditis and Sjögren disease, which are associated with the development of marginal cell lymphoma at these anatomic sites (Kinlen, 1985; Mackay & Rose, 2001). These autoimmune disease states may therefore serve as good causal models of marginal zone lymphoma (Table 5).

Another important aspect of developing biomarkers to study the etiology of lymphoma is the application of tools that examine the status of the immune system. The immune system can be considered to be composed of an innate system, which recognizes broad groups of potential pathogens, and an adaptive system which recognizes specific infections as a result of prior exposure. Helper T cells within this system are ordered into two major types. TH1 lymphocytes secrete interleukin (IL)2, interferon-γ, IL12, IL18 and tumour necrosis factor, potentiating cell-mediated immunity and response to bacterial and viral infection (Figure 2). An excess of this response is associated with

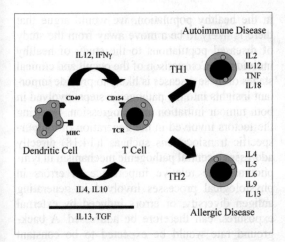

Figure 2. Modulation by infection. Non-specific infections may modulate the TH1/TH2 ratio and consequently modulate risk of childhood acute lymphoblastic leukaemia and autoimmune diseases

organ-specific autoimmune disease. The opposing system is termed TH2 and is associated with the production of IL4, IL6, IL9, IL10 and IL13, promoting humoral immunity and resistance to parasitic infections (Figure 2). An excess of the TH1 response is associated with autoimmune disease and possibly paediatric acute lymphoblastic leukaemia, whereas an excess of the TH2 response is associated with allergy. Interestingly, these types of response are derived from the same precursor cell. Variation in the pro-inflammatory pathway or in the ratio of the TH1/TH2 response may significantly affect the risk of developing lymphoproliferative disease. Thus, altered TH1/TH2 status could be an important biomarker of early effect for lymphoma (Table 4). Further, polymorphisms in cytokine genes affecting these pathways may be important factors in defining the individual risk of developing lymphoma and could serve as biomarkers of susceptibility (Table 4).

Viruses, immunosuppression and lymphoma
The two major causes of severe immunosuppression associated with lymphoma are transplantation and infection with HIV. In both settings, lymphoma is manifest as a predominantly aggressive variant of diffuse large B-cell lymphoma occurring at extranodal sites, frequently affecting the central

nervous system (Obrams & Grufferman, 1991; Ballerini *et al.*, 1993). There is also usually an excess of tumours occurring as a consequence of Epstein–Barr virus (EBV) infection, particularly following transplantation. It has been suggested that minor degrees of immunodeficiency may mediate the development of lymphoma (Cunningham-Rundles *et al.*, 1991). There is, however, no current definition of 'minimally immunosuppressed' or any way of reliably identifying such a state in epidemiological studies. However, from the evidence of lymphoma in HIV and drug-associated immunodeficiency, it would be predicted that EBV-driven lymphoma would be the result. This is usually not the case, raising questions about the general applicability of lymphoma induced by HIV or transplantation as causal models of non-Hodgkin lymphoma in the general population (Table 5).

Causal models of lymphoma related to chemical exposure
There are a number of potential causal models in which occupational or environmental chemical exposures are implicated, including exposure to organophosphate insecticides, organochlorines and a range of solvents (Hardell & Axelson, 1998; Mao *et al.*, 2000; Fabbro-Peray *et al.*, 2001) (Table 5). However, using these as causal models in molecular epidemiological studies is difficult because there are few people with sufficient singular exposure and the association with non-Hodgkin lymphoma is not established. We do, however, have some understanding of the metabolism of these agents and of key genes and their polymorphic variants involved in these processes. Variants that affect the activity of these gene products could be studied using PCR. Significant associations with these variants would suggest that an exposure mediated by that enzyme pathway is important in the etiology of lymphoma (Sarmanová *et al.*, 2001). Examples of this would include variants of CYPIA1 and the Ah receptor which are known to metabolize or interact with dioxins and polychlorinated biphenyls (PCBs), exposure to which is implicated in the etiology of lymphoma. There are, of course, many other polymorphisms that could also be examined.

Utilising biomarkers in causal models of lymphoma in the population setting

Biomarkers of early effect

Low levels of cells with the same phenotype as chronic lymphoblastic leukaemia can be detected with increasing frequency as the population ages (Rawstron et al., 2000, 2001). Thus cells with a chronic lymphoblastic leukaemia phenotype may serve as early effect biomarkers for this disease, especially in its hidden or occult phase (Table 4). Another example of occult lymphoproliferative disease is monoclonal gammopathy of undetermined significance, 10% of which transforms to myeloma at 20 years (Pasqualetti et al., 1997). These preclinical stages could teach us a great deal about disease progression in lymphoma and myeloma. Further, as we noted earlier, 30–50% of apparently normal individuals have evidence of the t(14;18) typical of follicular lymphoma (Liu et al., 1994; Fuscoe et al., 1996; Paltiel et al., 2000). Despite the apparent contradictory nature of this observation, it is consistent with the results of studies on mice carrying a Bcl-2 trans-gene. In these mice, despite the constitutive expression of Bcl-2, there is a delay in the onset of true lymphoid tumours, compatible with the necessity for acquisition of additional genetic hits before the clinical phenotype develops. These observations are of particular importance for studies looking at the etiology of lymphoproliferative disease. With a natural history such as is described, the initial transforming event may have occurred many years previously, making the study of relevant exposures very difficult. However, the description of the preclinical disease phases opens the possibility of dissecting the disease process, allowing the epidemiological characterization of each of these phases. Early attempts at this have been carried out using PCR to investigate the epidemiological associations of t(14;18) occurring in the healthy population. However, these studies have been hampered by the potential for false-positive results and the lack of quantitivity with the technology used. Many of these problems have now been addressed, allowing more accurate studies to be developed.

Since occult B-cell chronic lymphoblastic leukaemia, monoclonal gammopathy of undetermined significance and t(14;18) are very common in the healthy population, we would argue that there is likely to be a move away from the study of diseased populations to the study of healthy individuals. Comparison of the occult and clinical stages of these diseases is likely to provide important insights into the pathogenic steps involved in both tumour initiation and progression. Studying the factors involved in the generation of tumour-specific translocations such as t(14;18) directly addresses a central pathogenic mechanism in lymphomas. The relative importance of errors in physiological processes involved in generating antigen diversity, or errors induced by external exposures, can therefore be addressed. A background rate would be expected to be constant between different populations. The definition of increased rates in exposed populations would be very important and would, for the first time, allow us to develop biomarkers of populations 'at risk'. We have focused on t(14;18), but other aberrant events such as TCRα/β rearrangements may be more useful as they do not affect the process of apoptosis and so may reflect more accurately the incidence of these events. Similarly, with the development of flow cytometry approaches for defining subclinical disease populations, we may more readily look at factors important in the etiology of chronic lymphoblastic leukaemia. Application of these potential biomarkers in the causal models listed in Table 5 and healthy controls could teach us a great deal.

Biomarkers of susceptibility

There are a number of large case–control studies of lymphoma currently nearing completion that have incorporated pathological review using the REAL classification and have also collected biological material. The adequate analysis of these studies will allow the criticisms aimed at previous studies to be addressed fully. In addition, the availability of biological material from cases and controls will allow the full evaluation of the genetic factors associated with lymphoma. This approach is beginning to examine the association between disease subtype and polymorphisms of enzymes involved in the key processes of carcinogen metabolism, immune response and DNA repair. Central to these studies is an analysis not only of the association between exposure and lymphoma causation but, in addition, the effect of genetic polymorphisms that can mediate the metabolism of these exposures and affect the frequency of intrinsic events. Single gene variants are unlikely to increase risk to a clinically significant degree, and current effort is directed at understanding how variants at many different genes may interact to give rise to an 'at risk phenotype' and so develop biomarkers of susceptibility.

Conclusion

We conclude that biomarkers of exposure, early effect and susceptibility could be used in causal models of leukaemia and lymphoma to elucidate further the etiology of these diseases. In these investigations, we predict that there will be a move away from the study of diseased populations to the study of healthy individuals 'at risk'. Biomarkers of susceptibility will continue to be studied in the case–control format, but in large pooled studies, such as the International Consortium of Investigators Working on Lymphoma Epidemiologic Studies (Inter-Lymph).

Acknowledgements

Martyn T. Smith and Christine F. Skibola were supported by the National Institute of Environmental Health Sciences (grants P42ES04705, P30 ES01896 and R01ES06721), the National Cancer Institute (grant RO1CA87014) and the National Foundation for Cancer Research Center for Genomics and Nutrition. James M. Allan and Gareth J. Morgan were supported by the Leukaemia Research Fund of Great Britain.

References

Aksoy, M. (1985) Benzene as a leukemogenic and carcinogenic agent. *Am. J. ind. Med.*, **8**, 9–20

Allan, J.M., Wild, C.P., Rollinson, S., Willett, E.V., Moorman, A.V., Dovey, G.J., Roddam, P.L., Roman, E., Cartwright, R.A. & Morgan, G.J. (2001) Polymorphism in glutathione *S*-transferase P1 is associated with susceptibility to chemotherapy-induced leukaemia. *Proc. natl Acad. Sci. USA*, **98**, 11592–11597

Alter, B.P. (1996) Fanconi's anemia and malignancies. *Am. J. Hematol.*, **53**, 99–110

Andersen, M.K., Johansson, B., Larsen, S.O. & Pedersen-Bjergaard, J. (1998) Chromosomal abnormalities in secondary MDS and AML. Relationship to drugs and radiation with specific emphasis on the balanced rearrangements. *Haematologica*, **83**, 483–488

Ballerini, P., Gaidano, G., Gong, J.Z., Tassi, V., Saglio, G., Knowles, D.M. & Dalla-Favera, R. (1993) Multiple genetic lesions in acquired immunodeficiency syndrome-related non-Hodgkin's lymphoma. *Blood*, **81**, 166–176

Bell, D.A., Liu, Y. & Cortopassi, G.A. (1995) Occurrence of *BCL*-2 oncogene translocation with increased frequency in the peripheral blood of heavy smokers. *J. natl Cancer Inst.*, **87**, 223–224

Biernaux, C., Loos, M., Sels, A., Huez, G. & Stryckmans, P. (1995) Detection of major *BCR*-abl gene expression at a very low level in blood cells of some healthy individuals. *Blood*, **86**, 3118–3122

Blount, B.C., Mack, M.M., Wehr, C.M., MacGregor, J.T., Hiatt, R.A., Wang, G., Wickramasinghe, S.N., Everson, R.B. & Ames, B.N. (1997) Folate deficiency causes uracil misincorporation into human DNA and chromosome breakage: implications for cancer and neuronal damage. *Proc. natl Acad. Sci. USA*, **94**, 3290–3295

Broeker, P.L., Super, H.G., Thirman, M.J., Pomykala, H., Yonebayashi, Y., Tanabe, S., Zeleznik-Le, N. & Rowley, J.D. (1996) Distribution of 11q23 breakpoints within the MLL breakpoint cluster region in de novo acute leukemia and in treatment-related acute myeloid leukemia: correlation with scaffold attachment regions and topoisomerase II consensus binding sites. *Blood*, **87**, 1912–1922

Choi, S.W., Kim, Y.I., Weitzel, J.N. & Mason, J.B. (1998) Folate depletion impairs DNA excision repair in the colon of the rat. *Gut*, **43**, 93–9

Cunningham-Rundles, C., Lieberman, P., Hellman, G. & Chaganti, R.S. (1991) Non-Hodgkin lymphoma in common variable immunodeficiency. *Am. J. Hematol.*, **37**, 69–74

Curtis, R.E., Boice, J.D., Jr, Stovall, M., Bornstein, L., Greenberg, R.S., Flannery, J.T., Schwartz, A.G., Weyer, P., Moloney, W.C. & Hoover, R.N. (1992) Risk of leukemia after chemotherapy and radiation treatment for breast cancer. *New Engl. J. Med.*, **326**, 1745–1751

Digweed, M., Reis, A. & Sperling, K. (1999) Nijmegen breakage syndrome: consequences of defective DNA double strand break repair. *Bioessays*, **21**, 649–956

Dölken, L., Schüler, F. & Dölken, G. (1998) Quantitative detection of t(14;18)-positive cells by real-time quantitative PCR using fluorogenic probes. *Biotechniques*, **25**, 1058–1064

Fabbro-Peray, P., Daures, J.P. & Rossi, J.F. (2001) Environmental risk factors for non-Hodgkin's lymphoma: a population-based case–control study in Languedoc-Roussillon, France. *Cancer Causes Control*, **12**, 201–212

Felix, C.A. (1998) Secondary leukemias induced by topoisomerase-targeted drugs. *Biochim. biophys. Acta*, **1400**, 233–255

Felix, C.A. (2001) Leukemias related to treatment with DNA topoisomerase II inhibitors. *Med. pediatr. Oncol.*, **36**, 525–535

Felix, C.A., Walker, A.H., Lange, B.J., Williams, T.M., Winick, N.J., Cheung, N.K., Lovett, B.D., Nowell, P.C., Blair, I.A. & Rebbeck, T.R. (1998) Association of CYP3A4 genotype with treatment-related leukemia. *Proc. natl Acad. Sci. USA*, **95**, 13176–13181

Fenech, M. (2001) The role of folic acid and Vitamin B12 in genomic stability of human cells. *Mutat. Res.*, **475**, 57–67

Frosst, P., Blom, H.J., Milos, R., Goyette, P., Sheppard, C.A., Matthews, R.G., Boers, G.J., den Heijer, M., Kluijtmans, L.A., van den Heuvel, L.P. & Rosen, R. (1995) A candidate genetic risk factor for vascular disease: a common mutation in methylenetetrahydrofolate reductase [Letter]. *Nature Genet.*, **10**, 111–113

Fuscoe, J.C., Setzer, R.W., Collard, D.D. & Moore, M.M. (1996) Quantification of t(14;18) in the lymphocytes of healthy adult humans as a possible biomarker for environmental exposures to carcinogens. *Carcinogenesis*, **17**, 1013–1020

Garfinkel, L. & Boffetta, P. (1990) Association between smoking and leukemia in two American Cancer Society prospective studies. *Cancer*, **65**, 2356–2360

Goossens, T., Klein, U. & Küppers, R. (1998) Frequent occurrence of deletions and duplications during somatic hypermutation: implications for oncogene translocations and heavy chain disease. *Proc. natl Acad. Sci. USA*, **95**, 2463–2468

Grignani, F., Valtieri, M., Gabbianelli, M., Gelmetti, V., Botta, R., Luchetti, L., Masella, B., Morsilli, O., Pelosi, E., Samoggia, P., Pelicci, P.G. & Peschle, C. (2000) PML/RAR alpha fusion protein expression in normal human hematopoietic progenitors dictates myeloid commitment and the promyelocytic phenotype. *Blood*, **96**, 1531–1537

Hagemeijer, A., de Klein, A., Wijsman, J., van Meerten, E., de Greef, G.E. & Sacchi, N. (1998) Development of an interphase fluorescent in situ hybridization (FISH) test to detect t(8;21) in AML patients. *Leukemia*, **12**, 96–101

Hardell, L. & Axelson, O. (1998) Environmental and occupational aspects on the etiology of non-Hodgkin's lymphoma. *Oncol. Res.*, **10**, 1–5

Harris, N.L., Jaffe, E.S., Diebold, J., Flandrin, G., Muller-Hermelink, H.K., Vardiman, J., Lister, T.A. & Bloomfield, C.D. (1999) The World Health Organization classification of neoplastic diseases of the hematopoietic and lymphoid tissues. Report of the Clinical Advisory Committee meeting, Airlie House, Virginia, November, 1997. *Ann. Oncol.*, **10**, 1419–1432

Hasle, H., Clemmensen, I.H. & Mikkelsen, M. (2000) Risks of leukaemia and solid tumours in individuals with Down's syndrome. *Lancet*, **355**, 165–169

Hayes, R.B., Yin, S.N., Dosemeci, M., Li, G.L., Wacholder, S., Travis, L.B., Li, C.Y., Rothman, N., Hoover, R.N. & Linet, M.S. (1997) Benzene and the dose-related incidence of hematologic neoplasms in China. Chinese Academy of Preventive Medicine–National Cancer Institute Benzene Study Group. *J. natl Cancer Inst.*, **89**, 1065–1071

Hayes, R.B., Songnian, Y., Dosemeci, M. & Linet, M. (2001) Benzene and lymphohematopoietic malignancies in humans. *Am. J. ind. Med.*, **40**, 117–126

Irons, R.D. & Stillman, W.S. (1996) The process of leukemogenesis. *Environ. Health Perspect.*, **104** (Suppl. 6), 1239–1246

Isaacson, P.G., Spencer, J. & Finn, T. (1986) Primary B-cell gastric lymphoma. *Hum. Pathol.*, **17**, 72–82

Kane, E.V., Roman, E., Cartwright, R., Parker, J. & Morgan, G. (1999) Tobacco and the risk of acute leukaemia in adults. *Br. J. Cancer*, **81**, 1228–1233

Kelsoe, G. (1998) V(D)J hypermutation and DNA mismatch repair: vexed by fixation. *Proc. natl Acad. Sci. USA*, **95**, 6576–6577

Kim, N. & Storb, U. (1998) The role of DNA repair in somatic hypermutation of immunoglobulin genes. *J. exp. Med.*, **187**, 1729–1733

Kim, Y.I., Pogribny, I.P., Basnakian, A.G., Miller, J.W., Selhub, J., James, S.J. & Mason, J.B. (1997) Folate deficiency in rats induces DNA strand breaks and hypomethylation within the p53 tumor suppressor gene. *Am. J. clin. Nutr.*, **65**, 46–52

Kinlen, L.J. (1985) Incidence of cancer in rheumatoid arthritis and other disorders after immuno-suppressive treatment. *Am. J. Med.*, **78**, 44–49

Kong, Q., Harris, R.S. & Maizels, N. (1998) Recombi-nation-based mechanisms for somatic hyper-mutation. *Immunol. Rev.*, **162**, 67–76

Krishnan, A., Bhatia, S., Slovak, M.L., Arber, D.A., Niland, J.C., Nademanee, A., Fung, H., Bhatia, R., Kashyap, A., Molina, A., O'Donnell, M.R., Parker, P.A., Sniecinski, I., Snyder, D.S., Spielberger, R., Stein, A. & Forman, S.J. (2000) Predictors of therapy-related leukemia and myelodysplasia following autologous transplantation for lym-phoma: an assessment of risk factors. *Blood*, **95**, 1588–1193

Kwong, Y.L., Ng, M.H. & Ma, S.K. (2000) Familial acute myeloid leukemia with monosomy 7: late onset and involvement of a multipotential pro-genitor cell. *Cancer Genet. Cytogenet.*, **116**, 170–173

Larson, R.A., Wang, Y., Banerjee, M., Wiemels, J., Hartford, C., Le Beau, M.M. & Smith, M.T. (1999) Prevalence of the inactivating 609 C→T poly-morphism in the NAD(P)H:quinone oxido-reductase (NQO1) gene in patients with primary and therapy-related myeloid leukemia. *Blood*, **94**, 803–807

Lee, G.R., Foerster, J., Lukens, J., Paraskevas, F., Greer, J.P. & Rodgers, G.M. (1999) *Wintrobe's Clinical Hematology*, Philadelphia, Lippincott Williams and Wilkins, pp. 56–71, 2209–2373

van Leeuwen, F.E. (1996) Risk of acute myelogenous leukaemia and myelodysplasia following cancer treatment. *Bailliere's clin. Haematol.*, **9**, 57–85

Liao, M.J. & Van Dyke, T. (1999) Critical role for Atm in suppressing V(D)J recombination-driven thymic lymphoma. *Genes Dev.*, **13**, 1246–1250

Little, J.B. (1993) Cellular, molecular, and carcino-genic effects of radiation. *Hematol. Oncol. Clin. North Am.*, **7**, 337–352

Liu, Y., Hernandez, A.M., Shibata, D. & Cortopassi, G.A. (1994) BCL2 translocation frequency rises with age in humans. *Proc. natl Acad. Sci. USA*, **91**, 8910–8914

Luthra, R., McBride, J.A., Cabanillas, F. & Sarris, A. (1998) Novel 5' exonuclease-based real-time PCR assay for the detection of t(14;18)(q32;q21) in patients with follicular lymphoma. *Am. J. Pathol.*, **153**, 63–68

Mackay, I.R. & Rose, N.R. (2001) Autoimmunity and lymphoma: tribulations of B cells. *Nature Immunol.*, **2**, 793–795

Mao, Y., Hu, J., Ugnat, A.M. &White, K. (2000) Non-Hodgkin's lymphoma and occupational exposure to chemicals in Canada. Canadian Cancer Registries Epidemiology Research Group. *Ann. Oncol.*, **11** (Suppl. 1), 69–73

Marcucci, G., Livak, K.J., Bi, W., Strout, M.P., Bloomfield, C.D. & Caligiuri, M.A. (1998) Detec-tion of minimal residual disease in patients with AML1/ETO-associated acute myeloid leukemia using a novel quantitative reverse transcription polymerase chain reaction assay. *Leukemia*, **12**, 1482–1489

McDonald, T.A., Waidyanatha, S. & Rappaport, S.M. (1993) Production of benzoquinone adducts with hemoglobin and bone-marrow proteins following administration of [^{13}C]benzene to rats. *Carcino-genesis*, **14**, 1921–1925

McDonald, T.A., Yeowell-O'Connell, K. & Rappaport, S.M. (1994) Comparison of protein adducts of benzene oxide and benzoquinone in the blood and bone marrow of rats and mice exposed to [^{14}C/^{13}C]-benzene. *Cancer Res.*, **54**, 4907–4914

McDonald, T.A., Holland, N.T., Skibola, C., Duramad, P. & Smith, M.T. (2001) Hypothesis: phenol and hydroquinone derived mainly from diet and gastro-intestinal flora activity are causal factors in leukemia. *Leukemia*, **15**, 10–20

Megonigal, M.D., Cheung, N.K., Rappaport, E.F., Nowell, P.C., Wilson, R.B., Jones, D.H., Addya, K., Leonard, D.G., Kushner, B.H., Williams, T.M., Lange, B.J. & Felix, C.A. (2000) Detection of leukemia-associated MLL-GAS7 translocation early during chemotherapy with DNA topoiso-merase II inhibitors. *Proc. natl Acad. Sci. USA*, **97**, 2814–2819

Melek, M., Gellert, M. & van Gent, D.C. (1998) Rejoining of DNA by the RAG1 and RAG2 proteins. *Science*, **280**, 301–303

Moorman, A.V., Roman, E., Willett, E.V., Dovey, G.J., Cartwright, R.A. & Morgan, G.J. (2001) Karyotype and age in acute myeloid leukemia. Are they linked? *Cancer Genet. Cytogenet.*, **126**, 155–161

Naoe, T., Takeyama, K., Yokozawa, T., Kiyoi, H., Seto, M., Uike, N., Ino, T., Utsunomiya, A., Maruta, A., Jin-nai, I., Kamada, N., Kubota, Y., Nakamura, H., Shimazaki, C., Horiike, S., Kodera, Y., Saito, H., Ueda, R., Wiemels, J. & Ohno, R. (2000) Analysis of genetic polymorphism in NQO1, GST-M1, GST-T1, and CYP3A4 in 469 Japanese patients with therapy-related leukemia/myelodysplastic syndrome and de novo acute myeloid leukemia. *Clin. Cancer Res.*, **6**, 4091–4095

Obrams, G.I. & Grufferman, S. (1991) Epidemiology of HIV associated non-Hodgkin lymphoma. *Cancer Surv.*, **10**, 91–102

Paltiel, O., Zelenetz, A., Sverdlin, I., Gordon, L. & Ben-Yehuda, D. (2000) Translocation t(14;18) in healthy individuals: preliminary study of its association with family history and agricultural exposure. *Ann. Oncol.*, **11** (Suppl. 1), 75–80

Pasqualetti, P., Festuccia, V., Collacciani, A. & Casale, R. (1997) The natural history of monoclonal gammopathy of undetermined significance. A 5- to 20-year follow-up of 263 cases. *Acta haematol.*, **97**, 174–179

Pasqualucci, L., Migliazza, A., Fracchiolla, N., William, C., Neri, A., Baldini, L., Chaganti, R.S., Klein, U., Küppers, R., Rajewsky, K. & Dalla-Favera, R. (1998) BCL-6 mutations in normal germinal center B cells: evidence of somatic hypermutation acting outside Ig loci. *Proc. natl Acad. Sci. USA*, **95**, 11816–11821

Pasqualucci, L., Neumeister, P., Goossens, T., Nanjangud, G., Chaganti, R.S., Küppers, R. & Dalla-Favera, R. (2001) Hypermutation of multiple proto-oncogenes in B-cell diffuse large-cell lymphomas. *Nature*, **412**, 341–346

Pogribny, I.P., Muskhelishvili, L., Miller, B.J. & James, S.J. (1997) Presence and consequence of uracil in preneoplastic DNA from folate/methyl-deficient rats. *Carcinogenesis*, **18**, 2071–2076

Ramsden, D.A., Paull, T.T. & Gellert, M. (1997) Cell-free V(D)J recombination. *Nature*, **388**, 488–491

Rawstron, A.C., Fenton, J.A., Ashcroft, J., English, A., Jones, R.A., Richards, S.J., Pratt, G., Owen, R., Davies, F.E., Child, J.A., Jack, A.S. & Morgan, G. (2000) The interleukin-6 receptor alpha-chain (CD126) is expressed by neoplastic but not normal plasma cells. *Blood*, **96**, 3880–3886

Rawstron, A.C., Kennedy, B., Evans, P.A., Davies, F.E., Richards, S.J., Haynes, A.P., Russell, N.H., Hale, G., Morgan, G.J., Jack, A.S. & Hillmen, P. (2001) Quantitation of minimal disease levels in chronic lymphocytic leukemia using a sensitive flow cytometric assay improves the prediction of outcome and can be used to optimize therapy. *Blood*, **98**, 29–35

Rinsky, R.A., Smith, A.B., Hornung, R., Filloon, T.G., Young, R.J., Okun, A.H. & Landrigan, P.J. (1987) Benzene and leukemia. An epidemiologic risk assessment. *New Engl. J. Med.*, **316**, 1044–1050

Ross, D. (1996) Metabolic basis of benzene toxicity. *Eur. J. Haematol.*, **60** (Suppl.), 111–118

Rossi, G., Pelizzari, A.M., Bellotti, D., Tonelli, M. & Barlati, S. (2000) Cytogenetic analogy between myelodysplastic syndrome and acute myeloid leukemia of elderly patients. *Leukemia*, **14**, 636–641

Rothman, N., Smith, M.T., Hayes, R.B., Traver, R.D., Hoener, B., Campleman, S., Li, G.L., Dosemeci, M., Linet, M., Zhang, L., Xi, L., Wacholder, S., Lu, W., Meyer, K.B., Titenko-Holland, N., Stewart, J.T., Yin, S. & Ross, D. (1997) Benzene poisoning, a risk factor for hematological malignancy, is associated with the NQO1 609 C→T mutation and rapid fractional excretion of chlorzoxazone. *Cancer Res.*, **57**, 2839–2842

Rowley, J.D. (1998) The critical role of chromosome translocations in human leukemias. *Annu. Rev. Genet.*, **32**, 495–519

Sainty, D., Liso, V., Cantù-Rajnoldi, A., Head, D., Mozziconacci, M.J., Arnoulet, C., Benattar, L., Fenu, S., Mancini, M., Duchayne, E., Mahon, F.X., Gutierrez, N., Birg, F., Biondi, A., Grimwade, D., Lafage-Pochitaloff, M., Hagemeijer, A. & Flandrin, G. (2000) A new morphologic classification system for acute promyelocytic leukemia distinguishes cases with underlying PLZF/RARA gene rearrangements. Groupe Français de Cytogénétique Hématologique, UK Cancer Cytogenetics Group and BIOMED 1 European Community-Concerted Action 'Molecular Cytogenetic Diagnosis in

Haematological Malignancies'. *Blood*, **96**, 1287–1296

Sarmanová, J., Benesová, K., Gut, I., Nedelcheva-Kristensen, V., Tynková, L. & Soucek, P. (2001) Genetic polymorphisms of biotransformation enzymes in patients with Hodgkin's and non-Hodgkin's lymphomas. *Hum. mol. Genet.*, **10**, 1265–1273

Savitz, D.A. & Andrews, K.W. (1997) Review of epidemiologic evidence on benzene and lymphatic and hematopoietic cancers. *Am. J. ind. Med.*, **31**, 287–295

Siegel, D., McGuinness, S.M., Winski, S.L. & Ross, D. (1999) Genotype–phenotype relationships in studies of a polymorphism in NAD(P)H:quinone oxidoreductase 1. *Pharmacogenetics*, **9**, 113–121

Skibola, C.F., Smith, M.T., Kane, E., Roman, E., Rollinson, S., Cartwright, R.A. & Morgan, G. (1999) Polymorphisms in the methylenetetrahydrofolate reductase gene are associated with susceptibility to acute leukemia in adults. *Proc. natl Acad. Sci. USA*, **96**, 12810–12815

Smith, M.T. (1996) The mechanism of benzene-induced leukemia: a hypothesis and speculations on the causes of leukemia. *Environ. Health Perspect.*, **104** (Suppl. 6), 1219–1225

Smith, M.T. (1999) Benzene, NQO1, and genetic susceptibility to cancer. *Proc. natl Acad. Sci. USA*, **96**, 7624–7626

Smith, M.T. & Zhang, L. (1998) Biomarkers of leukemia risk: benzene as a model. *Environ. Health Perspect.*, **106** (Suppl. 4), 937–946

Smith, M.T., Zhang, L., Wang, Y., Hayes, R.B., Li, G., Wiemels, J., Dosemeci, M., Titenko-Holland, N., Xi, L., Kolachana, P., Yin, S. & Rothman, N. (1998) Increased translocations and aneusomy in chromosomes 8 and 21 among workers exposed to benzene. *Cancer Res.*, **58**, 2176–2181

Smith, M.A., Rubinstein, L., Anderson, J.R., Arthur, D., Catalano, P.J., Freidlin, B., Heyn, R., Khayat, A., Krailo, M., Land, V.J., Miser, J., Shuster, J. & Vena, D. (1999) Secondary leukemia or myelodysplastic syndrome after treatment with epipodophyllotoxins. *J. clin. Oncol.*, **1**, 569–577

Smith, M.T., Wang, Y., Kane, E., Rollinson, S., Wiemels, J.L., Roman, E., Roddam, P., Cartwright, R. & Morgan, G. (2001) Low NAD(P)H:quinone oxidoreductase 1 activity is associated with

increased risk of acute leukemia in adults. *Blood*, **97**, 1422–1426

Snyder, R. (2000) Overview of the toxicology of benzene. *J. Toxicol. environ. Health A*, **61**, 339–346

Solé, F., Espinet, B., Sanz, G.F., Cervera, J., Calasanz, M.J., Luño, E., Prieto, F., Granada, I., Hernández, J.M., Cigudosa, J.C., Diez, J.L., Bureo, E., Marqués, M.L., Arranz, E., Ríos, R., Martínez Climent, J.A., Vallespí, T., Florensa, L. & Woessner, S. (2000) Incidence, characterization and prognostic significance of chromosomal abnormalities in 640 patients with primary myelodysplastic syndromes. Grupo Cooperativo Español de Citogenética Hematológica. *Br. J. Haematol.*, **108**, 346–356

Stewart, G.S., Maser, R.S., Stankovic, T., Bressan, D.A., Kaplan, M.I., Jaspers, N.G., Raams, A., Byrd, P.J., Petrini, J.H. & Taylor, A.M. (1999) The DNA double-strand break repair gene hMRE11 is mutated in individuals with an ataxia-telangiectasia-like disorder. *Cell*, **99**, 577–587

Storb, U., Shen, H.M., Michael, N. & Kim, N. (2001) Somatic hypermutation of immunoglobulin and non-immunoglobulin genes. *Philos. Trans. R. Soc. London. Ser. B: biol. Sci.*, **356**, 13–19

Taccioli, G.E., Rathbun, G., Oltz, E., Stamato, T., Jeggo, P.A. & Alt, F.W. (1993) Impairment of V(D)J recombination in double-strand break repair mutants. *Science*, **260**, 207–210

Takata, M., Sasaki, M.S., Sonoda, E., Morrison, C., Hashimoto, M., Utsumi, H., Yamaguchi-Iwai, Y., Shinohara, A. & Takeda, S. (1998) Homologous recombination and non-homologous end-joining pathways of DNA double-strand break repair have overlapping roles in the maintenance of chromosomal integrity in vertebrate cells. *EMBO J.*, **17**, 5497–5508

Traver, R.D., Horikoshi, T., Danenberg, K.D., Stadlbauer, T.H., Danenberg, P.V., Ross, D. & Gibson, N.W. (1992) NAD(P)H:quinone oxidoreductase gene expression in human colon carcinoma cells: characterization of a mutation which modulates DT-diaphorase activity and mitomycin sensitivity. *Cancer Res.*, **52**, 797–802

Valentine, J.L., Lee, S.S., Seaton, M.J., Asgharian, B., Farris, G., Corton, J.C., Gonzalez, F.J. & Medinsky, M.A. (1996) Reduction of benzene metabolism and toxicity in mice that lack CYP2E1 expression. *Toxicol. appl. Pharmacol.*, **141**, 205–213

Waidyanatha, S., Yeowell-O'Connell, K. & Rappaport, S.M. (1998) A new assay for albumin and hemoglobin adducts of 1,2- and 1,4-benzoquinones. *Chem.-biol. Interact.*, **115**, 117–139

Wiemels, J.L., Pagnamenta, A., Taylor, G.M., Eden, O.B., Alexander, F.E. & Greaves, M.F. (1999) A lack of a functional NAD(P)H:quinone oxidoreductase allele is selectively associated with pediatric leukemias that have MLL fusions. United Kingdom Childhood Cancer Study Investigators. *Cancer Res.*, **59**, 4095–4099

Wiemels, J.L., Alexander, F.E., Cazzaniga, G., Biondi, A., Mayer, S.P. & Greaves, M.F. (2000) Microclustering of TEL-AML1 translocation breakpoints in childhood acute lymphoblastic leukemia. *Genes Chromosomes Cancer*, **29**, 219–228

Wiemels, J.L., Smith, R.N., Taylor, G.M., Eden, O.B., Alexander, F.E. & Greaves, M.F. (2001) Methylenetetrahydrofolate reductase (MTHFR) polymorphisms and risk of molecularly defined subtypes of childhood acute leukemia. United Kingdom Childhood Cancer Study Investigators. *Proc. natl Acad. Sci. USA*, **98**, 4004–4009

Willman, C.L. (1999) Molecular evaluation of acute myeloid leukemias. *Semin. Hematol.*, **36**, 390–400

Wong, K.F. & Kwong, Y.L. (1999) Trisomy 22 in acute myeloid leukemia: a marker for myeloid leukemia with monocytic features and cytogenetically cryptic inversion 16. *Cancer Genet. Cytogenet.*, **109**, 131–133

Xu, Y., Yang, E.M., Brugarolas, J., Jacks, T. & Baltimore, D. (1998) Involvement of p53 and p21 in cellular defects and tumorigenesis in Atm$^{-/-}$ mice. *Mol. cell. Biol.*, **18**, 4385–4390

Yeowell-O'Connell, K., Rothman, N., Waidyanatha, S., Smith, M.T., Hayes, R.B., Li, G., Bechtold, W.E.,

Dosemeci, M., Zhang, L., Yin, S. & Rappaport, S.M. (2001) Protein adducts of 1,4-benzoquinone and benzene oxide among smokers and nonsmokers exposed to benzene in China. *Cancer Epidemiol. Biomarkers Prev.*, **10**, 831–838

Zhang, L., Rothman, N., Wang, Y., Hayes, R.B., Li, G., Dosemeci, M., Yin, S., Kolachana, P., Titenko-Holland, N. & Smith, M.T. (1998a) Increased aneusomy and long arm deletion of chromosomes 5 and 7 in the lymphocytes of Chinese workers exposed to benzene. *Carcinogenesis*, **19**, 1955–1961

Zhang, L., Wang, Y., Shang, N. & Smith, M.T. (1998b) Benzene metabolites induce the loss and long arm deletion of chromosomes 5 and 7 in human lymphocytes. *Leuk. Res.*, **22**, 105–113

Zhang, L., Eastmond, D.A. & Smith, M.T. (2002) The nature of chromosomal aberrations detected in humans exposed to benzene. *Crit. Rev. Toxicol.*, **32**, 1–42

Zhu, C., Bogue, M.A., Lim, D.S., Hasty, P. & Roth, D.B. (1996) Ku86-deficient mice exhibit severe combined immunodeficiency and defective processing of V(D)J recombination intermediates. *Cell*, **86**, 379–389

Corresponding author:

Martyn T. Smith
Division of Environmental Health Sciences,
School of Public Health,
216 Earl Warren Hall,
University of California,
Berkeley, CA 94720-7360, USA
martynts@uclink4.berkeley.edu

Mechanisms of Carcinogenesis: Contributions of Molecular Epidemiology
Patricia Buffler, Jerry Rice, Robert Baan, Michael Bird and Paolo Boffetta, eds
IARC Scientific Publications No. 157
International Agency for Research on Cancer, Lyon, 2004

Mechanistic Considerations in the Molecular Epidemiology of Head and Neck Cancer

Paul Brennan and Paolo Boffetta

Summary

Head and neck cancer occurs through a complex multistage process that is likely to involve a combination of carcinogen exposure and genetic susceptibility. The primary cause of head and neck cancer are alcohol consumption and cigarette smoking, although the carcinogenic mechanism for these agents is unclear. Molecular epidemiological studies of head and neck cancer can help to clarify the carcinogenic process in several ways, including identification of metabolizing genes which increase the risk of head and neck cancer, identification of DNA adducts in target cells and analysis of specific gene mutations and their relationship with exposure. This review summarizes current knowledge on the molecular epidemiology of head and neck cancer and attempts to identify those areas where future studies may prove fruitful.

Descriptive epidemiology of head and neck cancers

Head and neck cancers form a related group of cancers including neoplasms originating from the oral cavity, pharynx, larynx and esophagus. Together they account for about 10% of all cancers worldwide, although their incidence varies widely. For example, the incidence of cancers of the oral cavity and pharynx varies over 20-fold between high-risk areas (e.g. France, Switzerland, Italy, Spain, India, black people in the USA) and low-risk populations (e.g. China, Nordic countries, the United Kingdom). The highest rates in the world among men are recorded in France; those in women are from India (Parkin et al., 1997). In all populations, rates in men exceed those in women by a factor of 4–10. There is variation in subsites, too: cancers of the oropharynx and hypopharynx account for at least as many cases as cancer of the oral cavity in high-risk European populations, whereas in India and the USA, cancers of the tongue, floor of the mouth and other parts of the oral cavity are more common.

The geographical distribution of esophageal cancer is also characterized by very wide variations within relatively small areas. Very high rates (over 50/100 000) are recorded in both genders from northern Iran and the provinces of eastern China, in certain areas of Kazakhstan and among men from Zimbabwe. Intermediate rates in men (10–50/100 000) occur in eastern Africa, southern Brazil, the Caribbean, most of China (with the exception of southern provinces), regions of central Asia, northern India and southern Europe, as well as in black people from the USA (Parkin et al., 1997). In men, rates are 2–10-fold higher than in women. Squamous-cell carcinoma is the predominant type in most human populations, particularly in populations at very high risk. In many high-risk areas, the incidence of esophageal cancer has decreased during recent decades. The opposite pattern has been shown in low-risk populations, such as northern Europeans and white people in the USA. This increase is mainly accounted for by an increase of adenocarcinoma of the lower esophagus; the incidence of squamous-cell carcinoma remained stable (Blot & McLaughlin, 1999).

More than 90% of cancers of the larynx are squamous-cell carcinomas, and most originate from the supraglottic and glottic regions of the organ. The incidence in men is high (10/100 000 or more) in southern and central Europe, southern Brazil, Uruguay and Argentina and among black people in the USA; the lowest rates (< 1/100 000) are recorded in South-east Asia and central Africa (Parkin *et al.*, 1997). The incidence in women is below 1/100 000 in most populations. Rates have not changed markedly during the last two decades.

Areas of high incidence for head and neck cancers in non-western populations are largely explained by local habits such as chewing of betel quid in southern Asia and consumption of very hot mate in South America (Castelletto *et al.*, 1994; Blot *et al.*, 1996; Balaram *et al.*, 2002). The cause behind the extremely high incidence of esophageal cancer in North-east Iran is unclear, although it may be due to consumption of opium (Ghadirian *et al.*, 1985). The main risk factors for head and neck cancers in Western countries are alcohol and tobacco consumption, which, in individual studies, have been found to account for between 75% and 90% of the disease (Blot *et al.*, 1996). The risk of head and neck cancer increases rapidly with the amount of both tobacco and alcohol consumption, and the effect of alcohol has been observed among both smokers and non-smokers (Talamini *et al.*, 1990). Most studies appear to show a dose–response relationship with tobacco consumption, with increased risks of the order of 3–10-fold compared with never-smokers. An increase in risk has been observed with both duration and quantity of tobacco consumption, and decreases in risk are found after quitting smoking. Similarly, a dose–response relationship is observed with increasing alcohol consumption.

However, it is not apparent that absolute levels of tobacco or alcohol consumption can explain the large differences between countries. For example, in European Union countries, male/female combined head and neck cancer rates vary by over fourfold with high rates being observed in Spain and France, and low rates in Greece, Finland and Sweden (Table 1). Measures of tobacco consumption do not correlate with overall rates of head and neck cancer, whether measured by lung cancer rates for the same year ($r = -0.03$) or per-capita adult cigarette consumption with a 5-year time lag ($r = -0.06$) or a 25-year time lag ($r = -0.2$) (Table 1). These results are surprising, given the strong relationship between cigarette smoking and head and neck cancers in individual-level studies, and suggest that the relationship between tobacco consumption and risk of head and neck cancers is not a simple dose–response one but may also be subject to other factors. The correlation between lung cancer rates in 1995 and national smoking levels in 1970 is relatively strong ($r = 0.62$, $p < 0.05$), which provides some validation for this type of comparison. Conversely, alcohol consumption with a 25-year lag does correspond well with overall rates of head and neck cancer ($r = 0.78$), especially for oropharyngeal and laryngeal cancer, although several anomalies are present. For example, average alcohol consumption in 1970 was almost twice as high in Italy as in Ireland or in Denmark, but their rates of head and neck cancer are similar. Conversely, average alcohol and tobacco consumption in Greece is similar to or greater than levels of tobacco and alcohol consumption in northern European countries including Ireland, Belgium and Denmark, but the incidence of head and neck cancer is approximately half. Site-specific rates also show strong differences due to other factors.

Assuming the national data on alcohol and tobacco consumption are reasonably accurate and not confounded by age- and sex-specific differences, these inconsistencies point to factors other than amount of alcohol and tobacco consumed being important in head and neck cancers. Possible factors include:

• different patterns of tobacco and alcohol consumption and types of tobacco or alcoholic beverage between European populations;
• differing prevalence of other risk factors, including dietary or infectious factors;
• different genetic susceptibility between populations including genetic factors for metabolism of alcohol and tobacco components, as well as other factors including DNA-repair efficiency and cell-cycle control.

The observational evidence for each of these groups will be investigated. Two aspects of the epidemiological evidence of alcohol and tobacco carcinogenicity on head and neck cancers are of

Table 1. Correlation between head and neck cancer incidence rates/100 000 in 1995 and national cigarette and alcohol consumption levels in 1970 and 1990 in EU countries

Country	All head and neck cancers	Oral/ pharynx	Larynx	Oeso- phagus	Lung	Cig 1970	Cig 1990	Alcohol 1970	Alcohol 1990
France	28.3	16.9	5.2	6.3	24.8	1850	2170	21	14
Spain	21.9	12.0	6.7	3.2	26.5	2243	2347	16	11
Portugal	17.7	8.3	6.2	3.2	17.7	1362	2211	14	14
Italy	14.7	6.6	5.7	2.4	33.5	1850	1997	18	10
Belgium	14.3	6.2	5.3	2.8	42.3	2455	2350	11	12
Denmark	14.0	7.3	3.2	3.4	38.2	1937	1860	9	12
Ireland	14.6	6.2	2.5	5.9	28.4	2377	2388	9	12
Austria	12.9	7.4	3.4	2.0	26.8	2347	2073	14	13
United Kingdom	12.6	4.2	2.4	6.0	36.2	3057	2109	7	9
Finland	9.6	6.0	1.4	2.3	22.5	1776	1923	6	8
Greece	7.3	2.8	3.6	0.9	30.5	2575	3355	11	11
Sweden	7.2	4.5	1.0	1.8	16.5	1723	1650	7	6
Correlations between head and neck cancer and markers of alcohol/tobacco consumption									
All head and neck cancers	0	0	0	−0.03	−0.20	−0.06	0.78**	0.64*
Oral/pharynx		0	0	−0.20	−0.34	−0.16	0.76**	0.54
Larynx			0	0.15	−0.17	0.27	0.80**	0.64
Esophagus				0.14	0.23	−0.15	0.14	0.30

Columns 2–7: All incidence data are from EUCAN and are for 1995.
Columns 7 and 8: Cig = per-capita cigarette consumption in 1970 and 1990, respectively. Column 9 and 10: Alcohol = estimated average alcohol consumption (in litres) in 1970 and 1990, respectively. Alcohol and mortality data are from WHO.
Netherlands excluded due to unreliable cigarette smoking statistics. Luxembourg excluded due to small denominator population.
* correlation coefficient significant at 0.05, ** significant at 0.01.170

particular interest with respect to mechanistic information and will be discussed in more detail: the possible effect of acetaldehyde, the main metabolite of ethanol, and the different effect of black and blond tobacco products.

Tobacco and alcohol consumption
Mechanisms of alcohol carcinogenicity
The mechanism by which alcohol is a risk factor for head and neck cancer is unclear, especially as ethanol in its pure form does not act as a carcinogen in experimental models (IARC, 1988). One potential reason why alcoholic beverages are carcinogenic is that alcohol may act merely as a solvent for tobacco carcinogens (Seitz *et al.*, 1998; Wight & Ogden, 1998). This is, however, unable to account fully for the risk observed with alcoholic drinks independent of tobacco smoke, as several studies with a sufficiently large sample

size have been able to illustrate an increased risk among never-smokers.

Impurities or contaminants in alcoholic drinks have also been suggested to represent the main carcinogenic agent. For example, polycyclic aromatic hydrocarbons (PAHs) are found in strong, dark liquors such as whiskey, and *N*-nitrosodiethylamine has been detected in some beers. If contaminants in alcoholic beverages represent the primary risk factor, this would suggest that type of alcoholic beverage would be an important risk factor. The relationship between different types of alcoholic beverage and cancers of the head and neck is, however, inconsistent. A recent population-based cohort study in Denmark reported a threefold increased risk of head and neck cancer associated with alcohol from beer or spirits, but no increased risk with a similar level of alcohol from wine (Gronbaek *et al.*, 1998). This finding is in general agreement with two studies from the USA (Kabat & Wynder, 1989; Mashberg et al., 1993), although a study based in northern Italy reported a strong increased risk among heavy drinkers of wine for cancers of the oral cavity, pharynx and esophagus (La Vecchia et al., 1999). One reason for these inconsistent findings may be that studies conducted in one area are unable to recruit a sufficiently large number of individuals who drink alcoholic beverages other than the main local type (e.g. beer drinkers in Italy or wine drinkers in Denmark). Conversely, it may be that moderate consumption of wine entails no increased risk of head and neck cancers, whereas moderate consumption of beer and spirits entails a considerable increase in risk.

A further possibility is that acetaldehyde, the primary metabolite of ethanol, is the cause of the carcinogenic effect of alcoholic beverages, although direct evidence that acetaldehyde is a cause of head and neck cancer in humans is hard to establish.

Acetaldehyde forms adducts with DNA in human cells in vitro (Vaca et al., 1998) as well as in rats chronically exposed to ethanol (Rintala et al., 2000). In experimental models, inhalation of acetaldehyde has been shown to cause tumours of the respiratory tract, particularly adeno-carcinomas and squamous-cell carcinomas of the nasal mucosa in rats and laryngeal carcinomas in hamsters. Overall, the IARC has determined that there is sufficient evidence in experimental animals for the carcinogenicity of acetaldehyde (IARC, 1988). In a study of 24 alcohol abusers and 12 controls, the average level of lymphocyte DNA adducts of acetaldehyde was sevenfold higher in patients than in controls (Fang & Vaca, 1997). Autoantibodies against acetaldehyde-modified proteins (oxidized epitopes) were detected in blood and bone marrow of alcohol abusers (Rolla et al., 2000; Latvala et al., 2001). In one study, autoantibody levels were higher in patients with alcohol-induced liver disease than in non-drinking controls as well as in heavy drinkers without liver disease (Viitala et al., 2000). Overall, these studies strongly suggest that DNA damage occurs in humans after heavy alcohol consumption. It is plausible that host factors,

including polymorphism in enzymes implicated in the oxidation of ethanol and acetaldehyde, modulate the extent of such damage. Future studies, with proper design and adequate sample size, should aim to:

- investigate DNA adducts in target cells (e.g. head and neck mucosa);
- clarify the relationship between alcohol intake, DNA damage and subsequent steps in carcinogenesis;
- measure newly discovered acetaldehyde adducts in relation to alcohol intake (Hecht et al., 2001);
- develop biomarkers integrating exposure over a longer time, such as protein adducts (Hecht et al., 2001).

Binge drinking is likely to lead to short peaks of acetaldehyde exposure, whereas frequent moderate consumption is likely to lead to constant exposure at a much lower level. The biological significance of this, and whether one type of exposure is likely to represent a greater risk for head and neck cancer, is not well known.

Carcinogenicity of black and blond tobacco

Black (air-cured) tobacco has traditionally been used in Latin American and Mediterranean countries in preference to blond (flue-cured) tobacco, which is the predominant type in most industrialized countries. It is plausible that black and blond tobacco represent potentially different risks of head and neck cancer, because the concentrations of several carcinogens differ substantially between black and blond tobacco; notably, there is a higher level of N-nitrosamines and aromatic amines in black tobacco smoke (Boffetta, 1993; De Stefani et al., 1993; Sancho-Garnier & Theobold, 1993).

Three case–control studies have reported on oral cancer and tobacco type (Table 2). A case–control study from Uruguay on 425 oropharyngeal cases and 427 hospital controls reported a threefold increased risk of both oral cancer (95% confidence interval [CI], 1.8–4.9) and pharyngeal cancer (95% CI, 1.8–4.9) (De Stefani et al., 1998). A case–control study in three areas of Brazil comprising 784 cases of oral, pharyngeal and laryngeal cancer and 1578 controls found no

Table 2. Case–control studies investigating the risk associated with black or blond tobacco smoking and head and neck cancer

		Blond tobacco	Black tobacco
Oral cancer	Merletti *et al.* (1989)	Men: 1.0	1.0 (0.4–2.6)
		Women: 1.0	2.3 (0.3–15.2)
	De Stefani *et al.* (1998)	1.0	3.0 (1.8–4.9)
	Schlect *et al.* (1999)	8.0 (4.3–14.9)	10.1 (5.2–19.6)
Pharynx	Tuyns *et al.* (1988) (hypopharynx)	1.0	2.16 (1.1–4.2)
	De Stefani *et al.* (1998)	1.0	3.0 (1.8–4.9)
	Schlect *et al.* (1999)	5.9 (2.2–15.3)	10.6 (3.6–30.6)
Larynx	Tuyns *et al.* (1988)	1.0	1.98 (1.2–3.2)
	Schlect *et al.* (1999)	10.2 (3.7–27.9)	17.8 (6.3–50.4)
	De Stefani (1987)	1.0	2.5
	Schlect *et al.* (1999)	10.2 (3.7–27.9)	17.8 (6.3–50.4)
Esophageal cancer	Castellsague *et al.* (1999)	Men: 1.0	2.0 (1.5–2.7)
		Women: 1.0	3.4 (0.9–13.0)

difference between use of commercial cigarettes or hand-rolled black tobacco for oral cancer, although the risk of pharyngeal cancer was approximately twice as high in black tobacco smokers (Schlecht *et al.*, 1999). Also of relevance is a multicentre case–control study of hypopharyngeal and laryngeal cancer in six regions of Italy, Spain, Switzerland and France based on 1147 male cases and 3057 controls (Tuyns *et al.*, 1988). Higher risks of both hypopharyngeal and laryngeal cancer were observed for smokers of black tobacco only, as compared with blond tobacco only, with those who smoked both types of tobacco having intermediate risks. Finally, the results of five previous studies on esophageal cancer and tobacco type conducted in South America have recently been combined into a pooled analysis comprising 830 cases and 1779 controls (Castellsague *et al.*, 1999). An increased risk of black tobacco as opposed to blond tobacco was observed in both men and women.

These results indicate an increased risk of black tobacco in head and neck cancers, particularly for pharyngeal, laryngeal and esophageal cancer. The findings for oral cancer are equivocal, however, and may even point to an absence of effect in two of the three studies. Overall, however, these findings may help to explain why tobacco consumption levels *per se* fail to correlate strongly with incidence rates for head and neck cancer, as perhaps the most important exposure for tobacco consumption is type of tobacco. Although this hypothesis is appealing, an alternative possibility is that black tobacco consumption is simply a marker of other risk factors for head and neck cancer including poor social class, high alcohol consumption and poor diet. All studies attempted to adjust their findings for some or all of these factors, but there is still the possibility that residual confounding may explain the increased risk observed for black tobacco. An evaluation of the mechanistic evidence for the role of black tobacco in head and neck cancer is therefore essential.

Additional evidence on the carcinogenicity of black and blond tobacco comes from studies on proteins and DNA adducts. Aromatic DNA adducts were analysed by the ^{32}P-postlabelling method in 41 people with laryngeal cancer (Szyfter *et al.*, 1994). The levels of aromatic DNA adducts were $5.72/10^8$ nucleotides in tumour tissue and $3.74/10^8$ nucleotides in non-tumour tissue.

Smokers had higher levels of adducts in tumour tissue. DNA adduct levels in tumour and non-tumour tissue correlated with the levels found in leukocytes ($r = 0.87$ and 0.86, respectively).

Studies also measured 7-alkylguanine adducts among 44 people with laryngeal cancer (Szyfter et al., 1996). The adducts included 7-methyl-guanine and 7-hydroxyethylguanine. Smoking level correlated with the adduct level and among heavy smokers, $61.8/10^8$ nucleotides alkylguanine adducts were found, compared with 23.2 and $11.3/10^8$ nucleotides among moderate and non/ex-smokers, respectively. The adduct levels in leukocytes of patients and control subjects were about $5–14/10^8$ nucleotides. The levels of 7-alkylguanine did not correlate with the level of aromatic adducts.

A number of studies have shown a higher level of haemoglobin adducts formed by aromatic amines such as 4-aminobiphenyl and heterocyclic amines such as 2-amino-1-methyl-6-phenylimi-dazo(4,5-b)pyridine (PhIP) in smokers of black tobacco as compared with smokers of blond tobacco (Bartsch et al., 1993). A similar phenomenon is plausible for DNA adducts, although the characteristics of the adducts specific to black tobacco smoke have not been fully established (Vineis et al., 1996). Elevated levels of protein adducts have been associated with an increased risk of urinary bladder cancer (Vineis, 1992), a neoplasm that has a well-established association with smoking of black tobacco. Similar data are lacking for head and neck cancer, although adducts can be detected in the oral mucosa (Stone et al., 1995), and a correlation between their levels and tobacco smoking has been shown (Jones et al., 1993). In one study, levels of in-vitro benzo[a]pyrene diol epoxide-induced DNA adducts in lymphocytes were higher in cases of head and neck cancer than in controls (Li et al., 2001). There is a need to investigate whether adducts (either to protein or DNA) specific to black tobacco products do represent a risk factor for head and neck cancer.

As with adducts, studies of urinary mutagenicity have shown a greater effect after smoking of black tobacco as compared with blond tobacco (Bartsch et al., 1990), and this has also been associated with bladder cancer risk (Malaveille et al., 1989). Comparable data for head and neck cancer are lacking.

In conclusion, studies of markers of exposure to tobacco have the potential to contribute to the study of differences in carcinogenicity of types of tobacco on head and neck organs, but currently available data offer limited information.

Interaction with dietary factors and human papillomaviruses

A diet which is deficient in fruit and vegetables is a recognized risk factor for head and neck cancer, accounting for possibly 10–15% of cases (WCRF, 1997). Increased risks have been found with decreasing consumption of fresh fruit and vegetables, as well as vitamins A and C. Conversely, it is possible that frequent dietary consumption of salted meat and fish, as well as pickled vegetables, may represent a risk factor. An area that has received little attention is the effect of alcohol in conjunction with a diet deficient in fruit and vegetables. It has been postulated that mucous lesions caused by niacin or riboflavin deficiency may enhance the topical action of alcohol, possibly by enhancing the action of carcinogenic compounds.

Benign lesions of the head and neck including laryngeal papillomas and oral verrucal papillary lesions illustrate the potential for human papillomaviruses (HPV) to infect squamous tissue of the head and neck. These raise the possibility that oncogenic HPV may be involved in the development of some cases of head and neck cancer. The two types of studies that have been most useful for investigating this relationship are serological studies based on blood samples taken before onset of disease, and large case series investigations of the presence of HPV DNA in tumour tissue.

The most informative serological studies for head and neck cancer are based on a network of large serum banks in Norway, Finland and Sweden, containing samples from approximately 900 000 subjects (Dillner et al., 1995; Bjorge et al., 1997; Mork et al., 2001). By linking these serum banks to national cancer registries it is possible to identify almost 100% of cases, allowing the conduct of nested case–control studies. In a recent analysis of 292 people with oral, pharyngeal or laryngeal cancer and 1568 matched controls, an increased risk of 2.2 (95% CI, 1.4–3.4) was observed for HPV-16 and all head and neck cancer sites combined. No increased risk was observed for HPV-18, HPV-33 or HPV-73. The increased risk for HPV-16 was most apparent for the oropharynx (odds ratio, 14.4; 95% CI, 3.6–58.1), tongue (2.8; 95% CI, 1.2–6.6) and larynx (2.4; 95% CI, 1.0–5.6). Paraffin-embedded tumour tissue was available from 160 of the cases, allowing PCR analysis for HPV DNA, which was detected in 15 cases (9%) including 9/18 (50%) oropharyngeal cases, 4/29 (14%) tongue cancer cases and 1/32 (3%) laryngeal cancer cases. Three separate studies from the same group were based on 57 cases of esophageal cancer and 171 matched controls in Norway, 39 cases and 330 controls in Finland and 121 cases and 302 controls in Sweden. An increased association was observed between HPV-16 and esophageal cancer in both the Norwegian sample (odds ratio, 6.6; 95% CI, 1.1–71) and the Finnish sample (14.6; 95% CI, 1.8–117), although not in the Swedish samples (1.0; 95% CI, 0.5–2.0) (Dillner *et al.*, 1995; Bjorge *et al.*, 1997; Lagergren *et al.*, 1999).

The largest case series of head and neck cancer investigated for HPV DNA is a series of 253 cases in the USA (Gillison *et al.*, 2000). The presence of the HPV genome was tested using PCR-based assays, Southern blot hybridization and in-situ hybridization. Overall, HPV was detected in 62 (25%) of the cases, with HPV-16 making up 90% of positive cases. HPV detection was most common in the oropharynx (57% of cases) and moderately frequent in the larynx (19%), oral cavity (12%) and hypopharynx (10%).

These studies indicate a role for oncogenic HPV in head and neck cancers, although several questions remain. First, the association between HPV and survival is of interest although it is unclear whether stage of disease may also be associated with the sensitivity of HPV detection. Similarly, the relationship between serology and site-specific infection rates is unclear, and a site-specific marker of HPV infection would be extremely useful. Previous case series of oral cancers have included HPV analysis of oral DNA obtained from scrapings, although little correlation has been found with HPV in tumour tissue. Such a marker would allow an analysis of HPV head and neck infection in various populations.

Genetic susceptibility factors

Figure 1 illustrates in a simplified manner some of the gene families that may be involved in head and neck carcinogenesis. As well as behavioural genes, which may lead to increased alcohol or tobacco consumption, phase I and II metabolizing genes such as *ADH*, *CYP* and *NAT* are likely to be important in determining the level of internal carcinogenic dose. The subsequent development of DNA mutations, repair of these errors or cell apoptosis may also be regulated by DNA-repair genes or tumour-suppressor genes. The efficiency of DNA repair and tumour suppression may vary greatly between individuals, providing further opportunities for differences in risk.

Alcohol metabolism

Alcohol is metabolized to acetaldehyde by alcohol dehydrogenases (ADH) and, to a lesser extent, by cytochrome P450 2E1. Subsequent conversion of acetaldehyde to acetic acid is catalysed by aldehyde dehydrogenases (ALDH). The majority of alcohol and aldehyde metabolism is carried out in the liver, although metabolism involving ADH, CYP2E1 and ALDH has also been demonstrated in the upper aerodigestive tract. Of the three genes responsible for ADH enzymes, *ADH2* and *ADH3* are polymorphic, with enzymes encoded by the *ADH3*1* and *ADH2*2* alleles representing 'fast' metabolizers. The *ADH3*1* allele, which increases oxidation by about 2.5-fold, is present in approximately 60% of white people, resulting in about 10–30% of individuals being homozygous for the *ADH3*2/2* slow genotype. The *ADH2*1* and *ADH2*2* alleles differ greatly in oxidation efficiencies, with the *ADH2*1/1* genotype having only 1% and 0.5% of the oxidation capability of the *ADH2*1/2* and *ADH2*2/2* genotypes, respectively. The *ADH2*1* allele is more common in white people, with approximately 90% being homozygous for the slow *ADH2*1/1* genotype, and approximately 10% being *ADH2*1/2* heterozygotes (Borras *et al.*, 2000).

Given that fast alcohol metabolizers will receive a greater peak exposure to acetaldehyde than slow metabolizers after a comparable intake of alcohol, a prime hypothesis is that possession of *ADH3*1* alleles and *ADH2*2* alleles will

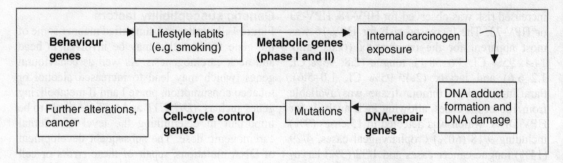

Figure 1. Potential role of genetic susceptibility in the pathway of head and neck cancer.

confer increased risks for head and neck cancer. Nine case–control studies investigating this hypothesis have been published, seven for *ADH3* and two for *ADH2*, and the results are presented in Table 3. The first two studies provided some supportive evidence for an increased risk of the *ADH3*1/1* genotype in oral and pharyngeal cancer, but the subsequent five studies have all found no evidence of an increased risk. The second study (Harty *et al.*, 1997) was particularly appealing because of the apparent evidence it provided for a gene–environment interaction. Heavy alcohol drinkers with the fast *ADH3*1/1* genotype were at a 10-fold increased risk of oral/pharyngeal cancer (odds ratio, 40.1; 95% CI, 5.4–296) compared with heavy drinkers with the *ADH3*2/2* genotype (odds ratio, 4.4; 95% CI, 0.6–33.3). These results were, however, based on small numbers and do not appear to have been replicated in later studies. No data are available for esophageal cancer and *ADH3* polymorphism.

The two Japanese studies for *ADH2* both indicate a higher risk among head and neck cancer cases for the slow *ADH2*1/1* genotype, which is contrary to the hypothesis (Table 3). In a study of 94 esophageal cancer patients and 70 controls, an over sixfold increased risk was observed for *ADH2*1/1* and a 70% increased risk for *ADH2*1/2* (Hori *et al.*, 1997). In a case–control study of alcoholics, a similar sixfold increase in risk was observed for oral and laryngeal cancer and *ADH2*1/1* when compared with *ADH*1/2* or *ADH*2/2*, and a twofold increase in risk for esophageal cancer (Yokoyama *et al.*, 2001).

As previously described, acetaldehyde is subsequently metabolized to acetic acid by the aldehyde dehydrogenase 2 enzyme encoded by *ALDH2*. The gene contains an inactive *ALDH2*2* allele, resulting in homozygotes who are unable to oxidize acetaldehyde and heterozygotes who do so inefficiently. This leads to homozygous and heterozygous *ALDH2*2* individuals who experience a build-up of acetaldehyde resulting in a toxic reaction including flushing, increased heart rate and nausea. Indeed, it is likely that possession of one or two *ALDH2*2* alleles leads to a reduced alcohol intake and consequently a reduced risk of alcohol-related cancers. The *ALDH2*2* allele is very rare in white populations, although common in Asian populations. Four Japanese studies have investigated the relationship between *ALDH2* and head and neck cancers. One study among alcoholics identified a strong relative risk associated with the heterozygote genotype compared with the fully functional *ALDH2*1/1* genotype for oral, laryngeal and esophageal cancer (Yokoyama *et al.*, 2001). One study of oral cancer cases and controls identified no association for either the non-functional or the heterozygote genotype (Katoh *et al.*, 1999). Two other Japanese studies of esophageal cancer patients identified no association with the functional homozygote or non-functional homozygote, although a strong increased risk was observed with the heterozygote genotype. These results therefore suggest a possible increase in risk of head and neck cancer associated with possessing one inactive *ALDH2*2* allele but not two inactive alleles. Indeed, it is plausible that possession of two inactive alleles is protective against head and neck cancer as it leads to lower alcohol consumption as a result of the strong side-effects experienced.

Table 3. Polymorphism in alcohol-metabolizing genes ADH2, ADH3 and ALDH2 and head and neck cancer

Reference (population)	Genotype	Cases/controls	Oral/pharynx	Larynx	Esophagus
ADH3					
Coutelle et al. (1997) (French alcoholics)	*1/1 v 1/2 or 2/2	21: Oro-pharyngeal 18: Laryngeal 37: Controls	2.6 (0.7–10)	6.1 (1.3–28.6)	
Harty et al. (1997) (Puerto Rico)	*1/1 v 2/2 *1/2 v 2/2	137: Oro-pharyngeal 146: Controls	1.67 (0.62–3.33) 1.4 (0.77–2.5)		
Bouchardy et al. (2000) (France)	*1/1 v 2/2 *1/2 v 2/2	121: Oro-pharyngeal 129: Laryngeal 172: Controls	1.1 (0.6–2.2) 0.7 (0.4–1.4)	0.7 (0.4–1.4) 1.0 (0.5–1.8)	
Sturgis et al. (2001) (USA)	*1/1 v 2/2 *1/2 v 2/2	229: Oro-pharyngeal 575: Controls	0.81 (0.52–1.28) 1.04 (0.73–1.47)		
Olshan (2001) (USA)	*1/1 v 2/2 *1/2 v 2/2	173: Oro-pharyngeal + Laryngeal 194: Controls	0.9 (0.4–1.9) 0.8 (0.4–1.7)		
Schwartz et al. (2001) (USA)	*1/1 v 2/2 *1/2 v 2/2	333: Oral 541: Controls	1.1 (0.7–1.5) 1.3 (1.0–1.8)		
Zavras (2002) (Greece)	*1/1 v 2/2 *1/2 v 2/2	93: Oral 99: Controls	1.25 (0.45–3.3) 1.25 (0.6–2.0)		
ADH2					
Hori et al. (1997) (Japan)	*1/1 v *2/2 *1/2 v 2/2	94: Esophageal 70: Controls			6.2 (2.6–14.7) 1.7 (0.9–3.0)
Yokoyama et al. (2001) (Japanese alcoholics)	*1/1 v *1/2 or *2/2	16: Oro-pharyngeal 18: Laryngeal/hypopharyngeal 112: Esophageal 526: Controls	5.48 (1.77–17.0)	6.57 (1.62–21.3)	2.64 (1.62–4.31)
ALDH2					
Hori et al. (1997) (Japan)	*2/2 v *1/1 *1/2 v 1/1	90: Esophageal 70: Controls			0.9 (0.2–3.6) 4.4 (2.5–5.7)
Katoh et al. (1999) (Japan)	*2/2 v *1/1 *1/2 v 1/1	92: Oral 147: Controls	0.35 (0.57–2.17)* 1.18 (0.65–2.13)*		
Yokoyama et al. (2001) (Japanese alcoholics)	*1/2 v 1/1	16: Oro-pharyngeal 18: Laryngeal/hypopharyngeal 112: Esophageal 526: Controls	20.8 (6.62–55.5)	28.9 (8.66–96.6)	13.5 (8.06–22.6)
Matsuo et al. (2001) (Japan)	*1/1 v *2/2 *1/2 v 2/2	102: Esophageal 241: Controls			0.80[a] (0.09–6.88) 3.72[a] (1.88–7.36)

[a] Adjusted for alcohol consumption.

A similar explanation may underly the increased risk associated with the *ADH2* slow genotype (*ADH2*1/1*). The one study on *ADH2* conducted in the Japanese general population did not adjust for alcohol consumption (Hori *et al.*, 1997). These findings point to the necessity for careful control of alcohol consumption in the analysis of genetic studies for *ADH2* and *ALDH2*.

Overall, the available incidence excludes a role of *ADH3* polymorphism in susceptibility to alcohol-related head and neck cancer, although polymorphism of *ADH2* and *ALDH2* may play a role. These results are therefore compatible with an effect of acetaldehyde in head and neck carcinogenesis.

A better understanding of the possible role of acetaldehyde in head and neck cancer requires larger studies that incorporate a joint analysis of all alcohol and aldehyde dehydrogenase genes simultaneously. This will require studies of a sufficient sample size to investigate possible gene–gene and gene–environment interactions.

Mechanistic studies are also required to clarify the role of individual *ADH* and *ALDH* genes in acetaldehyde exposure, including an assessment of combinations of these genes. An assessment of acetaldehyde levels with different patterns of alcohol consumption, including binge drinking as well as moderate chronic consumption, would also be of interest. Finally, the roles of *ADH* and *ALDH* genes should also be assessed with respect to intermediate markers including acetaldehyde adducts in head and neck tissue.

CYP2E1
A further metabolizing gene of strong interest for head and neck cancers is *CYP2E1*, which is induced by ethanol and involved in the metabolism of ethanol as well as several tobacco procarcinogens including nitrosamines. Two functional polymorphisms have been identified (*Rsa*1 and *Dra*1) although the prevalence is rather low (approximately 10% heterozygotes and less than 1% homozygotes in white people). Of the *Rsa*1 polymorphism, the *c2* allele is thought to have a lower enzyme activity than the *c1* allele, although the functional relevance of the two *Dra*1 alleles (*C* and *D*) is unclear. Six studies have reported on

CYP2E1 and head and neck cancer. Approximately a twofold increased risk has been associated with the *c2* homozygous or heterozygous genotype in some studies (Hung *et al.*, 1997; Bouchardy *et al.*, 2000; Tan *et al.*, 2000) but not in others (Table 4) (Matthias *et al.*, 1998; Morita *et al.*, 1999). Of the two studies that reported on the *Dra*1 polymorphism, one reported a twofold increased risk with one or two *C* alleles (Bouchardy *et al.*, 2000), but this was not found in the second study (Matthias *et al.*, 1998).

Tobacco metabolism
As previously discussed, a prime hypothesis for head and neck cancer is that smokers of black tobacco experience higher cancer risk than smokers of blond tobacco because of the increased exposure to *N*-nitrosamines and aromatic amines which are found in higher concentrations in black tobacco. Aromatic and heterocyclic amines require metabolic activation to interact with DNA. After *N*-acetylation, the *N*-hydroxyaromatic and *N*-hydroxyheterocyclic amines are further activated (via *O*-acetylation) by *N*-acetyltransferases to acetoxy intermediates, which react with DNA to form DNA adducts. Two *N*-acetyltransferase genes, *NAT1* and *NAT2*, involved in both *N*- and *O*-acetylation, are highly polymorphic with variants that strongly influence the rate of activity. *NAT2* polymorphism has been identified as being involved in bladder cancer, another cancer that is related to aromatic amines and black tobacco consumption, with an increased prevalence of *NAT2* slow genotypes in bladder cancer cases (Vineis *et al.*, 2001). *NAT1* is thought to be expressed mainly in extrahepatic tissues with some studies reporting higher *N*-acetyltransferase activity with the *NAT1*10* allele compared with *NAT1*4*, the other common *NAT1* allele. Five case–control studies have investigated a role for *NAT1* polymorphism in head and neck cancer, with only one small study among Japanese oral cancer cases reporting an increase in risk for the fast *NAT1*10/10* allele, or the intermediate *NAT1*10/4* allele (Table 5). *NAT2* is also highly polymorphic, with *NAT2*4*, *NAT2*12* and *NAT2*13* being the main fast-metabolizing alleles. Five case–control studies have also investigated the relationship between *NAT2*

Table 4. Cytochrome P450 genes *2E1* and *1A1* and head and neck cancer

Reference (population)	Gene	Cases/controls	Oral/pharynx	Larynx	Esophagus
Hung *et al.* (1997) (Taiwan)	*Rsa*1 *c2/c2* v *c1/c1* *c2/c1* v *c1/c1*	Oral: 43 Controls: 123	1.8 (0.3–10.7) 1.8 (0.9–3.8)		
Tan *et al.* (2000) (China)	*Rsa*1 *c2/c2 + c1/c2* v *c1/c1*	150: Esophageal 150: Controls			3.2 (2.5–4.1)
Matthias *et al.* (1998) (Germany)	*Dra*1 *CC* or *CD* v *DD* Rsa1 *c2/c2 + c1/c2* v *c1/c1*	126: Oral + Pharyngeal 272: Laryngeal 219: Controls	*Dra*1 1.0 (0.5–2.0) *Rsa*1 1.0 (0.5–1.9)	*Dra*1 0.9 (0.5–1.7) *Rsa*1 1.0 (0.6–1.8)	
Morita *et al.* (1999) (Japan)	*Rsa*1 *c2/c2 + c1/c2* v *c1/c1*	45: Laryngeal 69: Laryngeal 164: Controls	1.0 (0.5–1.9)	1.0 (0.6–1.8)	
Katoh *et al.* (1999) (Japan)	*Rsa*1 *c2/c2* v *c1/c1* *c2/c1* v *c1/c1*	92: Oral 147: Controls	0.77 (0.19–3.10) 1.43 (0.83–2.49)		
Bouchardy *et al.* (2000) (France)	*Dra*1 *CC* or *CD* v *DD* *Rsa*1 *c2c2* or *c1c2* v *c1c1*	121: Oro-pharyngeal 129: Laryngeal 172: Controls	*Dra*1 2.0 (1.0–3.9) *Rsa*1 2.6 (1.0–6.6)	*Dra*1 1.8 (1.0–3.5) *Rsa*1 1.4 (0.5–4.0)	

and head and neck cancer. Three studies of *NAT2* and oropharyngeal cancer have all found some evidence of an increased risk of slow *NAT2* genotypes, although this was only significant in the French case–control study (Jourenkova-Mironova *et al.*, 1999). Two further studies that reported on laryngeal cancer and esophageal cancer found no evidence of an increase in risk with slow acetylation.

DNA-repair genes

Phenotypic measures of DNA-repair capacity using measurements in cultured lymphocytes and host-cell reactivation assays have been very productive in confirming that people with head and neck cancer do experience substantial DNA-repair deficiency which is unrelated to exposure (Cheng *et al.*, 1998; Sturgis *et al.*, 1999). Individuals with reduced DNA-repair capacity also appear to have high levels of carcinogen–DNA adducts in their tissues (Duell *et al.*, 2000;

Matullo *et al.*, 2001). The challenge is now to identify the genotypes responsible for DNA-repair deficiency in head and neck cancer. A few small studies have recently reported results for some DNA-repair candidate genes that appear to indicate that they are likely to modulate the risk of cancers related to tobacco and alcohol.

A study of 203 head and neck cancer cases and 424 controls reported increased risks associated with an *XRCC1* allele on exon 6, with the risk being most prominent for oral and pharyngeal cancer (odds ratio, 2.5; 95% CI, 1.2–5.0) (Sturgis *et al.*, 1999). A subsequent analysis of two *XPD* polymorphisms in roughly the same population identified a slightly increased risk for the homozygous genotype of one of these polymorphisms (*35931C*) (odds ratio, 1.55; 95% CI, 0.96–2.52) (Sturgis *et al.*, 2000). Other DNA-repair candidate genes that have been identified include *XRCC2*, *XRCC9*, *ERCC1*, *LIG3*, *POLB*, *APEX*, *UCGT1A1*, *PCNA*, *MPG*, *OGG1* and *AGT*, although there is

Table 5. Polymorphism of N-acetyltransferase genes NAT1 and NAT2 and head and neck cancers

Reference (population)	Gene	Cases/controls	Oral/pharynx	Larynx	Esophagus
NAT1					
Katoh et al. (1998) (Japan)	*10/10 v *4/4 *4/10 v 4/4	62: Oral 122: Controls	3.3 (1.31–8.56) 3.7 (1.60–8.46)		
Henning et al. (1999) (Germany)	*4 v NAT*X *10 v NAT*X	255: Laryngeal 510: Controls		1.04 (0.80–1.35) 0.99 (0.74–1.33)	
Olshan et al. (2000) (USA)	*10/10 v *4/4 *4/10 v *4/4	182: Oro-pharyngeal + Laryngeal 202: Controls	0.6 (0.2–1.5) 1.2 (0.7–1.9)		
Jourenkova-Mironova et al. (1999) (France)	* X/X v *X/4 or *4/4	121: Oro-pharyngeal 129: Laryngeal 172: Controls	1.2 (0.7–2.1)	1.0 (0.6–1.7)	
Fronhoffs et al. (2001) (Germany)	*10 v NAT1*4	143:Oro-pharyngeal 148: Laryngeal 300: Controls	1.0 (0.7–1.4)	1.2 (0.8–1.7)	
NAT2					
Katoh et al. (1998) (Japan)	*slow/slow v *4/4 *slow/4 v 4/4	62: Oral 122: Controls	2.3 (0.8–7.2) 1.3 (0.7–2.4)		
Henning et al. (1999) (Germany)	*4 v *X *5B v *X *6A v *X	255: Laryngeal 510: Controls		1.17 (0.91–1.50) 0.91 (0.73–1.14) 0.96 (0.74–1.22)	
Jourenkova-Mironova et al. (1999) (France)	Slow v intermediate or rapid	121: Oro-pharyngeal 129: Laryngeal 172: Controls	1.7 (1.0–3.0)	0.9 (0.5–1.6)	
Morita et al. (1999) (Japan)	Slow v rapid Intermediate v rapid	145: Oro-pharyngeal + Laryngeal 164: Controls	1.53 (0.74–3.16) 1.69 (1.04–2.74)		
Lee et al. (2000) (Taiwan)	Slow v rapid Intermediate v rapid	90: Esophageal 254: Controls			0.60 (0.30–1.19) 0.80 (0.46–1.33)

NAT2*4 represents a rapid phenotype; NAT2*5B and 6A represent slow phenotypes.
NAT1*10 represents a fast metabolizer.

currently no information on their role in tobacco-related carcinogenesis.

Cell-cycle control genes

Although tumour-suppressor genes such as *TP53* are primarily of interest in cancer because they are frequently mutated (see below), approximately 70% of head and neck cancers do not exhibit *TP53* mutations (Hernandez-Boussard *et al.*, 1999). One hypothesis for tumours that occur in the absence of *TP53* mutation is that common polymorphisms may result in limited efficiency in tumour suppression. The *TP53* gene exhibits a polymorphism at codon 72 involving a single base change. The functional significance of this variation is unclear, but one report has indicated a higher risk with the Pro/Pro genotype as opposed to the Arg/Arg genotype in a case–control study of esophageal cancer in Taiwan (odds ratio, 2.3; 95% CI, 0.9–4.4) (Lee *et al.*, 2000). Other polymorphic tumour-suppressor genes that are frequently mutated in tobacco-related cancers include *p16* and *cyclin D1* (see below). One polymorphism of *CCND1* (G870A) is thought to be associated with an increased likelihood that DNA-damaged cells progress through the G_1/S cell-cycle checkpoint. A recent case–control study of 233 head and neck cancers and 248 controls reported an increase in risk of head and neck cancer with the *AA* genotype compared with the *GG* genotype (odds ratio, 1.77; 95% CI, 1.04–3.02) (Zheng *et al.*, 2001).

Acquired genetic alterations

Knowledge of the genetic alterations occurring in the development of head and neck cancer has greatly increased in recent years. The estimated number of accumulated genetic events needed for the development of head and neck cancer is in the range of 5–10 (Renan, 1993). Figure 2 depicts a model of head and neck carcinogenesis. As in the case of other human neoplasms, such models represent an oversimplification, since multiple pathways are possible, involving alterations in different genes and at different times.

Cytogenetic alterations in head and neck cancer have been identified in studies of tumour-cell cultures and comparative genomic hybridization (Cowan *et al.*, 1993; van Dyke *et al.*,

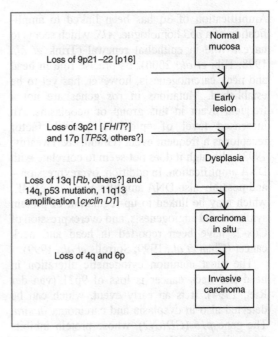

Figure 2. Model of development of head and neck cancer, with main genetic alterations (modified from Sidransky, 2001). Genes that may be involved are indicated in square brackets.

1994; Brzoska *et al.*, 1995). Alterations of specific genes have been associated with some of these cytogenetic abnormalities. Among the proto-oncogenes, amplification of *cyclin D1*, a key component of cell-cycle machinery, seems to be the main event involved in 11q13 amplification, although other genes were also reported to be co-amplified. *Cyclin D1* amplification, which occurs in approximately 30% of head and neck cancers (Berenson *et al.*, 1989), is associated with overexpression and with tumour progression (Jares *et al.*, 1994). As discussed below, inactivation of p16 and Rb, two negative regulators of the cyclin D1 pathway, is also a frequent event in head and neck cancer, suggesting that alteration in the G_1/S check-point is a critical mechanism in head and neck carcinogenesis. No information is available on whether amplification of *cyclin D1* is associated with either environmental exposures or genetic susceptibility factors.

The role of proto-oncogenes other than *cyclin D1* in head and neck cancer is not well known.

Amplification of 3q has been linked to amplification of a *p53* homologue, *AIS*, which seems to have a role in epithelial renewal (Trink *et al.*, 1998; Hibi *et al.*, 2000). Its precise role in head and neck carcinogenesis, however, has yet to be established. Mutations in *ras* genes are not a frequent event in this group of neoplasms. An increased level of epidermal growth factor receptor is a frequent event (Grandis & Tweardy, 1993), although it does not seem to correlate with DNA amplification. In addition, overexpression – and possibly also DNA amplification – of eIF4E, which may be linked to up-regulation of protein synthesis and angiogenesis, and overexpression of Cox-2, have been reported in head and neck cancer (Chan *et al.*, 1999; Sorrells *et al.*, 1999).

The most common cytogenetic alteration in head and neck cancer is loss of 9p21 (van der Riet, 1994). It is an early event, which can be detected also in dysplasia and carcinoma *in situ*. The gene *p16* (*CDKN2*), whose protein inhibits the cyclin D1/CDK4 complex, is located in this region. Inactivation of *p16* occurs through various mechanisms: chromosome loss, homozygous deletion (25%), methylation at 5'CpG (25%, leading to block of transcription) or mutation (10–15%) (Cairns *et al.*, 1995; Merlo *et al.*, 1995). In particular, loss of *p16* is a frequent event in head and neck cancer, including early lesions (Reed *et al.*, 1996; Papadimitrakopoulou *et al.*, 1997). No information is available on the association between *p16* loss or other forms of inactivation and exposure to environmental agents or genetic susceptibility factors.

Loss of 3p21 is also a frequent and early event in head and neck cancer. A possible role has been suggested for *FHIT*, although mutations have not been described very frequently in these tumours (Mao, L. *et al.*, 1996). Loss of 17p occurs in 60% of advanced head and neck cancers (Boyle *et al.*, 1993). On the other hand, *TP53* mutation is a rare event in the case of 17p loss, suggesting that a second tumour-suppressor gene may be present in 17p. The prevalence of *TP53* mutation in head and neck cancer is of the order of 35% and the pattern of mutations derived from the IARC *TP53* database (http://www.iarc.fr/TP53/index.html) is summarized in Figure 3.

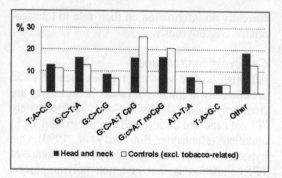

Figure 3. Types of *TP53* mutation in head and neck and control cancers.

Cancers of head and neck show an intermediate *TP53* mutation profile between tobacco-related and non-related cancers, and the degree of similarity with tobacco-related cancers increases from the oral cavity to the pharynx and the larynx. When tobacco-specific mutations, defined as G:C→T:A transversions at codons 157, 248 or 273 were grouped together, the odds ratio of such a type of mutation, using non-tobacco related cancers as control group, was 2.2 (95% CI, 1.4–3.5) (Table 6). On the other hand, the odds ratio for mutations which can be interpreted as resulting from spontaneous deamination of methylated cytosine or other endogenous mechanisms (G:C→A:T transitions at CpG sites at codons 175, 245, 248, 273 and 282) is 0.5 (95% CI, 0.4–0.6). Most of the mutations were investigated in patients from western Europe and North America; the similarities with the mutation spectrum of lung cancer are stronger for these cancers than for those of Asian countries. The smoking status was known for 220 head and neck cancer patients; 188 of them were ever-smokers. When their mutation pattern was compared with that of never-smokers, an increased odds ratio was noticed for tobacco-related mutations and a decreased odds ratio for endogenous mutations (Table 7). Data were too sparse to allow an analysis by amount of smoking. Alcohol drinking was known for 98 patients; their mutations did not show a specific pattern (Table 7). In a few studies, mutations in *TP53* have been analysed in tumours characterized for presence of HPV. An analysis of the results of four studies, including 140 cases of oral and other head and neck cancers (Brachman

Table 6. Odds ratio of presence of specific *TP53* mutations, by site within the head and neck compared with non-tobacco-related cancers

	Head and neck		Oral cavity		Oropharynx		Hypopharynx		Larynx	
	OR	95% CI	OR	95% CI	OR	95% CI	OR	95% CI	OR	95% CI
Tobacco-related mutations[a]	2.2	1.4–3.5	2.2	1.2–4.2	4.7	2.2–10	1.0	0.1–7.2	2.2	1.0–5.1
Endogenous mutations[b]	0.5	0.4–0.6	0.6	0.4–0.9	0.4	0.2–0.8	0.4	0.1–1.0	0.3	0.1–0.5

OR, odds ratio adjusted for geographic region; CI, confidence interval
[a] G:C→T:A transversion at codons 157, 248 or 273.
[b] G:C→A:T transitions at CpG sites at codons 175, 245, 248, 273, or 282.

Table 7. Odds ratio of presence of specific *TP53* mutations, by tobacco smoking and drinking habits. Results of logistic regression analysis

	Tobacco smoking		Alcohol drinking	
	OR$_s$	95% CI	OR$_d$	95% CI
Tobacco-related mutations[a]	2.4	0.7–8.3	0.7	0.1–7.3
Endogenous mutations[b]	0.5	0.2–0.9	0.4	0.1–1.0

OR$_s$, odds ratio of mutation in smokers versus nonsmokers, adjusted for geographic region and head and neck tumour site; CI, confidence interval; OR$_d$, odds ratio of mutation in drinkers versus non-drinkers, adjusted for geographic region and head and neck tumour site.
[a] G:C→T:A transversion at codons 157, 248 or 273.
[b] G:C→A:T transitions at CpG sites at codons 175, 245, 248, 273 or 282.

et al., 1992; Mao, E.J. *et al.*, 1996; Scholes *et al.*, 1997; Koh *et al.*, 1998) did not reveal a different prevalence of *TP53* mutation in HPV-positive and HPV-negative tumours (Mantel-Haenszel odds ratio, 0.6; 95% CI, 0.3–1.4), suggesting that *TP53* mutation and HPV infection are independent events in the development of head and neck cancer. Information on the possible role of other environmental carcinogens in causing head and neck cancer is limited. A separate study of 253 patients with newly diagnosed or recurrent head and neck cancer detected HPV in 62 (25%) of 253 cases (95% CI, 19%–30%) (Gillison *et al.*, 2000). High-risk, tumorigenic type HPV-16 was identified in

90% of the HPV-positive tumours. Poor tumour grade (odds ratio, 2.4; 95% CI, 1.2–4.9) and oropharyngeal site (odds ratio, 6.2; 95% CI, 3.1–12.1) independently increased the probability of the presence of HPV. As compared with HPV-negative oropharyngeal cancers, HPV-positive oropharyngeal cancers were less likely to occur among moderate to heavy drinkers (odds ratio, 0.17; 95% CI, 0.05–0.61) and smokers (odds ratio, 0.16; 95% CI, 0.02–1.4), had a characteristic basaloid morphology (odds ratio, 18.7; 95% CI, 2.1–167), were less likely to have *TP53* mutations (odds ratio, 0.06; 95% CI, 0.01–0.36) and had improved disease-specific survival (hazard ratio, 0.26; 95% CI,

0.07–0.98). These results would appear to suggest that HPV-positive oropharyngeal cancers comprise a distinct molecular, clinical and pathological disease entity with a different prognosis, although this needs to be repeated in other samples. In one study of 187 cases of oral cancer from Taiwan, the overall prevalence of mutation was 49%, and there was no difference between chewers of betel quid and other cases (Hsieh *et al.*, 2001).

Mutations in transforming growth factor-β receptor, which may lead to abrogation of negative cell-cycle regulation, have been reported in head and neck cancer (Wang *et al.*, 1997). Homozygous deletion and inactivation of PTEN have been reported in 10% of head and neck cancers, and may reflect the underlying phenomenon of 10q loss. Mutations in this gene are, however, rare in head and neck cancer (Okami *et al.*, 1998; Shao *et al.*, 1998). Although 13q loss is frequent in head and neck cancer, inactivation of Rb is not a frequent event, suggesting that other tumour-suppressor genes may be present in this region (Yoo *et al.*, 1994). Loss of 8p (several regions), 7q31 and 18q have been reported, although no genes have been identified thus far that may be linked to head and neck cancer (Papadimitrako-poulou *et al.*, 1998; Wang *et al.*, 1998; Ishwad *et al.*, 1999; Sunwoo *et al.*, 1999).

In conclusion, despite the increase in the understanding of genetic mechanisms underlying the development of head and neck cancer in the last decade, we still have limited information on the interplay between exposure to environmental carcinogens, host susceptibility factors and acquired alterations. The presence and pattern of mutations in *TP53* is the only example of an attempt to correlate risk factors and genetic events. Future studies investigating the pattern of genetic alterations should incorporate valid information on exposure to environmental factors and susceptibility markers.

References

Balaram, P., Sridhar, H., Rajkumar, T., Vaccarella, S., Herrero, R., Nandakumar, A., Ravichandran, K., Ramdas, K., Sankaranarayanan, R., Gajalakshmi, V., Munoz, N. & Franceschi S. (2002) Oral cancer in southern India: the influence of smoking, drinking, paan-chewing and oral hygiene. *Int. J. Cancer*, **98**, 440–445

Bartsch, H., Caporaso, N., Coda, M., Kadlubar, F., Malaveille, C., Skipper, P., Talaska, G., Tannenbaum, S.R. & Vineis, P. (1990) Carcinogen hemoglobin adducts, urinary mutagenicity, and metabolic phenotype in active and passive cigarette smokers. *J. natl Cancer Inst.*, **82**, 1826–1831

Bartsch, H., Malaveille, C., Friesen, M., Kadlubar, F.F. & Vineis, P. (1993) Black (air-cured) and blond (flue-cured) tobacco cancer risk. IV: Molecular dosimetry studies implicate aromatic amines as bladder carcinogens. *Eur. J. Cancer*, **29A**, 1199–1207

Berenson, J.R., Yang, J. & Mickel, R.A. (1989) Frequent amplification of the bcl-1 locus in head and neck squamous cell carcinomas. *Oncogene*, **4**, 1111–1116

Bjorge, T., Hakulinen, T., Engeland, A., Jellum, E., Koskela, P., Lehtinen, M., Luostarinen, T., Paavonen, J., Sapp, M., Schiller, J., Thoresen, S., Wang, Z., Youngman, L. & Dillner, J. (1997) A prospective, seroepidemiological study of the role of human papillomavirus in esophageal cancer in Norway. *Cancer Res.*, **57**, 3989–3992

Blot, W.J. & McLaughlin, J.K. (1999) The changing epidemiology of esophageal cancer. *Semin. Oncol.*, **26** (Suppl. 15), 2–8

Blot, W.J., McLaughlin, J.K., Devesa, S.S. & Fraumeni, J.F., Jr (1996) Cancers of the oral cavity and pharynx. *Cancer Epidemiol. Prev.*, **32**, 666–680

Boffetta, P. (1993) Black (air-cured) and blond (flue-cured) tobacco and cancer risk. V: Oral cavity cancer. *Eur. J. Cancer*, **29A**, 1331–1335

Borras, E., Coutelle, C., Rosell, A., Fernandez-Muixi, F., Broch, M., Crosas, B., Hjelmqvist, L., Lorenzo, A., Gutierrez, C., Santos, M., Szczepanek, M., Heilig, M., Quattrocchi, P., Farres, J., Vidal, F., Richart, C., Mach, T., Bogdal, J., Jornvall, H., Seitz, H.K., Couzigou, P. & Pares, X. (2000) Genetic polymorphism of alcohol dehydrogenase in Europeans: the ADH2*2 allele decreases the risk for alcoholism and is associated with ADH3*1. *Hepatology*, **31**, 984–989

Bouchardy, C., Hirvonen, A., Coutelle, C., Ward, P.J., Dayer, P. & Benhamou, S. (2000) Role of alcohol dehydrogenase 3 and cytochrome P-4502E1 genotypes in susceptibility to cancers of the upper aerodigestive tract. *Int. J. Cancer*, **87**, 734–740

Boyle, J.O., Hakim, J., Koch, W., van der Riet, P., Hruban, R.H., Roa, R.A., Correo, R., Eby, Y.J., Ruppert, J.M. & Sidransky, D. (1993) The incidence of p53 mutations increases with progression of head and neck cancer. *Cancer Res.*, **53**, 4477–4480

Brachman, D.G, Graves, D., Vokes, E., Beckett, M., Haraf, D., Montag, A., Dunphy, E., Mick, R., Yandell, D. & Weichselbaum, R.R. (1992) Occurrence of p53 gene deletions and human papilloma virus infection in human head and neck cancer. *Cancer Res.*, **52**, 4832–4836

Brzoska, P.M., Levin, N.A., Fu, K.K., Kaplan, M.J., Singer, M.I., Gray, J.W. & Christman, M.F. (1995) Frequent novel DNA copy number increase in squamous cell head and neck tumors. *Cancer Res.*, **55**, 3055–3059

Cairns, P., Polascik, T.J., Eby, Y., Tokino, K., Califano, J., Merlo, A., Mao, L., Herath, J., Jenkins, R., Westra, W., Rutter, J.L., Buckler, A., Gabrielson, E., Tockman, M., Cho, K.R., Hedrick, L., Bova, G.S., Isaacs, W., Koch, W., Schwab, D. & Sidransky, D. (1995) Frequency of homozygous deletion at p16/CDKN2 in primary human tumors. *Nature Genet.*, **11**, 210–212

Castelletto, R., Castellsague, X., Munoz, N., Iscovich, J., Chopita, N. & Jmelnitsky, A. (1994) Alcohol, tobacco, diet, mate drinking, and esophageal cancer in Argentina. *Cancer Epidemiol. Biomarkers Prev.*, **3**, 557–564

Castellsague, X., Muñoz, N., De Stefani, E., Victora, C.G., Castelletto, R., Rolon, P.A. & Quintana, M.J. (1999) Independent and joint effects of tobacco smoking and alcohol drinking on the risk of esophageal cancer in men and women. *Int. J. Cancer*, **82**, 657–664

Chan, G, Boyle, J.O., Yang. E.K., Zhang, F., Sacks, P.G, Shah, J.P., Edelstein, D., Soslow, R.A., Koki, A.T., Woerner, B.M., Masferrer, J.L. & Dannenberg, A.J. (1999) Cyclooxygenase-2 expression is up-regulated in squamous cell carcinoma of the head and neck. *Cancer Res.*, **59**, 991–994

Cheng, L., Eicher, S.A., Guo, Z., Hong, W.K., Sptiz, M.R. & Wei, Q. (1998) Reduced DNA repair capacity in head and neck cancer patients. *Cancer Epidemiol. Biomarkers Prev.*, **7**, 465–468

Coutelle, C., Ward, P.J., Fleury, B., Quattrocchi, P., Chambrin, H., Iron, A., Couzigou, P. & Cassaigne, A. (1997) Laryngeal and oropharyngeal cancer, and alcohol dehydrogenase 3 and glutathione S-transferase M1 polymorphisms. *Hum. Genet.*, **99**, 319–325

Cowan, J.M., Beckett, M.A. & Weichselbaum, R.R. (1993) Chromosome changes characterizing *in vitro* response to radiation in human squamous cell carcinoma lines. *Cancer Res.*, **53**, 5542–5547

De Stefani, E., Correa, P., Oreggia, F., Leiva, J., Rivero, S., Fernandez, G, Deneo-Pellegrini, H., Zavala, D. & Fontham, E. (1987) Risk factors for laryngeal cancer. *Cancer*, **60**, 3087–3091

De Stefani, E., Barrios, E. & Fierro, L. (1993) Black (air-cured) and blond (flue-cured) tobacco and cancer risk. III: Oesophageal cancer. *Eur. J. Cancer*, **29A**, 763–766

De Stefani, E., Boffetta, P., Oreggia, F., Mendilaharsu, M. & Deneo-Pellegrini, H. (1998) Smoking patterns and cancer of the oral cavity and pharynx: a case–control study in Uruguay. *Oral Oncol.*, **34**, 340–346

Dillner, J., Knekt, P., Schiller, J.T. & Hakulinen, T. (1995) Prospective seroepidemiological evidence that human papillomavirus type 16 infection is a risk factor for oesophageal squamous cell carcinoma. *Br. med. J.*, **311**, 1346

Duell, E.J., Wiencke, J.K., Cheng, T.J., Varkonyi, A., Zuo, Z.F., Ashok, T.D., Mark, E.J., Wain, J.C., Christiani, D.C. & Kelsey, K.T. (2000) Polymorphisms in the DNA repair genes XRCC1 and ERCC2 and biomarkers of DNA damage in human blood mononuclear cells. *Carcinogenesis*, **21**, 965–971

Fang, J.L. & Vaca, C.E. (1997) Detection of DNA adducts of acetaldehyde in peripheral white blood cells of alcohol abusers. *Carcinogenesis*, **18**, 627–632

Fronhoffs, S., Bruning, T., Ortiz-Pallardo, E., Brode, P., Koch, B., Harth, V., Sachinidis, A., Bolt, H.M., Herberhold, C., Vetter, H. & Ko, Y. (2001) Real-time PCR analysis of the N-acetyltransferase NAT1 allele *3, *4, *10, *11, *14 and *17 polymorphism in squamous cell cancer of head and neck. *Carcinogenesis*, **22**, 1405–1412

Ghadirian, P., Stein, G.F., Gorodetzky, C., Roberfroid, M.B., Mahon, G.A., Bartsch, H. & Day, N.E. (1985)

Oesophageal cancer studies in the Caspian littoral of Iran: some residual results, including opium use as a risk factor. *Int. J. Cancer*, **35**, 593–597

Gillison, M.L., Koch, W.M., Capone, R.B., Spafford, M., Westra, W.H., Wu, L., Zahurak, M.L., Daniel, R.W., Viglione, M., Symer, D.E., Shah, K.V. & Sidransky, D. (2000) Evidence for a causal association between human papillomavirus and a subset of head and neck cancers. *J. natl Cancer Inst.*, **92**, 709–720

Grandis, J.R. & Tweardy, D.J. (1993) Elevated levels of transforming growth factor alpha and epidermal growth factor receptor messenger RNA are early markers of carcinogenesis in head and neck cancer. *Cancer Res.*, **53**, 3579–3584

Gronbaek, M., Becker, U., Johansen, D., Tonnesen, H., Jensen, G. & Sorensen, T.I. (1998) Population based cohort study of the association between alcohol intake and cancer of the upper digestive tract. *Br. med. J.*, **317**, 844–847

Harty, L.C., Caporaso, N.E., Hayes, R.B., Winn, D.M., Bravo-Otero, E., Blot, W.J., Kleinman, D.V., Brown, L.M., Armenian, H.K., Fraumeni, J.F., Jr & Shields, P.G. (1997) Alcohol dehydrogenase 3 genotype and risk of oral cavity and pharyngeal cancers. *J. natl Cancer Inst.*, **89**, 1698–1705

Hecht, S.S., McIntee, E.J. & Wang M. (2001) New DNA adducts of crotonaldehyde and acetaldehyde. *Toxicology*, **166**, 31–36

Henning, S., Cascorbi, I., Munchow, B., Jahnke, V. & Roots, I. (1999) Association of arylamine N-acetyltransferases NAT1 and NAT2 genotypes to laryngeal cancer risk. *Pharmacogenetics*, **9**, 103–111

Hernandez-Boussard, T., Rodriguez-Tome, P., Montesano, R. & Hainaut, P. (1999) IARC p53 mutation database: a relational database to compile and analyze p53 mutations in human tumors and cell lines. *Hum. Mutat.*, **14**, 1–8

Hibi, K., Trink, B., Patturajan, M., Westra, W.H., Caballero, O.L., Hill, D.E., Ratovitski, E.A., Jen, J. & Sidransky, D. (2000) AIS is an oncogene amplified in squamous cell carcinoma. *Proc. natl Acad. Sci. USA*, **97**, 5462–5467

Hori, H., Kawano, T., Endo, M. & Yuasa, Y. (1997) Genetic polymorphisms of tobacco- and alcohol-related metabolizing enzymes and human eso-phageal squamous cell carcinoma susceptibility. *J. clin. Gastroenterol.*, **25**, 568–575

Hsieh, L.L., Wang, P.F., Chen, I.H., Liao, C.T., Wang, H.M., Chen, M.C., Chang, J.T. & Cheng, A.J. (2001) Characteristics of mutations in the p53 gene in oral squamous cell carcinoma associated with betel quid chewing and cigarette smoking in Taiwanese. *Carcinogenesis*, **22**, 1497–1503

Hung, H.C., Chuang, J., Chien, Y.C., Chern, H.D., Chiang, C.P., Kuo, Y.S., Hildesheim, A. & Chen, C.J. (1997) Genetic polymorphisms of CYP2E1, GSTM1, and GSTT1; environmental factors and risk of oral cancer. *Cancer Epidemiol. Biomarkers Prev.*, **6**, 901–905

IARC (1988) *IARC Monographs on the Evaluation of Carcinogenic Risks to Humans*, Vol. 44, *Alcohol Drinking*, Lyon, IARC*Press*

Ishwad, C.S., Shuster, M., Bockmuhl, U., Thakker, N., Shah. P., Toomes, C., Dixon, M., Ferrell, R.E. & Gollin, S.M. (1999) Frequent allelic loss and homozygous deletion in chromosome band 8p23 in oral cancer. *Int. J. Cancer*, **80**, 25–31

Jares, P., Fernandez, P.L., Campo, E., Nadal, A., Bosch, F., Aiza, G., Nayach, I., Traserra, J. & Cardesa, A. (1994) PRAD-1/cyclin Dl gene amplification correlates with messenger RNA overexpression and tumor progression in human laryngeal carcinomas. *Cancer Res.*, **54**, 4813–4817

Jones, N.J., McGregor, A.D. & Waters, R. (1993) Detection of DNA adducts in human oral tissue: correlation of adduct levels with tobacco smoking and differential enhancement of adducts using the butanol extraction and nuclease P1 versions of 32P postlabeling. *Cancer Res.*, **53**, 1522–1528

Jourenkova-Mironova, N., Wikman, H., Bouchardy, C., Mitrunen, K., Dayer, P., Benhamou, S. & Hirvonen, A. (1999) Role of arylamine *N*-acetyltransferase 1 and 2 (*NAT1* and *NAT2*) genotypes in susceptibility to oral/pharyngeal and laryngeal cancers. *Pharmacogenetics*, **9**, 533–537

Kabat, G.C. & Wynder, E.L. (1989) Type of alcoholic beverage and oral cancer. *Int. J. Cancer*, **43**, 190–194

Katoh, T., Kaneko, S., Boissy, R., Watson, M., Ikemura, K. & Bell, D.A. (1998) A pilot study testing the association between N-acetyltransferases 1 and 2 and risk of oral squamous cell carcinoma in Japanese people. *Carcinogenesis*, **19**, 1803–1807

Katoh, T., Kaneko, S., Kohshi, K., Munaka, M., Kitagawa, K., Kunugita, N., Ikemura, K. & Kawamoto, T. (1999) Genetic polymorphisms of tobacco- and alcohol-related metabolizing enzymes and oral cavity cancer. *Int. J. Cancer*, **83**, 606–609

Koh, J.Y., Cho, N.P., Kong, G., Lee, J.D. & Yoon, K. (1998) p53 Mutations and human papillomavirus DNA in oral squamous cell carcinoma: correlation with apoptosis. *Br. J. Cancer*, **78**, 354–359

Lagergren, J., Wang, Z., Bergstrom, R., Dillner, J. & Nyren, O. (1999) Human papillomavirus infection and esophageal cancer: a nationwide seroepidemiologic case–control study in Sweden. *J. natl Cancer Inst.*, **91**, 156–162

Latvala, J., Parkkila, S., Melkko, J. & Niemela, O. (2001) Acetaldehyde adducts in blood and bone marrow of patients with ethanol-induced erythrocyte abnormalities. *Mol. Med.*, **7**, 401–405

La Vecchia, C., Franceschi, S., Favero, A., Talamini, R. & Negri, E. (1999) Alcohol intake and cancer of the upper digestive tract. Pattern of risk in Italy is different from that in Denmark. *Br. med. J.*, **318**, 1289–1290

Lee, J.M., Lee, Y.C., Yang, S.Y., Shi, W.L., Lee, C.J., Luh, S.P., Chen, C.J., Hsieh, C.Y. & Wu, MT. (2000) Genetic polymorphisms of p53 and GSTP1, but not NAT2, are associated with susceptibility to squamous-cell carcinoma of the esophagus. *Int. J. Cancer*, **89**, 458–464

Li, D., Firozi, P.F., Chang, P., Wang, L.E., Xiong, P., Sturgis, E.M., Eicher, S.A., Spitz, M.R., Hong, W.K. & Wei, Q. (2001) In vitro BPDE-induced DNA adducts in peripheral lymphocytes as a risk factor for squamous cell carcinoma of the head and neck. *Int. J. Cancer*, **93**, 436–440

Malaveille, C., Vineis, P., Estève, J., Ohshima, H., Brun, G., Hautefeuille, A., Gallet, P., Ronco, G., Terracini, B. & Bartsch, H. (1989) Levels of mutagens in the urine of smokers of black and blond tobacco correlate with their risk of bladder cancer. *Carcinogenesis*, **10**, 577–586

Mao, E.J., Schwartz, S.M., Daling, J.R., Oda, D., Tickman, L. & Beckmann, A.M. (1996) Human papilloma viruses and p53 mutations in normal premalignant and malignant oral epithelia. *Int. J. Cancer*, **69**, 152–158

Mao, L., Fan, Y.H., Lotan, R. & Hong, W.K. (1996) Frequent abnormalities of FHIT, a candidate tumor suppressor gene, in head and neck cancer cell lines. *Cancer Res.*, **56**, 5128–5131

Mashberg, A., Boffetta, P., Winkelman, R. & Garfinkel, L. (1993) Tobacco smoking, alcohol drinking, and cancer of the oral cavity and oropharynx among U.S. veterans. *Cancer*, **72**, 1369–1375

Matsuo, K., Hamajima, N., Shinoda, M., Hatooka, S., Inoue, M., Takezaki, T. & Tajima, K. (2001) Gene–environment interaction between an aldehyde dehydrogenase-2 (ALDH2) polymorphism and alcohol consumption for the risk of esophageal cancer. *Carcinogenesis*, **22**, 913–916

Matthias, C., Bockmuhl, U., Jahnke, V., Jones, P.W., Hayes, J.D., Alldersea, J., Gilford, J., Bailey, L., Bath, J., Worrall, S.F., Hand, P., Fryer, A.A. & Strange, R.C. (1998) Polymorphism in cytochrome P450 CYP2D6, CYP1A1, CYP2E1 and glutathione *S*-transferase, GSTM1, GSTM3, GSTT1 and susceptibility to tobacco-related cancers: studies in upper aerodigestive tract cancers. *Pharmacogenetics*, **8**, 91–100

Matullo, G., Palli, D., Peluso, M., Guarrera, S., Carturan, S., Celentano, E., Krogh, V., Munnia, A., Tumino, R., Polidoro, S., Piazza, A. & Vineis, P. (2001) XRCC1, XRCC3, XPD gene polymorphisms, smoking and (32)P-DNA adducts in a sample of healthy subjects. *Carcinogenesis*, **22**, 1437–1445

Merletti, F., Boffetta, P., Ciccone, G., Mashberg, A. & Terracini, B. (1989) Role of tobacco and alcoholic beverages in the etiology of cancer of the oral cavity/oropharynx in Torino, Italy. *Cancer Res.*, **49**, 4919–4924

Merlo, A., Herman, J.G., Mao, L., Lee, D.J., Gabrielson, E., Burger, P.C., Baylin, S.B. & Sidransky, D. (1995) 5′ CpG island methylation is associated with transcriptional silencing of the tumour suppressor p16/CDKN2/MTS1 in human cancers. *Nature Med.*, **1**, 686–692

Morita, S., Yano, M., Tsujinaka, T., Akiyama, Y., Taniguchi, M., Kaneko, K., Miki, H., Fujii, T., Yoshino, K., Kusuoka, H. & Monden, M. (1999) Genetic polymorphisms of drug-metabolizing enzymes and susceptibility to head-and-neck squamous-cell carcinoma. *Int. J. Cancer*, **80**, 685–688

Mork, J., Lie, A.K., Glattre, E., Hallmans, G., Jellum, E., Koskela, P., Moller, B., Pukkala, E., Schiller, J.T., Youngman, L., Lehtinen, M. & Dillner, J. (2001) Human papillomavirus infection as a risk factor for squamous-cell carcinoma of the head and neck. *New Engl. J. Med.*, **344**, 1125–1131

Okami, K., Wu, L., Riggins, G., Cairns, P., Goggins, M., Evron, E., Halachmi, N., Ahrendt, S.A., Reed, A.L., Hilgers, W., Kern, S.E., Koch, W.M., Sidransky, D. & Jen, J. (1998) Analysis of PTEN/ MMAC1 alterations in aerodigestive tract tumors. *Cancer Res.*, **58**, 509–511

Olshan, A.F., Weissler, M.C., Watson, M.A. & Bell, D.A. (2000) GSTM1, GSTT1, GSTP1, CYP1A1, and NAT1 polymorphisms, tobacco use, and the risk of head and neck cancer. *Cancer Epidemiol. Biomarkers Prev.*, **9**, 185–191

Olshan, A.F., Weissler, M.C., Watson, M.A. & Bell, D.A. (2001) Risk of head and neck cancer and the alcohol dehydrogenase 3 genotype. *Carcinogenesis*, **22**, 57–61

Papadimitrakopoulou, V., Izzo, J., Lippman, S.M., Lee, J.S., Fan, Y.H., Clayman, G., Ro, J.Y., Hittelman, W.N., Lotan, R., Hong, W.K. & Mao, L. (1997) Frequent inactivation of p16INK4a in oral premalignant lesions. *Oncogene*, **14**, 1799–1803

Papadimitrakopoulou, V.A., Oh, Y., El-Naggar, A., Izzo, J., Clayman, G. & Mao, L. (1998) Presence of multiple incontiguous deleted regions at the long arm of chromosome 18 in head and neck cancer. *Clin. Cancer Res.*, **4**, 539–544

Parkin, D.M., Whelan, S.L., Ferlay, J., Raymond, L. & Young, J., eds (1997) *Cancer Incidence in Five Continents Vol. VII* (IARC Scientific Publications No. 143), Lyon, IARC*Press*

Reed, A.L., Califano, J., Cairns, P., Westra, W.H., Jones, R.M., Koch, W., Ahrendt, S., Eby, Y., Sewell, D., Nawroz, H., Bartek, J. & Sidransky, D. (1996) High frequency of p16 (CDKN2/MTS-1/INK4A) inactivation in head and neck squamous cell carcinoma. *Cancer Res.*, **56**, 3630–3633

Renan, M.J. (1993) How many mutations are required for tumorigenesis? Implications from human cancer data. *Mol. Carcinog.*, **7**, 139–146

Rintala, J., Jaatinen, P., Parkkila, S., Sarviharju, M., Kiianmaa, K., Hervonen, A. & Niemela, O. (2000) Evidence of acetaldehyde–protein adduct formation in rat brain after lifelong consumption of ethanol. *Alcohol Alcohol.*, **35**, 458–463

Rolla, R., Vay, D., Mottaran, E., Parodi, M., Traverso, N., Arico, S., Sartori, M., Bellomo, G., Klassen, L.W., Thiele, G.M., Tuma, D.J. & Albano, E. (2000) Detection of circulating antibodies against malondialdehyde–acetaldehyde adducts in patients with alcohol-induced liver disease. *Hepatology*, **31**, 878–884

Sancho-Garnier, H. & Theobald, S. (1993) Black (aircured) and blond (flue-cured) tobacco and cancer risk II: Pharynx and larynx cancer. *Eur. J. Cancer*, **29A**, 273–276

Schlecht, N.F., Franco, E.L., Pintos, J., Negassa, A., Kowalski, L.P., Oliveira, B.V. & Curado, M.P. (1999) Interaction between tobacco and alcohol consumption and the risk of cancers of the upper aero-digestive tract in Brazil. *Am. J. Epidemiol.*, **150**, 1129–1137

Scholes, A.G., Liloglou, T., Snijders, P.J., Hart, C.A., Jones, A.S., Woolgar, J.A., Vaughan, E.D., Walboomers, J.M. & Field, J.K. (1997) p53 Mutations in relation to human papillomavirus type 16 infection in squamous cell carcinomas of the head and neck. *Int. J. Cancer*, **71**, 796–799

Schwartz, S.M., Doody, D.R., Fitzgibbons, E.D., Ricks, S., Porter, P.L. & Chen, C. (2001) Oral squamous cell cancer risk in relation to alcohol consumption and alcohol dehydrogenase-3 genotypes. *Cancer Epidemiol. Biomarkers Prev.*, **10**, 1137–1144

Seitz, H.K., Poschl, G. & Simanowski, U.A. (1998) Alcohol and cancer. *Recent Dev. Alcohol.*, **14**, 67–95.

Shao, X., Tandon, R., Samara, G., Kanki, H., Yano, H., Close, L.G., Parsons, R. & Sato, T. (1998) Mutational analysis of the PTEN gene in head and neck squamous cell carcinoma. *Int. J. Cancer*, **77**, 684–688

Sidransky, D. (2001) Head and neck cancer. In: DeVita, V.T., Jr, Hellman, S. & Rosenberg, S, eds, *Cancer: Principles and Practice of Oncology*, 6th Ed., Philadelphia, Lippincott Williams and Wilkins

Sorrells, D.L., Ghali, G.E., Meschonat, C., DeFatta, R.J., Black, D., Liu, L., De Benedetti, A., Nathan, C.A. & Li, B.D. (1999) Competitive PCR to detect eIF4E gene amplification in head and neck cancer. *Head Neck*, **21**, 60–65

Stone, J.G., Jones, N.J., McGregor, A.D. & Waters, R. (1995) Development of a human biomonitoring assay using buccal mucosa: comparison of smoking-related DNA adducts in mucosa versus biopsies. *Cancer Res.*, **55**, 1267–1270

Sturgis, E.M., Castillo, E.J., Li, L., Zheng, R., Eicher, S.A., Clayman, G.L., Strom, S.S., Spitz, M.R. & Wei, Q. (1999) Polymorphisms of DNA repair gene XRCC1 in squamous cell carcinoma of the head and neck. *Carcinogenesis*, **20**, 2125–2129

Sturgis, E.M., Zheng, R., Li, L., Castillo, E.J., Eicher, S.A., Chen, M., Strom, S.S., Spitz, M.R. & Wei, Q. (2000) XPD/ERCC2 polymorphisms and risk of head and neck cancer: a case–control analysis. *Carcinogenesis*, **21**, 2219–2223

Sturgis, E.M., Dahlstrom, K.R., Guan, Y., Eicher, S.A., Strom, S.S., Spitz, M.R. & Wei, Q. (2001) Alcohol dehydrogenase 3 genotype is not associated with risk of squamous cell carcinoma of the oral cavity and pharynx. *Cancer Epidemiol. Biomarkers Prev.*, **10**, 273–275

Sunwoo, J.B., Sun, P.C., Gupta, V.K., Schmidt, A.P., El-Mofty, S. & Scholnick, S.B. (1999) Localization of a putative tumor suppressor gene in the sub-telomeric region of chromosome 8p. *Oncogene*, **18**, 2651–2655

Szyfter, K., Hemminki, K., Szyfter, W., Szmeja, Z., Banaszewski, J. & Yang, K. (1994) Aromatic DNA adducts in larynx biopsies and leukocytes. *Carcinogenesis*, **15**, 2195–2199

Szyfter, K., Hemminki, K., Szyfter, W., Szmeja, Z., Banaszewski, J. & Pabiszczak, M. (1996) Tobacco smoke-associated N7-alkylguanine in DNA of larynx tissue and leucocytes. *Carcinogenesis*, **17**, 501–506

Talamini, R., Franceschi, S., Barra, S. & La Vecchia, C. (1990) The role of alcohol in oral and pharyngeal cancer in non-smokers, and of tobacco in non-drinkers. *Int. J. Cancer*, **46**, 391–393

Tan, W., Song, N., Wang, G.Q., Liu, Q., Tang, H.J., Kadlubar, F.F. & Lin, D.X. (2000) Impact of genetic polymorphisms in cytochrome P450 2E1 and glutathione S-transferases M1, T1, and P1 on susceptibility to esophageal cancer among high-risk individuals in China. *Cancer Epidemiol. Biomarkers Prev.*, **9**, 551–556

Trink, B., Okami, K., Wu, L., Sriuranpong, V., Jen, J. & Sidransky D. (1998) A new p53 homologue. *Nature Med.*, **4**, 747–748

Tuyns, A.J., Esteve, J., Raymond, L., Berrino, F., Benhamou, E., Blanchet, F., Boffetta, P., Crosignani, P., del Moral, A., Lehmann, W., Merletti, F., Pequignot, G., Riboli, E., Sancho-Garnier, H., Terracini, B., Zubiri, A. & Zubiri, L. (1988) Cancer of the larynx/hypopharynx, tobacco and alcohol: IARC international case–control study in Turin and Varese (Italy), Zaragoza and Navarra (Spain), Geneva (Switzerland) and Calvados (France). *Int. J. Cancer*, **41**, 483–491

Vaca, C.E., Nilsson, J.A., Fang, J.L. & Grafstrom, R.C. (1998) Formation of DNA adducts in human buccal epithelial cells exposed to acetaldehyde and methylglyoxal *in vitro*. *Chem.-biol. Interact.*, **108**, 197–208

Van der Riet, P., Nawroz, H., Hruban, R.H., Corio, R., Tokino, K., Koch, W. & Sidransky, D. (1994) Frequent loss of chromosome 9p21-22 early in head and neck cancer progression. *Cancer Res.*, **54**, 1156–1158

Van Dyke, D.L., Worsham, M.J., Benninger, M.S., Krause, C.J., Baker, S.R., Wolf, G.T., Drumheller, T., Tilley, B.C. & Carey, T.E. (1994) Recurrent cytogenetic abnormalities in squamous cell carcinomas of the head and neck region. *Genes Chromosomes Cancer*, **9**, 192–206

Viitala, K., Makkonen, K., Israel, Y., Lehtimaki, T., Jaakkola, O., Koivula, T., Blake, J.E. & Niemela, O. (2000) Autoimmune responses against oxidant stress and acetaldehyde-derived epitopes in human alcohol consumers. *Alcohol clin. exp. Res.*, **24**, 1103–1109

Vineis, P. (1992) The use of biomarkers in epidemiology: the example of bladder cancer. *Toxicol. Lett.*, **64–65**, 463–467

Vineis, P., Talaska, G., Malaveille, C., Bartsch, H., Martone, T., Sithisarankul, P. & Strickland, P. (1996) DNA adducts in urothelial cells: relationship with biomarkers of exposure to arylamines and polycyclic aromatic hydrocarbons from tobacco smoke. *Int. J. Cancer*, **65**, 314–316

Vineis, P., Marinelli, D., Autrup, H., Brockmoller, J., Cascorbi, I., Daly, A.K., Golka, K., Okkels, H., Risch, A., Rothman, N., Sim, E. & Taioli, E. (2001) Current smoking, occupation, N-acetyltransferase-2 and bladder cancer: a pooled analysis of genotype-based studies. *Cancer Epidemiol. Biomarkers Prev.*, **10**, 1249–1252

Wang, D., Song, H., Evans, J.A., Lang, J.C., Schuller, D.E. & Weghorst, C.M. (1997) Mutation and downregulation of the transforming growth factor beta type II receptor gene in primary squamous cell carcinomas of the head and neck. *Carcinogenesis*, **18**, 2285–2290

Wang, X.L., Uzawa, K., Miyakawa, A., Shiiba, M., Watanabe, T., Sato, T., Miya, T., Yokoe, H. & Tanzawa, H. (1998) Localization of a tumour-suppressor gene associated with human oral cancer on 7q31.1. *Int. J. Cancer*, **75**, 671–674

WCRF (1997) *Food, Nutrition and the Prevention of Cancer: A Global Perspective*, Washington DC, American Institute for Cancer Research, World Cancer Research Fund

Wight, A.J. & Ogden, G.R. (1998) Possible mechanisms by which alcohol may influence the development of oral cancer – a review. *Oral Oncol.*, **34**, 441–447.

Yoo, G.H., Xu, H.J., Brennan, J.A., Westra, W., Hruban, R.H., Koch, W., Benedict. W.F. & Sidransky, D. (1994) Infrequent inactivation of the retinoblastoma gene despite frequent loss of chromosome 13q in head and neck squamous cell carcinoma. *Cancer Res.*, **54**, 4603–4606

Yokoyama, A., Muramatsu, T., Omori, T., Yokoyama, T., Matsushita, S., Higuchi, S., Maruyama, K. &

Ishii, H. (2001) Alcohol and aldehyde dehydrogenase gene polymorphisms and oropharyngolaryngeal, esophageal and stomach cancers in Japanese alcoholics. *Carcinogenesis*, **22**, 433–439

Zavras, A.I., Wu, T., Laskaris, G., Wang, Y.F., Cartsos, V., Segas, J., Lefantzis, D., Joshipura, K., Douglass, C.W. & Diehl, S.R. (2002) Interaction between a single nucleotide polymorphism in the alcohol dehydrogenase 3 gene, alcohol consumption and oral cancer risk. *Int. J. Cancer*, **97**, 526–530

Zheng, Y., Shen, H., Sturgis, E.M., Wang, L.E., Eicher, S.A., Strom, S.S., Frazier, M.L., Spitz, M.R. & Wei, Q. (2001) Cyclin D1 polymorphism and risk for squamous cell carcinoma of the head and neck: a case–control study. *Carcinogenesis*, **22**, 1195–1199

Corresponding author:

P. Brennan
Unit of Environmental Cancer Epidemiology,
International Agency for Research on Cancer,
150 cours Albert-Thomas,
69372 Lyon cedex 08, France,
brennan@iarc.fr

Future Studies and
Design Considerations

Mechanisms of Carcinogenesis: Contributions of Molecular Epidemiology
Patricia Buffler, Jerry Rice, Robert Baan, Michael Bird and Paolo Boffetta, eds
IARC Scientific Publications No. 157
International Agency for Research on Cancer, Lyon, 2004

Issues of Design and Analysis in Studies of Gene–Environment Interactions

Paolo Vineis, Paul A. Schulte, Tania Carreón, A. John Bailer and
Mario Medvedovic

The nature–nurture debate has given way to the fundamental realization that both genes and environment play a role in disease, especially cancer. Interaction has been defined in several ways, for example as 'the coparticipation of two or more agents in the same causal mechanism leading to disease development' (Yang & Khoury, 1997). According to a more generally accepted definition, interaction occurs when the effect of multiple factors differs from the effect predicted on the basis of the separate effects of each of the factors.

Interactions need to be explicitly considered in the design and analysis of epidemiological studies. If only the association between a genotype and disease is examined, the effect of biological interaction cannot be appreciated (Khoury et al., 1993). Epidemiologists need to measure relevant risk factors, in addition to genotypes. Also, it is likely that each exposure interacts with genes along a pathway (typically DNA-repair genes), so multiple interactions are likely to be the norm. Evidence for a three-way interaction was shown by Taylor et al. (1998) for NAT2 and NAT1 genotypes and smoking as risk factors for bladder cancer. Depending on the type of model for gene–environment interaction, risk estimates can vary dramatically. At least five different types of gene–environment interaction have been described (Khoury & Wagener, 1995). These have generally been considered with dichotomous conditions: a single susceptibility genotype (present or absent) and a single environmental factor (present or absent). For example, in one analysis (Ottman, 1996), the risk to an exposed person with a rare (1% prevalence) susceptibility genotype ranges from 8% (under a multiplicative model of interaction) to 95.6% (when we assume that the exposure has no effect in the susceptible, but the genotype raises risk in unexposed as well as exposed people).

Various study designs have been identified for the detection of gene–environment interaction. These include case-only designs, case–control study designs using unrelated controls, case–control designs using related controls, case–control designs using relatives of cases and population- or hospital-based controls, twin study designs family study designs and combined segregation and linkage analyses.

To assess gene–environment interaction, data could be displayed in a 2×4 table, where exposure is classified as being either present or absent and the underlying susceptibility genotype is also classified as present or absent. Using unexposed subjects with no susceptibility genotype as the reference group, odds ratios can be computed for all other groups (Khoury et al., 1993; Botto & Khoury, 2001). Power and sample size are critical in the statistical analysis of these models of interaction. A moderate number of cases and controls is required to detect an interaction when both the exposure frequency and the proportion of susceptible individuals are close to 50%. However, a large sample size is required, although not necessarily attainable, when the exposure frequency is very low or very high, or when the proportion of risk-increasing alleles at the susceptibility locus is very rare or very common (Hwang et al., 1994). Even larger numbers are needed if more than one genetic and environmental factor are to be studied. Statistical models to assess interaction have been developed, but rarely applied, beyond the $2 \times 2 \times 2$ design because sample sizes in the cells become small and hence limit the power of the study (Selvin, 1991). Assessment of interaction can also be affected by exposure and genotype misclassification. A modest error in exposure assessment may result in substantial increases in sample size requirements, and this problem is compounded by even small errors in genotype assessment (Rothman *et al.*, 1993; Garcia-Closas *et al.*, 1999; Clayton & McKeigue, 2001).

Alternatively, frequency matching for known environmental risk factors with a low prevalence in the population has been proposed to gain power in the study of gene–environment interactions (Stürmer & Brenner, 2000). In the meantime, matching is far less efficient than an unmatched design, and statistical adjustment can achieve unbiased estimates without such loss of efficiency.

New study designs: the case-only design

Epidemiological studies usually involve the comparison of different subpopulations, for example subjects exposed or not exposed to an environmental agent, or cancer patients and healthy controls (for design issues in molecular epidemiological studies, see Schulte & Perera 1993; Toniolo *et al.*, 1997). Given the recent emphasis on gene–environment interactions, which seem to be the norm and not the exception in the study of chronic diseases including cancer, a different study design has been proposed, which avoids the use of a comparison series. This 'case-only' design is based only on the study of patients affected by the disease at issue, and is valuable only for the investigation of interactions, in particular gene–environment interactions (Khoury & Flanders, 1996; Umbach & Weinberg, 1997; Yang *et al.*, 1999). The basic idea is that, in the presence of interaction, the association between a certain exposure and a genetic trait departs from a predefined model, and to test such a hypothesis just the case series is sufficient. If the odds ratio for disease associated with exposure in the absence of the genetic trait of interest (ExOR) is 5, and the odds ratio for disease associated with the genetic trait in the absence of the exposure (GeOR) is 2, then under a multiplicative model we expect that the combination of the two will be 10 (the reasons for choosing a multiplicative model will be discussed below). The simple mathematics of the case-only design are shown, with an example, in Table 1.

The limitations of such an approach are obvious, but its advantages are not trivial. The first limitation is related to the impossibility of studying the exposure and the genetic trait independently; in other words, the etiological role of exposure must have been ascertained already. The case-only approach allows the researcher to establish, under a plausible interaction model, whether the genetic trait modifies the effect of the exposure. In the example, we already know that smoking is a well-established cause of bladder cancer, and the object of the case-only analysis was to study interaction with the *NAT2* genotype. A second limitation is related to the selection of the cases. If, for any reason, the frequency of the genetic trait among the cases does not reflect the expected frequency – irrespective of the etiological relationship in question – then any inference based on the case-only approach will be biased. This occurs, for example, if prevalent cases are

Table 1. Aggregated data from case–control studies on the *NAT-2* genotype and the risk of bladder cancer

Conventional analysis

Gene	Exposure	Controls	Cases	OR
0	0	225	215	
0	1	412	601	1.53
1	0	214	233	
1	1	400	950	2.18
Interaction:	2.18/1.53 = 1.43 (95% CI, 1.04–1.96)			

Case-only approach

	g = 0	g = 1
e = 0	215	233
e = 1	601	950

Odds ratio (for interaction) = 1.46 (95% CI, 1.18–1.80)

From Marcus *et al.* (2000)
Exposure: ever-smokers (e = 1) or never smokers (e = 0); genetic trait: slow acetylator (g = 1) or rapid acetylators (g = 0).
OR, odds ratio; CI, confidence interval

recruited: since some genetic traits modify life expectancy, we will find more subjects with a certain allele among those still alive. This is clearly shown by the apolipoprotein E *e4* polymorphism: since in smokers the presence of this polymorphism considerably increases the risk of dying from cardiovascular disease, the recruitment of prevalent (i.e. surviving) patients with myocardial infarction will be associated with an abnormally low prevalence of the *e4* allele, particularly among nonsmokers. Clearly, this second limitation can be overcome by recruiting incident cases. A third limitation is related to an association between the genetic trait and the exposure among the controls: for example, if the genetic trait induces the subjects to drink more alcohol (as in the case of the *ADH2* polymorphism), then any 'interaction' found in the cases only is uninterpretable. If the assumption of independence between genetic and environmental factors is violated, the case-only design will perform poorly, causing multiplicative interactions to be highly distorted (Albert *et al.*, 2001).

Let us now consider the advantages of this design. The case-only approach allows us to study interaction with at least the same statistical power as the more conventional case–control design; in fact, the power is usually greater because of the lack of controls: their variability is in fact eliminated (Khoury & Flanders, 1996). Also, confidence intervals tend to be narrower with this approach. The case-only design starts with the plausible assumption of independence between exposure and genotype in the population, and requires fewer case subjects than a case–control design. As a rule of thumb, to study interaction in a case–control design, we need approximately four times more subjects than in a design aiming to investigate one exposure only. To attain at least the same statistical power in the case-only approach, we need the same number of cases, but controls are not needed. A second advantage is related to the well-known difficulties associated with the choice of controls in epidemiological studies. In a population-based study, controls should be a random sample of the source population from which the cases originated, and, in a hospital-based design, controls are patients

admitted for diseases other than the one under investigation. In the former design, one frequent drawback is the low response rate (often around 50% or less) of the population controls; in the latter, the most common problem is the non-comparability of cases and controls (Wacholder *et al.*, 1992). The case series is usually less affected by low response rates, and its representativeness of all cases of the disease in question is more easily attained. Therefore, a study design based on cases only has several advantages. It should be clear, however, that it allows us to explore just one specific scientific enquiry; whether some characteristic (usually a genetic trait) modifies the effect of another (usually an environmental exposure). In addition, it is worth noting that in the absence of knowledge – from other sources – about the role played by the exposure, it is impossible to conclude whether the effect of exposure is adverse in genetic subgroup 1 versus subgroup 2 or protective in subgroup 2 versus subgroup 1.

Now comes the key question, i.e. what is the expected value for the interactive term we model in the context of the case-only study? In the example in Table 1, we assumed that the null hypothesis of no interaction corresponds to a multiplication of the odds ratios for the environmental trait and the genetic trait separately. Other models for the lack of interaction have been proposed, for example an additive model. While, according to the multiplicative model, the null hypothesis of no interaction is OR(joint) = ExOR × GeOR, according to the additive model, OR(joint) = ExOR + GeOR − 1 (Rothman *et al.*, 1980). In general, it has been stressed that any statistical model can be used to generate the null hypothesis, depending on the underlying biological hypotheses. For example, exposures that act on the same target can have less than additive effects if they compete for a receptor (an example could be polycyclic aromatic hydrocarbons and dioxins in relation to the Ah receptor). Conversely, an agent that impairs DNA repair can interact more than multiplicatively with an agent that mutates a cell-cycle gene. However, the multiplicative model is a special case that deserves a central role. The fact that the odds of disease (when the environmental and genetic traits are jointly assessed) equals the product of the exposure-only and genetic trait-only odds ratios indicates the statistical independence, i.e. lack of effect modification. If the multiplicative model is not taken by default as the expression of the null hypothesis, a different statistical treatment of the data would be required, including techniques for analysing special designs such as the case–control study, the absence of interaction is expressed by the same GeOR in exposed and unexposed populations, i.e. the same odds of disease related to genetic trait regardless of exposure status. In the case-only approach the same concept is expressed by an 'interaction odds ratio' (Table 1) of 1.0. However, there can be good biological reasons to express the null hypothesis under a non-multiplicative mathematical model. Although the case-only study is used to assess departures from multiplicative effects, it does not allow the investigation of the independent effects of the exposure alone or the genotype alone.

New methodological problems: population stratification

In a pooled analysis of the studies on *CYP1A1* polymorphisms and the risk of lung cancer (Vineis *et al.*, 2003), the odds ratios shown in Table 2 have been observed for the *CYP1A1*2* (MspI) polymorphism.

It is clear that, although mixing ethnicities conceals any relationship (odds ratios are lower than 1 and not statistically significant), when we consider Caucasians and Asians separately, there is an association at least with the homozygous genotype in Caucasians. This phenomenon is an example of confounding, since Asians have a much higher frequency of the variant genotype, in comparison with Caucasians, and have a different baseline risk of lung cancer, thus fulfilling the criteria for confounding (in this case negative confounding, since the association disappears when mixing the populations).

Population stratification occurs when any factor – genetic or environmental – with a variable frequency between ethnic groups with different risks of disease appears to be related to disease;

Table 2. Odds ratios for the *CYP1A1*2* (MspI) polymorphism

	Heterozygotes	Homozygotes
All ethnicities		
OR	0.88	0.88
95% CI	0.77–1.01	0.68–1.14
Caucasians		
OR	1.02	2.36
95% CI	0.84–1.24	1.16–4.81
Asians		
OR	1.06	1.14
95% CI	0.81–1.41	0.78–1.69

From Vineis *et al.* (2003)
OR, odds ratio; CI, confidence interval

this is noted even if there is no causal relationship. Wacholder *et al.* (2000) have shown that population stratification can cause a spurious allele–disease association, but is likely to occur rarely. This phenomenon is observed when allele frequency and disease rates not only differ substantially across ethnic groups, but also correlate strongly with each other and the true risk factor that is responsible for the disease rate difference. However, the true risk factor may be unknown, and so investigators may fail to account for it. For epidemiologists, this is nothing new, being just an issue of confounding. However, it is a particularly important type of confounding in the era of the genome project and of extensive studies on genes and disease. As Altshuler *et al.* (1998) have stressed, if we do not stratify by ethnicity we risk to attribute to genes a causal responsibility that is in fact related to other characteristics associated with ethnicity, such as other genetic traits or environmental exposures. For example, African-Americans tend to smoke more than white Americans, have a higher prevalence of hypertension and also have a different distribution of many genetic polymorphisms. Therefore, in an unstratified study, in which 'population admixture' occurs, one could find a spurious association between smoking-related diseases or hypertension and some polymorphisms; the association would disappear after stratification by ethnicity. However, the problem is not so simple. In fact, it is probably not sufficient to stratify by ethnicity, since genetic heterogeneity also occurs within ethnic groups.

There is currently a debate whether bias from population stratification (the mixture of individuals from heterogeneous genetic backgrounds) undermines the credibility of epidemiological studies designed to estimate the association between genotype and risk of disease. However, Wacholder *et al.* (2000) found only a small bias from stratification in a well-designed case–control study of genetic factors that ignored ethnicity among non-Hispanic white Americans of European origin. In general, there are good reasons to argue that population admixture can only rarely distort the estimates.

- In the example above, it is very unlikely that the investigators will ignore the simple white/Asian stratification.
- The greater the degree of admixture within a population, and the smaller the difference in allele frequency or baseline disease risk, the less likely it is that population stratification will lead to confounding (Wacholder *et al.*, 2000).
- When important confounding caused by population stratification does occur, it should be controllable by the usual design and analytical features employed by epidemiologists.

Finally, genetic studies are becoming more and more sophisticated, and the genetic background of populations can be investigated in several ways, for example by stratifying by microsatellite polymorphisms as markers of genetic heterogeneity within a population. Devlin *et al.* (2001) have proposed complex statistical methods. For example, the genomic control method exploits the fact that the population substructure generates 'overdispersion' of statistics used to assess association. By testing multiple polymorphisms throughout the genome, only some of which are pertinent to the disease of interest, the degree of overdispersion generated by population substructure can be estimated and taken into account.

New issues related to the statistical analysis of data on biomarkers
Analysis of multiple markers: lessons from the past
The analysis of multiple molecular and genetic markers presents many problems generally known to epidemiologists and statisticians, but rarely experienced at the levels likely to be seen in the future. These include difficulty in data reduction, collinearity, multiple comparisons and assessment of interaction. With high-throughput technologies, markers will likely be highly correlated and, in variables that are not correlated, associations between markers and disease may occur by chance alone.

The range of statistical methods used in studies involving the use of multiple markers follows what one would expect from the type of epidemiological study designs that are used. Many of the studies examining the association between a single biomarker and exposure are simple quantifications as incorporated in simple linear regression models or using correlation coefficients (both the Pearson and Spearman rank coefficients have been used). Multiple regression is often used when a set of biomarkers is being studied to determine if relationships exist with a particular exposure. These studies are typically exploratory and sometimes use variable selection methods, such as step-wise selection, backward elimination or forward selection (Neter *et al.*, 1996). The multiple regression models also accommodate other characteristics or risk factors in these analyses (e.g. age, smoking status, alcohol, gender). Other regression models have been employed in addition to the linear and multiple regression models for describing a continuous exposure variable as a function of biomarkers and other variables. In the analysis of the relationship of biomarkers to disease, logistic regression models (for disease/non-disease status responses) and Cox regression models for survival time analyses have been used.

Finally, simple comparisons have been conducted between biomarker concentrations in two or more exposure (or disease) groups using both parametric (*t*-tests, ANOVA models) and nonparametric (Wilcoxon rank sum tests, categorical data analysis) statistical methods. These methods focus on whether groups that can be identified by other means (e.g. workers exposed to styrene versus workers not exposed) differ with regard to concentrations of biomarkers. In contrast, the regression models provide an estimate of the magnitude of the relationship between biomarkers and disease/survival/exposure status variables (e.g. estimated relative risks, odds ratios, regression coefficients).

The problems associated with building regression models may be magnified in biomarker studies because an investigator may try to select the best regression model from a large number of predictor variables. If the predictor variables in this set are highly interrelated (e.g. if one or more variables can be well predicted from the other predictor variables – that is, if collinearity is present), then the order in which variables enter the model will be very important and will determine the resulting 'best' model in many of the variable selection methods. In addition, collinearity may cause the values of parameter estimates to be suspect, causing potential misinterpretations of the strength and possibly the direction of relationship between a predictor variable and the response of interest. If the direction of the relationship between predictor variables defined by a particular marker and a response is altered by the presence of other variables, then the interpretation of the marker is completely confused. If care is not exercised, an investigator might claim that a marker is clearly linked to a disease when the observed relationship is an artefact of this markers' high degree of association with other predictive variables. Thus the effect of one variable cannot be interpreted separately when high degrees of collinearity are present.

Since the use of molecular biology may yield a host of risk factors for consideration in an epidemiological investigation, data reduction methods might be appropriate at early stages of an analysis. For example, Miettinen (1976) advocated the determination of discriminant scores from the linear combination of confounders that optimally discriminates between disease states. Scores on this derived function were used to define strata for further analysis. Although it is not currently used in epidemiological analysis to

any great degree, the logic and pattern of this analytical strategy appears promising for studies of molecular biomarkers. It is important to distinguish statistical approaches used for molecular markers in a causal pathway from those used for markers not in the pathway. The former should not be treated as confounders.

An alternative form of correlated data arises when multiple measurements of a response variable are taken on each subject, as is often encountered in prospective cohort studies. In this situation, repeated measurements on the response variable exhibit a correlation. The magnitude of this correlation may decrease for observations that are distant in time. Thus, not only must the change in the mean response as a function of covariates be modelled, but the nature of the correlation in the responses must be considered. This type of correlated data pattern is most commonly encountered in longitudinal study designs. Analysis of such data requires the use of mixed models or generalized estimating equations (see Diggle *et al.*, 1994 for more details and description of these methods).

One concern debated in the epidemiological literature is the adjustment of tests and confidence intervals to reflect the fact that a family of inferential statements are of interest (Savitz & Olshan, 1995). If no relationship exists between a disease and collection of risk factors and confounders, then individual tests that suggest a relationship may be 'significant' due to sampling variability. It would be unfortunate if a potentially important marker were to be ignored at an early stage of development because of reliance on adjustments linked to multiple comparisons. In contrast, if markers are used as prognostic factors, then inclusion of unimportant markers may lead to predictive models that are unnecessarily complex and perhaps less generalizable to contexts. So, how does the question of multiple comparisons pertain to multiple data on molecular and genetic markers? Our view is one of balance: we want to avoid missing out on potentially important markers but we want to keep parsimony as an ultimate goal for models. Therefore, a possible compromise would be to consider multiple comparison methods employed with relatively large overall family-wise error rates during early phases of model development. This exercise would be conducted with the knowledge and appreciation of the investigator. We feel that this may be an area where the 'art' of statistical inference must be appreciated as much as the 'science'.

In approaching the analysis of large data sets involving products of high-throughput technologies, lessons can be learned from past analysis of mutational spectra. The data that arise in studies of mutational spectra are classifications of people into a set of possible genotypes. Thus these data are primarily categorical, and the statistical analyses reflect this focus. The general analysis conducted in these studies involves the comparison of a spectrum of mutations for exposed diseased people with the spectrum of mutations for unexposed diseased people. The rigour of analyses of spectral data ranges from informal comparisons of relative frequencies of genotypes between two groups to more complicated tests of homogeneity that address issues of the sparseness of mutational spectral data (i.e. some genotypes are quite rare, occurring with very low frequencies). The tests of homogeneity include the chi-squared test of homogeneity, Fisher's exact test and multi-category generalizations of this test. One of the more common tests used to determine differences in mutational spectra between two groups is an approximate exact test given by Adams and Skopek (1987). This procedure employs Monte Carlo computer simulations, generating data tables that assume an underlying hypergeometric distribution to determine a p value for the test of spectral equality. The p value corresponds to the proportion of simulated data tables that indicate greater differences than those seen in the observed data table. This procedure works well in sparse data tables (Piegorsch & Bailer, 1994), and computer programmes are available for calculating this test (Cariello *et al.*, 1994). In general, however, attention to how mutational spectra change in some systematic way, perhaps as a function of exposure, has not been the focus of inquiry.

It is worth noting that the classification strategies for comparisons of mutational spectra are overwhelmed by the sheer volume of data produced by the new high-throughput technologies.

Thus, multivariate analysis options are very popular for these data. Different multivariate techniques, such as analysis of principal components and cluster analysis, have been used in one of the earliest high-output technologies, two-dimensional electrophoresis (2DPAGE) gels. Many of the current issues associated with the analysis of gene and expression microarrays were first encountered in animal studies comparing 2DPAGE gels from treated and untreated animals (Anderson *et al.*, 1987). Critical for epidemiological purposes is how gels from multiple study subjects are compared either with a master set of data or with a comparison group. In order to address successfully comparative effects involving potentially hundreds of biological mechanisms, databases are required in which data from numerous studies are directly accessible as a homogeneous whole. One approach used very large databases of relational structure, in which each protein spot on each gel is stored as a discrete record. A system has been used to retrieve statistical data in real time for one spot across a set of 12 305 gels containing 8 099 806 spot measurements (Anderson & Anderson, 1996). More recent examples of complex serum proteomic patterns have been described (Petricoin *et al.*, 2002). Such analyses of proteomic spectra, generated by mass spectroscopy, may provide a useful tool for diagnosis based on the pattern independent of the identity of the proteins or peptides.

Observations related to the analysis of large datasets on gene expression and polymorphism

New high-throughput technologies, such as gene and expression microarrays, will present a number of issues that amplify the challenges of combining genetic and environmental variables. The large amount of data will be a challenge in terms of validity, reduction, summarization, analysis and interpretation. Many early studies have shown different sets of genes perturbed for similar exposures. This may be due to a lack of standardization of approach to guide analysis and interpretation. Studies where expression of genes is measured under different conditions need rules for determining what is an outlier (a potentially important deviation in expression). In the context of data on gene expression, this is sometimes described as the challenge of detecting 'signal', a true difference in expression, among the 'noise' of natural variability in gene expression. There is a need to determine whether variability of experience for each gene can be measured in the same or a different scale. Replication is necessary to determine whether tested genes have the same natural scales of measurement. Even if the scale of measurement is appropriate for different genes, the question arises whether an effective method has been used for detecting outliers (Wittes & Friedman, 1999). Other fundamental questions will need to be answered before interpretations of the deluge of data will begin to be possible. These include the ability to define empirically 'housekeeping' genes, to identify reproducible artefacts and to distinguish homeostatic from pathological perturbations.

Microarray technologies: DNA microarrays are glass slides on which a large number of DNA probes, each corresponding to a specific mRNA species, are placed at predefined positions. DNA probes are either synthesized *in situ* (Lockhart *et al.*, 1996) or are pre-synthesized and then spotted on the slide (DeRisi *et al.*, 1997). RNA is extracted from the biological sample, reverse transcribed into cDNA and labelled in the process. The labelled cDNA, representing the transcriptome of the biological sample, is hybridized on the microarray. The amount of label cDNA that hybridizes to each probe on the microarray is proportional to the relative abundance of the corresponding cDNA. The expression of all genes is then quantified by intensity of the colour used to label the RNA. The most common experimental protocol used with spotted microarrays consists of labelling two RNA extracts with different colours and co-hybridizing the samples to the same microarray. Although this approach introduces some restrictions on the experimental design (Kerr & Churchill, 2001), the overall principles of the two major technologies are the same. Quantification of individual gene expressions proceeds by various normalization procedures whose role is to remove systematic biases, and rescaling the

measurements on different arrays to be directly comparable. The development of an appropriate normalization procedure is still an active research topic (Hill *et al.*, 2001; Colantuoni *et al.*, 2002).

Applications of microarrays: Although the most common application of microarrays is in monitoring gene expression, other applications, corresponding to the analysis of genomic DNA, encompass analysis of the loss of heterozygosity (Pinkel *et al.*, 1998; Pollack *et al.*, 1999) and genotyping and re-sequencing applications (Iwasaki *et al.*, 2002; Warrington *et al.*, 2002). Data on gene expression generated using microarrays are generally used to identify genes that are expressed differentially under different experimental conditions, to identify groups of genes with similar expression profiles across different experimental conditions (co-expressed genes) and to classify the biological sample on the basis of the pattern of expression of all or a subset of genes on the microarray. Identified differentially expressed genes have been used successfully to hypothesize which pathways are involved in a particular biological process. The same is the case with groups of co-expressed genes identified in a cluster analysis. Additionally, clusters of co-expressed genes can be used to hypothesize the functional relationship of a clustered gene and as a starting point for dissecting regulatory mechanisms underlying the co-expression. Expression-based classification has been used successfully to classify tumour tissues as well as to characterize new tumour subtypes.

Detecting differentially expressed genes across different experimental conditions

Statistical methods for identifying differentially expressed genes have come a long way from initial heuristic attempts (Schena *et al.*, 1996), realizing that rigorous statistical analysis of replicated data is needed (Claverie, 1999), to sophisticated statistical modelling using frequentist and Bayesian approaches. Generic statistical methods of the analysis of variance (Kerr *et al.*, 2000) and mixed models (Wolfinger *et al.*, 2001) are complemented by specialized maximum likelihood approaches (Ideker *et al.*, 2000a) and Bayesian-flavoured approaches (Baldi & Long, 2001; Efron *et al.*, 2001; Tusher *et al.*, 2001). Although consensus about the optimal method has still not been reached, the intense statistical research is a promising sign. One of the most daunting issues in the process of identifying differentially expressed genes is the difficult problem of multiple comparisons. Presently, expression levels of up to more than 20 000 different genes can be assessed on a single microarray. Searching for genes whose change in expression is statistically significant corresponds to testing 20 000 hypotheses simultaneously. The traditional significance level of $\alpha = 0.05$, unadjusted for multiple comparisons, will yield on average 1000 falsely implicated genes. On the other hand, the traditional Bonferroni adjustment will result in an adjusted significance level of $\alpha = 0.0000025$. Such a level is virtually unattainable in simple experiments with very few experimental replicates. The false discovery rate (FDR) adjustment (Benjamini & Hochberg, 1995) keeps a balance between the specificity and the sensitivity of analysis of microarray data (Tusher *et al.*, 2001). In contrast to traditional adjustments that control the probability of a single false positive in the whole experiment, the FDR approach controls the proportion of false positives among the implicated genes. For example, if 20 genes are selected using FDR = 0.05, on average one of them will be a false positive regardless of the total number of genes. The traditional (e.g. Bonferroni) adjustment will limit the probability of a single false positive to 0.05, resulting in an over-conservative testing procedure.

Identifying clusters of co-expressed genes

Overview of clustering approaches: The high-dimensional nature of microarray data has prompted the widespread use of various multi-variate analytical approaches aimed at identifying and modelling patterns of expression behaviour. In this context, patterns of expression behaviour are defined by groups of genes with similar expression levels under different experimental conditions. The major premise of interpreting results of such analyses is that co-expression is the result of some underlying commonality between mechanisms of expression regulation of such genes. The results of

the cluster analysis can be used either to infer common biological function of co-expressed genes or to serve as a starting point for dissecting the common mechanism of co-regulation that drives the observed co-expression. Since the advent of microarray technology, virtually all traditional clustering approaches have been applied in this context, and numerous new clustering approaches have been developed.

Hierarchical clustering procedures were the first to be applied in the analysis of microarray data (Eisen *et al.*, 1998). Such methods rely on the calculation of pair-wise distances or similarities between the gene profiles. Various correlation coefficients are the most commonly used measures of similarity. Hierarchical agglomerative methods generally proceed by grouping genes on the basis of such pair-wise measures of similarity, and one of the several ways of establishing distance between groups of genes still using pair-wise distance measures (single linkage corresponding to the minimum pair-wise distance between genes in two different groups, complete linkage corresponding to the maximum distance, *k*-nearest neighbours principle corresponding to the *k*th largest distance and average linkage corresponding to the average distance) (Everitt, 1993).

Partitioning approaches, on the other hand, work by iteratively re-assigning profiles in a pre-specified number of clusters with the goal of optimizing an overall measure of fit. Two most commonly used traditional approaches are the *k*-means algorithm and the self-organizing map method, first applied in this context by Tavazoie *et al.* (1999) and Tamayo *et al.* (1999), respectively. One of the problems with clustering methods that are based on pair-wise distances of expression profiles is that, at least in the initial steps, data from only two profiles are used at a time. That is, the information about relationships between the two profiles and the rest of the profiles is not taken into account, although these relationships can be very informative about the association between them. The major drawback of partitioning approaches is the need to specify the number of clusters.

In a model-based approach to clustering, the probability distribution of observed data is approximated by a statistical model. Parameters in such a model define clusters of similar observations. The cluster analysis is performed by estimating these parameters from the data. In a Gaussian mixture model approach (McLachlan & Basford, 1987), similar individual profiles are assumed to have been generated by the common underlying 'pattern' represented by a multivariate Gaussian random variable (Yeung *et al.*, 2001; Ghosh & Chinnaiyan, 2002; McLachlan *et al.*, 2002). In the situation where the number of clusters is not known, this approach relies on the ability to identify the correct number of mixture components. A mixture-based method for clustering expression profiles that produces clusters by integrating over models with all possible numbers of clusters was developed by Medvedovic and Sivaganesan (2002). This method is based on the Bayesian non-parametric approach and Dirichlet process mixtures (Ferguson, 1973). The joint distribution of the data is modelled by a specific hierarchical Bayesian model and the posterior distribution of clusterings is generated using a Gibbs sampler.

Assessing statistical significance of observed patterns: A reliable assessment of reproducibility of observed expression patterns and gene clusters is one of the burning issues in cluster analysis. Since cluster analysis has generally been used as a tool for exploratory analysis, not for hypothesis testing, establishing the statistical significance of observed results has not been a priority. The problem is exacerbated by the heuristic nature of most clustering procedures and the complexity of the clustering space. Even for model-based approaches, designing the appropriate null distribution for establishing the statistical significance of specific features of created clusters is usually difficult. Two exceptions are the significance of the existence of the overall clustering structure and the significance of pair-wise associations between individual profiles. In both situations, the null distributions can be constructed by simulating 'randomized' data sets and comparing the observed distribution of the overall measure of the model fit, or pair-wise similarities, to their distribution in 'randomized' data. In the finite mixture model approach, the confidence in obtained

patterns and the confidence in individual assignments to particular clusters are assessed by estimating the confidence in corresponding parameter estimates. Assuming that the number of mixture components is correctly specified, this approach offers reliable estimates of confidence in assigning individual profiles to particular clusters. All conclusions are then made assuming that the correct number of clusters is known. Consequently, estimates of the model parameters do not take into account the uncertainty in choosing the correct number of clusters. The ability of Bayesian approaches to assess directly the probability of any particular feature of the constructed clusters seems to be an obvious advantage in these situations.

Modelling experimental variability
Precision of measurements of gene expression generally varies across different genes. A portion of such variability is attributable to the association between the absolute expression levels and the variance of the corresponding estimate. Such variability can also be introduced artificially when the numbers of replicated measurements used to calculate gene expression vary for different genes. When identifying differentially expressed genes, this heterogeneous variability is taken into account by analysing each gene separately (Wolfinger *et al.*, 2001) or by modelling gene-specific variability due to different levels of expression directly (Baggerly *et al.*, 2001; Newton *et al.*, 2001). Unfortunately, such precise characterizations of experimental variability have not been common in the context of cluster analysis. Disregarding information about such variability can result in a biased clustering, and the Bayesian mixture model, which can model gene-specific variability directly, has been shown to perform better in such situations (Medvedovic & Sivaganesan, 2002).

Reducing the dimensionality of the data
Traditional statistical approaches to identifying the coordinate system in which most of the variability in the data is associated with only a few coordinates, such as analysis of principal components, have been applied in the analysis of microarray data. The reduction of dimensionality can be applied to either the number of genes or to the

number of experiments. Genes are considered replicates and experimental conditions variables when the intention is to cluster genes over a lower-dimensional space. The reverse is the case when the intention is to reduce the number of genes to be used in the microarray-based classification problem. In this case, the number of non-zero components that can be used as gene surrogates is limited by the number of microarrays. Yeung and Ruzzo (2001) demonstrated that such reduction in dimensionality of the experimental condition space may or may not be beneficial when clustering genes. Principal component reduction of the number of genes seems to have been more beneficial when constructing efficient classifiers of tumour samples (West *et al.*, 2001). Other variance decomposition approaches, such as partial least squares (Nguyen & Rocke, 2002) and correspondence analysis (Fellenberg *et al.*, 2001), have also been applied in such analyses with apparent success. In particular, the method of partial least squares appears to have certain advantages over that of principal components when reducing the number of genes to be used in the classification of tumours, because it chooses an alternative coordinate system that accentuates the relationship between projections and the grouping of microarrays. Another approach to identifying the most informative projections of the data on a low-dimensional space (one or two dimensions) that is yet to be applied in this context is the method of projection pursuit. In contrast to the principal components approach, which assumes that projection on the plane determined by a few largest principal components separates data well because of the large spread, projection pursuit searches directly for the projection that best separates data.

Drawing conclusions about co-regulation on the basis of co-expression

Transcriptional regulation is one of crucial mechanisms used by a living system to regulate protein levels. It is estimated that 5–10% of the genes in eukaryotic genomes encode transcription factors (Brivanlou & Darnell, 2002) that are dedicated to the complex task of deciding where, when and which gene is to be expressed. Mechanisms applied by these factors range from the recruit-

ment and activation of the transcriptional pre-initiation complex to necessary modulations of local chromatin structure. Two major determinants of gene expression specificity seem to be the composition of their *cis*-regulatory modules and the presence or absence and phosphorylation status of *trans*-acting regulatory factors that interact with DNA regulatory modules and each other. However, the exact nature of the interactions between various components of the regulatory mechanism is still largely unknown. Identification of co-expressed genes by a cluster analysis of gene expression profiles has often been used as a first step in identifying factors regulating expression of different genes (Chu *et al.*, 1998; Tavazoie *et al.*, 1999). On the other hand, using information about presence of known regulatory elements can be applied to refine the cluster analysis of expression profiles and the simultaneous identification of known regulatory elements causing such co-regulation (Pilpel *et al.*, 2001).

An indirect indication of co-regulation of co-expressed genes is the tendency of co-expressed genes to participate in the same biological pathway (Tavazoie *et al.*, 1999) as well as their tendency to code for proteins that interact with each other (Fuchs *et al.*, 2001). In both of these situations, the mechanism of co-regulation might not be at the level of common *cis*-regulatory elements, yet the need for co-regulation and the actual presence of these elements are obvious. In fact, it has been shown that the particular regulatory mechanism of expression can sometimes be a better determinant of the protein function than even its three-dimensional structure. All these suggest that analytical methods capable of integrating information about regulatory sequences, biological pathways and protein–protein interactions and expression data generated in microarray experiments will be better able to create biologically meaningful clusters of genes than data on clustering expression alone.

Gene expression-based classification

Classification of biological samples on the basis of their transcriptome profile has been shown to have a tremendous potential for clinical applications in the areas of tumour classification and toxicity screens of potential drug compounds (Thomas *et al.*, 2001; Waring *et al.*, 2001a,b). Dudoit *et al.* (2002) carried out a comprehensive comparison of the performance of traditional classification methods with microarray data-based tumour classification. Among other things, their results support the need to base classifiers on statistical theory. For example, they showed that the maximum likelihood-based classifier clearly outperforms a popular heuristic equivalent described by Golub *et al.* (1999). Because of the large number of variables (genes) used to classify a relatively small number of samples (tumours), most traditional statistical approaches require subsetting of the genes. Genes are usually selected on the basis of their association with the disease state. However, when designing a support vector-machine classifier, Ramaswamy *et al.* (2001) argued that the maximum precision is achieved when all genes are used.

Modelling genetic networks

The traditional approach to characterizing roles of different cellular components has been to collect information on a single gene, a single protein or a single interaction at a time. However, some characteristics of behaviour of the complex network of biochemical interactions defining the living system are unlikely to be recovered by such localized approaches (Ideker *et al.*, 2001). For example, the functional role of a gene whose expression is regulated by several transcription factors cannot be fully understood without simultaneously monitoring for the presence or activation status of all of them. The ability of modern high-throughput assays to generate simultaneously measurements on a large number of molecules participating in such a network allows us to tackle the problem of reconstructing the whole networks. The complete strategy for such an analysis consists of a mathematical model describing interactions of various components of the network, experimental approaches to perturb the network, biological assays for quantifying the effects of such perturbation and the inference procedures for estimating parameters of the assumed model (Ideker *et al.*, 2000b).

Mathematical models of genetic networks

Mathematical models describing dynamics of biochemical networks include the deterministic ordinary differential equation-based models of kinetics of coupled chemical reactions; stochastic generalization of such models following the Gillespie algorithm for simulation approach to the chemical master equations (McAdams & Arkin, 1997, 1998, 1999; Kierzek, 2002); Boolean network models which reduce the information on the abundance of various interacting molecules to a binary variable representing on/off (0/1, present/absent) states (D'haeseleer *et al.*, 2000); and hierarchical Bayesian models (Friedman *et al.*, 2000). All of these mathematical models have certain advantages and disadvantages, depending on the goal of the analysis, available data and the knowledge about interactions of various molecules in the network. The specification of an ordinary differential equation model requires detailed knowledge of the interactions to be modelled, and is intended for examination of the overall dynamics of the system when individual relationships between components of the network are more or less known. In this context, the data are more commonly used for checking the predictions based on such models than for reconstructing the networks themselves. The same is true of various stochastic approaches to simulating behaviour of such networks. Stochastic approaches are likely to offer a more realistic result in biochemical networks involving molecules of very low abundance, as is the case in regulation of gene expression (McAdams & Arkin, 1997, 1998). In contrast, the Boolean network (Toh & Horimoto, 2002) model approach offers a relatively straightforward approach to reconstructing the topology of the network based on discretized data. However, it has been argued that the binary 0/1 representation of network components is inadequate in many situations (McAdams & Arkin, 1998). Finally, hierarchical Bayesian models, Bayesian networks in particular, seem to be capable of capturing the rich topological structure, integrating components operating on various scales and the stochastic component both of the underlying biological processes and of the noise inherent in the data. In this statistical approach, the behaviour of the network is expressed as the joint probability distribution of measurements that can be made on elements of the network. The structure of the network is described in terms of the directed acyclic graph (DAG) (Cowell *et al.*, 1999). Nodes in the network correspond to the elements of the network, and directed edges specify the dependences between the components. A DAG specifies the dependence structure of the network through the Markov assumption that the node is statistically independent of its non-descendants, given its parents. Well-established inferential procedures allow for the data-driven reconstruction of the network topology and specific interactions, together with the corresponding measures of confidence in the estimated structure and model parameters (Heckerman, 1998). The ability to incorporate various levels of prior knowledge through the informative priors about the structure and the local probability distributions (Heckerman *et al.*, 1995) allows Bayesian networks to serve potentially as the model of choice for encoding the current knowledge and the analysis of new data on the background of the current knowledge. Predictions about the future behaviour of the network can take into account all sources of uncertainties: uncertainty about the estimated parameters of the networks, structure of the network and the stochastic nature of the biological system modelled by the network. The application of Bayesian networks for constructing genetic networks based on microarray data has been demonstrated (Friedman *et al.*, 2000). The combined approach of clustering gene expression profiles first and then fitting a probabilistic network using average cluster profiles (Toh & Horimoto, 2002) as well as the use of probabilistic Boolean networks, which share properties of Boolean and Bayesian networks (Shmulevich *et al.*, 2002), have also been described in this context.

Integrating current knowledge and various types of data in the analysis of experimental data

Formal methods of integrating accumulated knowledge and information in the analysis have been developed. Zien *et al.* (2000) integrated the existing pathway information with microarray data and developed a method for scoring likelihood of whole pathway involvement in the process under investigation based on the expression levels of genes involved in the pathway. Holmes and Bruno (2000) developed the gene clustering procedure based on the statistical model that integrates microarray data and the genomic regulatory sequence data models. Barash and Friedman (2001) developed a similar approach using higher-level information about known regulatory motifs in the genomic data. Ideker *et al.* (2001) demonstrated how to use joint proteomic and functional genomic data after perturbing a biological system to restore the underlying network of molecular interactions. They used a maximum likelihood approach to identify genes with significantly changed expression levels (Ideker *et al.*, 2000a) and a Boolean network model for modelling the network (Ideker *et al.*, 2000b). Benefits of integrating genomic, functional genomic and proteomic data have been demonstrated (Ge *et al.*, 2001; Matthews *et al.*, 2001; Vidal, 2001; Boulton *et al.*, 2002).

In terms of human studies, tumours represent naturally perturbed genomic systems. Concurrent genomic and functional genomic investigations of tumours by high-throughput microarray approaches can be used to dissect genetic networks involved in the process of tumour genesis. In this context, microarrays can be used to characterize both the genomic aberrations and the gene expression in different tumours. Several models mentioned above are capable of integrating such information into a single powerful analysis.

Implications for future research

The combination of genetic and environmental variables, always somewhat problematic, has been made more so by new biotechnologies. The design, analysis and interpretation of studies with genetic and environmental variables are among the issues that require consideration. The rationale for such studies must be considered first. Do they represent the judicious use of scarce resources or the diversion of disease prevention efforts? The potential conflict is between a focus on mechanistic studies at the expense of research on preventive or control efforts. Clearly both activities have their value. With limited budgets, it may be more appropriate to use research funds to effect the greatest health benefit. However, powerful new technologies have great promise if properly explored and harnessed.

As new information about the underlying molecular and genetic determinants becomes available, we are faced with questions about their impact on disease definition, classification and diagnosis. The high-throughput technologies have the potential to define subcategories of disease, and this could contribute considerably to the understanding of disease etiology if the subcategories have distinct etiologies. Even more important is the potential for new definitions of disease. In the biological sciences, speculation exists that a new molecular-based theoretical biology will emerge and lead to the identification of the coordinated action of the products of multiple genes. Such coordinated functions can be viewed as a genetic circuit representing the cellular 'wiring diagrams' – the collections of different gene products that together are required to execute a particular function (Palsson, 1997). Others have referred to it as a genome-operating system that translates any alteration in the quantity and configuration of a cellular protein into a signal that causes up- or down-regulation of either individual proteins or batteries of proteins (Strohman, 1997). In addition to the molecular, biochemical, physiological and medical analyses of the elements and hierarchies that constitute a person and are involved in disease, there may be a need to add a systems science approach to disease definition (Palsson, 1997; Strohman, 1997). Seemingly diverse diseases such as cancer, atherosclerosis and arthritis might have common cellular and molecular features (Satyanarayana & Schoskes, 1997). A better classification system might be one that links clinical observations with cellular and molecular biological data. In addition, artificial neural networks are being explored increasingly as alternatives to discriminant analyses in evaluating diagnostic parameters (e.g. presence of chest pain, serum creatine kinase concentration) and the best diagnosis available (e.g. whether myocardial infarction was present or not) (Schultz, 1996). This approach may also allow for the inclusion of multiple molecular markers, although the importance of comprehensive and extensive training sets for such methods cannot be overstated. The impact of these developments on epidemiological research is unknown, but they are likely to have an effect. Disease definitions may change and, hence, so will diagnostic procedures and ultimately therapeutic approaches (Gyorkos & Coupal, 1995; Crooke, 1996; Strohman, 1997). What constitutes a case or a control for epidemiological studies might be based on probabilities or distributions rather than on the presence or absence of a particular disease end-point (as in analyses conducted in studies of receiver operating characteristics).

Conclusions

We have addressed some of the new problems encountered in studies of genetic epidemiology and of gene–environment interactions. New study designs are emerging. We have considered the case-only approach, which has been proposed specifically for gene–environment interactions. It is clear that innovative study designs have both advantages and disadvantages. The case-only approach has greater power than the case–control approach, but it also has limitations such as the implicit multiplicative frame and the assumption of independence of gene and exposure.

Old methodological problems have been rediscovered in the case of gene–environment interactions. One is the so-called problem of 'population stratification'. For epidemiologists, this is the well-known problem of confounding, which is not necessarily an insurmountable obstacle in studies of gene–environment interactions. For example, the greater the degree of admixture within a population and the smaller the difference in allele frequency or baseline disease risk, the less likely it is that population stratification will lead to confounding. In addition, when important confounding caused by population stratification does occur, it should be controllable by the usual design and analytical features employed by epidemiologists.

Finally, we have considered a number of different statistical approaches to the analysis of extremely complex data sets such as those produced in the context of gene expression. The ingenuous nature of statistical solutions, aiming at overcoming the 'multiple comparisons' issue, summarizing large data sets and allowing reasonable and sound causal inferences, is notable. Unfortunately, most of these approaches still need to be validated and are far from being applicable in normal research practice.

Acknowledgements
This work has been partially funded with a grant of the Compagnia di San Paolo to the ISI Foundation and with a grant from the European Union (QLK4-CT-1999-00927). We are grateful to Colin Begg for thoughtful comments.

References

Adams, W.T. & Skopek, T.R. (1987) Statistical test for the comparison of samples from mutational spectra. *J. mol. Biol.*, **194**, 391–396

Albert, P.S., Ratnasinghe, D., Tangrea, J. & Wacholder, S. (2001) Limitations of the case-only design for identifying gene–environment interactions. *Am. J. Epidemiol.*, **154**, 687–693

Altshuler, D., Kruglyak, L. & Lander, E. (1998) Genetic polymorphisms and disease. *New Engl. J. Med.*, **338**, 1626

Anderson, N.G. & Anderson, N.L. (1996) Twenty years of two-dimensional electrophoresis: past, present, and future. *Electrophoresis*, **17**, 443–453

Anderson, N.L., Giere, F.A., Nance, S.L., Gemmell, M.A., Tollaksen, S.L. & Anderson, N.G. (1987) Effects of toxic agents on the protein level: quantitative measurement of 213 mouse liver proteins following xenobiotic treatment. *Fundam. appl. Toxicol.*, **8**, 39–50

Baggerly, K.A., Coombes, K.R., Hess, K.R., Stivers, D.N., Abruzzo, L.V. & Zhang, W. (2001) Identifying differentially expressed genes in cDNA microarray experiments. *J. comput. Biol.*, **8**, 639–659

Baldi, P. & Long, A. D. (2001) A Bayesian framework for the analysis of microarray expression data: regularized t-test and statistical inferences of gene changes. *Bioinformatics*, **17**, 509–519

Barash, Y. & Friedman, F. (2001) Context-specific Bayesian clustering for gene expression data. In: *Proceedings of the Fifth Annual International Conference on Computational Molecular Biology (RECOMB 2001)*

Benjamini, Y. & Hochberg, Y. (1995) Controlling the false discovery rate: a practical and powerful approach to multiple testing. *J. R. Statist. Soc. Ser. B*, **57**, 289–300

Botto, L.D. & Khoury, M.J. (2001) Commentary: facing the challenge of gene–environment interaction: the two-by-four table and beyond. *Am. J. Epidemiol.*, **153**, 1016–1020

Boulton, S.J., Gartner, A., Reboul, J., Vaglio, P., Dyson, N., Hill, D.E. & Vidal, M. (2002) Combined functional genomic maps of the *C. elegans* DNA damage response. *Science*, **295**, 127–131

Brivanlou, A.H. & Darnell, J.E., Jr (2002) Signal transduction and the control of gene expression. *Science*, **295**, 813–818

Cariello, N.F., Piegorsch, W.W., Adams, W.T. & Skopek, T.R. (1994) Computer program for the analysis of mutational spectra: application to *p53* mutations. *Carcinogenesis*, **15**, 2281–2285

Chu, S., DeRisi, J., Eisen, M., Mulholland, J., Botstein, D., Brown, P. O. & Herskowitz, I. (1998) The transcriptional program of sporulation in budding yeast. *Science*, **282**, 699–705

Claverie, J.M. (1999) Computational methods for the identification of differential and coordinated gene expression. *Hum. mol. Genet.*, **8**, 1821–1832

Clayton, D. & McKeigue, P.M. (2001) Epidemiological methods for studying genes and environmental factors in complex diseases. *Lancet*, **358**, 1356–1360

Colantuoni, C., Henry, G., Zeger, S. & Pevsner, J. (2002) Local mean normalization of microarray element signal intensities across an array surface: quality control and correction of spatially systematic artifacts. *Biotechniques*, **32**, 1316–1320

Cowell, R.G., Dawid, P.A., Lauritzen, S.L. & Spiegelhalter, D.J. (1999) *Probabilistic Networks and Expert Systems*, New York, Springer

Crooke, S.T. (1996) New drugs and changing disease paradigms. *Nature Biotechnol.*, **14**, 238–241

Devlin, B., Roeder, K. & Wasserman, L. (2001) Genomic control, a new approach to genetic-based association studies. *Theor. Popul. Biol.*, **60**, 155–66

DeRisi, J.L., Iyer, V.R. & Brown, P.O. (1997) Exploring the metabolic and genetic control of gene expression on a genomic scale. *Science*, **278**, 680–686

D'haeseleer, P., Liang, S. & Somogyi, R. (2000) Genetic network inference: from co-expression clustering to reverse engineering. *Bioinformatics*, **16**, 707–726

Diggle, P.J., Liang, K.-Y. & Zeger, S.L. (1994) *Analysis of Longitudinal Data*, New York, Oxford University Press

Dudoit, S., Fridlyand, J. & Speed, T.P. (2002) Comparison of discrimination methods for the classification of tumors using gene expression data. *J. Am. Stat. Assoc.*, **97**, 77

Efron, B., Tibshirani, R., Storey, J.D. & Tusher, V. (2001) Empirical Bayes analysis of a microarray experiment. *J. Am. Stat. Assoc.*, **96**, 1151–1160

Eisen, M.B., Spellman, P.T., Brown, P.O. & Botstein, D. (1998) Cluster analysis and display of genome-wide expression patterns. *Proc. natl Acad. Sci. USA*, **95**, 14863–14868

Everitt, B.S. (1993) *Cluster Analysis*, London, Edward Arnold

Fellenberg, K., Hauser, N.C., Brors, B., Neutzner, A., Hoheisel, J.D. & Vingron, M. (2001) Correspondence analysis applied to microarray data. *Proc. natl Acad. Sci. USA*, **98**, 10781–10786

Fellenberg, K., Hauser, N.C., Brors, B., Hoheisel, J.D. & Vingron, M. (2002) Microarray data warehouse allowing for inclusion of experiment annotations in statistical analysis. *Bioinformatics*, **18**, 423–433

Ferguson, T.S. (1973) A Bayesian analysis of some nonparametric problems. *Ann. Stat.*, **1**, 209–230

Friedman, N., Linial, M., Nachman, I. & Pe'er, D. (2000) Using Bayesian networks to analyze expression data. *J. comput. Biol.*, **7**, 601–620

Fuchs, T., Glusman, G., Horn-Saban, S., Lancet, D. & Pilpel, Y. (2001) The human olfactory subgenome: from sequence to structure and evolution. *Hum. Genet.*, **108**, 1–13

Garcia-Closas, M., Rothman, N. & Lubin, J. (1999) Misclassification in case–control studies of gene–environment interactions: assessment of bias and sample size. *Cancer Epidemiol. Biomarkers Prev.*, **8**, 1043–1050

Ge, H., Liu, Z., Church, G.M. & Vidal, M. (2001) Correlation between transcriptome and interactome mapping data from *Saccharomyces cerevisiae*. *Nature Genet.*, **29**, 482–486

Ghosh, D. & Chinnaiyan, A.M. (2002) Mixture modelling of gene expression data from microarray experiments. *Bioinformatics*, **18**, 275–286

Golub, T.R., Slonim, D.K., Tamayo, P., Huard, C., Gaasenbeek, M., Mesirov, J.P., Coller, H., Loh, M.L., Downing, J.R., Caligiuri, M.A., Bloomfield,

C.D. & Lander, E.S. (1999) Molecular classification of cancer: class discovery and class prediction by gene expression monitoring. *Science*, **286**, 531–537

Gyorkos, J.L. & Coupal, L. (1995) Bayesian estimation of disease prevalence and the parameters of diagnostic tests in the absence of a gold standard. *Am. J. Epidemiol.*, **141**, 263–272

Heckerman, D. (1998) A tutorial on learning with Bayesian networks. In: Jordan, M.I., ed., *Learning in Graphical Models*, Dordrecht, Kluwer Academic Publishers, pp. 301–354

Heckerman, D., Geiger, D. & Chickering, D. (1995) Learning Bayesian networks: the combination of knowledge and statistical data. *Machine Learning*, **20**, 197–243

Hill, A.A., Brown, E.L., Whitley, M.Z., Tucker-Kellogg, G., Hunter, C.P. & Slonim, D.K. (2001) Evaluation of normalization procedures for oligonucleotide array data based on spiked cRNA controls. *Genome Biol.*, **2**, 55

Holmes, I. & Bruno, W.J. (2000) Finding regulatory elements using joint likelihoods for sequence and expression profile data. *Proc. int. Conf. Intell. Syst. mol. Biol.*, **8**, 202–210

Hwang, S.-J., Beaty, T.H., Liang, K.-Y., Coresh, J. & Khoury, M.J. (1994) Minimum sample size estimation to detect gene–environment interaction in case–control designs. *Am. J. Epidemiol.*, **140**, 1029–1037

Ideker, T., Thorsson, V., Siegel, A.F. & Hood, L.E. (2000a) Testing for differentially-expressed genes by maximum-likelihood analysis of microarray data. *J. comput. Biol.*, **7**, 805–817

Ideker, T., Thorsson V. & Karp R.M. (2000b) Discovery of regulatory interactions through perturbation: inference and experimental design. *Pacific Symp. Biocomput.*, 305–316

Ideker, T., Thorsson, V., Ranish, J.A., Christmas, R., Buhler, J., Eng, J.K., Bumgarner, R., Goodlett, D.R., Aebersold, R. & Hood, L. (2001) Integrated genomic and proteomic analyses of a systematically perturbed metabolic network. *Science*, **292**, 929–934

Iwasaki, H., Ezura, Y., Ishida, R., Kajita, M., Kodaira, M., Knight, J., Daniel, S., Shi, M. & Emi, M. (2002) Accuracy of genotyping for single nucleotide polymorphisms by a microarray-based single nucleotide polymorphism typing method involving hybridization of short allele-specific oligonucleotides. *DNA Res.*, **9**, 59–62

Kerr, K.M. & Churchill, G.A. (2001) Experimental design for gene expression microarrays. *Biostatistics*, **2**, 183–201

Kerr, K.M., Martin M. & Churchill, G.A. (2000) Analysis of variance for gene expression microarray data. *J. comput. Biol.*, **7**, 819–837

Kierzek, A.M. (2002) STOCKS: stochastic kinetic simulations of biochemical systems with Gillespie algorithm. *Bioinformatics*, **18**, 470–481

Khoury, M.J. & Flanders, W.D. (1996) Non-traditional epidemiologic approaches in the analysis of gene–environment interaction: case–control studies with no controls! *Am. J. Epidemiol.*, **144**, 207–213

Khoury, M.J. & Wagener, D.K. (1995) Epidemiological evaluation of the use of genetics to improve the predictive value of disease risk factors. *Am. J. hum. Genet.*, **56**, 835–844

Khoury, M.J., Beaty, T.H. & Cohen, B.H. (1993) *Fundamentals of Genetic Epidemiology*, New York, Oxford University Press

Lockhart, D.J., Dong, H., Byrne, M.C., Follettie, M.T., Gallo, M.V., Chee, M.S., Mittmann, M., Wang, C., Kobayashi, M., Horton, H. & Brown, E.L. (1996) Expression monitoring by hybridization to high-density oligonucleotide arrays. *Nature Biotechnol.*, **14**, 1675–1680

Lowrance, W.W. (2001) The promise of human genetic databases. *Br. med. J.*, **322**, 1009–1010

Marcus, P.M., Hayes, R.B., Vineis, P., Garcia-Closas, M., Caporaso, N.E., Autrup, H., Branch, R.A., Brockmöller, J., Ishizaki, T., Karakaya, A.E., Ladero, J.M., Mommsen, S., Okkels, H., Romkes, M., Roots, I. & Rothman, N. (2000) Cigarette smoking, *N*-acetyltransferase 2 acetylation status, and bladder cancer risk: a case-series meta-analysis of a gene–environment interaction. *Cancer Epidemiol. Biomarkers Prev.*, **9**, 461–467

Matthews, L.R., Vaglio, P., Reboul, J., Ge, H., Davis, B.P., Garrels, J., Vincent, S. & Vidal, M. (2001) Identification of potential interaction networks using sequence-based searches for conserved protein–protein interactions or 'interologs'. *Genome Res.*, **11**, 2120–2126

McAdams, H.H. & Arkin, A. (1997) Stochastic mechanisms in gene expression. *Proc. natl Acad. Sci. USA*, **94**, 814–819

McAdams, H.H. & Arkin, A. (1998) Simulation of prokaryotic genetic circuits. *Annu. Rev. biophys. biomol. Struct.*, **27**, 199–224

McAdams, H.H. & Arkin, A. (1999) It's a noisy business! Genetic regulation at the nanomolar scale. *Trends Genet.*, **15**, 65–69

McLachlan, J.G. & Basford, E.K. (1987) *Mixture Models: Inference and Applications to Clustering*, New York, Marcel Dekker

McLachlan, G.J., Bean, R.W. & Peel, D. (2002) A mixture model-based approach to the clustering of microarray expression data. *Bioinformatics*, **18**, 413–422

Medvedovic, M. & Sivaganesan, S. (2002) Bayesian infinite mixture model based clustering of gene expression profiles. *Bioinformatics*, **18**, 1194–1206

Miettinen, O.S. (1976) Stratification by a multivariate confounder score. *Am. J. Epidemiol.*, **104**, 609–620

Neter, J., Kutner, M.H., Nachtsheim, C.J. & Wasserman, W. (1996) *Applied Linear Statistical Models*, 4th Ed., Chicago, Irwin

Newton, M.A., Kendziorski, C.M., Richmond, C.S., Blattner, F.R. & Tsui, K.W. (2001) On differential variability of expression ratios: improving statistical inference about gene expression changes from microarray data. *J. comput. Biol.*, **8**, 37–52

Nguyen, D.V. & Rocke, D.M. (2002) Tumor classification by partial least squares using microarray gene expression data. *Bioinformatics*, **18**, 39–50

Ottman, R. (1996) Gene–environment interaction: definitions and study designs. *Prev. Med.*, **25**, 764–770

Palsson, B.O. (1997) What lies beyond bioinformatics? *Nature Biotechnol.*, **15**, 3–4

Petricoin, E.F., Ardekani, A.M., Hitt, B.A., Levine, P.H., Fusaro, V.A., Steinberg, S.M., Mills, G.B., Simone, C., Fishman, D.A., Kohn, E.C. & Liotta, L.A. (2002) Use of proteomic patterns in serum to identify ovarian cancer. *Lancet*, **359**, 572–577

Piegorsch, W.W. & Bailer, A.J. (1994) Statistical approaches for analyzing mutational spectra: some recommendations for categorical data. *Genetics*, **136**, 403–416

Pilpel, Y., Sudarsanam, P. & Church, G.M. (2001) Identifying regulatory networks by combinatorial analysis of promoter elements. *Nature Genet.*, **29**, 153–159

Pinkel, D., Segraves, R., Sudar, D., Clark, S., Poole, I., Kowbel, D., Collins, C., Kuo, W.L., Chen, C., Zhai,

Y., Dairkee, S.H., Ljung, B.M., Gray, J.W. & Albertson, D.G. (1998) High resolution analysis of DNA copy number variation using comparative genomic hybridization to microarrays. *Nature Genet.*, **20**, 207–211

Pollack, J.R., Perou, C.M., Alizadeh, A.A., Eisen, M.B., Pergamenschikov, A., Williams, C.F., Jeffrey, S.S., Botstein, D. & Brown, P.O. (1999) Genome-wide analysis of DNA copy-number changes using cDNA microarrays. *Nature Genet.*, **23**, 41–46

Ramaswamy, S., Tamayo, P., Rifkin, R., Mukherjee, S., Yeang, C.H., Angelo, M., Ladd, C., Reich, M., Latulippe, E., Mesirov, J.P., Poggio, T., Gerald, W., Loda, M., Lander, E.S. & Golub, T.R. (2001) Multiclass cancer diagnosis using tumor gene expression signatures. *Proc. natl Acad. Sci. USA*, **98**, 15149–15154

Rothman, K.J., Greenland, S. & Walker, A.M. (1980) Concepts of interaction. *Am. J. Epidemiol.*, **112**, 467–470

Rothman, N., Stewart, W.E., Caporaso, N.E. & Hayes, R.B. (1993) Misclassification of genetic susceptibility biomarkers: implications for case–control studies and cross-population comparisons. *Cancer Epidemiol. Biomarkers Prev.*, **2**, 299–303

Satyanarayana, K. & Schoskes, D.A. (1997) A molecular injury–response model for the understanding of chronic diseases. *Mol. Med. Today*, **3**, 331–334

Savitz, D. & Olshan, A.F. (1995) Multiple comparisons and related issues in the interpretation of epidemiologic data. *Am. J. Epidemiol.*, **142**, 904–908

Schena, M., Shalon, D., Heller, R., Chai, A., Brown, P.O. & Davis, R.W. (1996) Parallel human genome analysis: microarray-based expression monitoring of 1000 genes. *Proc. natl Acad. Sci. USA*, **93**, 10614–10619

Schulte, P.A. & Halperin, W. (1987) Genetic screening and monitoring of workers. In: Harrington, M., ed., *Recent Avenues in Occupational Health*, Vol. 3, Edinburgh, Churchill Livingstone, pp. 135–154

Schulte, P.A. & Perera, F.P. (1993) *Molecular Epidemiology: Principles and Practices*, San Diego, Academic Press

Schultz, E.K. (1996) Artificial neural networks: laboratory aid or sorcerer's apprentice? *Clin. Chem.*, **42**, 496–497

Selvin, S. (1991) *Statistical Analysis of Epidemiological Data*, New York, Oxford University Press

Shmulevich, I., Dougherty, E.R., Kim, S. & Zhang, W. (2002) Probabilistic Boolean networks: a rule-based uncertainty model for gene regulatory networks. *Bioinformatics*, **18**, 261–274

Strohman, R.C. (1997) The coming Kuhnian revolution in biology. *Nature Biotechnol.*, **15**, 194–200

Stürmer, T. & Brenner, H. (2000) Potential gain in efficiency and power to detect gene–environment interactions by matching in case–control studies. *Genet. Epidemiol.*, **18**, 63–80

Tamayo, P., Slonim, D., Mesirov, J., Zhu, Q., Kitareewan, S., Dmitrovsky, E., Lander, E.S. & Golub, T.R. (1999) Interpreting patterns of gene expression with self-organizing maps: methods and application to hematopoietic differentiation. *Proc. natl Acad. Sci. USA*, **96**, 2907–2912

Taylor, J.A., Umbach, D.M., Stephens, E., Castranio, T., Paulson, D., Robertson, C., Mohler, J.L. & Bell, D.A. (1998) The role of *N*-acetylation polymorphisms in smoking associated bladder cancer: evidence of a gene–gene–exposure three way interaction. *Cancer Res.*, **58**, 3603–3610

Tavazoie, S., Hughes, J.D., Campbell, M.J., Cho, R.J. & Church, G.M. (1999) Systematic determination of genetic network architecture. *Nature Genet.*, **22**, 281–285

Thomas, R.S., Rank, D.R., Penn, S.G., Zastrow, G.M., Hayes, K.R., Pande, K., Glover, E., Silander, T., Craven, M.W., Reddy, J.K., Jovanovich, S.B. & Bradfield, C.A. (2001) Identification of toxicologically predictive gene sets using cDNA microarrays. *Mol. Pharmacol.*, **60**, 1189–1194

Tibshirani, R., Hastie, T., Narasimhan, B. & Chu, G. (2002) Diagnosis of multiple cancer types by shrunken centroids of gene expression. *Proc. natl Acad. Sci. USA*, **99**, 6567–6572

Toh, H. & Horimoto, K. (2002) Inference of a genetic network by a combined approach of cluster analysis and graphical Gaussian modeling. *Bioinformatics*, **18**, 287–297

Toniolo, P., Boffeta, P., Schuker, D.E.G., Rothman, N., Hulka, B. & Pearce, N., eds (1997) *Application of Biomarkers in Cancer Epidemiology* (IARC Scientific Publications No. 142), Lyon, IARC*Press*

Tusher, V.G., Tibshirani, R. & Chu, G. (2001) Significance analysis of microarrays applied to the ionizing radiation response. *Proc. natl Acad. Sci. USA*, **98**, 5116–5121

Umbach, D.M. & Weinberg, C.R. (1997) Designing and analysing case–control studies to exploit independence of genotype and exposure. *Stat. Med.*, **16**, 1731–1743

Vidal, M. (2001) A biological atlas of functional maps. *Cell*, **104**, 333–339

Vineis, P., Veglia, F., Benhamou, S., Butkiewicz, D., Cascorbi, I., Clapper, M.L., Dolzan, V., Haugen, A., Hirvonen, A., Ingelman-Sundberg, M., Kihara, M., Kiyohara, C., Kremers, P., Le Marchand, Loic, Ohshima, S., Pastorelli, R., Rannug, A., Romkes, M., Schoket, B., Shields, P., Strange, R.C., Stucker, I., Sugimura, H., Garte, S., Gaspari, L. & Taioli, E. (2003) CYP1A1 T^{3801} C polymorphism and lung cancer: a pooled analysis of 2451 cases and 3358 controls. *Int. J. Cancer*, **104**, 650–657

Wacholder, S., Silverman, D.T., McLaughlin, J.K. & Mandel, J.S. (1992) Selection of controls in case–control studies. II. Types of controls. *Am. J. Epidemiol.*, **135**, 1029–1041

Wacholder, S., Rothman, N. & Caporaso, N. (2000) Population stratification in epidemiologic studies of common genetic variants and cancer: quantification of bias. *J. natl Cancer Inst.*, **92**, 1151–1158

Waring, J.F., Ciurlionis, R., Jolly, R.A., Heindel, M. & Ulrich R.G. (2001a) Microarray analysis of hepatotoxins *in vitro* reveals a correlation between gene expression profiles and mechanisms of toxicity. *Toxicol. Lett.*, **120**, 359–368

Waring, J.F., Jolly, R.A., Ciurlionis, R., Lum, P.Y., Praestgaard, J.T., Morfitt, D.C., Buratto, B., Roberts, C., Schadt, E. & Ulrich, R.G. (2001b) Clustering of hepatotoxins based on mechanism of toxicity using gene expression profiles. *Toxicol. appl. Pharmacol.*, **175**, 28–42

Warrington, J.A., Shah, N.A., Chen, X., Janis, M., Liu, C., Kondapalli, S., Reyes, V., Savage, M.P., Zhang, Z., Watts, R., DeGuzman, M., Berno, A., Snyder, J. & Baid, J. (2002) New developments in high-throughput resequencing and variation detection using high density microarrays. *Hum. Mutat.*, **19**, 402–409

West, M., Blanchette, C., Dressman, H., Huang, E., Ishida, S., Spang, R., Zuzan, H., Olson, J.A., Jr, Marks, J.R. & Nevins, J.R. (2001) Predicting the clinical status of human breast cancer by using gene expression profiles. *Proc. natl. Acad. Sci. USA*, **98**, 11462–11467

Wittes, J. & Friedman, H.P. (1999) Searching for evidence of altered gene expression: a comment on statistical analysis of microarray data. *J. natl Cancer Inst.*, **91**, 400–401

Wolfinger, R.D., Gibson, G, Wolfinger, E.D., Bennett, L., Hamadeh, H., Bushel, P., Afshari, C. & Paules, R.S. (2001) Assessing gene significance from cDNA microarray expression data via mixed models. *J. comput. Biol.*, **8**, 625–637

Yang, Q. & Khoury, M.J. (1997) Evolving methods in genetic epidemiology. III. Gene–environment interaction in epidemiologic research. *Epidemiol. Rev.*, **19**, 33–43

Yang, Q., Khoury, M.J., Sun, F. & Flanders, W.D. (1999) Case-only design to measure gene–gene interaction. *Epidemiology*, **10**, 167–170

Yeung, K.Y. & Ruzzo, W.L. (2001) Principal component analysis for clustering gene expression data. *Bioinformatics*, **17**, 763–774

Yeung, K.Y., Fraley, C., Murua, A., Raftery, A.E. & Ruzzo, W.L. (2001) Model-based clustering and data transformations for gene expression data. *Bioinformatics*, **17**, 977–987

Zien, A., Kuffner, R., Zimmer, R. & Lengauer, T. (2000) Analysis of gene expression data with pathway scores. *Proc. int. Conf. Intell. Syst. mol. Biol.*, **8**, 407–417

Corresponding author:

Paolo Vineis
Dipartimento di Scienze Biomediche
e Oncologia Umana,
Università di Torino, via Santena 7,
10126 Torino, Italy
paolo.vineis@unito.it

Mechanisms of Carcinogenesis: Contributions of Molecular Epidemiology
Patricia Buffler, Jerry Rice, Robert Baan, Michael Bird and Paolo Boffetta, eds
IARC Scientific Publications No. 157
International Agency for Research on Cancer, Lyon, 2004

Emerging Biomarker Technologies

Laura Gunn and Martyn T. Smith

Summary
New technology offers great potential for advances in cancer biomarker research. Here, we describe a number of new technologies and discuss their potential for use in molecular cancer epidemiology. The successful sequencing of the human genome has revealed several new insights, including the fact that the human genome consists of only 40 000 genes and is highly variable, with approximately 60 000 functional polymorphisms. High-throughput genomic technologies continue to facilitate the identification and analysis of mutations and polymorphisms in key genes and expand the spectrum of available genomic biomarkers. The next major challenge is the identification of novel proteins and understanding the structure, function and interaction of proteins and other molecules – information that cannot be obtained from genomics alone. Emerging technologies including arrays, proteomics and nanotechnology provide new platforms for high-throughput, highly sensitive, functional assays. These technologies will complement existing and emerging genomic technologies and result in the identification of new biomarkers of cancer risk. They will, however, require extensive validation in epidemiological studies.

Introduction
Recent breakthroughs in biotechnology offer the possibility of developing a new series of biomarkers of cancer risk. Many of these technologies are based on the analysis of DNA, such as high-throughput genomics (the study of the human genome), whereas others are based on the analysis of RNA and proteins, such as microarrays and proteomics. The basis of the genomic technologies is the polymerase chain reaction (PCR), which allows the amplification of small amounts of DNA for high-throughput analysis of human genetic variation and, through the use of

fluorescent probes, the quantitation of specific gene expression using real-time PCR (Bieche et al., 1999; Eads et al., 1999). DNA chips and microarrays have further expanded the power of genomic research by allowing global gene expression to be studied (Ghosh, 2000; Chan & Huang, 2001; Hippo et al., 2002).

Although key in identifying genetic predisposition, genomic methodologies alone cannot identify other biomolecular processes responsible for changes in protein expression and function involved in carcinogenesis. The sequencing of the human genome has revealed fewer genes than we originally imagined (Venter et al., 2001). Thus, the diversity of mammalian proteins cannot be explained solely on the basis of genetics but is a result of post-transcriptional and post-translational modifications as well. Therefore, to understand a normal cellular phenotype and phenotypic changes involved in the neoplastic transformation of a cell, cancer research is expanding to include genomics' sister technology, proteomics.

Proteomics, the analysis of complete complements of proteins, includes not only the identification and quantification of proteins, but also the determination of their localization, modifications, interactions, activities and, ultimately, their function (Fields, 2001). These characteristics, which are integral to cellular function, determine the phenotypic fate of a cell. Distinct changes in these characteristics occur during the neoplastic transformation of a cell; therefore expression analysis on the protein level is necessary to elucidate functional changes during carcinogenesis that are not identifiable at the genomic level.

Proteomics will complement existing biomarker technologies, providing information lacking in genomic-based analyses. These emerging proteomic and genomic methodologies emphasize high throughput (Germer et al., 2000; MacBeath & Schreiber, 2000; Buetow et al.,

2001; Ranade *et al.*, 2001) and multiplexing capabilities (Armstrong *et al.*, 2000; Iannone *et al.*, 2000; Bray *et al.*, 2001; Nicewarner-Pena *et al.*, 2001; Srinivas *et al.*, 2001). As a result, future technologies will measure > 50 000 end-points on a drop of blood using proteomics and high-throughput cellular analysis as well as identifying all genetic polymorphisms related to susceptibility using high-throughput genomics. The purpose of this chapter is to review these emerging technologies and to discuss their potential application in molecular cancer epidemiology. Further details of these technologies are available on the company websites listed in Table 1.

Genomic technologies

Genomics is the study of the human genome, of which a draft sequence was recently completed (Lander *et al.*, 2001; Venter *et al.*, 2001). This large-scale sequencing effort has provided several new insights, including the fact that humans have only around 40 000 genes (Venter *et al.*, 2001), and has driven the development of various high-throughput technologies. In addition, it has revealed the large amount of variation between humans, with over 1.5

million genetic polymorphisms being described. Of these, more than 60 000 are thought to result in functional changes in proteins (Sachidanandam *et al.*, 2001). Thus genomics has opened up the possibility of studying human genetic variation in epidemiological studies using high-throughput technologies. However, although it is theoretically possible to study 60 000 polymorphisms in an epidemiological cohort, in practice this poses many technical challenges. These include the multiplexing of thousands of polymorphism assays with high precision and the statistical analysis of the data in the face of multiple comparisons (Risch & Teng, 1998; Patil *et al.*, 2001). A detailed discussion of available technologies for studying genetic polymorphisms and some of the drawbacks associated with them was provided by Syvanen (2001). It is our personal experience that real-time PCR with TaqMan probes (Livak, 1999) or melting curve analysis (Germer & Higuchi, 1999; Germer *et al.*, 2000) provides a highly robust system for use in epidemiological studies, and we have the capacity to study hundreds of samples per day with this technology. The advantages and disadvantages of this technology are presented in Table 2.

Table 1. Selected examples of company websites related to emerging biomarker technologies

Technology/application	Company/affiliation	Web address
SNPs	Applied Biosystems	www.appliedbiosystems.com
	Luminex	www.luminexcorp.com
	Orchid Biosciences	www.orchid.com
	Genelex	www.genelex.com
Arrays	Affymetrix	www.affymetrix.com
	Sequenom	www.sequenom.com
	Genomic Solutions	www.genomicsolutions.com
	Packard Bioscience	www.packardbioscience.com
Proteomics	Ciphergen	www.ciphergen.com
	Oxford GlycoSciences	www.ogs.com
	Protiveris	www.protiveris.com
Nanotechnology	Surromed	www.surromed.com
	Foresight Institute	www.foresight.org
Microcantilevers	Protiveris	www.protiveris.com

SNPs, single nucleotide polymorphisms

Table 2. Emerging technology applications: advantages and disadvantages

Technology	Application	Advantages	Disadvantages
Genomics			
Real-time PCR	Translocation detection/ frequency quantification, SNP analysis	Quantitative, sensitive, simplicity of assay	Expensive probes
Pyrosequencing	SNP analysis	High throughput, quantitative, may be used for pooled samples, may sequence up to 50 bases	Expensive, difficult to multiplex
Invader	SNP analysis	Does not use PCR	May require large amounts of DNA
MALDI-TOF	SNP analysis	High throughput, reactions cost effective	Requires highly purified product, expensive instrument
cDNA microarray	Gene expression	High throughput	Limited application in epidemiological studies, expensive
Proteomics			
2-DE	Protein expression profiling, novel protein identification	High resolution, currently available	Not sensitive for low-abundance proteins, limited throughput
Mass spectrometry	Protein characterization	Provides structural information	Expensive instrument
Protein chips (SELDI)	Protein expression profiling, protein interaction profiling, protein characterization and biomarker discovery	Small sample volume required, 2-DE analysis not required, uses affinity capture to overcome problems with 2-DE	Expensive instrument, not yet widely available
Nanotechnology			
Nanobarcodes	Functional assays (i.e. immunoassays, protein expression, gene expression)	Multiplexing, sample recovery	Not yet validated for epidemiological studies, not commercially available
Microcantilevers	Functional assays (i.e. immunoassays, protein expression, gene expression)	Potentially low production costs, array potential, high throughput	

PCR, polymerase chain reaction; SNP, single nucleotide polymorphism; MALDI-TOF, matrix-assisted laser desorption ionization-time of flight; 2-DE, 2-dimensional gel electrophoresis; SELDI, surface-enhanced laser desorption/ionization

Quantitative real-time PCR

The analysis of known polymorphisms or mutational events in epidemiological studies requires highly specific, relatively low-cost technology. One such technology is real-time or quantitative PCR. Real-time PCR may be used to detect a variety of genetic changes ranging from single nucleotide polymorphisms (SNPs) (Livak, 1999; Breen *et al.*, 2000; Germer *et al.*, 2000), translocations (Dolken *et al.*, 1998; Luthra *et al.*, 1998; Curry *et al.*, 2001), changes in methylation status (Eads *et al.*, 2000) and gene expression (Olsson *et al.*, 1999; Amabile *et al.*, 2001; Seeger *et al.*, 2001). Although not considered to be truly 'high throughput', it offers the highly sensitive, specific, quantitative analysis necessary for epidemiological studies.

Real-time PCR is comparable with conventional PCR in that it uses sense and antisense primers to amplify a targeted sequence of DNA. TaqMan employs an additional, non-extendable oligonucleotide probe, which is positioned between the two primers during the annealing phase of amplification. The oligonucleotide probe is labelled with a fluorescent reporter dye such as 6-carboxy-fluorescein (FAM) at the 5' end and a quencher fluorescent dye such as 6-carboxy-tetramethyl-rhodamine (TAMRA) at the 3' end. When the probe is intact, fluorescence resonance energy transfer to TAMRA quenches the FAM emission. During the extension phase of amplification, the *Taq* polymerase extends the primer to the region of the probe, at which point the 5' exonuclease property of *Taq* cleaves the reporter dye from the probe. This results in an increase in fluorescent signal that is proportional to the amount of amplification product. The increase in reporter molecules is measured by real-time dedicated instruments, such as the ABI Prism 5700 or 7700 Sequence Detection Systems (PE Applied Biosystems) or the Roche LightCycler. After each cycle, fluorescence signal is measured, resulting in an amplification plot in which the point at which the fluorescence crosses a defined threshold, C_t, is proportional to the starting copy number. The C_t values of positive-control samples are used to generate a standard curve, from which it is possible to calculate the copy number of unknown samples. Methods for the quantitative

detection of chromosomal rearrangements using the above TaqMan technology have been reported. For example, numerous methods for the analysis of translocations found in leukaemia and lymphoma have been described (Dolken *et al.*, 1998; Luthra *et al.*, 1998; Olsson *et al.*, 1999; Amabile *et al.*, 2001; Seeger *et al.*, 2001).

Other genomic-based assays including the Invader assay, pyrosequencing and mass spectrometry (MS) are currently being developed or adapted for high-throughput SNP analysis (reviewed in Syvanen, 2001) The advantages and disadvantages of these technologies are presented in Table 2.

cDNA microarrays

cDNA microarrays are based on cDNA or oligonucleotides immobilized on to a chip (Figure 1). The chips may be used to examine differential gene expression in high-throughput or global gene expression (Ghosh, 2000; Chan & Huang, 2001; Hippo *et al.*, 2002). To date, these arrays have found limited application in epidemiology but are being widely used in other applications, such as toxicogenomic studies (Jelinsky & Samson, 1999; Nuwaysir *et al.*, 1999). There are numerous problems associated with using cDNA arrays in epidemiological studies (Table 2). The first is the fact that they are used to analyse RNA arising from gene expression. Unfortunately, by its very nature, RNA is unstable. Thus, most epidemiological studies that have collected biological samples have not collected material that contains stabilized RNA for analysis. Further, there is the expense – each sample could cost hundreds of dollars to analyse by microarray. Finally, if one had all the money in the world and a plentiful supply of RNA, there remains the problem that microarrays generate large amounts of (often conflicting) data requiring sophisticated statistical analysis. Fortunately, the rapidly expanding field of bioinformatics may overcome this last problem (Weinstein *et al.*, 2002).

An example of a successful application of array technology is the emerging field of toxicogenomics (reviewed by Nuwaysir *et al.*, 1999), which is the use of arrays to study altered gene expression due to exposure to a toxicant. By using

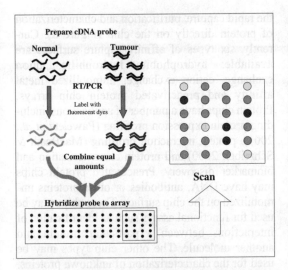

Figure 1. cDNA microarray. Fluorescent cDNA probes are generated by RT-PCR. cDNAs from control and tumour samples are combined in equal amounts and hybridized to oligonucleotides or cDNA bound to the chip. The chip is scanned and a ratio is generated reflecting differential gene expression.

experimental animals or cell cultures, highly controlled experiments can be performed that may help molecular epidemiologists appropriately target which genes to study and to understand which tissues act as the best surrogates for the target tissue.

Proteomic technologies

In light of the fact that the human genome consists of approximately 40 000 genes (Venter *et al.*, 2001), a fraction of what was originally expected, it has become clear that mammalian systems are too complex to be determined by genes alone. Alternative splicing, as well as over 200 post-translational modifications, affect a protein's structure, function, stability and interactions with other molecules (Banks *et al.*, 2000). It is therefore likely that a number of different proteins may be expressed by a single gene. Although proteomics has traditionally focused on quantitative analysis of protein expression, more recently it has expanded to include structural analysis and identification of protein (Srinivas *et al.*, 2001). Application of proteomic technologies to cancer research will provide

new biomarkers which reflect functional changes in protein expression within the causal pathway of cancer (Paweletz *et al.*, 2000; Jones *et al.*, 2002).

Proteomic research has recently been adapted to high throughput, highly sensitive technologies; however, much is based on methodology that has been used for decades. 2-Dimensional gel electrophoresis (2-DE) and MS have been and are still used today for the analysis and identification of proteins differentially expressed in healthy and neoplastic tissue. However, new technologies, particularly protein arrays, have increased throughput and sensitivity and may overcome many of the limitations of traditional proteomic methods (reviewed in Lee, 2001) (Table 2).

2-Dimensional gel electrophoresis and mass spectrometry

2-DE is used to identify proteins on the basis of two different properties: isoelectric point and molecular weight. Proteins are first denatured and then separated on the basis of charge by isoelectric focusing. The proteins are then further separated by migration through a polyacrylamide gel on the basis of molecular mass. By staining with silver or fluorescent stain, 2500–3000 proteins may be visualized on a single gel. The gel is scanned by densitometry and analysed by software (such as PDQuest, Melanie3). Ratio analysis is used to detect quantitative changes in proteins between two samples. In addition, protein databases and reference maps have been compiled (see, for example, www.expasy.ch). Therefore, spot profiles generated by 2-DE may be compared with one another as well as with reference maps available on the internet to identify differences in proteins expressed.

Gel 'spots' generated by 2-DE may also be purified and analysed by MS. Matrix-assisted laser desorption ionization (MALDI) is one type of MS used for the identification of proteins (Hillenkamp *et al.*, 1991; Bergman *et al.*, 2000). In MALDI-TOF (time of flight) (Krutchinsky *et al.*, 2000; Shevchenko *et al.*, 2000), proteins or peptides are co-precipitated with a light-absorbing matrix compound. Within the mass spectrometer, short pulses of laser light are passed through the matrix and peptide substance, resulting in the transfer of the peptides to the gas phase of the mass spectrometer. Ionization of the gaseous peptide results in the release of molecules which accelerate towards a detector that records the arrival of the ions, thus providing a time-of-flight analysis of the peptide mass. The mass of the molecule can be determined by the time of flight. This process results in a peptide map. A number of individual peptide-mass maps are generated, creating a mass spectrum which can be compared with peptide databases to find matching proteins.

2-DE and MS, used in combination, provide a reliable methodology for analysis of differential protein expression in healthy and different stages of neoplastic tissue which may identify early protein biomarkers of cancer. Higher-throughput versions of these methods are being developed which will facilitate their use for cancer proteomics (Hutchens & Yip, 1993; Lopez *et al.*, 2000).

Limitations of 2-dimensional gel electrophoresis and mass spectrometry: Despite their utility in cancer proteomics, these methodologies are limited in the spectrum of proteins they may be used to identify. 2-DE is not sensitive enough for low-abundance proteins which may be masked by the presence of high-abundance proteins. It is also not sensitive for the detection of low-molecular-weight or membrane proteins, or highly acidic or alkaline proteins (Harry *et al.*, 2000). In addition, the isolation of target cell populations is necessary for heterogeneous populations of cells, such as tumours or blood samples. This may require the use of additional sample manipulation such as microdissection or flow cytometry. Many of these limitations have been overcome by emerging technologies, particularly surface-enhanced laser desorption/ionization (SELDI), which combines chip technology and MS.

Protein chips
Protein chips overcome a number of the limitations of other proteomic methodologies by employing SELDI, a technology made widely available by Ciphergen Biosystems (Fremont, CA) (Merchant & Weinberger, 2000). SELDI-based protein chips use affinity capture to bind proteins with unique biochemical properties which allow

the rapid capture, purification and characterization of protein directly on the chip (Figure 2). Currently, six types of affinity capture surfaces are available: hydrophobic, hydrophilic, anion exchange, cation exchange, immobilized metal affinity and preactivated protein chip arrays. Protein chips have a number of applications, including protein expression profiling (Paweletz *et al.*, 2001), protein interaction profiling (MacBeath & Schreiber, 2000) and protein characterization and biomarker discovery. Preactivated protein chips may have DNA, antibodies or other proteins immobilized on the chip surface. These chips may be used for functional assays such as identification of interactions between a particular protein and another molecule. The other chip types may be used for the characterization of unknown proteins. The technology used to characterize unknown proteins is essentially the same as that described for MS. The SELDI process does not require sample purification or labelling. A crude sample may be applied directly to the chip, followed by washes to remove unbound protein or other impurities. The laser is then applied to the bound sample directly on the chip which then sends ions through the time-of-flight tube and is thus called SELDI-TOF-MS (Figure 3). A mass spectrum is generated, and may be compared with available databases.

The future is now: nanobarcodes and nanotechnology
Nanobarcodes
Nanobarcodes™, originally described by Michael Natan and his group at Surromed (Mountain View, CA) are cylindrical metal nanoparticles. The composition can be varied along the particle length in a stripe-like fashion similar to a supermarket barcode (Nicewarner-Pena *et al.*, 2001). Their identification is based on differential reflectivity, which can be determined by light microscopy. They can be functionalized with proteins, nucleic acids or organic chemicals, and serve essentially as a platform for chemistry that can be performed on a solid phase, i.e. gene expression analysis, protein expression, immunoassays and other functional assays. Because the number of stripes, the identity of metals used in their composition and the particle shape may all be varied, trillions of unique

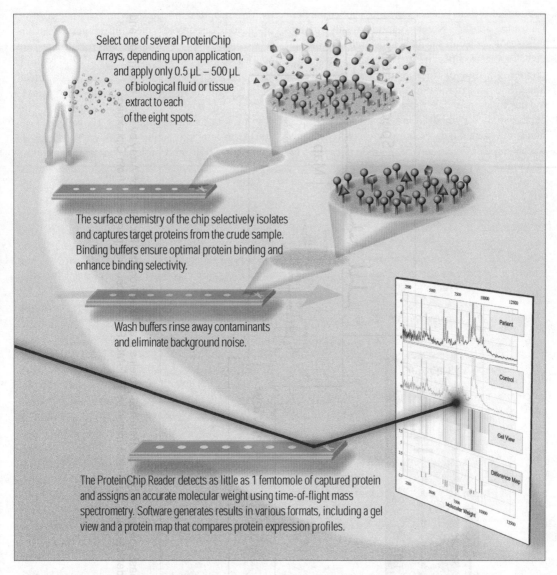

Select one of several ProteinChip Arrays, depending upon application, and apply only 0.5 µL – 500 µL of biological fluid or tissue extract to each of the eight spots.

The surface chemistry of the chip selectively isolates and captures target proteins from the crude sample. Binding buffers ensure optimal protein binding and enhance binding selectivity.

Wash buffers rinse away contaminants and eliminate background noise.

The ProteinChip Reader detects as little as 1 femtomole of captured protein and assigns an accurate molecular weight using time-of-flight mass spectrometry. Software generates results in various formats, including a gel view and a protein map that compares protein expression profiles.

Figure 2. Overview of Ciphergen ProteinChip® technology. Crude samples are applied, bound, washed and analysed directly on the chip. Reproduced with permission from Ciphergen.

'flavours' may be produced. Their size will allow literally thousands of these particles tailored for different end-points to be 'multiplexed' within a tiny amount of sample. In addition, nanobarcode particles are magnetic and can therefore be recovered from the sample, thus conserving the sample volume and simplifying analysis of complex mixtures.

Another potential high-throughput technology is volumetric capillary cytometry, which is being developed as Microvolume Laser Scanning Cytometer (MLSC) by Surromed. This technology is used for multiparameter cellular analysis, particularly immunological assays. It can quantify and classify hundreds of immune cell populations in small volumes of unprocessed biological fluids

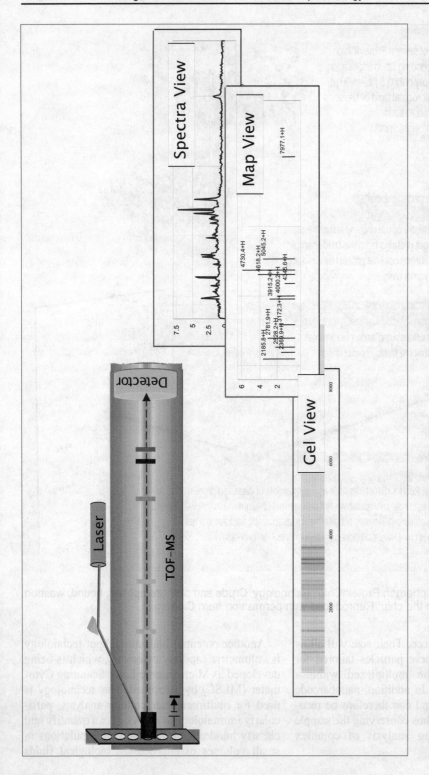

Figure 3. Time of flight (TOF) mass spectrometry (MS). Retained proteins are eluted from the ProteinChip® Array by laser desorption and ionization. Ionized proteins are detected and mass determined by TOF-MS. Reproduced with permission from Ciphergen.